EMERGENCY CARE
Assessment and Intervention

EMERGENCY CARE
Assessment and Intervention

Edited by

Carmen Germaine Warner, R.N., P.H.N.

Instructor, San Diego State University, College of Extended Studies;
Consultant, Nursing Education and Community Health Programs,
San Diego, California

SECOND EDITION

with 226 illustrations

THE C. V. MOSBY COMPANY

Saint Louis   1978

SECOND EDITION

Copyright © 1978 by The C. V. Mosby Company

All rights reserved. No part of this book may be reproduced in any manner without written permission of the publisher.

Previous edition copyrighted 1974

Printed in the United States of America

The C. V. Mosby Company
11830 Westline Industrial Drive, St. Louis, Missouri 63141

Library of Congress Cataloging in Publication Data

Main entry under title:

Emergency care.

   Includes bibliographical references and index.
   1. Medical emergencies. I. Warner, Carmen
Germaine, 1941-
RC86.7.E56   1978   616′.025   77-18285
ISBN 0-8016-4744-4

CB/CB/B 9 8 7 6 5 4 3 2 1

Contributors

Ralph D. Anderson, Jr., M.D.
Assistant Clinical Professor, University of California, San Diego, School of Medicine, La Jolla, California

Ronald L. Bouterie, M.D., F.A.C.S.
Surgical Consultant, Naval Regional Medical Center; Former Director, Surgical Education, Mercy Hospital and Medical Center, San Diego, California

Karen O. Butler, R.N., B.S.
Patient Education Coordinator, Mercy Hospital and Medical Center, San Diego, California

David L. Chadwick, M.D.
Medical Director, Children's Hospital and Health Center, San Diego, California

John R. Cote, Pharm.D.
Coordinator, Clinical Pharmacy Service, Yale-New Haven Hospital; Lecturer, Yale University School of Medicine, New Haven, Connecticut; Assistant Clinical Professor, University of Connecticut, School of Pharmacy, Storrs, Connecticut

Roger T. Crenshaw, M.D.
Codirector, The Crenshaw Clinic, San Diego, California; Instructor, Human Sexuality, University of California, San Diego, School of Medicine, La Jolla, California; Cochairperson, Western Region, American Association of Sex Educators, Counselors and Therapists

Theresa L. Crenshaw, M.D.
Codirector, The Crenshaw Clinic, San Diego, California; Clinical Instructor, Department of Reproductive Medicine, University of California, San Diego, School of Medicine, La Jolla, California;
Cochairperson, Western Region, American Association of Sex Educators, Counselors and Therapists

Stewart E. Dadmun, M.D., F.A.C.P.
Associate Clinical Professor of Medicine, University of California, San Diego, School of Medicine, La Jolla, California

Barbara J. Edwards, R.N.
Mental Health Coordinator, Department of Defense/CHAMPUS, San Diego, California

Tom Elo, M.D.
Assistant Professor, Division of Emergency Medicine; Director of Paramedic Training, University of Oregon Health Sciences Center, Portland, Oregon

Mildred K. Fincke, B.S.N.Ed.
Administrative Director, Emergency/Ambulatory Services, Allegheny General Hospital, Pittsburgh, Pennsylvania

Hugh A. Frank, M.D., F.A.C.S.
Clinical Professor, Department of Surgery, University of California, San Diego, School of Medicine, La Jolla, California

Gordon R. Freeman, M.D.
Associate Professor of Otolaryngology, University of California, San Diego, School of Medicine, La Jolla, California

Robert T. Gordon, M.D., F.A.C.O.G.
Clinical Instructor, Department of Obstetrics and Gynecology, University of California, San Diego, School of Medicine, La Jolla, California

Richard C. Gross, M.D.
Assistant Clinical Professor of Medicine, Division of Metabolic Disease, University of California, San Diego, School of Medicine, La Jolla, California

James D. Herrick, M.Sc.
Director of Pharmacy Services, United Hospitals, Inc., St. Paul, Minnesota; Assistant Professor, School of Pharmacy, University of Minnesota, Minneapolis, Minnesota

Mitchell, Schmidt, D'Amico, McCabe, and Stutz
Attorneys-at-Law, San Diego, California

Lawrence T. Moore, M.D., D.M.D., F.A.C.S.
Assistant Clinical Professor of Surgery, Division of Plastic Surgery, University of California, San Diego, School of Medicine, La Jolla, California

John R. Morse, M.D., F.A.C.C.
Associate in Cardiology, Department of Medicine, Mercy Hospital and Medical Center, San Diego, California; Assistant Clinical Professor of Medicine, University of California, San Diego, School of Medicine, La Jolla, California

Stephen P. Murphy, M.B., B.Ch.
Assistant Clinical Professor, Department of Anesthesiology, University of California, San Diego, School of Medicine; Chairman, Emergency Department, Scripps Memorial Hospital; Chairman, Paramedic and Base Station, Scripps Memorial Hospital, La Jolla, California

Doris Nelson, R.N., B.S.
Assistant Director, Emergency Services Department, Dallas County Hospital District, Dallas, Texas

Melvin A. Ochs, M.D., A.C.E.P.
Chairman, Emergency Services, Bay General Community Hospital; Instructor, Emergency Medical Technology, and Basic Emergency Nursing Programs, Southwestern College, Chula Vista, California

†William L. Orris, M.D.

Richard M. Peters, M.D.
Professor of Surgery, Department of Surgery, University of California, San Diego, La Jolla, California

---

†Deceased.

Randolph A. Read, M.D.
Adjunct Professor of Law, School of Law, University of San Diego, San Diego, California

Michael F. Rodi, M.D., A.A.O.S.
Assistant Clinical Professor of Orthopaedic Surgery, University of California, San Diego, School of Medicine, La Jolla, California

Thomas N. Rusk, M.D.
Associate Clinical Professor of Psychiatry, University of California, San Diego, School of Medicine, La Jolla, California

Jeffrey A. Sandler, M.D.
Assistant Professor of Medicine, Division of Metabolic Diseases, University of California, San Diego, School of Medicine, La Jolla, California

Sharon Lynn Sherman, Esq.
Mitchell, Schmidt, D'Amico, McCabe, and Stutz, Attorneys-at-Law, San Diego, California

Alan E. Shumacher, M.D., F.A.A.P.
Associate Medical Director and Director, Neonatal Intensive Care Unit, Children's Health Center, San Diego, California; Assistant Clinical Professor of Pediatrics, University of California, San Diego, School of Medicine, La Jolla, California

Jack C. Sipe, M.D.
Assistant Professor of Neurosciences, University of California, San Diego, School of Medicine, La Jolla, California; Neurologist, Veterans Administration Hospital, San Diego, California

David E. Smith, M.D.
Staff Surgeon, Trauma Branch, Surgical Service, Naval Regional Medical Center, San Diego, California

Randall W. Smith, M.D.
Assistant Professor of Neurosurgery, University of California, San Diego, School of Medicine, La Jolla, California

W. T. Soldmann, Jr., M.D.
Retired: General Practice, Obstetrics and Gynecology

Gordon Sproul, M.D.
Cardiovascular Surgeon, San Diego, California

Richard R. Uhl, M.D.
Associate Clinical Professor of Anesthesia, University of California, San Diego, School of Medicine, La Jolla, California

R. W. Virgilio, M.D.
Head, Trauma Branch, Department of Surgery, Naval Regional Medical Center, San Diego, California

Carmen Germaine Warner, R.N., P.H.N.
Instructor, San Diego State University, College of Extended Studies; Consultant, Nursing Education and Community Health Programs, San Diego, California

Mary Maude Winter, R.N.
Clinical Instructor, Senior Tutor, Nursing Department, Western Australian Institute of Technology, Western Australia

To you, the health profession, for your concern and devotion regarding quality emergency care.

To all the contributors who gave of themselves, making this book a reality.

In memory of my beloved father whose gift to me, I now give to you.

Foreword

Because emergency care is administered in such a wide variety of settings by personnel from diverse educational backgrounds, the organization of a comprehensive textbook on this subject presents major challenges.

The need for such a book, however, is evident. When hospitals instituted intensive care units and coronary care units, where continuous, precise monitoring could be offered under the supervision of expertly prepared physicians, nurses, and technicians, assurance that the patient could survive the initial period of trauma or seizure *with minimal suffering and loss of function* became a logical objective.

Achievement of this goal is a tremendous task, supported not only by primary training received in early adulthood, but also by continuing education as well. Proficiencies once developed have to be maintained, and the constant generation of new techniques, electronic devices, and other equipment compounds the overall effort.

Until very recently, a brief course in first aid was considered adequate training for those charged with transporting the sick and injured. Now, however, courses are being created in all aspects of emergency care.

For all those who provide emergency care—firemen, policemen, ambulance attendants, school nurses, industrial nurses, and the physicians and nurses in the emergency department of the hospital—continuing education is critical. Interdisciplinary courses are preparing physicians, nurses, and allied health professionals to work together as highly coordinated teams. Skill in communicating with patients and their families, the ability to talk with people undergoing stress and to intervene in the crisis when necessary, is taught alongside more technical procedures.

Emergency Care: Assessment and Intervention is an important contribution to the encouragement of the interdisciplinary approach.

The latest concepts in the intervention of trauma and some entirely new material on the topic of aquatic medicine are prominent features. The reader will find the book a valuable resource for basic as well as continuing education.

Shirley L. Brandt, R.N., M.A.

Assistant Clinical Professor,
Department of Community Medicine;
Director of Nursing Programs,
Office of Continuing Education in the
Health Sciences, University of California,
San Diego, School of Medicine,
La Jolla, California

Preface

The quality of emergency health care has become an increasing concern of emergency personnel over the past several years. With the 1972 passage of Public Law 92-603 providing for the creation of professional standards review organizations and the development and funding of health systems agencies, the quality of emergency care has been questioned by patients, hospitals, health personnel, and government. It is realized that often the actual performance of this vital function is inadequate, and legislation is now requiring accountability.

This book is an attempt to assist those responsible for providing quality emergency care to address this need with confidence and skill.

In the past, emergency department personnel and those performing prehospital emergency intervention had minimal or no specialized education and were confronted with situations in which lives were lost or disability prolonged because immediate proper care could not be initiated.

Fortunately, personnel now have the opportunity to acquire and utilize advanced education and performance skills. The Emergency Department Nurses' Association, recognizing the need for advancement, has established committees that have developed a core curriculum accompanying educational materials and an examination that provides certification for the "emergency nurse specialist." Continuing education for emergency physicians is following the same trend for advancement and upgrading.

With an increased emphasis on prehospital emergency care, utilizing paramedics as well as nursing personnel, the effectiveness of accessible quality care has saved many lives, resulting in the acceptance and support of such programs by the consumer.

Administering immediate appropriate emergency care will save lives and assist in the reduction of hospital costs and length of stay. Aspects of good preventive health maintenance, patient and family teaching, along with recognition and use of referral agencies, will reduce repeat visits and misunderstanding of prescribed intervention.

It is hoped that this book will enable all emergency personnel to counter some of the dissatisfaction with the current health delivery system.

Greater authority and direct responsibility must be accepted by everyone. Immediate proper emergency care must be the ultimate goal of every member of the emergency care team.

The second edition of this book has been prepared with minimal delay and frustration thanks to the cooperation and enthusiasm of many. The contributors, sharing their talents and expertise, have proven to be an asset to the advancement of emergency care.

A very special and unique addition has been provided by James D. Herrick and John R. Cote who, with their pharmacological knowledge, have reviewed every chapter to assure consistency and accuracy throughout the book. This was an incredible undertaking, and their patience and perseverance have been commendable. Again I am proud to honor the talents of Sue Adornato, an extremely creative medical illustrator, and Pat Summers, a typist whose meticulous manner has contributed to the quality of this book.

It is with great pleasure that I share with you the second edition of this book. A considerable amount of knowledge, dedication, and sensitivity has gone into its preparation, and it is an honor to be associated with all those involved.

Carmen Germaine Warner

Contents

CHAPTER 1

Elements of an emergency medical care system

Stephen P. Murphy, M.B., B.Ch.

Emergency health care—the phrase has such a fine ring to it! Like pure water and clean milk, we assume that it is there when we need it, if we only call. Yet for most of the country, this is not a reality. What should be available as a system of emergency care is rather a nonsystem born of a long line of ignoble ancestors, the great progenitor of the line being apathy. The "don't care" attitude seems to be at every level of government and health care when it comes to emergency medical care. Everyone agrees that such care should be available somewhere, but somebody else has the key! Emergency medical care is work; and only hard, long and consistent effort combined with planning will result in an effective emergency medical care system. There are no shortcuts, no easy ways, and no quickie systems.

Another progenitor of poor emergency medical care is esprit de corps, a fine, high-sounding title for interdepartmental jealousy. "Our people are better than your people." "We don't like to get our uniforms bloody. They cost too much to clean so we wait for the ambulance driver to arrive." We spend our time instead measuring skidmarks, kicking broken glass into the gutter, and directing traffic, while the victim chokes to death in vomitus. This is esprit de corps at its finest. A blood brother of such esprit de corps is hospital chauvinism. "My hospital is bigger and better than yours; it has five hundred beds." "My hospital is better than yours because we don't go to the same church." "My hospital has university affiliation and yours doesn't."

Another ancestor is pride. "We already have the best in the state. Leave it alone; it is working. We don't need to be improved." This, in a sense, is a combination of apathy and chauvinism and is revealed in the haughtiness of local government officials when there is any suggestion that the present system could be improved.

And lastly there is ignorance. No one knows how bad the system is because no one ever tries to find out. No data are gathered; no reports are made; no complaints are voiced; no figures are published. Such ignorance is perhaps the saddest of all excuses for poor emergency care.

What should be our philosophy of emergency medical care? What guiding principles should we use? Brought to its conclusion, in my view, emergency medical care is more a sensible awareness than a "thing."

1

It is a series of beliefs and attitudes which, when held by all the people in an area, will result in a total system of emergency medical care (just as a commitment to law and order, when held by the citizens in an area, will result in a first-rate police and judicial system). An emergency medical care system will evolve when the basic techniques and attitudes of effective emergency medical care are taught from earliest childhood in the school system as part of preparation for living. When children are taught effective self-help according to the principles of good health, when they are introduced at an early age into the organization and functioning of an effective emergency medical care system, when they are taught how to ask for help or how to access the system, and when they are taught how to give help to their neighbors, then an effective total system will follow. This should be our goal. However, throughout most of the country, rather than starting at the grade school level, we have to start at the political level and work our way down. This must be done so that we at least put together a basic system from elements now in existence; through persistent public relations efforts and the use of the media, we then try to get the word to the people.

Until the granting of state and federal funds is contingent upon the development of an effective emergency system, each county will have to generate its own enthusiasm and its own answers to problems. This depends upon leadership. One cannot imagine a committee's leading the Rough Riders of the Spanish-American Civil War as they charged up San Juan Hill. They were led by Teddy Roosevelt, who swung his saber and charged up the hill with his men following. Emergency medical care will never be as dramatic as this, but somebody, some person, has to be the leader of this effort. Too many committee members come to meetings and never open the file until the next meeting. It takes somebody to get on the phone, day after day, to irritate, to browbeat, to encourage, to coordinate, to facilitate, and to motivate the various elements in a beginning emergency medical care system. Once the patterns have been established, then much of the work is self-generating and automatic. But during the initial efforts, success or failure depends upon the efforts of a person, not a committee.

ORGANIZATION

Emergency medical care is a community, not a medical, responsibility. The community reaction to this responsibility must be based upon the political elements in the community, such as the board of supervisors, the mayor, or the city council. Experience shows that there is a direct relationship between political interest and involvement and the effectiveness of the emergency medical care committee. Following the National Safety Act of 1966, whereby each county had to appoint an emergency medical care committee, many counties appointed two or three doctors as the committee and left them like castaways on a desert island, cut off from all input and all effective governmental and administrative help—a paper committee on a paper island, surrounded by a sea of apathy. Their success was zero. During its formative years in San Diego County, the Emergency Medical Care Committee had to do everything. It had to develop, evaluate, advise, and operate the beginning system. It operated only with volunteer help. However, as the system developed and with federal grant money, full-time paid staff were acquired, and the Emergency Medical Care Committee then achieved its correct role, which is to give advice on program development, evaluation, and assignment of responsibilities. The role of the full-time staff is established by local political bodies (Fig. 1-1).

Medical personnel can provide leadership and technical expertise; they cannot

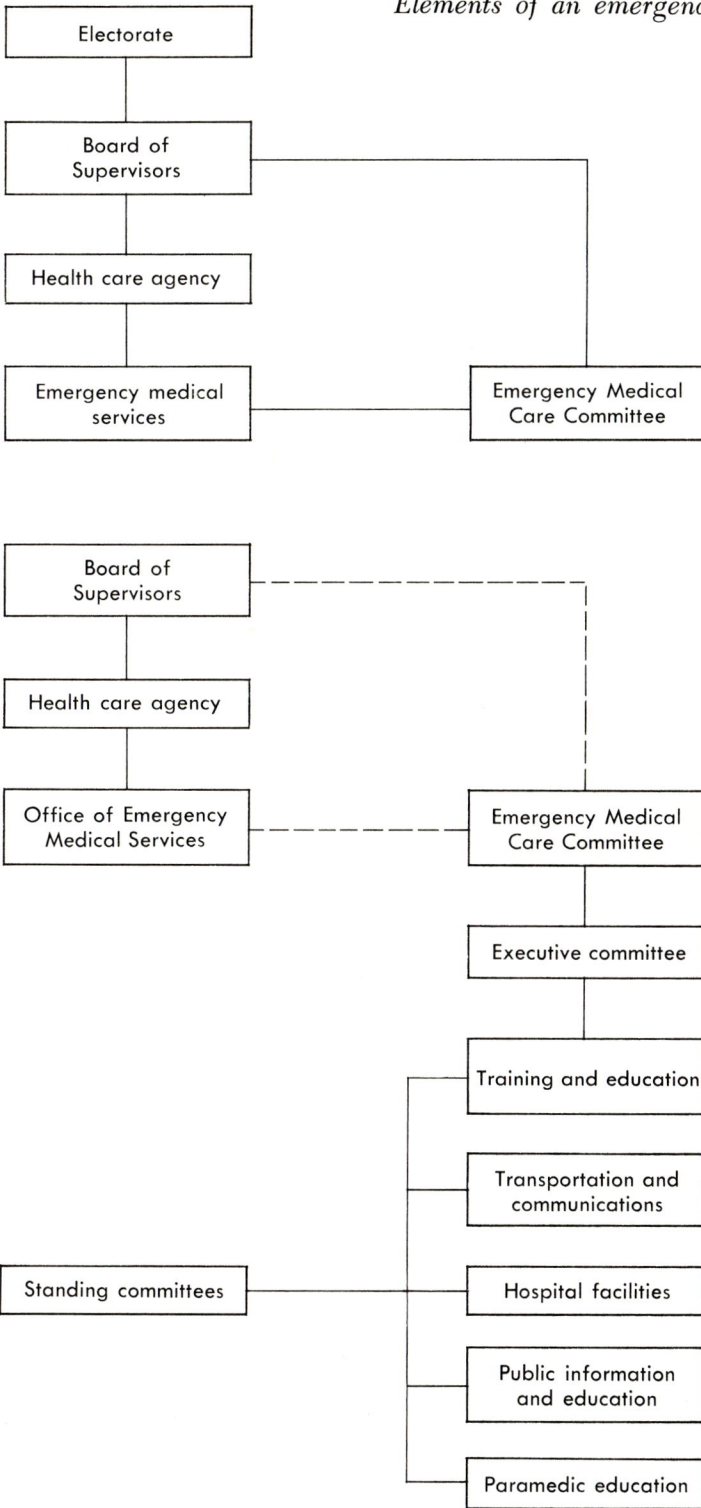

Fig. 1-1. Organizational chart, emergency medical services, San Diego County, January, 1977.

put together a system unless they act with the backing of the political elements in their area and within the limits of authority given them by the political leaders. The second most important element in developing a viable system, which must be immediately brought to bear, is the involvement of all agencies that have legitimate responsibilities in the provision of emergency medical services with the emergency medical care committee. This brings in virtually every element in the community. Approximately 24 separate elements exist in most organized communities:

County government
City government
Law enforcement agencies
Fire agencies
Park and recreation departments
Forestry services
Military services
Coast Guard (if applicable)
Educational facilities (universities, community colleges, and so forth)
Comprehensive health planning association
Highway patrol
Hospitals and health facilities
Medical community and the various elements that have had historical interest in emergency medical care (that is, the Committee on Trauma of the American Academy of Orthopaedists, the Committee on Trauma of the American College of Surgeons, and the vital American College of Emergency Physicians)
The nursing profession (and especially its Emergency Department Nurses' Association)
The American Heart Association
The American National Red Cross
Consumer representation of responsible citizens who are knowledgeable of the needs of the community such as clergymen and local political leaders (There should be one representative on the committee from each of the geographic areas.)
Emergency mental care associations and activities (a most important element, which needs to be part of the system, especially since the problems of drug addiction and drug overdose are so prevalent currently)
Communication media
Office of emergency services
Search and rescue organizations
Pharmaceutical industry
Local telephone company

If all the agencies listed above are included, the committee will be large and unwieldy. However, to make the committee smaller by omitting some of these elements will rebuff many agencies and individuals who have great interest in serving. Therefore, as the committee grows, the need for an executive committee will become apparent. In San Diego County we have broken down the large committee and assigned individual members to subcommittees, which usually meet monthly; the chairmen of these subcommittees form the Emergency Medical Care Executive Committee. The big EMCC must meet quarterly to assist in policy development and planning, but the subcommittees meet as directed by the executive committee, with a minimum of quarterly meetings. For the first ten years the big committee met bimonthly, but with the increasing scope of the operation, the complexity of the system, and the size of the EMCC, it became unwieldly, and a more effective and flexible system was developed with the executive committee as its head.

The third essential for an effective system is professional administration. This system cannot be developed or operated on volunteer time. Although most committee members will donate time, they also have responsibilities to their own departments or agencies, their practices, their livelihoods and their families that will prevent them from devoting large portions of their time to the development of the system. Implicit in the acknowledgement by local government that an effective emergency medical care system is necessary is their willingness to appoint and pay for full-time, professional help. However, this is no job for the old political war horse waiting for retirement. Rather, it is a job for an energetic, young, innovative, professional public administrator who can see the rare opportunity to build a reputation, in the success of his efforts. Many programs now have medical directors who are experienced administrators.

To organize and run a system, any system, in government requires data. The collection of data is an important component of an EMS system. Data are needed to help us decide where ambulances should be based, how they are to be staffed and equipped, what types of cases are being transported and treated, what the problems are, and how they are being solved. The development of data collection and evaluation by the coordinator of emergency medical care is one of the first and most important functions. This is the tool by which one measures needs and evaluates successes or shortcomings. The federal government funding for the development of emergency medical services systems requires the development of standardized record-keeping systems and evaluations of programs. Although many cities and counties, especially county departments of health, already gather data related to emergency medical care, the statistics frequently lack relevance to problems of the system as a whole, because the design and evaluation of the data are related to the sponsoring department rather than to emergency medical care. Therefore, a system of data collection and evaluation designed specifically for the emergency medical care system is essential.

COMMUNICATIONS

Without question, centralized communications and dispatch are intrinsic to the development of an emergency medical services system. All the organizational structure is useless if an ambulance cannot be dispatched to the appropriate area to help with the patient. Emergency medical care might be summarized as the success of a community in getting good, effective care to the man bleeding to death in a gutter. All the efforts in organization, education, communications, political input, and data gathering come to a focus on that individual, and they are useless if proper care is not forthcoming. The connecting link between the victim in the gutter and the system is the communications network. The citizen who sees the need must have knowledge of how to activate the system. He must have a universal number to call. The call should be routed to a centralized receipt and dispatch center where well-trained and experienced communicators can assess the request for help, and dispatch the appropriate resource to aid the emergency victim. Much of the success of emergency medical care efforts depends on factors of speed—speed of discovery, speed of access, and speed of response—although efforts at increasing the speed of response might be more productive if looked at from the point of eliminating causes of delay. The well-known studies that have shown a three-time increase in rural versus urban mortality and morbidity from comparable injuries can be roughly translated into terms of delay—delay in getting help to the victim and delay in getting the victim to help.

Effective emergency medical communication is a difficult and costly element in the system. The much discussed "911" system being developed will take years to complete and will cost many millions of dollars. Once completed, it will be of great help to the citizen in need, since it will mean that a single three-digit telephone number will automatically result in routing the call to the appropriate agency where trained operators will assess the need and correctly assign the effective help.

Centralized dispatch of ambulances, police, and fire units also implies that the emergency response services in a community are willing to bury some of their differences for the public good. Police and fire agencies tend to hang on to their communications nets with great tenacity and ferocity and generally tend to be adamant in their refusal to share some of their communications capability and dispatch. Yet this joint dispatch is desperately needed throughout the country.

Hospital radios are a form of communication that can be effectively used by an emergency medical care system. For approximately 11 years the hospitals in San Diego County have had their own emergency radio net. At first this was little more than a citizen band–type system with little power and no net discipline; it was rarely used. After the FCC refused to reassign this radio band for hospital use nationwide some years ago, the county government microwave net was offered to the hospitals as an alternative method of communicating. With the hospitals' agreement the county took on the job and allocated two bands to the hospitals—one for emergency and the other for administrative use. The arrangement is a great improvement, since net discipline is imposed by the communications department of the county. The net traverses the whole county with repeaters on the highest mountain tops, all of which are maintained by the county. It is no longer a weak line of sight system such as the Hospital Emergency Administrative Radio (H.E.A.R.) system, but rather it has ample power both in transmitters and repeaters, located to penetrate even the remote and deep canyons. The hospital sets cost approximately $2,500 and are placed in the emergency department with repeaters in the administrator's office. The present system is a great improvement over its more exclusive predecessor· The ambulances (98) have a two-way communication capability with the emergency department of any hospital in the county both for advice and to alert the hospital to prepare for the arrival of the emergency patient. The radio is in addition to the basic department radios (fire, police, or private ambulance) that all these vehicles already carry.

TRANSPORTATION

The basic element of emergency medical care transportation is four-wheeled vehicles. In San Diego County we have developed the phase concept of emergency

medical care transportation, beginning with the standard patrol car. All police officers are trained as EMT-1s. They operate 17 van ambulances. They provide approximately 12,000 emergency medical transportation functions a year. There are few drawbacks to the system since the geographical location of our hospitals is such that most of these vehicles are never more than ten minutes away from a certified primary emergency facility (PEF). Consequently, the police have been able to function very well over the years with dual-purpose vehicles. However, because of the increasing training, capability, and awareness, police are now using van ambulances rather than dual-purpose station wagons. The ambulances function both as patrol cars and ambulances.

The police ambulance is a first response system. These vehicles are on constant, 24-hour duty in traffic and patrol divisions. Only when needed do they function as ambulances. They are equipped to the standards of the American College of Surgeons with resuscitation equipment, splints, suction, and so on. The primary function of the first response team is to be first on the scene; hence, "first response" personnel assess the situation immediately (triage), initiate effective resuscitation, and call for appropriate help if there are multiple injuries. If victims of a major accident are being treated, then the second response vehicle is called.

The second response system, which is a real ambulance manned by two fully trained Emergency Medical Technicians 1 (EMT-1), has no function other than emergency medical care. This is why it is called the "second response." The second response system should not be sent off for minor needs on long distances into the rural or urban area. It should not respond for simple problems like a broken wrist, a bloody nose, or a scalp laceration.

The third response is the mobile intensive care unit. Though much effort and interest have been generated internationally by the mobile cardiac care unit, I feel that this type of unit is much too limited in scope. Although coronary care should be a primary and well-publicized function of the mobile intensive care unit, it should not be limited to such care. Therefore, our efforts in this line are directed to having the mobile intensive care units staffed by paramedics; these units become, in effect, mobile emergency departments. They are large, walk-in vans with operating tables, endotracheal tubes, fluids, suction, backboards, and so forth. They have defibrillators, cardiac monitors, and all the necessary drugs to perform effective cardiac resuscitation and support.

The country generally seems to be fascinated by the idea that helicopters can answer the emergency medical care needs of a community. There are so many bad things about helicopters that their relative role in an emergency medical care system must be realistically appraised. Just as the British used to complain about the Americans in World War II—"They are oversexed, oversized, and over here"—one might say about helicopters that they are "overpublicized, overpriced, and over-repaired." They are very expensive to buy and operate. An effective airborne emergency evacuation system requires three helicopters because of the FAA-imposed repair maintenance time. Their mandatory downtime must be compensated for by other available aircraft. Bad flying weather also necessitates grounding periodically. The rougher and more northerly the area, the less flying time is available. Furthermore, the financially feasible aircraft are small. They have internal dimensions little bigger than a horizontal telephone booth, and the idea that one can perform effective emergency medical care while bouncing around in such a small area is ridiculous. All that a helicopter really provides is speed of evacuation and transportation. In every other way it is inferior to good

surface transportation. An emergency medical care system should end, rather than begin, with helicopters.

Once the basic ground system has been in operation, and only then, should a community consider the use of helicopters. In an area such as San Diego County, which is made up of mountain ranges, deep canyons, and vast areas of rough terrain with no level ground where a helicopter can land, the helicopter evacuation team is frequently dependent upon four-wheel drive vehicles or a man-carried litter to get the patient to the helicopter. The victim may have to be hand-carried out of a canyon and then carried for a mile or two through the forest to get to a place suitable for a helicopter landing zone. Therefore, four-wheel drive emergency medical evacuation vehicles are now in operation in the sheriff's department for use in rough country. Frequently, victims are taken by surface vehicles from the accident site to the helicopter, which then takes them to the appropriate hospital. Because of the limited transportation capability of a medical evacuation helicopter and the possibility of there being several victims, we depend upon four-wheel drive vehicles to get the remainder of victims to help. Therefore it is essential to put helicopters in their true, realistic, and pragmatic perspective when planning and designing the medical transportation part of a system. They can be part of an effective system—the transportation subsystem.

EMERGENCY MEDICAL CARE FACILITIES

Many years ago when the San Diego City Police began their ambulance program and we began to study the results of 24-hour patrol, it became apparent that the transportation phase alone was not the beginning and the end of an emergency medical care system. Patients were brought to the hospitals under resuscitation who had waited for up to an hour before effective emergency medical care could be instituted. The personnel in emergency departments were frequently absent, they were untrained, the equipment and organization were poor, and there were no radios. To improve this situation, it was proposed to the hospitals that they voluntarily agree to a classification system of their facilities under reasonable guidelines and criteria. At first the hospitals rejected this proposal. It took three years of hard and persistent effort to get the hospitals, and particularly their medical staffs, to realize the need for improvement.

Our classification system has now been

Table 1-1. Classification of emergency facilities

		Primary or comprehensive (PEF)	Auxiliary	First aid	No facilities (referral only)
M.D.	In ER 24 hours	✓			
	On call for ER 24 hours		✓		
	None on call			✓	✓
R.N.	In ER 24 hours	✓	✓		
	On call for ER 24 hours			✓	✓
Specialty panel	Yes	✓			
	No		✓	✓	✓
Hospital radio net	Yes	✓	✓		
	No			✓	✓
Minimum 4-bed ER	Yes	✓			
	No		✓	✓	✓
CPR supplies defibrillator and monitor in ER	Yes	✓	✓		
	No			✓	✓
Laboratory technician 24 hours	Yes	✓	✓		
	No			✓	✓
Blood bank	Yes	✓	✓		
	No			✓	✓
X-ray technician available in 15 minutes	Yes	✓	✓		
	No			✓	✓
OR available 24 hours	Yes	✓	✓		
	No			✓	✓
Anesthesia available in 30 minutes	Yes	✓			
	No		✓	✓	✓
Intensive care unit	Yes	✓			
	No		✓	✓	✓
Disaster plan	Yes	✓	✓	✓	✓
	No				
Medical audit	Yes	✓	✓	✓	✓
	No				
J.C.A.H. accreditation ER under hospital's utilization committee of staff	Yes	✓	✓	✓	
	No				

in operation for over six years, and it has been the only working system that can act as a guide for the rest of the country.

The criteria for classification of emergency facilities are shown in Table 1-1. The facilities are currently classified into four grades. The primary emergency facility is the highest grade. This is particularly distinguished by having 24-hour, on-board physician coverage in the emergency department, 24-hour capability in the operating, x-ray, laboratory, and blood bank areas, and a minimum of a four-bed intensive care unit.

General hospitals that do not wish to provide 24-hour, on-board physician coverage are classified as auxiliary facilities.

Currently, there are 22 hospitals scattered throughout San Diego County that are classified as primary emergency facilities. This is not a self-classification. Each year a team of two physicians, one of whom is an emergency room physician, one emergency room nurse, and one hospital administrator inspects each primary emergency facility (PEF). Classification and certification is from January 1 to December 31 on the recommendations of the Emergency Medical Care Committee. A certificate is presented to each hospital to be displayed in the emergency department. This certificate is signed by the chairman of the Emergency Medical Care Committee and the inspection committee.

Although inspection imposes considerable strain on physicians' time to check out these hospitals, I believe that yearly inspection is most important, because people tend to become lax about their performance unless they realize that their shortcomings will be reported and commented on. Should a hospital not achieve classification of primary emergency facility even though the administration has requested it, and should the administration feel that the recommendations of the inspection committee were unfair and arbitrary, an appeal may be made to the Emergency

Medical Care Committee for a reappraisal and consideration.

CRITICAL CARE FACILITIES

In an effort to couple the high level of expertise and experience with the greatly expanded technology and the great increase in expense and sophistication of medical care, a number of communities have developed centralized critical care facilities. Typical of all these elements are the burn units. A single serious burn in any but the largest intensive care units is such a great drain on personnel and resources that other patients may be neglected. The sterility requirements alone pose a tremendous management problem. Therefore, concentrating specialized services in one hospital in a community is a conservation move. Again in the burn analogy, few of us see enough burns all the time to be expert at recognizing all the implications of the physiologic support of these people. We tend to be professional amateurs when dealing with them, and yet by concentrating all our expertise in one hospital, we then can take care of them properly. Similar centralization is occurring in other areas, such as poison control and trauma centers. These centers do not eliminate the primary care of the patient in the closest emergency department to stabilize and assess the situation; rather they are really "second stage" centers for the referral of cases from the medical community. I do not believe that assignment of cases to the specialized center should be done arbitrarily by ambulance attendants. Rather, all cases should first be taken to the closest primary (or similar comprehensive) facility, evaluated, and only then sent to the burn, trauma, or similar center after expert assessment in the emergency room. To do otherwise will subject the patients to longer ambulance trips prior to stabilization with consequent increase in morbidity and mortality. Such arbitrary transfer and bypass of intermediate areas will also increase the likelihood of lawsuits against the ambulance attendants.

Education of the medical community to the facilities' capabilities, not mandated criteria, is the key to proper utilization of specialized units. Critical care personnel need to talk to the medical community and the hospital staff to acquaint them with the services offered. No immediate impact will be seen, but as the use increases a gradual improvement in the statistics of survival should be seen.

DISASTER PREPAREDNESS

Disaster preparedness has been an immense element in every emergency medical care committee's responsibility. The emergency medical care functions of a county are responsible only for the emergency medical care component of a disaster preparedness program; they must not become responsible for overall disaster preparedness. This is a function of what was called Civil Defense or the Office of Emergency Services. Although the emergency medical care committee has some responsibilities, it does not have overall responsibility in disaster preparedness. It is, however, important that both functions are coordinated and that both functions have the closest daily working relationship with one another. Further, it is important that disaster exercises be organized on a six-month basis. These should not be in the obvious areas but moved around throughout the county so that all areas and organizations are exposed to a simulated disaster every year or so.

The government has recently realized that most airports have no facilities to handle even routine medical emergencies, let alone a disaster. This is in contradistinction to some of the larger European airports, which have fully developed, tent-type mobile hospitals available, preloaded into trucks, which can be immediately dispatched to a crash site at an airport, and comprehensive facilities can be developed

at the point of impact. Despite the fact that airports may not respond favorably to the possibility of a crash at their facilities, considering it poor public relations, it is imperative that medical and hospital organizations surrounding airports at least be realistic enough to put together their portion of the emergency medical care response to a possible crash.

EMERGENCY MENTAL HEALTH SERVICES

Throughout the original developmental period of emergency medical care concepts in San Diego County, aspects of emergency mental health care were relegated to the background, because it was felt that the spectacular highway accidents deserved more immediate concern. Possibly this is true. However, it must be realized that in these days of increasing drug abuse and drug overdose and with the increasing strain of modern urban life, terrible conditions can develop that need urgent care by the emergency medical care system personnel. The mental patient who seizes a gun and starts shooting people is not only a source of patients for the system but also is a problem in himself—he must be managed, transported, and cared for. The suicidal person who sits on the ledge of a building can tie up tremendous police and fire department resources as they try to talk him down from his ledge. The techniques used by police and fire personnel in talking to these people need to be practiced, rehearsed, and perfected in order to reduce the drain on emergency medical services that these incidents generate.

Emergency mental health services are assuming an increasingly important position in the emergency medical care picture. Each emergency medical care system should address the problem. So many private and public groups are involved in providing mental health services that one of the first functions of an emergency medical services office is to make a comprehensive study of all such activities. A plan should then be made to coordinate their work and reduce the duplication of activities in the emergency field. Problems of emergency medical care cross so many jurisdictions that a central office of emergency medical services should be established, preferably in the health department. Also, the problem of patient management needs to be given greater emphasis in the training of involved agencies.

EDUCATION AND TRAINING

The educational component of an emergency medical care system is now well organized. Standards for training personnel are developed and curricula are available.

Currently in southern California there are three layers of emergency medical care teaching. The first level is for the public safety personnel who are first responders. This course consists of a 30- to 40-hour basic course and includes a CPR component and also frequent refresher courses. In the city of San Diego the police ambulance crews are trained to the level of EMT-1, who have completed the 80-hour course or have passed the national certification examination. The EMT-2 is a paramedic who has received almost 1,000 hours of training. This program was pioneered at Harbor General Hospital in Los Angeles, California.

The Department of Transportation course and the Brady course of approximately 80 hours have been proposed as being adequate and feasible for EMT-1. We have not found this to be so, since our students who have challenged these courses have found that their greatest deficiencies are in terminology, basic anatomy, and physiology. This has been true despite the fact that one of the prerequisites of the course is receipt of the Advanced Red Cross First Aid card (which itself was not sufficient preparation for the EMT-1 course). In San Diego County each course has been expanded to 108 hours to

give students more intensive instruction in terminology and physiology and also to allow preceptorships at local emergency departments where they receive ten hours of training.

The highest level is the EMT-2, or paramedic. These people staff mobile intensive care units or special rescue vans, which are equipped more than the standard ambulance. These vans are equipped with endotracheal tubes, defibrillators, and so on, and the paramedics are allowed by law to give drugs intravenously and to initiate much more advanced medical techniques than are now performed by the EMT-1. We believe that with this three-level instruction a great number of individuals can be trained to the 40-hour level without imposing an unacceptable economic burden on the community. Selected personnel from fire, police, and lifeguard departments or from private ambulance services who have displayed aptitude at emergency medical care are trained to the EMT-1 level; of these, the most talented can be trained to the EMT-2 level and will man mobile intensive care units.

PUBLIC INFORMATION

Getting information to the public is one of the most difficult challenges facing the emergency medical care committee. The committee itself is composed of providers, and they are all interested and informed people. However, the general public must be given information on how to gain access to the system and what to do before help arrives. This has to be a continuing effort on the part of the committee, the community as a whole, and the media in particular. All sorts of resources must be used to keep this information in front of the public. One approach is requesting that the local telephone company place emergency telephone numbers in the front of the telephone directory. Information such as the location of local primary emergency facilities and the numbers to call for help can be included in monthly billings. Some emergency medical education should be included in the grade school so that as children develop and grow they become aware of how to use the system. In fact, emergency medical help needs to be brought into the public awareness as one of the emergency responses to the community—right alongside fire and police departments.

TECHNICAL ADVISORY COMMITTEE

Because of the technologic complexity involved in emergency medical care and the constant developments at all levels, one resource needs to be developed in each community and, eventually, at the state and national levels. This is a technical advisory committee composed of knowledgeable people involved in the various aspects of health care, communications, transportation, and so forth. One person in each specialty in medicine should be assigned by the specialty to represent its consensus of what constitutes optimal care. For instance, the local orthopedic society should assign someone representing its views to sit on the technical advisory committee of the county's emergency medical care committee. Any question concerning management of fractures or the use of new orthopedic equipment should be referred to this person. If necessary, this member can submit the question to the orthopedic society for final review and recommendations. These recommendations are then forwarded to the emergency medical care committee.

No single doctor should be held responsible for every possible aspect of emergency medical care. The field is too vast, too complicated, and too important. We should not expect an anesthesiologist, for example, to be an expert in fractures, or an orthopedist to be an expert in coronary care. Therefore, each of the major medical specialties should appoint someone to the technical advisory committee. In addition, there should be members from any other discipline that the committee feels it needs to help it perform its function and fulfill its responsibility to the community. These people should be appointed for a period of one year with the strong recommendation that it be a semipermanent responsibility, so that some continuity of effort and awareness can be developed in these individuals. Members should be knowledgeable, mature, responsible, and interested; they will become one of the most vital resources available to the educational elements of the emergency medical care system and to the evaluative function of the office of the coordinator.

SUMMARY

These, then, in very brief form are the elements of an emergency medical care system—its philosophy, its involvement, its development, and its operation. Awareness in recent years has increased tremendously, both at the local and national levels. Systems are being developed at a tremendous rate, both in number and in scope, and improvements at all levels and in all elements in the systems are constantly taking place. One can only hope that such a rate of development will continue and even increase.

CHAPTER **2**

Legal considerations

Sebastian D'Amico, Esq.
Sharon Lynn Sherman, Esq.

The purpose of this chapter is to set forth in summary fashion the basic principles of law most commonly confronting the personnel who work in an emergency department. The intended and proper use of this chapter should be as an awareness vehicle rather than as a technical-legal reference. Generally, local community standards dictate the legal parameters within which emergency departments should operate. Therefore, the advice of local counsel should be sought in defining those parameters.

The chapter begins with a discussion of the legal duty of, and the legal duty to, care that an emergency department must exercise toward all patients in general, and the extent of such duties when the patient has died or has been identified as a psychiatric patient. There follows a broad overview of the legal theories under which liability could attach to an emergency department in the course of performing its emergency treatment functions.

The chapter continues with a discussion of the need for maintaining accurate and complete records on all patients treated in the emergency department. One of the most important documents from a legal viewpoint, that which discloses the patient's consent to medical treatment, is reviewed.

Lastly, there is a detailed analysis of a patient's consent to medical treatment, and a discussion as to why such consent from the patient is required before any medical treatment may be given. The requirements of a valid consent from patients of different ages and mental capacities are set forth. Also included is a discussion of when the consent may be given by a third party, or when it may be implied due to an emergency situation.

DUTY OF CARE AND DUTY TO CARE

An emergency department must exercise toward any patient that degree of care, skill, and diligence generally used by hospitals in the community where the hospital is located, or that degree of care, skill, and diligence that is used by hospitals in similar communities.[1] There is, however, a growing tendency to abandon the community or similar community standard in favor of a national standard.[2] In addition to a general standard of care imposed, a heightened standard may be created by either express or implied contract between the patient and the hospital.[3]

A duty also exists to admit emergency patients once the hospital, whether public or private, has established an emergency department. The maintenance of an emergency department creates a reliance on the part of the public that medical care will be available whenever a true emergency presents itself.[4]

DUTY WHEN PATIENT HAS DIED

The rights to possession, custody, and control of a deceased patient for the purposes of disposition are controlled by state law.[5] State statutes in most cases require only that the attending physician complete a certificate upon the death of a patient.[6] The next of kin should be notified of the death immediately. The duty of the hospital to reveal to a patient that which, in his or her best interest, should be revealed extends after the patient's death to the next of kin.[7]

An autopsy should not be performed without obtaining the permission of the nearest relative, or without authority from the appropriate public office. State statutes usually list the parties from whom an authorization for an autopsy can be obtained.[8] Once a legal authorization to perform an autopsy has been granted, those persons are estopped from claiming otherwise.[9]

DUTY WITH PSYCHIATRIC PATIENT

The duty imposed by law on hospitals and emergency departments is the exercise of such reasonable care toward a patient as the patient's mental and physical conditions, if known, require.[10] The duty extends to hospital personnel and others to take reasonable preclusive measures to prevent harm due to a patient's mental incapacity.[11] If the patient is being transferred, this duty extends to securing adequate precautions to restrain the patient, including appropriate notice to the ambulance service regarding any potentially aggressive condition.[12] It is also the required duty of the emergency department to protect patients from their known conditions. Failure to take a personal medical history or failure to examine or review the contents

of an available history may result in liability for subsequent injuries, since such procedures are considered reasonable.[13]

BASIS FOR LIABILITY

An injured patient has alternative theories of recovery, either in tort or for breach of contract, if an emergency department has failed to perform its duties and render services according to accepted standards of skill and care appropriate to hospitals of like status.[14]

Tort

A tort in law consists of a violation of a duty imposed by general law or otherwise upon all persons occupying the relation to each other which is involved in a given transaction.[15]

A hospital's liability in tort for negligence as a result of a hospital's performing a medical service is based on either one of two theories: corporate negligence or vicarious liability under the doctrine of *respondeat superior*.[16] The concept of corporate negligence was set forth in the landmark case of *Darling v. Charleston Community Memorial Hospital*,[17] wherein the scope of duty of the hospital was defined in terms of the hospital's by-laws, state statutes, and accreditation rules, in addition to the standards of care followed by other hospitals in the general community.

Under the doctrine of *respondeat superior* an employer is liable for the tort of an employee committed within the scope of such employment. Hospitals have avoided liability in the past by raising either the defense of an independent contractor or that of a borrowed servant. However, some jurisdictions have limited the application of these defenses. The California Supreme Court, in the leading case of *Seneris v. Haas*,[18] held that if a hospital leads the patient to believe that a professional person is an employee, then it may be held liable for negligence. In *Matlick v. Long Island Jewish Hospital*,[19] the court completely abandoned the doctrine of borrowed servant by holding that a given employee can serve the mutual interests of two employers at the same time. Thus, specific areas of responsibility should be fully delineated as to each and every person performing services in the emergency department.

It should also be noted that the doctrine of *res ipsa loquitur* can be used by the courts to thrust upon the hospital charged the duty of producing evidence where the chief evidence of true cause of injury, whether culpable or innocent, is accessible to the hospital but inaccessible to the injured person.[20] This doctrine has been expanded and applied against all the physicians and hospital employees connected with a patient's course of medical treatment where the patient was, for a period of time, unconscious.[21]

Furthermore, this doctrine has been applied where the cause of injury is a mystery, if there is a reasonable inference that the hospital was negligent and such negligence caused the injury.[22]

As will be discussed, an action in tort may lie for assault and battery if medical treatment is performed on a patient without legal consent, or if the treatment exceeds the nature and scope of the consent that was given. Damages for such unauthorized treatment may be awarded without regard to whether or not negligence existed.

Contract

With respect to claims against hospitals arising out of contracts made by the emergency department, the rules of liability governing corporations generally are applied.[23] In the majority of jurisdictions exculpatory contracts (i.e., disclaimers of liability due to fault) between hospitals on one hand and patients on the other are invalid.[24] An emergency department can establish a contractual duty to cure if it assures the patient that a certain result

will be achieved or that a specific treatment will be given.

PATIENT RECORDS

From the time a patient enters the emergency department of a hospital until the time of discharge, a written record should be maintained showing personal history of the patient, diagnosis, a valid legal consent to treatment, and the actual emergency treatment and medication administered. This should be done not only to provide a basis for proper treatment but also to provide a foundation for strong medical testimony as a defense to any future allegations of malpractice.[25]

The record should be as accurate as time and circumstances permit. It should be complete and concise, yet include all essential details; it should also be easy to read and easy to fill out. Initial responsibility for maintenance of accurate emergency department records rests with the physician who examines the patient.[26]

The importance of complete and accurate records cannot be overemphasized. Failure to take a complete medical history upon hospital entry, where such would have disclosed a previous condition, is sufficient to impose liability.[27]

PATIENT CONSENT

All competent individuals have the right to determine what shall or shall not be done to their own bodies. Likewise, every patient has the right to consent or not to consent to treatment. Consequently, medical treatment in the absence of the patient's consent may give rise to liability on the part of the hospital and treating physicians on the theory of battery.[28] Battery is the unlawful touching of another person without consent.[29]

Even when consent has been granted, if the touching is of a different nature or scope from that to which consent was given, a cause of action for battery may still arise.[30] Thus, the "informed consent" of the patient must be acquired before treatment is proper. The term "informed consent" implies not only agreement by the patient to the proposed treatment, but also, that before agreeing, information about the risks inherent and alternatives to the treatment has been given to the patient.

There is no law or statute requiring that a signed, written consent be obtained from a patient prior to the performance of medical treatment.[31] Although oral consent may be valid, reliance upon it may complicate the problem of proving it was actually given. Where possible, the use of consent forms is preferable to oral consent, in order to minimize potential legal risks should the patient later charge he or she did not consent to a course of treatment.

One of the major problems confronting hospitals today is the use of blanket consent forms, that is, those which authorize the hospital to do anything on the patient's behalf which it deems necessary. Courts in general have viewed these forms as ambiguous and of little or no effect, especially if the form fails to designate the specific medical problem confronting the patient and nature of the authorized treatment.

Consent in an emergency

Every attempt should be made to comply with the general rules of consent set forth below. However, if such is not possible, there is an exception to the general rule. In an emergency situation the consent of the patient to treatment is implied.[32] "Emergency" in a medical situation is such as to render immediate treatment advisable because of an unexpected or sudden situation.[33] It connotes a situation wherein a certain course of treatment is required to save a life or to safeguard health.[34]

When an emergency is claimed, the determination should never be made by a nurse, orderly, aide, or clerk. If there is a reasonable doubt whether medical care beyond first aid is required, such determination should be made by a licensed physician.

Validity of consent

In an integrated society where individuals become inevitably dependent upon one another for the exercise of due care, the requirement for explanation is not too great a burden to impose upon those who possess the instruments of treatment and whose due care is vital to life itself.

The doctrine of informed consent imposes upon an emergency department's personnel a duty to disclose to the patient all relevant information concerning the proposed course of treatment including any collateral hazards attendant thereto. The purposes, nature, and risks of a proposed treatment should be reasonably explained so that the patient can give an intelligent consent. Disclosure of information regarding any hazardous consequences of a treatment may be withheld if full disclosure will be detrimental to the patient's total care and best interests.[35] However, some jurisdictions have established outer limits requiring full disclosure where surgical procedures bear a statistical probability of success of less than 50%.[36]

In determining the question of liability for nondisclosure for therapeutic reasons, courts will generally follow the rule applicable in medical malpractice actions whereby the question of negligence is decided by reference to the general practice followed by the medical profession in the locality under the same or similar circumstances.[37] In the case of a conscious adult this duty of disclosure is owed to the patient and not to the spouse or any other member of the family.[38] It is advisable also to procure the consent of a spouse if treatment involves either danger to life, sterilization, the impairment of sexual functions, or the death of an unborn child.

In summary, no hard and fast rule can be stated regarding the circumstances that will excuse the withholding of full disclosure, and each case will be determined on its own particular facts.[39]

Methods and elements of consent

Adults. The requirement of consent to administer medical treatment on a conscious adult can be met in several ways. Generally, consent may be obtained expressly from the patient either orally or in writing, keeping in mind the problems of proof discussed earlier in regard to oral consent. If the consent is not express, it may be implied from the action of a patient who knowingly accepts treatment. Also, consent may be implied by law when the patient, by age or condition, is unable to evidence acceptance.[40]

Also, if an adult is temporarily unable to give an informed consent because of unconsciousness resulting from trauma or sedation, consent may be obtained from another person, if that person was authorized previously to give such consent by the patient undergoing treatment.[41]

Minors. If the minor is younger than 14 years, consent must be obtained from either parent, if any, or legal guardian or a person *in loco parentis* (one standing in the place of a parent with a parent's rights, duties, and responsibilities).[42] The parent's consent must be an informed one.[43] In minors 14 years of age and older, consent is required from the minor patient and either parent, if any, or the legal guardian, or person standing *in loco parentis*. However, if such minor does not appear to be capable of understanding and executing an informed consent, then the rules for a minor under 14 years of age should be followed.

Under certain circumstances a minor 14 years of age or older may be considered emancipated, which means that the parents have relinquished control and their consent is not required. Factors that establish emancipation include marriage, the earning of one's own living, the maintenance of a home separate from one's par-

ents, and psychologic maturity.[44] Attempts should be made to comply with the rules regarding adults in the treatment of an emancipated minor. The fact of emancipation and the source of information should be carefully recorded.

Psychiatric patients. A finding of "mental illness," even by a judge or jury, does not raise a presumption that the patient is legally incompetent.[45] In the absence of a specific judicial finding of incompetence, a psychiatric patient retains the right to manage his or her own affairs.[46] Therefore, such a psychiatric patient has the right to consent, or refuse to consent, to a specific course of treatment.[47] If there has been a judicial determination of incompetence, implying that the patient is unable to understand the nature, purpose, and risks incident to a proposed medical treatment, consent must be obtained from a legally appointed guardian.[48] However, it should be noted that in some jurisdictions, in an emergency situation where the psychiatric patient is a danger to either himself or herself, or to others, stopgap emergency measures to reduce this danger may be introduced.[49] Also, the implied consent theory discussed above may be applied.

REFERENCES

1. *Foley v. Bishop Clarkson Hospital*, 195 Neb. 89, 173 N.W.2d 881 (1970). See also 40 Am. Jur.2d, *Hospitals & Asylums*, § 26 p. 869.
2. *Alden v. Providence Hospital*, 382 F.2d 163 (C.A.D.C. 1967).
3. 36 ALR 3d 440, § 3(e)451.
4. *Manlove v. Wilmington General Hospital*, 53 Del. 338, 169 A.2d 18 (1961).
5. 18 Am.Jur.2d, *Coroners or Medical Examiners*, § 6 p. 519.
6. West Cal. Health & Safety Code § 10202 (West 1970).
7. *Emmet v. Eastern Dispensary & Casualty Hospital*, 396 F.2d 931 (C.A.D.C. 1967).
8. *French v. Ochsner Clinic*, 200 So.2d 371 (La.App. 1967).
9. West Cal. Health & Safety Code § 7113 (West 1970).
10. *Vistisa v. Presbyterian Hospital & Medical Center of San Francisco, Inc.*, 67 Cal.2d 465, 432 P.2d 193 (1967).

11. *Rice v. California Lutheran Hospital,* 27 Cal.2d 296, 163 P.2d 860 (1945).
12. *Jones v. United States,* 272 F.Supp. 679, 399 F.2d 936 (2d Cir.N.Y. 1968).
13. *Macon-Bibb County Hospital Authority v. Appelton,* 123 Ga.App. 445, 181 S.E.2d 522 (1971).
14. *Greeson v. Sherman,* 265 F.Supp. 340 (D.C.Va. 1967).
15. Blacks Law Dictionary § 1660 (4th Ed.).
16. IIA Hospital Law Manual, *Negligence* (1968).
17. *Darling v. Charleston Community Memorial Hospital,* 33 Ill.2d 326, 211 N.E.2d 253 (1965), cert. denied, 383 U.S. 946 (1966).
18. *Seneris v. Haas,* 45 Cal.2d 811, 291 P.2d 951 (1955).
19. *Matlick v. Long Island Jewish Hospital,* 25 App.Div.2d 538, 267 N.U.S.2d 631 (1966).
20. *Ybarra v. Spangard,* 25 Cal.2d 486, 154 P.2d 687 (1944).
21. *Beaudoin v. Watertown Memorial Hospital,* 32 Wis.2d 132, 145 N.W.2d 166 (1966).
22. *Clark v. Gibbons,* 66 Cal.2d 399, 426 P.2d 525 (1967).
23. 40 Am.Jur.2d, *Hospitals & Asylums,* § 14 p. 860.
24. *Turkl v. Regents of University of California,* 50 Cal.2d 92, 383 P.2d 441 (1963).
25. 72 A.L.R.2d 396. See also *Joyner v. Alton Ochsner Medical Foundation,* 230 So.2d 913 (La.App. 1970).
26. Spencer, *Emergency Rooms in General Hospitals,* 25 No.Car. Med. J. 1 (Aug. 1964).
27. *Foley v. Bishop Clarkson Memorial Hospital, supra.*
28. *Rogers v. Lumberman's Mutual Casualty, Co.,* 119 So.2d 649 (La.App. 1960).
29. Black's Law Dictionary § 1660 (4th Ed.).
30. *Rogers v. Lumberman's Mutual Casualty, Co., supra.*
31. *Bradford v. Winter,* 30 Cal.Rptr. 243, 215 Cal.App.2d 448 (1963).
32. *Cobbs v. Grant,* 104 Cal.Rptr. 505, 502 P.2d 1 (1972).
33. *Moran v. Board of Medical Examiners,* 187 P.2d 878 (1947).
34. R. C. Morris & A. R. Moritz, *Doctor and Patient and the Law* (5th Ed. 1971).
35. *Falgo v. Leland Stanford, Jr. University Board of Trustees,* 154 Cal.App.2d 560, 317 P.2d 170 (1957).
36. *Hunter v. Brown,* 4 Wash.App. 899, 484 P.2d 1162 (1971).
37. *Brown v. Colm,* 114 Cal.Rptr. 128, 11c3d 639 (1974).
38. *Nishi v. Hartwell,* 52 H.A. 188, 473 P.2d 116 (1970).
39. *Watson v. Clutts,* 262 N.C. 153, 136 F.E.2d 617 (1964).
40. *Clemens v. Regents of University of California,* 8 Cal.App.3d 1, 87 Cal.Rptr. 108 (1970).
41. *Failure to Inform is Medical Malpractice,* 23 Vanderbuilt L.Rev. 754 (1970).
42. *Cobbs v. Grant, supra.*
43. *Brown v. Wood,* 202 So.2d 125 (Fla.App.Ct. 1967).
44. *Bach v. Long Island Jewish Hospital,* 48 Misc.2d 207, 267 Nys.2d 289 (Supp.Ct. 1966).
45. Cal. Welfare & Institution Code, § 5368.
46. *Sengstack v. Sengstack,* 4 N.Y.2d 502, 151 N.E.2d 887 (1958).
47. *Winters v. Miller,* 446 Fed.2d 65 (2d Cir. 1970), *Cert. denied,* 404 U.S. 985 (1971).
48. *Consent to Surgical Operations,* 26 Albany L. Rev. 25 (1962). See also *Morris & Moritz, supra.*
49. Cal. Welfare & Institutions Code, §§ 5150 et seq.

CHAPTER **3**

Behavior responses in emergency situations

Carmen Germaine Warner, R.N., P.H.N.

Life and death on this planet now lie in Man's
    hands.
    At depth after depth we penetrate these phe-
      nomena which encompass us.
    Still beyond our grasp shimmer the ultimate
      truths.
    Unless we master these, how shall we learn—
      not to die—but to live?*

The tendency of emergency department personnel to view patients as problems to be rid of must be changed. The purpose of a good emergency department is to initiate diagnostic and therapeutic maneuvers that will speed total care of the patient to the most successful conclusion.

The philosophy of "get the patient to the floor, keep the emergency department clear" is the antithesis of what this vital area's direction should be. Personnel must take pride in the completeness of rapid assessment, the rapid initiation of critical support, and the final outcome as influenced by their efforts. The good practitioner discharges patients with minimal delay to the floor, to the intensive care unit, to surgery, or to their homes, but with all the necessary information available and all

necessary support already accomplished or instituted.

Perhaps one of the most neglected areas of emergency education is that of behavior and human relations. This aspect of care will determine whether the maximum of good evolves from an emergency department experience or whether there will be an everlasting animosity toward the hospital from patients and their families and friends.

Patients are *not* problems; they *have* problems. Many of these problems relate to fear, unfamiliar surroundings, and catastrophe to family groups. These important aspects must be handled with skill and knowledge.

ADMISSION

The first individual in contact with a patient or relative provides the initial impression, which is most vividly recalled. Routine admission questioning, though necessary, is often met by impatient answers and a lack of understanding as to the purpose. Priorities of immediate medical evaluation and care are automatically set by the patient, relatives, and friends. The need for basic information is overlooked.

---

*From Adams, A., and Newhall, N.: This is the American earth, San Francisco, 1968, Sierra Club Ballantine Books.

Personnel must view this reaction as normal. Information should be obtained as quickly as possible, making sure to explain its importance and effect on total patient care. If this is done in a gentle, honest fashion, greater cooperation will result.

It is not unusual for a patient to be admitted unaccompanied by family or friends. This can occur in accidents or home emergencies. Emergency personnel must recognize that it is essential to locate family or friends. The fear of hospitals is real, and this becomes intensified when the patient is alone. Law enforcement officials are often helpful in contacting the patient's relatives. When practitioners are unable to make contact, the patient should be informed.

Support and assistance in locating friends or family may prevent panic. For example, if an individual calls the emergency department to inquire about a missing person, or if someone is falsely directed to the hospital in order to meet a patient, the hospital personnel should either assist with the resolution of the problem or contact the sheriff or police. The missing individual might be in another hospital or could be completely safe, but unless the inquirer discovers this, a problem still exists. Although this is outside hospital routine, it is an important aspect in maintaining community good will.

In every emergency there are problems and needs to be met. Determining total patient needs requires more than physical evaluation. Interpretation of why the problem exists or how it might have originally occurred is fundamental in providing complete care.[1] Satisfaction results for all if a complete assessment is made upon admission.

PATIENT CONCERNS

People come to the emergency department because they have some medical concern. Personnel are unaware of what transpired prior to admission and are often uninterested or "too busy" to find out. Whether the problem is emotional or physical, it is real to the patient and frequently it is painful or frightening. Personnel often judge the validity of an admission and respond based on their individual feelings. This is not their decision. Their role is to be supportive and nonjudgmental and to assess the patient, recognizing preadmission history.

The patient, who is often left alone, deserves the courtesy of frequent checks to simply ask, "How are you feeling now?" "May I do something to make you comfortable?" Relaying progress or explaining any delay is essential. Personnel will find time to meet these basic, human needs only if they themselves are at ease. Unfortunately, personnel often are uneasy when confronted with crying, upset, or emotional patients. The ability to relate to these patients cannot be learned from a book; it must be a way of life. In addition to their individual well-being, patients often express concern about other situations. These situations affect cooperation with personnel, which in turn influences their own response to care.

Family members

Emergencies involving many victims often necessitate family separations. Several hospitals could be involved in caring for one family. If family members question the safety of others, personnel must be responsible for locating them. Patients demand respect of their emotional and social needs as well as physical attention. When patients inquire about others, they are primarily interested in their location and general condition. The exact condition is not paramount. The ability to establish indirect contact reduces anxiety and fears. Maintaining a basic communication level is comforting and beneficial. If a family member has died, personnel must assess how such news will affect the patient's condition; if adversely affected by this knowledge, other comfort measures should be used.

Out-of-town travelers are confronted with additional problems. Adults become concerned about family accommodations, financial arrangements, delays in planned travel time, and possible vehicle rescheduling. If the patient is a child, fear of strangers, fear of being left alone, discomfort, and unfamiliarity with procedures intensify a difficult situation.

Complete social assistance should be provided to lessen these difficulties. An explanation of the help provided family and friends should be shared with the patient. Difficulties and unanticipated situations will frequently arise, but if an honest explanation is provided, acceptance is more easily achieved. Care must be provided, addressing physical needs first, but concern for loved ones and their well-being must be recognized as an essential part of total patient care.

Other patients

It is not unusual for one patient to inquire about the status of another patient. Confidentiality and privacy should be respected at all times, but certain responses or ignoring the question will cause the patient unnecessary embarrassment and uneasiness.

The usual intent is not to obtain specifics but merely to express concern and to satisfy curiosity. These questions are often indirect queries about their own condition. If you are impatient and secretive, patients wonder if you are being dishonest with them. When this occurs, the element of trust is lost. A general response is sufficient, quite easy, and meaningful.

NONMEDICAL NEEDS

Personal customs, beliefs, and practices are part of everyone's life, and the practitioner must appreciate a heightened sensitivity in this area during stress. These

practices are often misinterpreted or misunderstood, and an element of disagreement or doubt may arise. Personnel must accept each person's right to individual feelings and practices.[2]

Religion is very basic and personal to a patient, especially during sickness or injury. Awareness of religious beliefs is important. Certain contacts and inquiries should be made if the patient is critical. If a religious belief or practice is unfamiliar, personnel should inquire about appropriate action. If a religious leader is with a patient, privacy must be maintained during the visit.

Certain beliefs do not permit the use of blood transfusions or certain diagnostic procedures. Personnel have the responsibility of informing all those involved of recommended care, available alternatives, and possible long- or short-term effects. The patient and his or her family must then make a conscientious decision. Such decisions demand respect.

In some beliefs special garments are worn and modesty is extremely important. For example, Mormons wear an undergarment under the usual underwear. This practice must be respected. Should removal be necessary, an explanation must be provided. Patients are often uncooperative because they are frightened or do not understand the situation.

Medals, charms, and jewelry frequently require removal. This should never be attempted without first explaining what you must do and why. The patient should be asked whether he or she prefers that these items be placed in security or attached to the gown. This element of decision-making is essential. It affords the patient an opportunity to participate in his or her own care. If personnel neglect patient input, the action is interpreted as demeaning and impersonal. Patients feel they are being treated like an object or a disease with no self-identity.

How can self-respect be maintained if

none is received from personnel? No wonder patients become angry, uncooperative, and demanding. A patient will try anything to be recognized as a real person with real needs.

When home discharge is not possible, valuables, including large sums of money or jewelry, must be secured according to established practices. The patient or relatives must understand completely what action has transpired.

Individuals may enter the emergency department with such items as contact lenses, false teeth, wigs or hair pieces, false eyelashes or fingernails, cosmetic breasts, artificial limbs, or other cosmetic belongings. These items usually have great personal value; should removal be required, patients and relatives must fully understand. Removal may cause embarrassment, and privacy must be extended as long as the patient's health is not affected.

A personal history is essential. Information regarding daily routine, allergies, type of employment, recreational activities, and usual body functions and habits must be obtained to determine what is normal for each individual. Comparisons become significant and assessment is made easier if such a history is available. Specific treatment might be influenced by the patient's type of employment. For example, someone whose income depends on heavy physical labor will require faster physical rehabilitation than someone who is a writer or oil painter. Likewise, a musician who has an injured hand obviously is more concerned about the final outcome and length of recovery than is a singer with the same injury.

A few moments of personal inquiry can affect long-term results. These moments are obviously ones well spent. The patient feels that you are really interested and becomes more vocal, sharing feelings and ideas that are important in total patient assessment and intervention.

HOW TO HANDLE FAMILY AND FRIENDS

It is not unusual for several relatives and friends to accompany a patient in an emergency. Their concern and desire that immediate attention be given their loved one are frequently displayed by an attitude of impatience or forcefulness. Large families, motorcycle groups, gypsies, and those accompanying victims of violence and sexual assault not only want to stay with the patient, but also often refuse to leave hospital grounds. They camp out in the hospital lobby, parking lot, cafeteria, or other social area.

Personnel must realize that family and friends have needs similar to the patient's, and these needs must be met.[3] It takes only a moment to inform the relatives or friends of the patient's progress and to relay any messages. This is the one thing friends and relatives wait for. They often sit with nothing on their mind except the patient. Too frequently they are extended no courtesy, understanding, or even pleasant words. No wonder they become impatient and verbal.

There is no reason why personnel cannot be flexible, recognizing the importance of caring for the entire person.[3] This includes friends and relatives. Patients must maintain communication with friends or family. If visitation privileges are allowed, permitting one person to stay for a short period of time, then allowing someone else to visit will alleviate anxiety and reduce potential problems. Recognizing everyone's feelings and being courteous in initiating a decision will save time and prevent misunderstandings. Personnel will establish a much more comfortable working environment through initiation of these little things.

Difficulties can arise with overprotective family members or friends. They may insist on helping to care for the patient, or they may just want to be close by. Asking such an individual to wait outside could initiate a strong reaction, ultimately affecting the patient. Instead, have this person sit down close to the patient, but out of traffic. This will minimize pending conflicts. The patient is obviously accustomed to such protective action, and the relative or friend has his or her needs met also. (Obviously, possibility of such action will depend totally on the patient's condition.)

Families manifest other behavior patterns that affect practitioner performance and patient care. By recognizing these patterns and understanding how to deal with them effectively, anxiety levels will be reduced, greater cooperation will be achieved, and a more comfortable atmosphere will develop. In addition to the overprotective family, there are emotional, deceptive, primitive-depriving, magical-thinking, fatalistic-authoritarian, religious, and best adapted families.[4] Each requires special understanding.

Families often become unhappy with a hospital, its procedures, personnel, and the care. Complaints mask the cry for help and the family's fright and anxiety. Relatives and friends feel overwhelmed and want to *do* something but are unable to. If personnel do not recognize this, relatives will become impatient and hurt, making the situation more difficult.

There are times when a patient's condition does not allow having friends and family in the room. This decision is to be made by personnel for the protection of the patient. An explanation of why such a decision was made and how it relates to the patient should be clearly understood by everyone. Time taken initially to handle this situation correctly will eliminate frustration and confusion later.

People who are confronted with an emergency attempt to cling to what is familiar and comfortable. A personal physician may represent this element of familiarity. If their own physician is not available, patients will accept personnel already in the emergency department, pro-

viding an attempt is made to meet their request and an explanation is provided should this be impractical. The patients will realize that what they are asking is impossible and that people are trying to do their very best. This is really what is important.

Sometimes patients decide where they wish to be treated and who will care for them. If a patient's condition will not be jeopardized by this request, it should be carried out. If the patient cannot tolerate transfer and the physician requested is unavailable, personnel must be firm in their decision to not transfer the patient. This reasoning must be explained with assurance that something will be done as quickly as possible. Usually, under these circumstances, the patient is unable to express feelings, and the relatives or friends are the ones in communication.

INTERPRETATION OF BODY MESSAGES

Patients in the emergency department will reflect the way they perceive physical self through unspoken messages—body messages. This projected physical self may include aspects of (1) anger, (2) fear, (3) confusion, (4) anxiety regarding self-function, sensation, mobility, (5) distrust, and (6) disbelief. Emergency personnel must be alert to these unspoken messages, recognize their meanings, and be prepared to deal with them. In the emergency department, patients reflect a variety of body messages through a changing concept of their individual body boundaries.

Basically, there are two major types of boundary disturbances manifested in hospitalized patients:

1. As a result of accident or injury, body walls change but the patient maintains the old body boundary, that is, traumatic amputation or other form of loss.
2. The patient changes a body boundary even though the body wall remains intact,[5] that is, a stroke patient.

Table 3-1. Indicators for assessing patient needs

Indicator	Action	Possible message
Eye movement (oculesics)	Rapid change in direction	Uneasiness Fear Confusion
	Staring	Shock Disbelief Displacement
	Lack of eye contact when speaking	Rejection Isolation Resentment
	Downward glances	Retreat Withdrawal
Body movement (kinesics)	Synchronized in speed with speech	Nervous Fear, if rapid movement noted Shock; lack of reality Stunned, if slow movement
	Extension of limbs and head	Relaxed Bored At ease Trust
	Contraction of limbs, head, and shoulders	Anxious Fearful Disapproval
	Direction body faces as compared to personnel	Retreat, withdrawn if faces toward wall Open and comfortable if facing personnel
	Use of hands or arms to cover head, face, eyes, and so forth	Hiding Withdrawal Need to be protected Need for protection
Spacial separation (proxemics)	Intimate distance 6-18 inches, actual contact	Consoled Comforted
	Personal distance, 2-4 feet	Communicate Relate messages Discuss problems
	Social distance, 4-7 feet	I'm personal Set up protection of self Distrust Assessing situation
Touching (haptics)	Reaching out Embracing Striking	Emotional intensity Grief, love Hatred
Time (chronemics)	Waiting overtime to see someone	The person who waits deems himself inferior to the person he is waiting for
	Interrupts conversation	Interrupter reflects greater importance than the interrupted
	Silence	Boredom, thought Deep affection; sorrow
Voice[6] (vocalics)	Linguistic message spoken in normal tone of voice	Depicts fair measurement of honesty
	Vocalic nonverbal message occurs when intense volume and emotion accompany message	Depicts defensiveness Hidden messages Cover-up

Personnel must recognize the signs and symptoms of patients who may feel either trapped or confused by existing boundaries. There are several indicators that will provide clues for assessing patient needs, and these must be recognized and applied upon admission (Table 3-1). These are to be recognized only as possible indicators and serve as a door-opening mechanism for assessing patient needs.

Further determinations will need to be made in the form of direct communication. It is the role of emergency personnel to provide a platform of trust and comfort so patients feel more at ease in discussing feelings and concerns regarding disturbances to their body boundaries.

Several factors affect patient adaptation to changes:

1. Nature of the threat
2. Meaning of the threat to the person
3. Coping abilities
4. Response from others significant to them
5. Assistance available to patient and family

Thus, in order for personnel to intervene appropriately, they must—

1. Know and understand the nature of the threat
2. Assess how the patient perceives the threat
3. Identify and reinforce the patient's coping abilities
4. Assist significant others
5. Coordinate care, be an interpreter and advocate if the patient needs their assistance, and mobilize community resources.[6]

These steps sound logical and simple, but unless effective tools are employed that will aid in determining certain factors, the effort will be futile. There are two components to the process of determining factor or data collecting. The first concerns observation. This input will come from both visible determinants and recognition and understanding of body messages. Data gathered through observation include the following:

1. Pain and its severity
2. Bodily features (loss of limb, obesity, edema, etc.)
3. Presence of equipment or supportive devices, that is, splints, IVs, monitors, tubes, and so forth
4. The patient's resulting change in appearance, sensation, function, control, and disturbed body boundaries

The second component deals with direct patient interviews. Some of the questions valuable in determining pertinent data might include the following:

1. Patient's perception of existing problems
2. What coping mechanisms are being incorporated
3. Existing relationships with family and friends
4. An overview of the patient's normal daily pattern
5. The patient's self-perception
6. What areas of concern the patient is focusing on (body parts and so forth)

This information can be of value as long as the interviewer does not overwhelm or intimidate the patient or family. Intimidation may occur without direct intent or awareness, and personnel should be alert to signs of withdrawal. An accessible checklist including active listening techniques may be of assistance. The following techniques may be of value:

1. Restating or paraphrasing techniques
2. Summarizing frequently
3. Responding to nonverbal body messages
4. Responding to feelings

Refraining from the use of certain communication barriers will also prove valuable, save time, and prevent misunderstandings. A few common communication barriers are listed below:

1. Making premature comments and evaluations
2. Making statements that are too general

3. Interrupting the patient or family
4. Talking instead of actively listening
5. Talking down to patients and family
6. Asking loaded questions
7. Placing the blame
8. Arguing
9. Displaying irritating listening habits
10. Repeatedly telling patients and family what to do

Recognizing and understanding the meaning of body messages and applying good active listening and communication skills will enable emergency personnel to contribute greatly to an accurate and rapid patient assessment.

DEATH AND DYING

Death in the emergency department is traumatic for everyone. The unexpected creates problems for those trying to cope with, accept, or even handle a difficult situation.

Although a great deal has been written about death and the dying patient[7] this area is rejected and overlooked more than any other aspect of health care. Because it deals with the unknown, there is always an intense feeling of discomfort. This uneasy situation is compounded when an emergency factor is added. Immediate demands on personnel provide an excuse for not handling death at the emotional, feeling level.

Each emergency department must reevaluate roles and responsibilities to allow more effective handling of such situations. Personnel must deal with their own feelings about and reactions to death, recognizing that these feelings are obvious to the patient's friends, relatives, and other personnel. It is not unusual for personnel to feel they have failed should a patient die. Individuals who recognize this must take the initiative to assist personnel as well as family and friends in expressing how they feel.

For relatives and friends the death of a loved one is a very disturbing time. They are anxious, frightened, panicky, and angry. They want everything to be done immediately and feel that everyone should be involved. They resent not being with the patient despite the confusion that would result.

Someone such as a medical social worker or patient representative should devote time to the friends and family of the deceased. There is no reason why they should be left alone. Imagine how agonizing that must be. Relatives need someone who will listen in a nonjudgmental, nonthreatening manner. They need someone who will be supportive and understanding. This effort will save time, anxiety, and confusion, and it will also reduce potential disturbance to all patients, personnel, and other family members.

Religious leaders should be involved in aiding the relatives of the deceased as often as possible to augment the supportive measures initiated by personnel.

Death is certain but unknown; this creates an element of fear. The way in which each person relates to the knowledge that death is certain is critical.[8] Inability to accept death, difficulty in recognizing comfort efforts from others, and inability to accept aspects of the unreal, the uncertain, and the unbelievable may occur during this critical period.

Phases of dying

There is a clearly outlined sequence of dying that may be observed in the emergency department. Certain aspects of this sequence should be recognized and applied when caring for a dying patient.

1. The patient's sensation, power of motion, and reflexes are lost first in the legs and gradually diminish in the arms.
2. As peripheral circulation fails, there is a drenching sweat, causing the body surface to cool regardless of room temperature.

3. The head of the dying patient is always turned toward the light.
4. The sensation of touch is diminished, yet the patient can sense pressure.
5. Pain may be present throughout the entire dying process.
6. Dying patients are often conscious to the very end.
7. Spiritual needs become very strong and arise most strongly during night hours.
8. There appears to be an apparent interval of peace which is present before death.[9]

Throughout the dying process, patients will often manifest certain distinct and real, common fears. These often may be an intense point of focus and whether addressed verbally or through body messages, personnel must be cognizant of their existence.

1. *Pain.* This is often acute and realistic. Every effort should be made to keep the patient as comfortable as possible.

2. *Loneliness.* Pain becomes most intense when a patient is left alone. "Please don't leave me alone" may be a silent cry that must be respected. Patients desperately fear sleep, not because they feel they might die but because they cannot tolerate the thought of being alone.

3. *Fear.* With the presence of fear, life and value of self have no meaning. This becomes a choking, overwhelming feeling that blocks out all rational thought.

An example of this horrifying feeling is clearly expressed in the pleading words of a dying student.

The dying patient is not yet seen as a person and thus cannot be communicated with as such. He is a symbol of what every human fears and what we each know at least academically, that we, too, must someday face. . . . We may ask for whys and wherefores, but we don't really expect answers. . . . If only we could be honest, both admit of our fears, touch one another. If you really care, would you lose so much of your valuable professionalism if you cried with me?

Just person to person? Then it might not be hard to die . . . in a hospital . . . with friends close by.[8]

Phases of mourning

Reactions to the death of a loved one develop in stages that vary in length. Individuals will respond in various ways at different times, but each person must be allowed to initiate this process at his or her own rate.

Lindemann[10] explains the existence of three phases of mourning.

Phase 1: Shock and disbelief. In phase 1 actual symptoms of distress occur, lasting 20 to 30 minutes. Such manifestations as a feeling of tightness in the throat, choking with shortness of breath, need for sighing, an empty feeling in the abdomen, and lack of muscular power are present. Feelings that everything is unreal accompany feelings of emotional distance and preoccupation with the image of the deceased.

Guilt is present at this time; self-accusations of failure to have done right accompany exaggeration of the importance of minor omissions.

Phase 2: Developing awareness. Personality disorganization and pain or despair because of yearning for the lost object occur during phase 2. There is weeping and a feeling of helplessness and identification with the deceased.

Phase 3: Resolving the loss. Reorganization takes place and new relationships are formed during the third phase.

Obviously, the phases of mourning only begin in the emergency department, but if personnel are patient, understanding, and supportive, the entire process will be easier for the relatives and friends of the deceased.

Personnel often become impatient with the time involved in procedural duties following a death. Information that must be secured includes the following: (1) when was the patient last seen by a doctor; (2) did the physical condition warrant death;

and (3) will the coroner need to be called? The family physician will need to be contacted unless already in attendance, and mortuary arrangements must be made. The manner in which these duties are performed is observed and criticized by the family.

If there are no relatives at the hospital or if the deceased has no identification, law enforcement officers must be contacted for assistance.

Steps in dealing with family and friends

Caring for a patient who is dying drains emergency personnel physically and emotionally. The need to get away and to be alone is very real. Yet this need often has to be set aside because family and friends are hurting and desire someone to be with them.

They feel alone and frightened. Personnel can provide critical support and understanding at this time when it will have its greatest impact.

1. Personnel should first of all just listen. Assessment, understanding and the ability to empathize will come. When these factors are present, there is no need to supply an answer.

2. Respect body messages, changing roles, and conversation when it becomes appropriate.

3. Gather pertinent data that will aid in understanding the family as individuals. This is an extremely critical factor when attempting to establish a mechanism for trust and rapport.

4. Develop the concept of shared care, where family and relatives are afforded the opportunity to participate in the caring process. Unnecessary pain should be avoided at all costs.

5. When death is imminent, the patient and family members should not be agitated for any reason. Little things must be respected. Everything should be explained, including the "whys, hows, and whens."[11]

Finally, the patient and family need *permission—permission to cry, to be angry, to express resentment*. Let them know it is okay to feel, to be themselves—maybe for the first times in their lives. *Give them permission to be free.*

LOSS OF BODILY FUNCTION

Certain emergencies involve immediate or potential loss of function. In instances such as a traumatic amputation, destruction of a limb, or total removal of an eye, the loss is apparent and can be dealt with. In other situations the outcome is not always obvious in the emergency department. A traumatic eye injury might not cause vision disturbance for weeks, and the use or restoration of a severed limb will depend on effective growth and healing processes. A badly lacerated face may or may not require plastic repair for cosmetic purposes. If plastic repair is necessary, it must be performed correctly the first time to eliminate the need for future revision. Severe back or neck injuries can cause permanent paralysis or function may be restored following initial trauma. A person with a stroke may achieve total rehabilitation or may never regain speech or specific body movement.

These situations demand a great deal from all personnel. Questions from family and patient are searching, pleading, and demanding of reassurance. Fear of the unknown, accompanied by disbelief, is often more difficult to cope with than the obvious.

Patients and relatives depend on personnel for warmth, sincerity, and guided direction.[2] Tension may be lessened with proper support. False hope is dangerous and should never be offered in an attempt to make an individual feel better. Honesty regarding the unknown, reassurance concerning appropriateness of care, and just being there will be extremely beneficial. Many times quiet listening rather than constant talking is most helpful.

HOSPITALIZATION

Not all emergency patients are discharged following care. Hospitalization is required on many occasions. Patients are often unprepared for admission and are faced with a number of concerns. Patients are worried about how hospitalization will affect job security and their families: "Will my boss hire someone else?" "What about the money I will lose while not working?" "What about the cost of this hospitalization?" "How will my family function without me?" "I don't want to stay in this unfamiliar place!" These are all common and very real concerns.

Many of these questions stem from fear of the unknown. Emergency department personnel must take the time to perform preadmission teaching for patient and family. Answering questions usually is sufficient to begin with because it provides confidence that you care and are willing to help.

Like children, patients will not ask more questions than they are ready for. Their usual thoughts are, "How long will I have to stay?" "When can my family visit me?" "What will they do to me?" Generally, straightforward answers will meet this first phase of adjustment. Being honest when a specific answer is not available will actually gain patient and family respect.

Personnel must be familiar with hospital policy and procedures in order to answer questions and perform preadmission teaching effectively. This orientation period is essential, because it establishes an atmosphere of cooperation and trust that will accompany the patient during the remainder of the hospital stay.

Hospitalization might be advised when the patient's physician is out of town or unable to see the patient prior to admission. Communication must be established in reference to required care. The final decision is based on the patient's condition, and when patient choice is possible, it should be part of the plan regarding hospitalization and who will initiate care. Cooperation is easy once the patient feels comfortable with suggested care and has been involved in the plan. If patients are presented with all possibilities and associated difficulties, they will be less likely to make unrealistic requests. Patient involvement is very important in the decision-making process.

Transferring patients

If hospitalization is required and the patient and family desire another hospital or other personnel, arrangements should be made for this transaction. The basic consideration should be the patient's condition. If a transfer would endanger the patient's life, it should be denied and the reasoning explained to all involved. In such situations the requested physician would come to the patient. A transfer would be arranged when the patient's condition is *stabilized*. This information should be shared with the family.

If the patient can tolerate a transfer, appropriate communication should be established among involved personnel so as to expedite the transfer. An accurate awareness of the patient's condition is a must. The receiving emergency department must be adequately informed and prepared. This requires time, but if done properly, the transfer can be done with minimal trauma.

Sometimes transfers are made to other facilities such as extended care facilities or to the home. This must be arranged as quickly as possible so as not to inconvenience those involved.

REACTIONS TO AN EMERGENCY

Emergencies, especially those dealing with health situations, initiate very normal responses. Emergency personnel, because of demands to meet physical needs, often do not take time to react to the total patient or the total family.

Fear

Fear is a common reaction felt by most patients. Hospitals are extremely frightening even when an admission is scheduled. When someone is suddenly confronted with an admission, this fear is greatly intensified. Often the cause and extent of illness or injury are unknown, and the resulting fear is felt by patient and family. Fears regarding the patient's condition and the complexity of care required demand answers that often are neglected. This neglect may result in demanding families, uncooperative patients, and reduced response to care.

Understanding that fear is present represents the first step toward better and more effective care. As personnel accept more responsibility for care of the total patient and increase their skills, they must automatically comfort the patient, listen to expressed and unexpressed needs, and provide the courtesy of explaining what is transpiring and establishing good communication. The patient's fear will be reduced by such measures. Cooperation and understanding by friends and relatives will likewise increase if the same courtesy is extended to them.

Hysteria

The emergency department personnel, who deal with so many things that are unpredicted, often must deal with individuals who panic and progress into a state of hysteria. The beginning stage of hysteria should be familiar to all personnel and should be properly handled in order to prevent further explosive reactions. When someone begins to panic, he or she often expresses a very contagious and quite disorganized type of behavior, which is called "blind flight" depression.[2] When this action is observed, every effort should be made to remove any audience, because the patient will almost never calm with relatives and additional personnel present. One person must stay with the patient and speak in a slow, clear voice, using short sentences of one or two words. This gentle, kind firmness is necessary, because hysterical individuals are seeking some type of firm foundation. Providing strength and understanding to such patients must be recognized as an important function of all

personnel. This action will prevent a situation from arising in which physical attention is necessary and will reduce involvement of other patients and family members.

Increased or excessive activity should be recognized and handled in a similar fashion. People often cry out loudly for help in subtle ways, yet most emergency personnel do not recognize this until the problem becomes severe.

Impatience

When time must be spent in a hospital, the waiting period, though only a few minutes, seems like hours. Any medical concern, regardless of its seriousness, is extremely important to those involved. In fact, this becomes their entire life and they feel the need for full attention. If these situations are not handled properly, patients and family become angry and hostile, which can result in disruptive behavior that is often upsetting to others.

These situations can be prevented if a few moments are taken at the very beginning to explain what will be happening to the patient and the degree to which personnel will be involved. If other patients require immediate attention, people will understand and cooperate, but first they must be extended common courtesy and respect. If personnel assume that others understand what is happening, or if they say to patients in an offhand manner, "I'll be right with you" and then rush out, patients will accept this as neither courteous nor respectful and will respond accordingly. The small amount of time it takes to treat patients as real persons is beneficial yet rarely initiated. This effort affords much more comfort than most technical procedures and is definitely appreciated.

A brief explanation of a procedure before you begin is common courtesy. The patient has the right to know what is being done and why. This holds true for the unconscious patient as well who, though unresponsive, might still hear. A gentle hand on the forehead or a touch of reassurance to the arm lessens many anxieties that manifest themselves in effective or ineffective responses. These actions take but a few seconds. They are so very simple to do, yet they are often neglected, and tension levels rise as a result.

Sadness

Much softer than the grief of death is the reaction of sadness and loneliness. The person expressing this quiet feeling receives less attention than does the crying person; this lack of attention only intensifies the situation. The cry for help is much softer, and the acceptance of help is much more difficult. These people can easily become depressed and completely withdrawn.

Usually persons experiencing sadness enter the emergency department by themselves and have few relatives or friends. A physical illness or injury only intensifies their current feelings and makes their situation extremely difficult. It is almost as if they do not have the strength to ask for help.

Workers other than medical personnel should be utilized in a counseling role; time should be spent just listening to the patient. These patients have an intense need to express their feelings, but they can do so only to someone who will not rush off. They need someone who will demonstrate a tranquil, accepting attitude. Numerous problems, other than physical complaints, will unfold if such opportunities are made available. This will lead to referrals, which are necessary if the total patient is to be cared for.

If the patient is depressed, personnel should respond with appropriate care and attention in addition to any physical measures necessary.

Confusion

Injury or illness may precipitate disorientation and confusion, which can be either intense or minimal. This factor should be considered in total evaluation and care.

The cause may be chemical, physical trauma, or as a result of mental collapse.

Minimal confusion could result from being in unfamiliar surroundings with unfamiliar people and equipment. It is extremely important that prior to the initiation of any procedure an explanation be given regarding what is to be done and its purpose. A patient who has the feeling of being overwhelmed by intense activity and the use of unfamiliar equipment actually has a reduced response to care. This fact should be considered and attended to accordingly. It should be the routine procedure for everyone to relate the why's and how's to all patients before any care is provided.

DEALING WITH VICTIMS OF VIOLENCE

Emergency departments across the country are seeing more and more victims of sexual assault and intrafamily violence. The incidence of child abuse, child molestation, spouse battering, and rape has received considerable publicity, and society has become extremely vocal. Victims of these assaults are being encouraged to seek emergency medical assistance and to elicit support from various community agencies.

Reverberations of this increased community awareness, support, and sympathy have resulted in greater honesty regarding the actual causes of black eyes, bodily bruises, and lacerations on certain concealed portions of the body. There are requests for greater availability of medical, legal, and social services, augmented by support from local law enforcement officials.

These requests are being expressed by local women's groups and commissions, while more advocate groups are making themselves available to victims during the physical examination.

This available resource should be utilized as these advocate groups often form critical linkages between existing systems. Their support and willingness to assist victims may often be most helpful, especially when other demands do not permit the emergency personnel's continual presence with victims and family.

Following are some additional functions that advocacy groups provide:
1. Counseling support
2. Explaining policy and procedures
3. Making appropriate referrals
4. Contacting friends and family
5. Providing transportation, shelter, and clothing
6. Establishing a mechanism of trust for the frightened, confused, lonely victim

Emergency personnel must clearly recognize and admit the many hidden correlations between victims of violence and other family members. A woman who comes to the emergency department following a battering incident will often be the mother of children who have been abused or molested. Continual, unreported, untreated family batterings could end in homicide.

The sexually assaulted woman or child often faces tremendous emotional and self-persecuting problems. These result in distrust and hatred toward men, with accompanying guilt and lack of self-confidence. Couples who have had to deal with an incident of rape find their relationship dissolves unless proper counseling and therapy are secured.

This cycle repeats itself from generation to generation unless proper intervention is taken to break and correct the problem. A child abused or molested when small grows up knowing violence as an accepted form of dealing with problems and frustration. Never being confronted with alternative patterns of behavior, the child follows this as a way of life.

If emergency personnel can begin to understand and identify these phenomena, they will be better prepared to make appropriate referrals and to initiate a break in this cycle of violence.

EMERGENCY DEPARTMENT MEDICAL SOCIAL WORKER

Every emergency department needs a full-time medical social worker to handle the numerous nonmedical situations that arise. As has been stressed previously in this chapter, other factors related to the social environment greatly influence patient and family response to care, overall cooperation, and adjustment to the emergency. Emergency department personnel are often unable to spend time dealing with concerns unrelated to medical and emotional demands. A medical social worker would benefit family, friends, and the patient.

A medical social worker with a foundation in counseling and interpersonal relations would be invaluable in the emergency department. This person could work effectively in all situations that might otherwise develop into misunderstandings between personnel and patients. Being able to listen—taking the time to hear what patients are *really* saying rather than what they are verbally saying—would provide clues for adjustment to necessary care.

When patients shared problems that would require the attention of persons outside the emergency department, referrals could be made at that time and any resulting questions answered as they arose. Knowledge of available resources, provided by the medical social worker, would stimulate a learning opportunity for other personnel.

Referral services dealing with lodging, transportation, and food are extremely important. When people from out of town are confronted with an emergency, their first concern rests with the patient. After appropriate care has been instituted, their attention is directed to lodging facilities. If their automobile has been damaged, how can they find transportation? How will they inform others or their personal physician? What about establishing communication with employers or others when travel time is delayed? These concerns need attention, and presently it is the family's responsibility, while upset and anxious, to follow through on their own. A medical social worker would alleviate most of these worries.

With any type of illness or injury, insurance and financial costs present a problem. If people have inadequate insurance and very little money, they will not be able to pay the hospital fee without some guidance and direction in locating alternative funds. The lack of money also presents a problem in securing food and lodging. The more assistance the family can receive in such areas, the easier it will be to adjust to any existing emergency.

Special problems arise for the person who lives alone and has no one who can help during convalescence. Assistance in locating transportation and finding someone to care for this person is of primary concern once medical needs are met. If a child who has lost both parents is admitted to the hospital, the resulting problems are frustrating because of minimal time allotment and lack of referral knowledge. There are so many contacts to be made that handling such situations is a full-time job.

When a death has occurred a medical social worker would be invaluable. The amount of paperwork involved, the number of telephone calls to be made, and the number of people who must be contacted would justify employing a medical social worker. The friends and family of the deceased need the help of a full-time worker. Emotional situations require time, comfort, and reassurance from someone who cares, who is patient, and who can spend the necessary time.

A medical social worker must be part of the emergency team if emergency care is to meet the crying needs of our communities. People are demanding, and must receive, appropriate care; they need *care,* not just treatment of their physical condition.

Intervention must involve the entire person and associated family members.

PATIENT REPRESENTATIVE IN THE EMERGENCY DEPARTMENT

In addition to the use of social service department personnel in the emergency department, there is increasing use of a hospital patient representative or ombudsman in the emergency department. This adds an entirely new dimension of patient care and concern in problem-solving aspects, representing the total needs of patients and family.

Emphasis is placed on the characteristics of a patient representative that enable him or her to provide appropriate linkages with other aspects of the health care delivery system:

Dependability
Sensitivity
Insight into personal and hospital-related problems
Ability to practice good judgment
Confidentiality
Counseling techniques
Awareness of referral agencies
Knowledge of the role, function, policy, and personnel of every area within the hospital
Tactfulness and adaptability in dealing with personnel, patients, and relatives
Problem-solving and decision-making techniques practiced in a discreet manner
Good communications skills

With all these expectations, one would anticipate the patient representatives to be super persons but, like all humans, they are vulnerable; all too often situations can be challenging and at times discouraging.

The myriad requests from emergency personnel differ each day, and because of the nature of the situation, immediate action is required—often during evening and night hours. Hospital patient representatives have helped with many emergency requests; some of their valuable functions include the following:

1. Counseling friends and relatives at times of impending death

2. Staying with a patient who requires constant observation and stimulation
3. Working with sexual assault and battered victims
4. Contacting family and friends of a patient who enters the emergency department alone
5. Assessing specific personnel and patient needs and existing case loads by routine visits
6. Assisting with patient, family, and medical personnel conferences
7. Preventing patients from feeling they are merely numbers on a first come–first serve basis
8. Establishing friendly contacts and verbal interchange
9. Helping patients express their needs and concerns
10. Orienting emergency department personnel to the goals of the patient representative program and how it can assist emergency department personnel in becoming more effective
11. Serving on various patient care committees

As personnel become more convinced that patient representatives are a valuable asset, the coordinated team-building concept that results will create a more effective, efficient, qualitative manner of delivering emergency care.

TEACHING

Care, counseling, and referral services are provided for the patient. The patient also has a role and must take an active part in care received and the resulting recovery. This involvement develops as a result of patient and family teaching.

Procedures

Any procedure, before it is initiated, must be explained to the patient. If a procedure necessitates cooperation from the patient or family, patient and family teaching must be instituted. Effective teaching involves explaining a procedure, demon-

strating it, and allowing return demonstration accompanied by any questions. This should be performed very slowly to ensure understanding. If personnel closely observe facial expressions, the degree of understanding can automatically be interpreted. Patients should not be discharged until complete understanding is established. If teaching is not provided, the patient will have questions that must be clarified with emergency department personnel later, or more likely, the patient will perform the task incorrectly or not at all. Obviously, this method requires more time, is more frustrating, and reduces the total effectiveness of intended care. It is much easier to provide correct teaching initially.

Sometimes information sheets with home instructions are provided to patients. These should be used in addition to, not in place of, one-to-one patient teaching.

All emergency departments have certain rules and policies that might seem arbitrary or strange to patients and their families. These policies are often seen as time consuming and unrelated to actual physical care. People often become quite irritated and vocal unless the purpose of all policies, including the benefits to the patient, is explained to them in a polite manner.

All practitioners are expected to cope with crises and emergency situations in addition to assisting the patient in solving individual problems.[11] Many secondary irritations facing a patient must be dealt with, and individual help in these problem-solving areas is important. Basic judgment is essential and should be the foundation for appropriate action. In all problem-solving and patient-teaching situations, personnel must never act rushed, pushed, or irritated. Time and effort are completely wasted when patients become uncomfortable, are hurried, or feel that personnel are needed elsewhere. They are not listening and will not understand any individual teaching under such conditions.

Patient teaching, whether it involves

home teaching in preparation for discharge or preadmission teaching in preparation for continued hospital care, plays a major part in reducing the patient's fear and anxiety. Response to treatment is much more appropriate and effective when explanation of the why's, where's, and when's is introduced first. In the long-term picture, responses are quicker, thus reducing length of care and total cost.

Primary prevention

Primary prevention is essential in future care and protection of our communities. Direction has to be shifted from care of illness to protection of wellness. The emergency department is an excellent place for this to occur. When a patient is discharged, both the patient and the family should be taught how to prevent such an illness or injury from recurring. If people are given credit for and information about managing their own lives and health, the preventive care aspects might be more effectively implemented. Indicating known cases of emergencies and how these can be prevented or detected earlier is part of the necessary preventive teaching. All personnel must work toward this long-range goal. If all practitioners are effective in their charge, the patient load will be significantly reduced.

Introducing patients and family to certain trends in emergency identification and record keeping will assist personnel in determining histories and making quick medical assessments. Certain medals and identification cards assist in this process, and information about these services should be made available for patient evaluation.

Applied behavior modification

Behavior modification is a technique used to change behavior. It uses positive reinforcement extensively and applies negative reinforcement and aversive stimulation in lesser amounts.

Nursing professionals are beginning to utilize behavior modification techniques. This practice can be applied to emergency situations and should be recognized as a valuable tool. Certain aspects of behavior modification can be applied directly to emergency situations.

Positive reinforcement. Positive reinforcement is usually equated with the concept of reward. It implies that the logic behind the practice must be emphasized along with the practice itself. This technique is used to promote an increased frequency of a specific desired response.

According to the patient's behavior or reaction to treatment, counseling, and so forth, emergency personnel may respond with approval, attention, positive interactions, encouragement, and support. These reinforcers all serve to increase the frequency of a certain desired behavior.

Negative reinforcement. The concept of negative reinforcement is often misconceived. It is not a form of punishment, but an actual reward. It differs from positive reinforcement in that positive reinforcement is the granting of something the patient perceives as good, while the reward in negative reinforcement is the removal of something the patient perceives as bad. The actual removal is the reward. Negative reinforcement provides a reward that allows relief from anxiety, attempting to increase the frequency of a desired behavior response.

The practice of patient and family teaching emphasizing the removal or discontinuation of patterns or concepts having a negative effect on health is an example of this reinforcement.

Aversive stimulation. Punishment, or aversive stimulation, is meant to decrease the frequency of undesired behavior responses, thus not classifying it as a reinforcement. This concept punishes undesired behavior by following it with variables the patient may perceive as undesirable, resulting in a decreased probability of recurrence.

Personnel utilizing the concept of alternatives may have to reinforce aversive stimulation if corrective behavior does not occur.[12]

Recognizing that patient contact is short term, the impact of behavior modification may be less intense. However, it can and should be an integral part of the professional expansion of the nursing process into the area of patient management.

LEGAL CONCERNS

Because lawsuits occur frequently, emergency personnel have become knowledgeable in this area, and individual hospitals have established certain policies to keep employees updated.

The legal implications of emergency care demand that all personnel (1) recognize the services emergency departments can perform versus what is expected by the community, (2) become knowledgeable of all cases in which a consent is required, and (3) appreciate the value of admission histories[13] (see Chapter 2).

SUMMARY

Emergency situations arise every day. Practitioners must be knowledgeable, confident, and able to handle these problems immediately. Unlike the practitioner who works in the intensive care or coronary care unit and is familiar with each patient and the necessary care, the emergency department practitioner must be qualified to attend any emergency—immediately—with very little warning or patient history available. Consequently, all emergency practitioners *must* be able to execute the most advanced life-saving procedures. Life should *never* be endangered by awaiting an order when a physician is not available. The lack of foresight on the part of hospital administrators and educators to upgrade emergency departments has been a cause for current public criticism and unrest. There is no reason why, with proper education and practice, personnel should

not be able to effectively care for everyone —immediately—thus reducing current mortality rates.

Special emergencies also demand a great deal of assessment and intervention. Specific knowledge and tact are needed, for example, with a patient who does not speak English, with the victim of a sexual assault, with a patient who has a contagious or venereal disease, with a patient who is inebriated or has overdosed, or in cases where the patient is being held in custody.

In addition, the importance of behavioral reactions is stressed. This is the string that ties all emergencies together and is the one single common denominator. People everywhere have the same basic concerns, hurts, and sensitivities. Recognizing this and responding appropriately will lessen the stress and anxiety which currently exist in all emergency departments.

REFERENCES

1. Messick, J. M., and Aguilera, D. C.: A schema: the psychiatric nurse on the community mental health team, J. Psychiatr. Nurs. 4:481-539, Sept.-Oct. 1966.
2. Mahoney, R. F.: Emergency and disaster nursing, New York, 1967, The Macmillan Publishing Co.
3. Hofling, C., Leininger, M., and Brigg, E.: Basic psychiatric concepts in nursing, ed. 2, Philadelphia, 1967, J. B. Lippincott Co.
4. Petrello, M., and Sanger, S.: Eight types of families and how they affect your job, Nursing '73 3(5):43-47, May 1973.
5. McCloskey, J. C.: How to make the most of body image theory in nursing practice, Nursing '76 6(5):68-72, May 1976.
6. Egolf, D. B., and Chester, S.: Speechless messages, Nurs. Digest 4(2):26-29, March-April 1976.
7. Kubler-Ross, E.: Death and dying, New York, 1969, The Macmillan Publishing Co.
8. Aguilera, D., and Messick, J.: Crisis intervention: theory and methodology, ed. 2, St. Louis, 1974, The C. V. Mosby Co.
9. Gray, R. V.: Dealing with death and dying, nursing '77 skillbook, Jenkintown, Penn., 1977, Intermed Communications.

10. Lindemann, E.: Symptomatology and management of acute grief, Am. J. Psychiatry **101**:141-148, Sept. 1944.
11. Rinear, E.: Dealing with death and dying, nursing '77 skillbook, Jenkintown, Penn., 1977, Intermed Communications.
12. Closurdo, J. S.: Behavior modification and the nursing process, Nurs. Digest, pp. 27-31, Fall 1976.
13. Bromberg, M. J.: Legal problems and safeguards in the emergency department, RN **36**(5):48-49, 66-76, May 1973.

CHAPTER 4

Emergency nursing: the backbone of the emergency department

Mildred K. Fincke, B.S.N.Ed.

More than 125 years ago Florence Nightingale made a statement to the effect that a minimum requirement of the hospital is that it should do no harm. This remark gives us a graphic picture of hospital medicine and hospital nursing in the nineteenth century. Nursing as conceived today was admittedly in its infancy during most of Miss Nightingale's lifetime, and she could not in the wildest flight of fancy have envisioned the complexity of either hospitals or nursing as they are today.

In the 1970's nurses became the largest group of professionals in the health care system. Within the profession now are many specialty nursing services, and as medical science progresses and its techniques improve, these specialty services increase. Specialization is not unusual in our modern age, but in medicine it is the inevitable result of the requirement for sophisticated methods and tools to achieve a significant and unarguable goal: the best possible health care for every single patient, in or out of a hospital.

EMERGENCY NURSING AS A SPECIALTY NURSING SERVICE

Nursing services are so diversified that it is impossible to be highly trained and proficient in all aspects of patient care. As a section of specialty nursing, emergency nursing is not a Johnny-come-lately. For many years emergency nurses have been aware that improvement of emergency services and recognition of their role were essential to quality health care in hospitals and communities throughout the country. In contrast to earlier times, today the degree of knowledge, ability, and skills emergency nurses possess is now recognized. Nurses are a part of the health team in the delivery of health services, and they have responded to what is required of them, standing firmly alongside other specialty services as adept professionals distinctively trained in emergency nursing services. Nurses are fully aware that many times the emergency department has been a community's only recourse for health care, for such obvious reasons as inadequate physician coverage and limited or even poor health services. However, the role of every emergency nurse has changed. She or he must be able to articulate and respond to the full needs of the patient, to define individual functional positions and relationships to other members of the health team, and to demonstrate all of this in practice.

Methods by which the emergency nurse can achieve this particular status are readily available. It must first be emphasized that the nurse is held accountable for nursing practice and care. Both moral and legal responsibility must be accepted for each action, and therefore the nurse must be fully prepared by education, experience, mental confidence, and dedication to nursing to accept this responsibility. There is no other choice. If the nurse does not have the qualifications, the competence, and the desire to practice emergency nursing within the standards, regulations, and physical bounds of a particular setting, she or he should not be practicing.

All the standards, requirements and mechanisms for quality practice are well documented and provided for the emergency nurse in textbooks and guidelines prepared by numerous organizations. They are the products of study, experience, acquired wisdom, hard work, and unflagging concern for the achievement of optimum emergency health care.

EMERGENCY DEPARTMENT NURSES' ASSOCIATION

In 1970 the Emergency Department Nurses' Association was organized with one purpose in mind—the improvement of emergency health care delivery. Professional competency through the development of standards and provision for continuing educational opportunities were viewed as primary vehicles to reach this goal.

In 1973 the Federation of Specialty Nursing Organizations was formed to bring nursing organizations together as a means of discussing issues that face nursing and nurses and of influencing constructive changes in health care. EDNA became a member, and in 1975 the "Standards of Emergency Nursing Practice" was published by the American Nurses' Association, as approved by the Executive Com-

mittee of the ANA Division of Medical and Surgical Nursing Practice and by the Board of Directors of EDNA. EDNA was subsequently approved by the ANA National Accreditation Board as an accrediting body to review educational programs and award continuing education credits.

Continuing education

As an accrediting body, EDNA developed a continuing education curriculum,[1] which covers the areas of responsibility of emergency nurses, including clinical and management topics. The curriculum is intended as a guideline for emergency nurses to upgrade their knowledge and skills. All competencies required of emergency nurses are in the form of behavioral objectives. The curriculum represents the comprehensive overview of emergency nurses.

Nursing is going through a cataclysmic identity crisis, and nurses themselves are demanding a larger role in patient care. Evidence of this change is seen in emergency nursing in its continuing education programs and efforts toward certification as a specialty.

Continuing education is essential, and farsighted emergency nurses are fully cognizant of this. They are not content to be just competent in their specialty. Nurses want to be progressively more skilled and more prepared to meet and deal with the demands and challenges of their profession. Experience, even with its admittedly solid basis of training to a high level of manual skills and accumulated knowledge, cannot take the emergency nurse to the peak of available potential. For the nurse who chooses to make emergency nursing a career, specialty clinical and administrative experience is necessary and should be provided; but to become a specialist and to continue to function in this capacity, one must devote substantial time to ongoing education, both didactic and clinical. Only by keeping the avenues of education open can nurses retain motivation for increased proficiency and skill.

Continuing education for emergency nurses is a never ending process. Standards of emergency nursing practice were developed to recognize existing practice and to guarantee quality service as established for emergency nursing. The seven standards are each followed by assessment factors.[2] Using these standards, the emergency nurse is accepting the responsibility and accountability for the delivery of quality emergency nursing care. However, there is still a need for individual nurses to demonstrate that they meet the set standards.

Certification

The Emergency Department Nurses' Association concurs with recent trends in nursing which postulate that certification of competence by examination is possible. EDNA takes the position that certification of excellence rests on successful completion of a competency-based examination. The certification process functions as a motivation toward excellence and a reward to the professional emergency nurse, and also as a guarantee to the public and to hospital administration that standards of competency are being observed and followed.

Certification is useless unless it is recognized as representing significant achievement in the specialty of emergency nursing. State legislators, hospital administrators, and emergency department nurses themselves must accept EDNA certification as a valid indicator of competence. EDNA proposes that a well-researched and meticulously validated examination developed by a recognized testing agency will satisfy even the strictest criteria applied by potential reviewers. On-the-job performance of certified emergency nurses will be the ultimate convincing evidence.

TREATING NONHOSPITALIZED PATIENTS

In response to the changing health needs of society, nursing practice during the last decade has evolved to incorporate a variety of expanded roles for nurses. Quality in medical services delivered to the public is praised continually by health professionals. Individuals and institutions are encouraged to develop new programs that will improve the efficiency and ensure the availability of health care to the community. In evaluating these services, there is found to be an increasing dependence on emergency departments to treat nonhospitalized patients. Identification of this trend has led many to seek equitable alternatives for the demands of the emergency setting.

One alternative is teaching emergency medical technicians to deal with the emergency outside the hospital, on the premise that it is imperative there be trained personnel to handle the second stage of care when the patient reaches the emergency department.

Once the patient reaches the emergency department, physicians and nurses must be aware of and accept their responsibility for the quality of emergency services to the patient in the community and in the hospital. Both physicians and nurses must be members of emergency medical councils in determining all parameters of the emergency medical systems within each community and its hospital. This is the only way the essentials and the scope of emergency medicine and emergency nursing can be explained, recognized, and implemented.

EDUCATION OF EMERGENCY NURSES

The role of nurses in the emergency health system begins at the undergraduate level. Emergency nursing should be a department in nursing schools, with chair status. The first part of the nurse's education exposes the student to the realistic setting of the emergency department and to the environment of the delivery of emergency health services. Basic elements of life-support procedures are an essential part of this curriculum, not only in theory but in clinical management. Even though this may not be the ultimate choice of the nurse as a particular specialty field of nursing, it is an integral part of training regardless of where a career may ultimately lead. (For instance, cardiopulmonary resuscitation, a basic element of life support, must be repeatedly reviewed and practiced for proficiency in the management of this procedure.) At the graduate level, continuing program courses to give in-depth training related to emergency nursing must be incorporated into university, college, and hospital settings.

The uniqueness of emergency nursing lies in the synthesis of basic social and biologic sciences into functions that promote health. The new trends in nursing roles are providing more complete and comprehensive care to emergency patients through an increased sharing of patient care activities between the nursing and the medical professional.

EMERGENCY NURSING FUNCTIONS

Emergency nursing functions are independent, interdependent, and collaborative, and every emergency nurse must know and stay within the legal limitations of established practice. Quality-assurance performance patterns are dependent upon reliable standardized documentation, and emergency nurses must be capable of recording and auditing their own nursing practice.

Defining the emergency nurse specialist or the expanded role of the emergency nurse practitioner does not mean relinquishing the traditional functions of care and comfort; rather it means integrating some medical functions with improved nursing skills in the best interests of the patient. Emergency nurses and emergency physicians must learn to work together with respect for their own and each other's special abilities. These changes do not diminish the importance of either group but work to the benefit of both and toward the upgrading of emergency health care.

It is evident that the quality of initial and definitive care must be improved and that the time interval between an incident and the various levels of care must be reduced. This can be done only through a total-system approach to emergency health services, involving large numbers of allied health care personnel. The success of any one individual is strongly dependent upon the skills and efforts of all the others. The manpower capabilities at all levels and the educational programs to assure the capabilities at each level are a major concern.

Through the commitment of emergency nurses to the improvement of emergency practice, nurses are realizing their own potential influence in the delivery of emergency health care and must be involved in decisions and policies that affect their own practice. Emergency nurses must be recognized as a vital link in the system. If they are to be held accountable, then they must be a part of team management. Consequently, nurses, along with emergency physicians, are asserting themselves in the planning and implementation of policy in emergency care and are exercising their abilities as practitioners. A well-organized and managed emergency department can be developed only by team effort, with administration, physicians, and paraprofessionals working as a unit.

Emergency nurse practitioner

The expanded role of the nurse as an emergency nurse practitioner in the emergency department is becoming a reality, slowly but certainly. This is due to the national trend in quality availability of medical care and to the cost effectiveness of the nurse practitioner in emergency medical services. The interest of the U. S. Department of Health, Education, and Welfare in nurse practitioners developed in the early 1970's when federal funds became available for their training. Under the Emergency Medical Services Training Grant in 1973, the Emergency/Primary Care Nurse Practitioner Program was developed at Allegheny General Hospital,

Pittsburgh, Pennsylvania. The purpose of this program is to give additional education and clinical experience that will prepare the emergency/primary care professional nurse to make certain decisions and perform certain functions and tasks previously undertaken only by physicians. These tasks include independent and dependent functions and delegated medical responsibility under supervision.

For many years emergency nurses have acted and worked as the physician's assistant in all aspects of emergency care. Their emergency knowledge and skills vary from cardiopulmonary resuscitation to interpreting laboratory reports, from recognizing numerous medical conditions and injuries to eliciting and recording pertinent medical history and assisting the physician in critiques on patient care. As mainstays of emergency care, emergency nurses provide continuity in the day-to-day functioning of the department. They are also knowledgeable and well trained in coordinating the services of the hospital, community, public health departments, home health care, social services, specialty ambulatory services, mental health/mental retardation agencies, psychiatric counseling services, and family planning services. Emergency nurses already have the expertise to use these services for the ultimate care of patients. By the very nature of their profession, nurses already have the basic qualifications and the ability to take a more active role in the actual treatment of patients. The expanded role of the emergency nurse will include taking histories of patients, performing physical examinations, carrying out treatment and procedures, counseling and teaching patients health maintenance, and making referrals for the continuity of care and lifesaving measures.

Preparation for practitioner function

To prepare professional emergency nurses to assume these additional responsi-

bilities, it was decided that participants in the Emergency/Primary Care Nurse Practitioner Program would be required to take core courses in normal anatomy, physiology, and pathophysiology. The course content and methods for implementation of the program were determined in a painstaking process. The course curriculum extends over a 40-week period and was written to prepare the RN for both emergency and primary care practice.

Training includes theory, lectures, and directed clinical practice, along with the laboratory and preceptorship training. Clinical experiences during this portion of the course are planned to give each participant opportunities to examine the well patient. Once participants have a firm understanding of what is normal, the pathophysiology is introduced. Here nurses learn the effects of various disease entities on normal functioning of the body and how to assess the patient who is no longer well. Pathophysiology is approached from a clinic manifestation viewpoint rather than a disease focus, since most of the patients in the emergency department present undiagnosed conditions. Emphasis is also placed on the ongoing assessment and management of patients with diagnosed chronic disease entities. Time is devoted to the assessment of children with common pediatric problems and of obstetrical and gynecological problems commonly seen in the emergency department. The final area covered is the assessment and management of the patient with an acute medical or surgical problem.

The program is divided so that the first 20 weeks focus on the theory and demonstration for clinical practice and the second 20 weeks focus on the practice and acquisition of clinic skills. During the second 20 weeks the program participants spend four days each week in their home hospitals under the guidance and direction of their physician preceptors. This gives them the opportunity to practice the skills they have learned as well as to acquire new ones. They continue to return to the site hospital one day each week for unusual experiences not generally encountered in their home hospitals. Some time is devoted to review and to reenforce areas needing more exposure. Perhaps one of the most important functions of the nurse practitioner is to relieve the physician of nonurgent care, thus lowering the financial cost of the patient in the hospital.

Responsibilities of an emergency nurse practitioner

The practitioner is a nurse whose skills are in the emergency-primary health care field. Since skills such as the physical examination have been traditionally medical, the practitioner is clinically responsible to the emergency physician, but as a nurse she is also responsible to nursing. It is expected that practitioners will function within their institutions where there is full-time emergency physician coverage. The emergency nurse practitioner is expected to facilitate care of the patient by laying the groundwork in more depth for the physician.

There are many demands placed on emergency nurses by the physician, by the consumer, by the community, and by their own co-workers. Policies and procedures of the emergency department dictate how well run the department will be, but a well-trained emergency nurse must be able to give emergency care, must be able to make an assessment, and must be able to proceed with sound plans of action. If emergency nurses today are to help the patient obtain the highest possible level of general health, then nurses giving this care must be knowledgeable in this field.

The number of people who rely on the emergency department instead of the physician's office for all aspects of health care is growing steadily. Not only have hospitals recognized this trend for some time, but health agencies, social agencies, and

health professionals see it as an inevitable result of the individual's inability to find a physician when needed for individual or family care. Because of the continuing scarcity and geographical maldistribution of physicians, these changes in the health care pattern must be accepted as fact, and members of the emergency health care team other than physicians must be equipped to handle some of the patient load. Emergency nurses are uniquely positioned to assume a more active role in actual patient care. The emergency nurse practitioner with additional education is prepared for an expanded role in emergency health care. The responsibilities and tasks this nurse is expected to assume can be identified as interdependent or independent functions to differentiate between those tasks that the nurse practitioner initiates without physician consultation and those in which both physician and nurse practitioner participate directly.

The professional role of the nurse practitioner in the emergency department will depend on where he or she practices. Statutory provisions governing the legal scope of nursing practice vary from state to state. State nurse practice acts are being broadened to define the role of certified registered nurse practitioners.

Emergency nurses are practitioners, leaders, teachers, counselors, and coordinators. As coordinators they can effectively implement and supplement efforts of administrators, physicians, paraprofessionals, and community agencies in the delivery of quality emergency health care.

SUMMARY

The emergency nurse is an integral and vital part of an emergency health care team. Should she or he be inadequate or incompetent, the effectiveness of the team diminishes or fails, and there is only one result—the patient suffers unnecessarily, or dies. Few professions other than medicine and nursing have inherent in them this direct relationship of cause and effect. When accepted, the job of dealing with human lives is a staggering obligation, and the emergency nurse must constantly prepare, educate, and train herself to be ready for it. After all, without the backbone of emergency nursing, like everything requiring a supporting element to keep it steady and efficiently functional, the emer- gency department cannot serve its patients in a way they have a right to expect from any health care agency.

REFERENCES

1. Emergency Department Nurses' Association Continuing Education Core Curriculum.
2. American Nurses' Association, Emergency Department Nurses' Association: Standards of emergency nursing practice, 1975.

CHAPTER 5

Triage and assessment

Doris Nelson, R.N., B.S.

Many hospitals, both large and small, throughout the country are utilizing some form of triage in their emergency departments. Triage is a system developed on the battlefield during World War II to assess the care required for the wounded and designate them to a specific area to receive that care.

Triage in hospitals has been prevalent for approximately 20 years, and many variations are being utilized. As the patient volume presenting to the emergency department on a 24-hour basis is constantly growing, hospitals have sought ways to care for these patients effectively and efficiently. In many hospitals, space to provide this care is limited. Staffing, from a physician, nursing, and a paraprofessional standpoint, is a crucial issue in meeting the consumer's needs in today's health care system.

Unfortunately, many patients abuse the system, and the volume of patients entering large emergency departments presents the danger that the acutely ill patient will go unrecognized and not be separated from patients with nonacute conditions. An effective triage system can accomplish some of the following:

1. Expedite the care of the patient through initial assessment skills by the triage person
2. Ensure that patient priorities are established according to the acuteness of the condition
3. Function as a referral center for patients not requiring emergency facilities, or for those desiring information from other community agencies
4. Decrease patient delays by initiating diagnostic procedures such as x-ray, laboratory, and pregnancy tests prior to seeing a physician (Many times there may be a delay due to the physician's being involved with more acutely ill patients.)
5. Function as a screening area for patients who need information
6. Promote patient rapport through demonstration of concern for patient problems immediately upon arrival in the emergency department
7. Improve family, visitor rapport as it relates to the patient through reassurance of family and maintenance of effective communications to them while the patient is being cared for in a treatment area, and they are being required to wait in the waiting room
8. Assume responsibility for notification of law enforcement agencies regarding reportable patient complaints, for example, gunshot wounds, rape victims, and battered children

9. Improve public relations among patients, visitors, families, law enforcement agencies, and community agencies
10. Provide opportunities for training of personnel and an effective instruction center for the development of assessment skills under supervision
11. Relieve congestion in critical treatment areas and improve traffic flow
12. Assist in more effective utilization of space and personnel through assignment of patients to specific treatment areas
13. Act as stimulus for the triage personnel in that the one who is triaging and initially assesses the patient's chief complaint should have the opportunity to review the patient's record on discharge or admission to the hospital in order to determine if his or her initial assessment of the patient's problem was accurate
14. Determine the allergies a patient may have and previous immunizations received
15. Document care provided by EMT and paramedics prior to hospital arrival
16. Obtain information and document unusual circumstances involving patient prior to arrival at hospital
17. Decrease anxiety levels and stress factor
18. Decrease the duplication of functions in relation to management of the medical care of the patient (An example of this would be that patients with surgical problems would be initially seen and treated by a surgeon.)
19. Provide for effective utilization of clinical facilities

CAPABILITIES

The capabilities required of triage personnel vary from hospital to hospital. Their functions are based on policies established by the nursing administrative coordinator in conjunction with hospital policy, the emergency department, the city, and the medical advisory committee. Many hospitals require that triage personnel demonstrate a thorough knowledge of the clinical signs and symptoms of disease and have at least two years clinical experience. The triage person should—

1. Be able to function at a maximum under stress
2. Possess the ability to make accurate and concise assessments regarding the care required by the patient
3. Demonstrate leadership qualities and abilities
4. Possess an excellent knowledge of all aspects of emergency care and the operation of the emergency department and other departments within the hospital
5. Have the ability to make quick decisions based on sound judgments
6. Be able to communicate effectively with the patient and maintain open lines of communication with other departments within the hospital and various community agencies
7. Possess ability to establish and maintain good visitor rapport
8. Possess ability to tactfully interpret the policies of the hospital
9. Maintain a close working relationship with ambulance personnel
10. Act as a resource person in training of other personnel and ambulance personnel
11. Be involved in patient and family teaching
12. Possess the ability to provide emotional support to the patient, family and friends
13. Maintain supervision of personnel assigned to the triage desk
14. Be cognizant of patient traffic flow, ensuring that the entrance into the emergency department is kept clear

to provide fast movement of acutely ill or injured patients to treatment areas

15. Possess the ability to recognize and prevent potentially explosive situations and situations that develop in relation to combative, inebriated, uncooperative, and unreasonable, demanding patients and visitors
16. Present a good image for the hospital
17. Work closely with the chaplain or the family's minister
18. Maintain good rapport with physicians
19. Arrange for transfer by ambulance of patients to other facilities when requested by a physician
20. Work closely with the social worker and patient coordinator in meeting the needs of the patient and family
21. Assist in discharge planning for the patient
22. Promote open communication lines with hospital security
23. Possess the organizational concepts and skills for decision making, problem solving, and awareness building.

DESIGN OF FACILITIES FOR TRIAGE

The triage desk should be located immediately within the entrance of the emergency department. It should be well lighted and designated by a sign. It should be adjacent to the entrance lobby to provide an area for ambulance stretchers and also for patients who may be waiting to talk to the triage person.

Plans should be made to provide an alternate triage system should the system not be usable due to internal problems such as floods, fire, tornado, or inadequate staff to perform this function.

Traffic flow of patients entering into the system must be maintained to decrease congestion and to provide the triage person visual accessibility to all patients entering the emergency department. Privacy of communication between the patient and the triage person should be maintained. This may be accomplished by utilizing a safety glass–enclosed booth, depending on the volume of patients.

In emergency departments that have a large volume (over 100 per eight-hour shift), the use of a glass-enclosed booth may not be practical. An open counter area may be more feasible. This, of course, would decrease the privacy desired when interviewing and assessing the patient's chief complaint.

The triage desk should have information and ambulance phone lines available and an effective intercom system to communicate with the treatment areas within the emergency department. The intercom system should have the capability of instituting a page system within the treatment area to alert the area of acutely ill or injured patients arriving in the treatment area.

A large waiting area should be adjacent to the triage desk to maintain effective communication regarding patients being cared for in the treatment area.

A wheelchair and stretcher area should be adjacent to the triage desk. Cabinet space for storage should be provided. A lavoratory is essential within this area since the triage person must maintain good hand-washing technique after caring for patients whose treatment requires physical contact, such as splinting fractures and controlling bleeding.

A family room with a phone should be near the triage desk. This area should be utilized for families of patients who are seriously ill or injured, or who have expired on arrival or within the emergency department. It is desirable that this family room be decorated similar to a home, with comfortable chairs, a couch, pictures on the wall, carpeting and coffee service available. It is essential that the area be large enough for those who become hysterical and highly emotional to be able to pass out on the floor without striking furniture and possibly injuring themselves.

It is also helpful to have a police room, which may also be designated the press room as needed, adjacent to the triage desk. Having this area adjacent to triage personnel gives the press easy access to information maintained at the desk. Also, when this room is in use as a police room, should a patient or visitor become uncooperative or violent, the person may be placed there out of the main entrance way where other patients may be waiting to be interviewed by the triage person.

SECURITY

In many hospitals, security is an essential element in the control of activities around the triage desk and at the emergency entrance. A security officer should be assigned to this area around the clock to control traffic flow both within and outside the entrance and to control uncooperative patients, visitors, and families. This person may also direct personnel to areas within the hospital.

TRAINING OF TRIAGE PERSONNEL

Some hospitals have permanent triage personnel. This may be satisfactory for small emergency departments with low volumes of patients. It is not recommended for large emergency departments because of the many stress factors that exist.

Previous clinical experience is essential, preferably in an emergency department setting or in a medical-surgical intensive care unit, as is an orientation to the facilities of the hospital and community agencies. The triage person must possess a thorough knowledge of the functions performed in the entire emergency department and the policies and procedures of all departments.

Assessment skills and a thorough knowledge of anatomy and physiology and signs and symptoms should be demonstrated during orientation to this position. How

well the individual takes case histories, that is, whether the proper feedback is obtained, is a good measure of these qualities. It is suggested that this not be an in-hiring position in order to thoroughly evaluate the individual who may be assigned to work in this position.

Many hospital emergency departments use all their nursing personnel as triage persons on a daily or weekly rotating basis. This has proven satisfactory and is a factor in relieving the stress that is present for some persons.

Triage personnel need to be able to understand the vocabulary of the patients. Personnel from New York may have many problems with patient interviews in Texas if they are unaware of the meaning of terminology the patient is using. During orientation to triage the person should be provided with a list of words most frequently used during patient interviews. For example, a patient may come to the emergency department with one or more of the following symptoms: clogs, bad blood, fireballs, harking up clogs, loss my nature, running range, cadillacs or cold rigors.

An orientation checklist for triage should consist of the following:
1. Assessment skills based on all body systems
2. Knowledge of policies and procedures in the emergency treatment area
3. Knowledge of patient coordinator's duties
4. Knowledge of chaplain's functions
5. Knowledge of ambulance services available in the community, the type of training and the capabilities of each
6. Knowledge of community agencies
7. Ability to deliver a baby
8. Knowledge of how to effectively handle medical advice information
9. Knowledge of duties and functions of the orderly, information clerk,

and registration clerk and ability to supervise them effectively

10. Knowledge of location of stretchers and wheelchairs
11. Knowledge of emergency admission and discharge policies
12. Knowledge of procedure for identification and documentation of allergies
13. Knowledge of location of all forms necessary at triage
14. Ability to splint fractures
15. Ability to bandage and control superficial bleeding
16. Knowledge of social service functions
17. Ability to handle problems that arise in relation to irate, uncooperative patients and visitors
18. Knowledge of functions of security department
19. Knowledge of intercom system and all communication systems within the hospital
20. Knowledge of telemetry systems available within the community
21. Knowledge of functions in time of disaster
22. Knowledge of information that may be released to the news media
23. Knowledge of idiosyncrasies present in relation to notification of next-of-kin in relation to injury of police officers, various company employees, personnel injured in airplane crashes, and the like
24. Knowledge of procedure to follow in admitting a VIP
25. In some institutions, a thorough knowledge of the hospital billing system and the insurance department
26. Knowledge of the visiting policy within the hospital
27. Knowledge of the clinic system

TYPES OF TRIAGE

Triage varies according to the particular institution in which it is employed. A vast difference in the duties and responsibilities may exist from institution to institution based on the level of skill of the person who is performing the triage and the policies established within the hospital. Listed below are some of the triage systems that exist throughout the country.

Physician triage

The patient is initially seen prior to registration by a physician who assesses whether emergency care is required at that time. He or she may also evaluate the patient as to priority of care. The physician may refer the patient to a private physician, the outpatient department for care, or treatment in the emergency department.

Some hospitals utilize a physician in a screening area to treat the "walk-in" patient with minor complaints such as rash, colds, and urinary tract infections. Using a screening area will decrease the volume of nonacute patients within the main emergency treatment area, thus providing for more room to care for the acutely ill patient.

Nurse triage

The triage nurse sees each patient upon entry into the emergency department, obtains a brief history concerning medical problems, allergies, and immunizations, and assesses the patient's chief complaint. At this time, the nurse may initiate a request for laboratory tests and roentgenogram. This system allows the nurse to counsel the patient, provides an opportunity for patient and family teaching, and assists the physician in rendering emergency care more expediently, thereby facilitating the evaluation of a larger volume of patients more quickly.

In some emergency departments where there are large volumes of patients, the emergency department is divided into medical services by area, staffed 24 hours a day by physicians of that specialty area. The nurse may make an initial assessment of the care, record it on the patient's emergency record, and designate the medical area he or she feels can best care for the patient.

Triage by code number

Numerous studies have been made of triage by code number. In most instances it is based on the patient's condition, using arbitrary figures from one to four:

1 A patient with a life-threatening illness

2 A patient with significant medical problems that could be detrimental if not treated within the next one to two hours

3 A patient whose condition is stable but will require care within the next four to six hours

4 A patient who has no significant medical problem and in many instances can be seen in the out-patient clinic or by a private physician the next day

Patients are seen by the physicians according to the code number system. In most instances this system is designated by a physician.

External triage

External triage refers to initial evaluation of the patient's problem prior to arrival of the patient at the treatment area. Radio-telemetry ambulance systems connected to the emergency department are an example of external triage. The patient's condition has been assessed by the paramedic personnel and the physician prior to the patient's arrival at the hospital. When the patient arrives in the emergency department, the triage person has been informed and is anticipating the patient's arrival, is aware of the patient's condition, and does not detain the patient for further assessment. This system serves to expedite the care of the patient and to improve patient care for those with immediate needs, by decreasing the time that may be taken by the triage person to assess the situation.

Another reason for external triage would be a disaster. Each emergency department should use some form of triage system in a disaster. It is advisable not to overextend the emergency department by trying to take care of every disaster victim who arrives. It is essential that the initial triage be performed outside the emergency department. The emergency department dock, using the overhang where the ambulances enter, is an ideal location. Preestablished clinical criteria should be followed by the person performing the triage, and alternate areas other than the emergency department should be available for the triaging of patients with nonacute conditions who require first aid, emotional support, or treatment for minor injuries such as fractures.

In a disaster with large volumes of patients involved, it is essential that all facilities be used to provide adequate care to all patients and not to overburden one facility. This, in most instances, can be accomplished through proper dispatching of ambulances through telephone communication with other hospitals. Many patients in time of disaster will arrive at the hospital by private conveyance; therefore the ambulance dispatch system is not totally reliable. Many cities with several hospitals within the city or county have established a hospital-based radio communication system that is very effective in ensuring that reception of patients into their facilities is distributed adequately to provide maximum care.

Internal triage

Internal triage exists once the patient arrives in the treatment area, based on the condition of the patient at the time, the type of care required, the time frame required to give the care necessary, and the facilities available within the emergency treatment area. Should a patient with a history of cardiac condition arrive in the emergency department with a crushing chest pain, a decision is made immediately to send the patient to the acute care room within the area, versus the patient who arrives with a history of flulike symptoms for a week. This patient may be required to wait until an examination room is available or be placed in an examining room with no special monitoring equipment.

INTERVIEW TECHNIQUES IN OBTAINING INFORMATION AND MAKING AN ASSESSMENT

Interviews are based on five major factors. These are the use of the eyes, ears, nose, hands, and good nursing knowledge. The method used is not important as long as it is a comprehensive, efficient system, keeping in mind that a history and inspection can be done concurrently. An adequate assessment can usually be obtained in less than five minutes from a relatively cooperative patient.

One of the most common mistakes made by personnel in taking a history is "giving" the patient a diagnosis. Everyone has heard at one time or another about patients with epigastric pain being asked, "Do you have a crushing substernal pain that radiates to your left shoulder causing nausea or vomiting, shortness of breath, and sweating?" If the patients with gastritis should happen to say "yes," they may find themselves in the coronary care unit. Many patients are very vague in describing symptoms. They know it hurts, but their ability to describe how it hurts is limited at times.

It is essential that triage personnel possess the communication skills necessary to elicit from the patient the information sought. The nurse must be aware of the socioeconomic environment of the patient and be able to relay questions the patient will understand and also to understand the patient's reply to questions.

It is not unusual for a patient to arrive in the emergency department, and when asked the nature of the problem, the patient says, "I don't know; that's what I came to find out." At times it can be difficult to obtain a good history. Probably one of the most difficult patient complaints to assess is abdominal pain. During the assessment triage personnel must answer the following questions: (1) Is the pain due to a viral condition such as gastroenteritis? (2) Does the patient have a surgical problem such as appendicitis or gallbladder disease or obstruction? (3) Is the patient having a miscarriage or possibly a ruptured ectopic pregnancy? Many patients have difficulty describing their symptoms.

Many times personnel will be unable to pinpoint the patient's problem after performing a thorough assessment and history taking. In a situation such as this, he or she triages the patient according to physical appearance and what are perceived to be his or her problems.

Another problem in the initial interview is communicating with the non-English-speaking patient, the hysterical or belligerent patient, or the patient who explains one problem because family or friends are present but who really manifests another condition. An example is the patient who suspects venereal disease—the young girl who arrives with her mother and complains of burning during urination or nausea and vomiting. The patient with suspected venereal disease will relate almost anything. Another example is the young girl who denies missing any menstrual periods because she does not want her mother to know. This patient may be considered as someone with a minor complaint when actually she is having a miscarriage or possible ruptured ectopic pregnancy.

Visitors can also be a problem during the initial patient interview. They wish to interject their comments concerning the patient's problem. At times they may wish to do all the talking, or they may scream, "Can't you see he is dying," although the patient has only a minor laceration. It is imperative, in order to avoid conflict and to provide the best possible care, to have the visitor physically removed from the triage area during the initial assessment.

Patients can be assessed rapidly by using a nursing assessment guide or sheet. It is recommended that the initial triage assessment sheet contain the most significant conditions and a more in-depth assessment sheet be filled out once the patient arrives in the treatment area. For those emergency departments that have divided clinical services the assessment sheet can be a general sheet, one specific to that clinical service, or one designed for a particular type of patient problem, such as the trauma patient in surgery.

For the initial triage assessment guide it sometimes may not be essential to complete the entire sheet. If the patient is having severe chest pain radiating down the left arm, difficulty breathing, and is cyanotic, that is all the information needed by the triage person at the time. The decision has been made that this patient has probably sustained a significant cardiac attack and should be triaged into an acute care room within the emergency treatment area.

Should three patients arrive simultaneously at the triage desk, each with multiple injuries, the immediate concern is to assess which patient needs the most immediate care. A detailed nursing assessment on each patient is not necessary at this time.

Initial nursing assessment can be of great significance as it relates to changes of the patient's condition during the emergency department stay and subsequent admission to the hospital.

Examples of some questions in history taking are as follows. Keep in mind the three important life-threatening emergencies—airway, breathing, and circulation—versus the less acute problems.

General questions

1. Is the pain sharp like a knife, or dull like an ache?
2. Did the pain wake you up?
3. Does it stay in one place or go somewhere else?
4. Did it come on suddenly or gradually?
5. Does it hurt all the time, or does it come and go?
6. Did you bump it or do something to cause the pain?
7. Is there anything you can do to make the pain better or worse?

Chest pain

1. Is it in the front or back?
2. Does the pain make it hard for you to breathe?
3. Does it get worse when you take a deep breath?
4. Have you been coughing?
5. Do you smoke?

Abdominal pain

1. Where is the pain? Can you point to it with one finger?
2. Have you vomited or felt like vomiting?
3. Have you had normal bowel movements lately or loose bowels?
4. Does eating, or what you eat, affect the pain?
5. Does it burn when you urinate, or pass your water?
6. Do you have a discharge from your penis/vagina?
7. When was your last menstrual period?

Trauma

1. Where were you in the car?
2. Were you hit from the front, side, or back?
3. Where was the gun? What type of gun was used?
4. Were you stabbed from above or below?
5. Were you standing upright, leaning over, or lying down?

Sensorium

1. Do you know where you are?
2. Do you remember what happened?
3. What time/day/month/year is it?
4. Do you know your address/phone number/Social Security number?

Examples of things that can be seen

1. Respiratory distress
2. Obvious bleeding or open wounds
3. Dried blood present in the mouth, nose, or ears
4. Level of consciousness
5. Color, skin condition, condition in general

6. Asymmetry of pupils, face, shoulders, arms, chest, pelvis, legs; obvious fractures
7. Physical activity
8. Emotional status
9. Obvious deformities

Examples of things that can be felt

1. Pulse, present and rate
2. Crepitus
3. Cold
4. Abnormal profusions
5. Induration
6. Resistance or guarding
7. Fragmented bone
8. Heat
9. Pressure point resulting in pain

Examples of things that can be smelled

1. Unusual odors on breath
2. Purulent infections
3. Rectal or urinary incontinence

An example of an initial interview and assessment sheet that could be used at the triage desk and that would encompass most clinical signs and symptoms of the vast majority of patients entering the emergency department is shown on pp. 53-55. An interview assessment sheet for a special clinical problem or disease can be developed as the assessment sheet for trauma patients on pp. 56-57.

Text continued on p. 57.

TRIAGE INITIAL NURSING ASSESSMENT

Name _____ Time _____

Chief complaint as stated by patient _____

_____

Allergies _____

Unusual problems _____ (i.e., deaf, mute, speaks no English, etc.) _____

Respiratory status

Breath sounds: Present ☐ Absent ☐ Normal rate ☐
Apnea ☐ Dyspnea ☐ Cheyne Stokes ☐ Kussmaul ☐ Retracting ☐
Hyperventilation ☐ Wheezing ☐ Stridor rales ☐
Symmetry of chest: Normal ☐ Abnormal ☐
Foreign body obstructing airway ☐

Circulatory status

	Absent	Present	
Pulse			
Carotid	_____	_____	Regular? Yes ☐ No ☐
Radial	_____	_____	Bradycardia? Yes ☐ No ☐
Femoral	_____	_____	Tachycardia? Yes ☐ No ☐
Pedal	_____	_____	Amplitude: Weak ☐ Strong ☐
			Cyanosis: Present ☐ Absent ☐

Bleeding status

Arterial wound present? No ☐ Yes ☐ Amount of bleeding: _____

Venous wound present? No ☐ Yes ☐ Amount of bleeding: _____
Hematoma present? Yes ☐ No ☐ Tarry stools? Yes ☐ No ☐ Open wound Yes ☐ No ☐

Location of open wound

Head _____Neck _____

Chest _____

Abdomen _____

Extremity _____

Continued.

TRIAGE INITIAL NURSING ASSESSMENT—cont'd

Bleeding status—cont'd

Closed wound with evidence of internal bleeding (location) _____

_____

Vaginal bleeding (amount of bleeding) _____

Epistaxis _____

Hematuria _____

Hematemesis _____

Pupillary examination

	Right	Left		Right	Left
Equality	____	____	Fixed	____	____
Position	____	____	Gaze	____	____
Constricted	____	____	Involuntary movement	____	____
Dilated	____	____			

Reaction to light
  Right? _____

  Left? _____

Neurologic status

Unconscious ☐ Conscious ☐ Agitated ☐ Confused ☐ Lethargic ☐
Oriented to time and place ☐ Hallucinating ☐
Consciousness level normal? Yes ☐ No ☐
Responds to command? Yes ☐ No ☐

Motor function

Spastic movement ☐ Decerebrate movement ☐ Spontaneous movement ☐ Gag reflex ☐

Strength
  Arms _____
  Hands _____
  Legs _____
  Feet _____

Pain status

	Location	Causative factor
Absent	_____	_____
Sharp	_____	_____
Dull	_____	_____
Radiating	_____	_____
Constant	_____	_____
Intermittent	_____	_____
Increasing	_____	_____

Sensory status

	Location	Causative factor
Normal	_____	_____
Numbness	_____	_____
Diminished	_____	_____

TRIAGE INITIAL NURSING ASSESSMENT—cont'd

Skeletal system

	Absent	*Present*	*Location*
Fracture			
Open	_____	_____	_____
Closed	_____	_____	_____

Dislocation? (location) _____

Tenderness? (location) _____

Limitation of movement? _____

Rotation of extremities? _____

_____

Swelling? _____

Deformity? _____

Skin status

Cyanotic ☐ Cold ☐ Clammy ☐ Dehydrated ☐ Urticaria ☐ Burned ☐ Hot ☐
Infected ☐ Ecchymosis ☐ Normal ☐ Edematous ☐ Crepitus ☐ Macules
Papules ☐ Abrasions ☐ Marks ☐ Pallor ☐ Yellow ☐

Emotional status

Apparently normal ☐ Crying ☐ Screaming ☐ Violent ☐ Quiet ☐

Nutritional and elimination status

Normal ☐ Anorexia ☐ Nausea ☐ Diarrhea ☐ Incontinent ☐ Dysuria ☐
Oliguria ☐ Anuria ☐ Vomiting ☐ Constipated ☐ Urine discolored ☐

Color of urine _____

Special problems

Overdose

  Drug _____ Amount _____

  Previous history _____

Ingestion

  Drug or material ingested _____ Amount _____

  Previous history _____

Seizure _____

  Previous history _____

_____

Other _____

_____

_____

_____

_____

TRAUMA PATIENT ASSESSMENT FORM*

Respiratory status

A. Respiration equal and full with good breath sounds bilaterally ☐
   Splinting of respirations ☐
   Diminished ☐ or Absent ☐ breath sounds left side
   Diminished ☐ or Absent ☐ breath sounds right side

B. Quality
   No dyspnea noted ☐
   Mild dyspnea noted ☐
   Moderate dyspnea noted ☐
   Severe dyspnea noted (with retractions) ☐
   Apnea ☐

C. Rate
   Less than 10/min ☐ 12-16 /min ☐ 16-24/min ☐ 26-30/min ☐ More than 50/min ☐

D. Presence of spontaneous respirations ☐

Cardiovascular status

A. Blood pressure _____

B. Pulse rate
   Below 50/min ☐ 50-60/min ☐ 60-80/min ☐ 80-100/min ☐ 100-120/min ☐ Above 120/min ☐ Asystole ☐ V-Fib ☐

C. Pulse
   Equal and full in all extremities ☐
   Pulse diminished in _____ extremity(ies) ☐
   Pulse absent in _____ extremity(ies) ☐

D. Bleeding
   No bleeding noted ☐
   Bleeding, oozing ☐
   Bleeding, pumping artery type ☐
   Hematoma over site of fracture or injury ☐

E. Extremity
   Pink ☐ Pale ☐ Blanched ☐ Blue ☐ Warm ☐ Cool ☐ Cold ☐

Neurologic status

A. Alert ☐ Lethargic ☐ Stuporous ☐ Obtunded ☐ Comatose ☐

B. Able to follow simple commands ☐
   Diminished response time in following simple commands ☐ Unable to follow simple commands ☐

C. Oriented to
   Time ☐ Place ☐ Person ☐ Self ☐
   Disoriented ☐

D. Movement
   Moving all extremities equally well ☐ Moving only upper extremities ☐ Moving only lower extremities ☐ Moving only left side extremities ☐ Moving only right side extremities ☐ Unable to assess because of injuries ☐ Purposeful movement in response to stimulation ☐

E. Posturing _____

   _____

F. Strength
   Hand grasps equal and strong ☐
   Left hand grasp stronger than right hand grasp ☐
   Right hand grasp stronger than left hand grasp ☐
   Unable to grasp hands ☐

G. Pupils
   Pupils equal and reacting to light ☐
   Left pupil reacting more than right pupil ☐
   Right pupil reacting more than left pupil ☐
   Pupils unreactive ☐ Dilated ☐ Constricted ☐

Pain status

Head _____

Neck _____

Abdomen _____

Extremities _____

Abdominal examination

A. Bowel sounds heard ☐ Absent bowel sounds ☐

B. No tenderness or guarding noted ☐ Abdomen tender ☐ Voluntary guarding ☐ Involuntary guarding ☐ Abdomen rigid and boardlike ☐

*Courtesy Helen A. Cusick, R.N., Inservice Instructor, Education and Training Department, Parkland Memorial Hospital, Dallas, Texas.

TRAUMA PATIENT ASSESSMENT FORM—cont'd

C. If N/G tube passed Clear returns ☐ Bile-colored returns ☐ Green returns ☐ Blood-tinged returns ☐ Bloody returns ☐

Other _____

D. If Foley inserted Clear returns ☐ Pinkish returns ☐ Bloody returns ☐

E. Result of peritoneal lavage
Clear ☐ Blood tinged ☐ Bloody ☐ Gross blood ☐

Injuries noted and severity

Head _____

_____

Neck _____

_____

Chest _____

_____

Abdomen _____

_____

Upper extremities _____

_____

Lower extremities _____

_____

SUMMARY

Triage personnel must possess good interviewing techniques and assessment skills and a sound clinical knowledge. They must be aware of every type of emergency situation involving a patient that can arise and must be able to interpret the needs of the patient through an adequate history and assessment. In 1856 Florence Nightingale said:

The most important practical lesson that can be given to nurses is to teach them what to observe—how to observe—what symptoms indicate improvement—what the reverse—which are of importance—which are of none—which are evidence of neglect—and what kind of neglect.

But if you cannot obtain the habit of observation one way or other, you had better give up being a nurse, for it is not your calling, however kind and anxious you may be.

ADDITIONAL READINGS

Jones, R. C.: Initial care of the injured patient. In Care of the trauma patient, New York, 1966, McGraw-Hill Book Co.

O'Boyle, C.: A new era in emergency services, Am. J. Nurs. **72:**1394, 1972.

Shires, T. G.: Psychological management of patients in emergencies. In Care of the trauma patient, New York, 1966, McGraw-Hill Book Co.

Slater, R. R.: Triage nurse in the emergency Department, Am. J. Nurs. **70:**128, 1970.

Thal, E. R., and Shires, T. G.: No at Parkland, Am. J. Nurs. **72:**2054, 1974.

CHAPTER **6**

Surface trauma and hemorrhage

Tom Elo, M.D.

Generally, wounds and their care present a unique opportunity and often a challenge to professional emergency department personnel, for it is in the emergency department that primary wound care begins and that definitive care many times is instituted. The healing course of many of the wounds depends on the adequacy of preparation and degree of cleanliness used in their management. In addition, it is necessary to ascertain the need for the use of tetanus and rabies prophylaxis. Other procedures including handling fish hooks, ring removal, and subungual hematomas, along with crucial steps in recognizing and managing various types of hemorrhage, are also presented in this chapter.

THE SKIN

In dealing with wounds of any type it is first necessary to take an overall view of the skin, the structure through which a foreign material must pass to be harmful to the human body.

The skin makes up about 15% of the dry weight of the body and is generally considered to consist of three major layers: (1) epidermis, (2) dermis, and (3) subcutis (Fig. 6-1).

The epidermis, the outer protective covering, is made up of epithelial cells

in varying stages of cornification. It is essentially impermeable to water and many other agents. It is the first line of defense against many bacteria and fungi. The epidermis is avascular and receives its nourishment from the small vessels in the dermis.

The dermis, or middle layer, constitutes the bulk of the skin and is composed of connective tissue (collagen), ground sub-

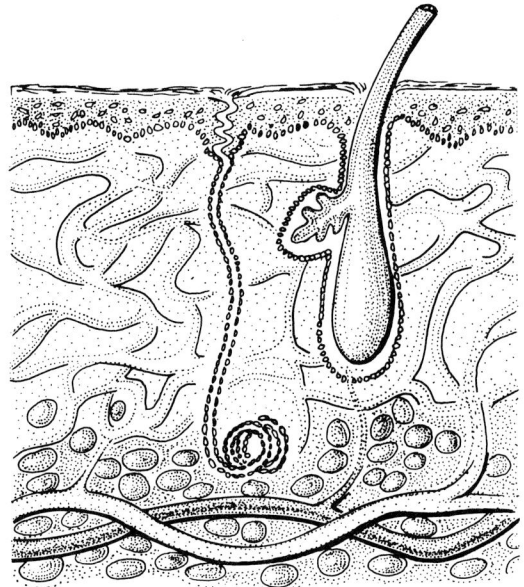

Fig. 6-1. Skin cross section.

58

stance, blood vessels, lymphatics, and nerves. The main function is to provide support for the epidermis and the skin appendages.

The subcutis, or lowest layer, is easily distinguished by the presence of fat. It also contains some of the lower parts of the sweat glands and hair follicles. In addition, it contains blood vessels, lymphatics, nerves, and connective tissue.

The major skin appendages are the hair and hair follicles, sweat glands (apocrine and exocrine), and nails.

Any or all of these layers or appendages may be involved in the wound depending upon the cause and physical factors operating at the time of injury.

EXAMINATION OF THE PATIENT

At the time the patient enters the emergency department, a quick triage and general assessment should be made as to airway problems and severe hemorrhage. The presence of either of these problems, of course, requires immediate attention. Following the initial rapid assessment a more detailed history and inspection of the patient and the wound are undertaken. A history indicates how the wound was inflicted and the physical factors involved. It is important to ascertain the time since the incident happened. In addition, it is helpful to know what first aid has been applied. The history of allergies and of past tetanus immunization is of utmost importance. Even while a history is being obtained, a rather thorough inspection of the wound can be made by checking such parameters as depth of the wound; nerve, vessel, or tendon involvement; bone injury; foreign bodies; and general extent of wound contamination.[1-4]

WOUND TYPES AND MANAGEMENT

After the history and examination are completed, definitive care of the wound may proceed. There are certain objectives that must be followed in the management of any wound. These include (1) healing by primary intention, (2) function maintenance or restoration, and (3) minimization of scarring and deformity.[2-6]

Healing

There are three means by which wounds may heal: (1) primary intention, (2) secondary intention (granulation), and (3) tertiary intention (delayed closure or secondary suture) (Fig. 6-2).

In primary intention wound healing the wound is initially and definitively closed at the first sitting. This leads to minimal scarring and deformity and is the preferred method by which wound healing should take place.

In secondary intention wound healing no attempt is made to close the wound. Instead, the wound is allowed to "granulate in" with resulting scar formation and subsequent contraction of that scar. This leads to greater deformity and possible loss of function of the area involved.

Finally, in the case of tertiary, or third, intention healing, suturing is delayed for several days because of infection or gross amounts of contamination. It is during this time that wound cleansing and debridement are carried out. Also during this period a minimal amount of granulation tissue forms. Scar formation is less than in secondary intention healing; however, it is greater than with primary closure.

Wounds heal from side to side (not end to end) and in phases, and it *is* necessary to inform patients of this. When sutures are first removed the scar appears fairly decent. Within a few days to weeks the scar usually turns erythematous, somewhat thick and lumpy, and is very sensitive to heat and cold. This is due to active fibroplasia, which can last for three to four months. After this the process slowly reverses itself. Up to six months later the nerve supply returns, the erythema fades, and the sensitivity gradually disappears. Usually the scar takes on its final appear-

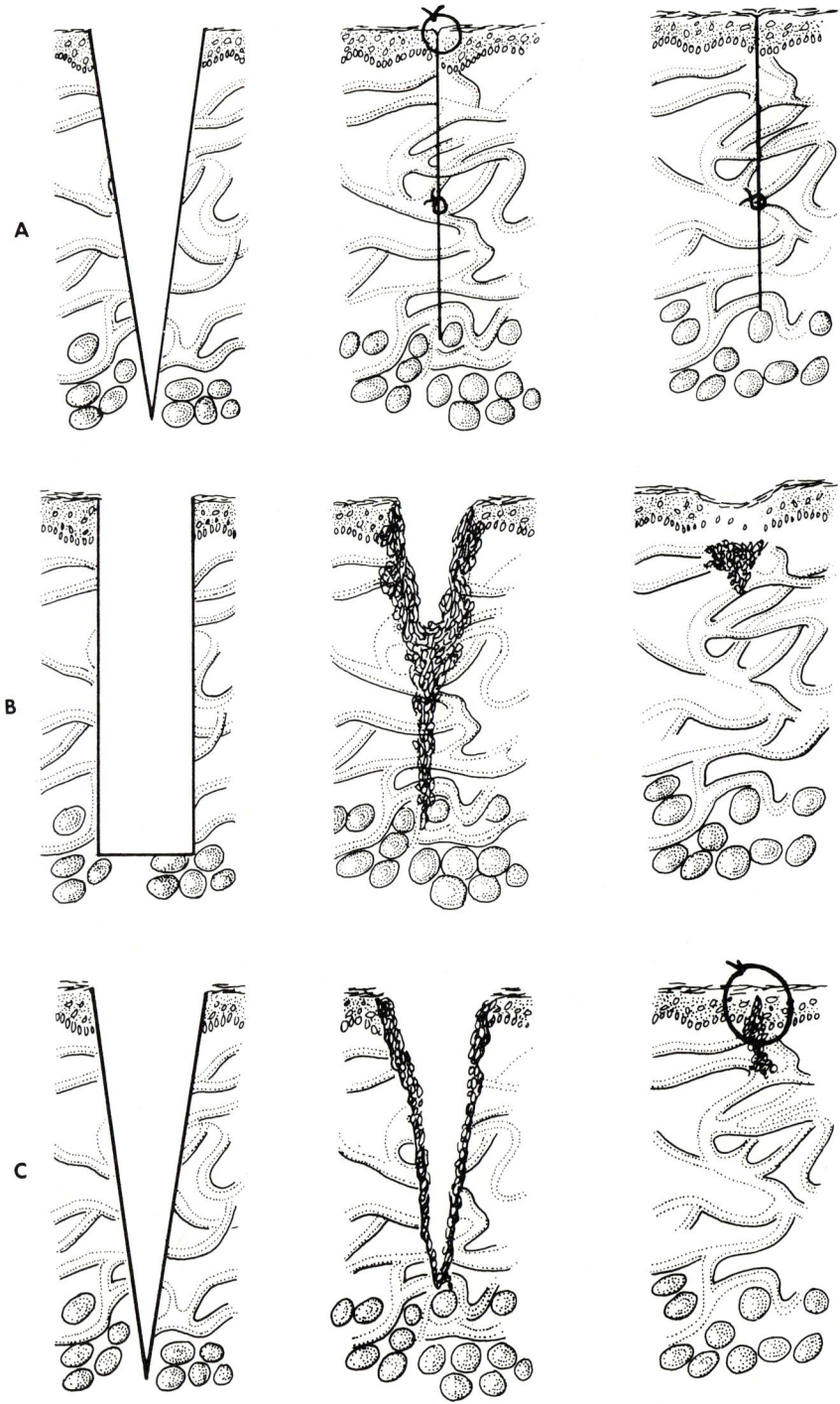

Fig. 6-2. A, Primary; **B,** secondary; and, **C,** tertiary intention wound healing.

ance from six months to a year after the injury.[2-6]

Wound cleansing and preparation

In the initial treatment of wounds, cleansing and preparation can make the difference between a clean, healed wound and an infected one. Techniques for preparation should be adhered to rigidly.

After a thorough evaluation of the wound the surrounding area of skin is shaved (never the eyebrows, however). An adequate area of preparation should be made, preferably 3.5 to 5 cm (1½ to 2 in) around the wound; sometimes more than this is necessary. Remember that hair grows back; there is no reason for an inadequate shave preparation. After the area is shaved, the skin surrounding the wound is thoroughly cleansed. This should take five to ten minutes by the clock. Betadine, Septisol, Chlorhexidine (for those sensitive to iodine), or the newer surgical scrub soaps are frequently used. Since products containing 3% hexachlorophene are linked to CNS toxic side effects and are now controlled under federal guidelines, their use is best avoided. The skin is then flushed with sterile water or saline. Then copious amounts of saline should be used to irrigate the wound itself. Scrubbing the wound with aseptic surgical soaps should be avoided. Soaking of most wounds (except puncture wounds) should not be undertaken because of subsequent maceration of the surrounding viable tissues. This may well hinder the closure and healing of the injured area. Ground-in foreign materials can be removed with a soft surgical brush; however, it may be necessary to anesthetize the area before doing this. Foreign material, if not removed, may result in permanent tatooing.

Following cleansing, preparation, and the administration of an anesthetic, all devitalized and contaminated tissue along with foreign material should be removed from the wound. This will facilitate closure and more rapid healing.[2-6]

Anesthesia

In the management of wounds and their closure, anesthesia is of utmost importance both to the patient and to the person treating the injury. The forms of anesthesia used in the emergency department include local infiltrations and regional blocks. By far the most common variety is the local infiltration of the tissues around the wound, usually with one of the "caine" drugs (e.g., lidocaine, procaine, mepivacaine). Concentrations of local anesthetic vary from 0.5% to 2%. Epinephrine is also contained in some preparations (1:200,000). This is not to be used when infiltrating areas such as the fingers, toes, ears, or nose because of possible compromise of the vascular supply to these areas.

Before infiltration the wound and surrounding area should be cleansed and prepared. The initial infiltration is made through a small skin wheal (Fig. 6-3). The needle is then advanced through the wheal and more anesthetic is injected. This procedure is followed throughout the wound. It is much less painful because each injection is made through an already anesthetized area. Usually a fairly small-gauge needle is used (24 to 26). Another method of infiltration is to use a long (3.5 to 5 cm., 1½ to 3 in) needle, make the initial wheal, insert the needle to its maximum length along the wound edge, and then inject the anesthetic as the needle is slowly withdrawn. This method is quite useful in lengthy linear lacerations.

Regional anesthesia includes digital

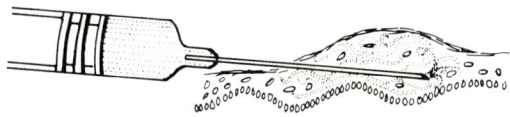

Fig. 6-3. Initial infiltration—wheal.

blocks and various nerve blocks (e.g., axillary, brachial plexus, foot and leg blocks). To accomplish these blocks a fundamental knowledge of the neuroanatomy of the area involved is essential. Then local anesthetic can be infiltrated around the nerves to produce anesthesia distal to the injection site. A detailed discussion of the blocks can be found in other sources.[7]

Lacerations

A laceration is a wound produced by tearing (Fig. 6-4). A similar wound made by smooth, sharp cutting is called an incisional wound. There are many causes of lacerations, ranging from auto accidents to knifings. Lacerations or incisions vary in length and especially in depth. They may involve subcutaneous tissues, fascial planes, tendons, nerves, muscles, and larger blood vessels. The deeper a laceration and the more structures involved, the more painstaking measures must be utilized to obtain closure while maintaining function and procuring as good a cosmetic result as possible. A most important rule to remember concerning the time elapsed between injury and closure is the "golden period" during which wound closure should take place. This golden period is generally within six to eight hours after injury. If the wound is in a very vascular area and the amount of contamination is small, the period may be extended to 12 hours. When contamination is heavy and there is some question as to the vascular supply, it is wise to cleanse the wound thoroughly and to use tertiary (delayed) closure as the method of choice for wound care.

Primary closure of the wound is undertaken after adequate cleansing of the surrounding tissues, irrigation of the wound, and administration of adequate anesthetic. The wound should be carefully inspected and all devitalized material debrided. Wound edges are generally trimmed back to a slant (Fig. 6-5). Another important rule to remember in the handling of lacera-

tions that involve the subcutaneous tissue and below is to close all dead space (Fig. 6-6). If this is not done, body fluids collect in this space and form a nidus for bacterial invasion and growth. In addition, seromas and abscesses may form in the dead space, which will require drainage.

A wide choice of suture material is available, for example, nylon, catgut, Mersilene, and Dexon. Silk is generally not used because of the fairly marked tissue reaction it causes. With the use of swaged needles, closure is made simpler. The suture needles should be of the stout, reverse cutting-edge type.

In suturing, wound edges should be everted and heights should be matched as closely as possible. A suture should be placed so that the depth is greater than the width; this should produce an everting closure (Fig. 6-7). To avoid scalloping or a bunching up appearance to the wound, one should suture the wound the same distance along each side. Textbooks frequently recommend "divide and conquer," thus halving the wound with each suture. Generally, the wound edges will not turn out to be equal in length and height with this technique.

Another important principle when there

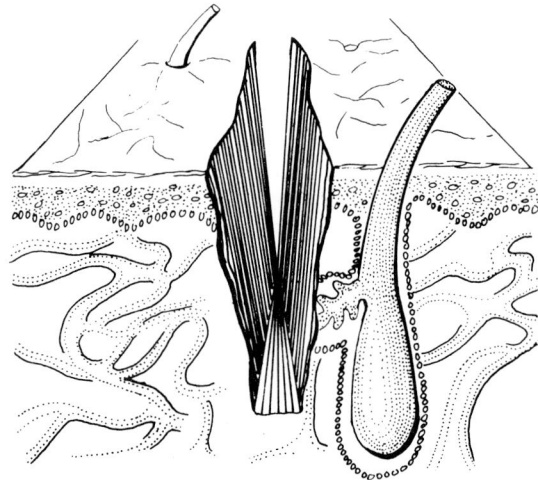

Fig. 6-4. Laceration.

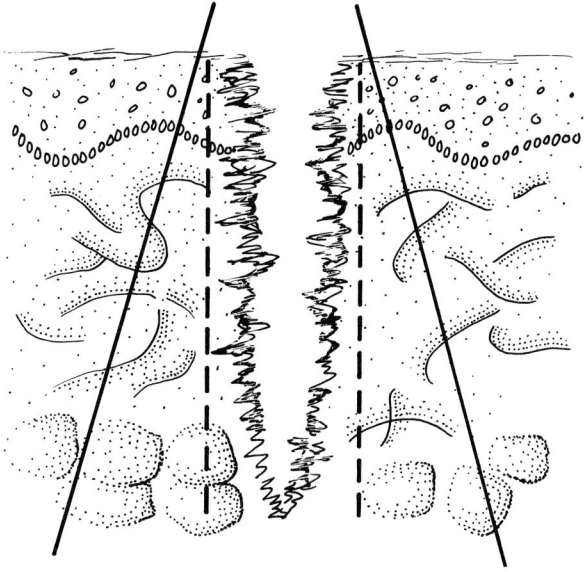

Fig. 6-5. Devitalized material debrided and wound edges trimmed back to a slant.

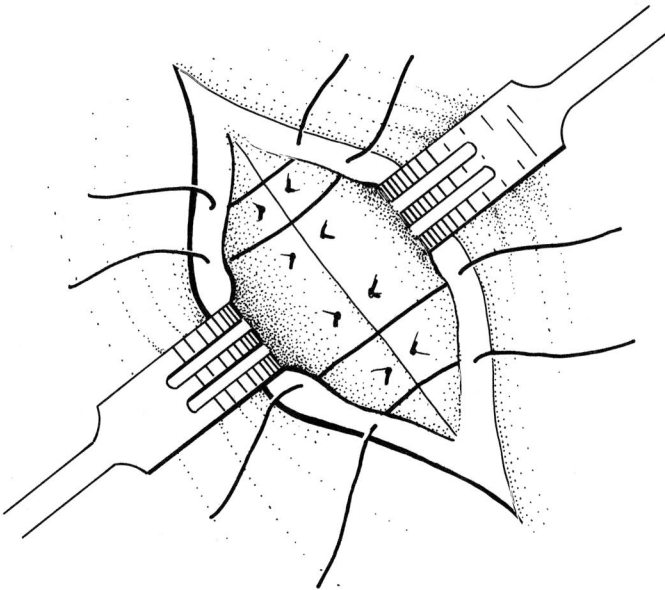

Fig. 6-6. Close all dead space.

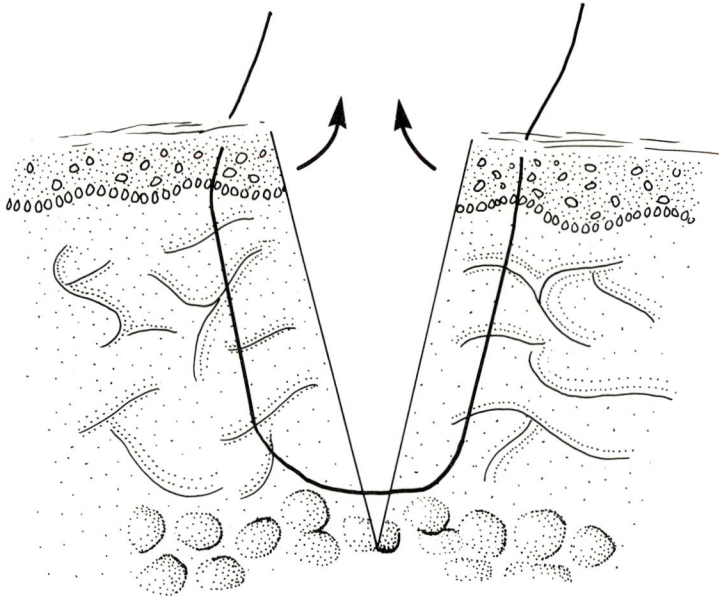

Fig. 6-7. Suture placed so depth is greater than width thus producing a slightly everted closure.

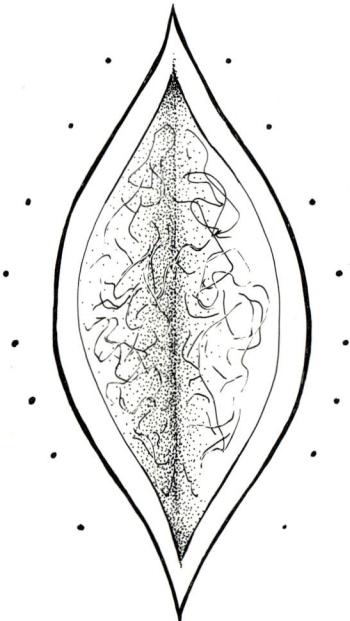

Fig. 6-8. Placement of sutures the same distance on each side.

is wound tension is that the greater the tension, the closer together the sutures should be placed and the closer they should be placed to the wound edge (Fig. 6-8). This should avoid marked tension on the wound.

Of course, deep wound closure is the best way to avoid high skin tension. These sutures should be placed at three areas: the fat-fascial junction, the fat-dermal junction, and the dermal epithelial junction.

If after the skin has been pulled together it appears there is a high and low side (this may occur especially in a wound that has been deeply sutured or one that cuts around planes), "locking the stitch" will correct this. Locking the stitch on the *low* side will depress the high side and raise the low side. It is not at all necessary to have the sutures tied on one side. It looks nice but it fails to give the needed equal height.[6]

At the present time many emergency personnel prefer to use Steristrips for skin

Table 6-1. Guideline for length of time between suturing and suture removal

Location of laceration	Suture removal (days)
Face	3 to 5
Scalp	6 to 8
Trunk	7 to 10
Extremities	7 to 10
If at joints*	12 to 16
Hands	7 to 10
Feet	7 to 10

*If lacerations occur over joints, it is necessary that the involved joint be splinted until the sutures are removed.

closure of facial wounds, providing that very little tension must be placed on the strips.[2-6]

Delayed closures of lacerations, or for that matter any wound, are handled the same way as primary closure up to the point of suturing. After the area is anesthetized, all devitalized tissue and foreign material are removed. The laceration is packed, possibly soaked, and then sutured, generally within two to six days. Suturing must occur during this time period because it becomes extremely difficult to mobilize wound margins after six to eight days. Many dog bites and especially human bites are handled in this manner.[2-6]

After closure of the laceration, a dry, sterile dressing is applied, generally over the top of a nonadherent layer of material. Dressings are changed regularly and usually cover the wound until sutures are removed, especially in areas of constant movement, stress, or rubbing. Sometimes hydrogen peroxide applied lightly to the suture line once or twice daily will keep serum and crusts from forming.

Protective splints should be applied when lacerations are over joints and sites involved in frequent movements and minor day-to-day trauma. They should be left in place until the sutures are removed and perhaps for several days after removal. To keep wound dressings clean, stockinette may be useful.

Time of suture removal varies within limits and generally is a matter of personal preference. A general guideline is presented in Table 6-1, which gives ranges for length of time between suturing and suture removal in various areas of the body.

Wound infections

Wound infections must be recognized and cared for with any type of injury. They usually show up within 24 to 48 hours after the injury, but in severely contaminated wounds infection may be noticed after 8 to 12 hours. Some of the signs and symptoms include local pain, erythema, swelling, and purulent exudates. Systemic findings are fever, lymphadenopathy, and lymphangitis. Treatment usually consists of thorough cleansing of the wound, removal of some (if not all) sutures, soaks, and systemic antibiotics. A culture of the wound should be taken. Frequent follow-ups are needed in these instances.[2, 3, 5]

Abrasions

An abrasion may be defined as a denudation of a portion of the body's skin (Fig. 6-9). It involves only a partial thickness of skin. If it involves the full skin thickness or deeper, it is referred to as an avulsion laceration or injury. The most frequent causes of abrasions are motorcycle and bicycle accidents. Unlike lacerations, abrasions tend to be very painful; they are similar to thermal burns. Local anesthesia or systemic analgesia may be necessary for their care.

Abrasions are managed by simple cleansing of the area with a surgical soap, followed by thorough rinsing with normal sterile saline. Then a layer of antibacterial ointment is applied, on top of which is placed a nonadhering, sterile, fine mesh material. Finally, a gauze dressing is used. The dressing is changed daily until a firm

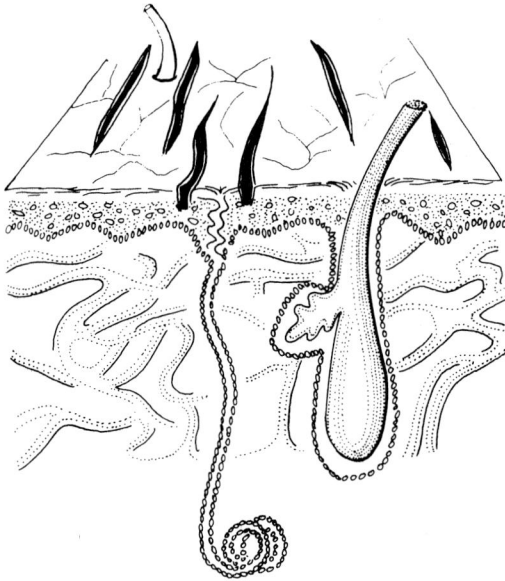

Fig. 6-9. Abrasion.

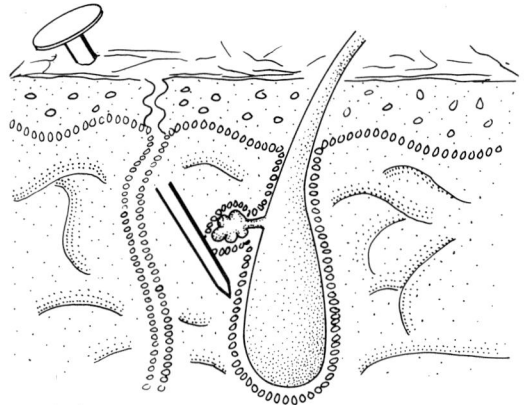

Fig. 6-10. Puncture wound.

eschar is formed. Complete healing generally takes from 12 to 16 days.

If the abrasion is extensive or quite painful, especially with cleansing, local anesthetic may be injected beneath the abrasion or applied topically in 4% strength impregnated into a sterile gauze. The latter method is painless; however, the gauze must be left in place for several minutes for anesthesia to be produced. This method is extremely useful in children.

All too frequently ground-in material is found in the abrasion. This must be removed; otherwise, a permanent tattoo may be formed. Generally, local anesthesia is used and the wound is scrubbed with a surgical brush and soap until the material is removed.

If the abrasion is of the full thickness variety, the wound will generally require a skin graft of some type. These patients should be referred to the proper personnel for treatment.

Fairly frequent follow-up visits are necessary to detect and prevent infection and assure minimal scarring.[2-5]

Puncture wounds

A puncture wound is a wound in which a foreign object, usually pointed or sharp, pierces the skin (Fig. 6-10). They are most commonly caused by stepping on nails, tacks, or staples and by accidental or intentional stabbing with ice picks, knives, or similar instruments. Wound depth and organ involvement are quite variable, ranging from superficial to deeply penetrating puncture wounds of the chest or abdomen.

Management depends on depth and degree of contamination. When both the skin and the penetrating object are known to be clean, the wound is soaked in a diluted surgical soap or paint, after which a sterile dressing is applied. Soaks are continued at home for two to four days with plain warm water. If contamination is present, the skin is thoroughly cleansed, the wound is soaked as above, and a local anesthetic is given. Following this the wound is opened, and devitalized tissue is removed. Finally, a thorough irrigation with normal saline is done, the wound is packed, and a sterile dressing is applied. Soaks are continued at home, and packing is removed in 24 to 48 hours. The wound is generally allowed to heal by secondary intention.

Deep puncture wounds of the chest, abdomen, or extremities are usually handled

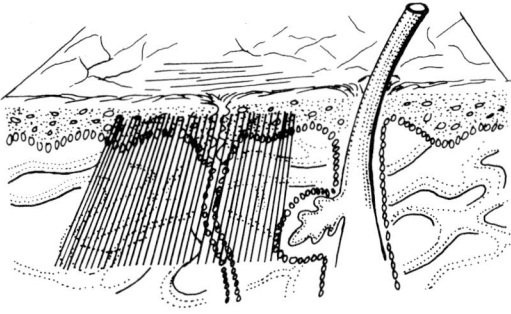

Fig. 6-11. Contusion.

in an operating room after initial therapy is carried out.

Puncture wounds are particularly prone to tetanus and other bacterial contamination; therefore it is necessary to check the patient's history of tetanus immunizations very closely. It may also be necessary to begin the patient on prophylactic antibiotics (penicillin G and gentamicin) if the puncture wound is thought to be highly contaminated. In this case follow-up care is mandatory.[1-5]

Contusions

Contusions, or bruises, are generally benign lesions resulting from blunt trauma to the superficial tissues. There is breakage of small blood vessels and extravasation of blood into the tissues (Fig. 6-11). These injuries are usually mildly to moderately painful, especially to touch, and usually require minimal care, such as ice packs or cool soaks and mild analgesia. Healing takes place in two to three weeks, with pain subsiding within a few days.[2,3,5]

Bites

There are two types of bites that deserve mention here: animal (dog, cat, fox, squirrel) and human. The animal bite is common, and dog bites occur most frequently. Bites are essentially puncture wounds in which both contamination and tissue injury are common; however, teeth may produce extensive lacerations. In ad-

dition, contusions and abrasions may be associated with the injury. The biggest problem associated with bites is infection. Carnivorous animals harbor many types of bacteria in their mouths, but none harbors more than does man.

The injuries are treated as contaminated puncture wounds except when lacerations are produced exposing muscle, nerves, or tendons or when the bite is on the face. In these instances suturing or delayed closure is necessary. Antibiotics (cephalosporins, penicillin) are frequently used prophylactically. Bites require frequent follow-up visits. Of utmost importance is the question of rabies and whether to begin antirabies immunizations. It is necessary to ascertain whether the bite was provoked or nonprovoked and exactly what type of animal did the biting, who (if anyone) owns the animal, and if the animal is vaccinated against rabies.

Human bites are worthy of separate mention because of the severe necrotizing infections frequently associated with them. Infections are caused by anaerobic and microaerophilic organisms harbored in the human mouth. These wounds are usually located on the knuckles. They require thorough cleansing and debridement and many times even admission to the hospital. Prophylactic antibiotics are used in all but the most trivial wounds. Close follow-up of these bites is a prerequisite to adequate therapy.[1-5,8]

Tetanus prophylaxis

Tetanus is a frequently fatal disease that can be almost totally prevented by active immunization. At the present time, approximately 200 or more cases per year are reported in the United States. This figure may be grossly low because many children are *not* being properly immunized, usually due to parental indiscretion. Most cases of tetanus generally occur in older individuals and in nonimmunized children. Recommendations listed here are from the Center for Disease Control (CDC), the American College of Surgeons (ACS), and the Public Health Service (PHS).

Tetanus is an acute CNS intoxication caused by the fixation of a toxin elaborated by the anaerobic *Clostridium tetani.* Once the toxin is fixed in the tissue, it is doubtful that it can be neutralized. The incubation period is from one day to 15 weeks, with the average about eight days.

Signs and symptoms include pain and tingling at the site of innoculation, which is quickly followed by spasticity of nearby muscle groups. This rapidly spreads to the jaw, along with neck stiffness, dysphagia, and irritability. Painful tonic-clonic convulsions precipitated by minor stimuli are common. Almost the entire time the patient is conscious. The mortality rate is high in a full-blown case.[9,10]

Primary immunization may begin in infants as young as 6 weeks of age with 0.5 ml of diphtheria toxoid, pertussis vaccine, and tetanus toxoid (DPT) (best in absorbed form) given intramuscularly or subcutaneously on three consecutive occasions at four- to six-week intervals. A reinforcing dose is given one year after the third injection. If the primary series is not completed—even if up to two years have elapsed between doses—the final response is not adversely affected, and the primary series need not be restarted from the beginning.

For those children over age 6 years and adults who have not been immunized, diphtheria-tetanus (DT) intramuscular injections are given on two consecutive occasions four to six weeks apart, with a reinforcing dose given one year after the second dose.

Booster immunization of DPT or DT in single doses of 0.5 ml intramuscularly is preferably given at the time of entrance into grade school. From then on, and for all other boosters, 0.5 ml of adult *DT* is given every ten years. Annual boosters should be avoided.

In dealing with injuries, booster immunizations are given according to the following schedule:

A. For minor injuries in fully immunized children and adults a booster is given only if the last immunization was administered more than ten years previously. Minor injuries include superficial wounds, clean but not extensive wounds, and minor burns.

B. For serious injuries (such as deep puncture wounds, contaminated wounds, crush injuries, animal bites, more severe burns) in fully immunized persons a booster is given unless there is *definite* evidence that an immunization injection has been given within the preceding 12 months.

C. In partially immunized individuals (i.e., those who have not completed the primary series plus the booster):
   1. For minor injuries the series is completed.
   2. For serious injuries the series is completed and tetanus immune globulin human (TIGH) is also given. Most recent articles are now advocating 500 units routinely. Larger doses have been found to be of no more benefit than the 500-unit injection. Equine antitoxin is virtually never given.
   3. Antibiotics, such as penicillin or its derivatives, are employed in very severe and extensive injuries in addition to TIGH and completion of the series.

D. In unimmunized persons:
   1. Begin and complete the series of immunizations in patients with minor injuries.
   2. For serious injuries TIGH, 500 units intramuscularly, is indicated, along with commencement of the basic series. Antibiotics are generally given also.

E. For those fully immunized persons with no booster in the last ten years and who are seen more than 24 hours after a serious injury, TIGH and a booster are given.

In cases of serious injury it is usually best to err on the side of giving TIGH because (1) the incubation period of tetanus can be as short as one day; (2) ten-year boosters may be inadequate in some instances; (3) the immunization history may be unreliable; and (4) there are rare failures of primary immunization doses (3.8 per 100 million).

Side effects or untoward reactions to tetanus toxoid or DT immunizations are extremely uncommon. However, a localized or generalized urticaria may occur. These may be easily controlled with antihistamines. Serious reactions such as anaphylaxis, erythema-multiforme, or the Stevens-Johnson syndrome are quite rare. Fatal reactions are virtually unheard of. There is no real contraindication to tetanus immunization except infection. In that case postpone immunization until the infection passes.[9-12]

Rabies prophylaxis

Although unknown numbers of cases of rabies are reported in humans each year in the world, rarely does anyone survive this most deadly disease (the first reported recovery was in Lima, Ohio, St. Rita's Hospital). Before 1960 over 5,000 cases of rabies in animals were being reported each year in the United States (this was estimated to be about one tenth of the actual number of cases). Since then the incidence has dropped to around 200 cases per year due to the marked increase in the use of antirabies vaccines for animals. Rabies in humans is now acquired from rabid wild animals. Animals most frequently affected by rabies are bats, dogs, foxes, skunks, and raccoons and sometimes horses, cattle, and cats. Rabies is *not* endemic in rodents, and bites by such species as rats, chipmunks, squirrels, and rabbits rarely, if ever, justify antirabies vaccination.

Fortunately, there is a method of vaccination against rabies, but because the effectiveness of postexposure rabies prophylaxis decreases with time, a prompt medical decision is necessary to begin or not.[13]

Incubation period for rabies varies from under ten days to about one year and sometimes more. Usually the variance is between 2 to 12 weeks. Symptoms at first are nonspecific with fever, headache, malaise, and abdominal pain. More specific symptoms are pain or paresthesias about the bite. Then behavioral or neurologic abnormalities gradually develop, including hyperactivity, hypersalivation, and pharynegal spasms. The clinical condition slowly deteriorates over four to ten days; the patient lapses into a coma; and death soon follows.[14]

The basic decision the physician must make is whether to give postexposure prophylaxis, which type, and how long.

Rabies is transmitted mainly by the bite of a rabid animal. However, contamination can occur with the combination of rabid saliva and an open wound, laboratory specimens, or by aerosols containing high concentrations of rabies virus.[14]

Every effort should be made to capture the offending animal should it be one of the species in which rabies is known to spread. This usually requires knowledge of the epizoology of rabies in that area. If the animal is captured, it should be observed closely for ten days, or if the animal is acting quite strangely, examination of the brain tissue by the state health department is in order.

The World Health Organization (WHO), the Center for Disease Control (CDC), and the Public Health Service recommend the following postexposure vaccination schedules.

Most often duck embryo vaccine (DEV) is used, but in certain cases antiserum must be started. NOTE: nerve tissue vaccine is not used at this time. Fortunately, there is now a human rabies immune globulin (HRIG) available in addition to the standard equine antirabies serum (EARS). The latter is inexpensive with a dose range from 40 to 100 Iμ/kg and with many side effects. The former is much more expensive, and the dose is 20 Iμ/kg. If the HRIG is not available locally, one may obtain it by calling the manufacturer directly anytime (day or night, seven days a week) at 1-214/631-6240.

If the offending animal was a dog or cat that escaped and the animal had *only licked* the victim, then a series of 14 doses of DEV with one dose per day and no further doses at 10 and 20 days after vaccination is indicated.

Whenever rabies immune globulin (HRIG or EARS) is given, duck embyro vaccine is *always* begun. The treatment of DEV is 23 doses of 1 ml each, given in the following ways:

1. One dose per day for 21 days; then boosters at 10 and 20 days after the last dose.
2. Two 1 ml doses a day for seven days, followed by one dose a day for seven days with boosters as listed above.[14]

Side effects from EARS occur in 40% of adults and 20% of children. With HRIG the incidence of side effects is low and the possibility of serum sickness is eliminated. Local reactions to duck embryo vaccine occur in nearly all persons with pain, swelling, and erythema. Systemic symptoms such as generalized urticaria, regional or generalized adenopathy, fever, headache, and sometimes nausea occur in 25% to 33% of those treated. Treatment with antihistamines is necessary; some antiemetics may help; but steroids should not be given because they reduce the immune responses. If severe reactions occur, then the possibility of discontinuing the DEV must be given careful consideration, taking into account the nature of the attack and the offending animal and the possibility of the patient's acquiring rabies. In these cases test the adequacy of immunization already given by examining the antibody titers already present.[13]

Following are the different treatment schedules to be followed:

A. Licks
   1. Victim licked on an open wound or mucous membrane by a possibly rabid animal.
      a. Begin vaccine at first signs of rabies in the offending animal.
      b. If the animal has signs suggestive of rabies at the time of licking, begin vaccine immediately, but stop treatment if the animal is normal on the fifth day after the exposure.
      c. If the animal is known to be rabid or has been killed, has escaped, or is lost, HRIG or EARS and the vaccine should be begun immediately.

B. Bites
   1. In mild exposure cases where the animal is healthy at the time of biting, begin vaccine at first signs of rabies in the biting animal.
   2. In mild exposures where the animal has signs suggestive of rabies at the onset, begin the vaccine immediately and stop treatment if the animal is normal on the fifth day after exposure.
   3. In mild cases of exposure where the animal is rabid, has escaped, or is lost, begin HRIG and vaccine immediately. This is especially true of wild wolves, jackals, foxes, and bats (high-risk animals).
   4. In severe exposures (multiple bites or bites about the face, head, fingers, or neck) where the animal is healthy at the time of biting, give HRIG immediately and start vaccine at the first sign of rabies in the biting animal.
   5. In severe exposures where the animal has signs suggestive or rabies, begin both HRIG and the vaccine immediately. If the animal is under observation and is normal on the fifth

day after exposure, the vaccine may be discontinued.

6. In severe cases where the animal is rabid, has escaped, or is lost (especially bats, foxes, jackals, wild wolves), begin the HRIG and vaccine immediately.

Preexposure prophylaxis can be given to those individuals at high risk to rabies exposure such as veterinarians, laboratory workers, and spelunkers. Current recommendations are as follows:

1. Three 1 ml injections of DEV given at weekly intervals with a 1 ml booster at three weeks

2. Two 1 ml injections of DEV 30 days apart with a 1 ml booster at six months.

About 85% to 95% of those immunized in this manner will develop antirabies antibodies. If one of the individuals is exposed to rabies, only a short series of five DEV injections (1 ml each day times five days) plus a booster at ten days is indicated. On the other hand, the nonresponsive individual must undergo the complete postexposure prophylaxis regimen.[14]

Embedded fishhook

An embedded fishhook, a common, generally nice-weather malady, has presented itself thousands of times to countless emergency departments. There are two methods for removal of the hook.

1. With anesthesia. Cleanse the area and infiltrate with local anesthetic (painful); then push the barb through the skin and either clip it off and withdraw the hook through the old wound or snip the shank and push the remainder of the hook through the new wound.

2. Without anesthesia. Soak the wounded area and, if possible, gently cleanse around the hook. Loop a strong piece of string over the curved portion of the hook. Wrap the loose ends firmly around one or two fingers of the right hand (Fig. 6-12, *A*). The left hand is used to press the area hooked

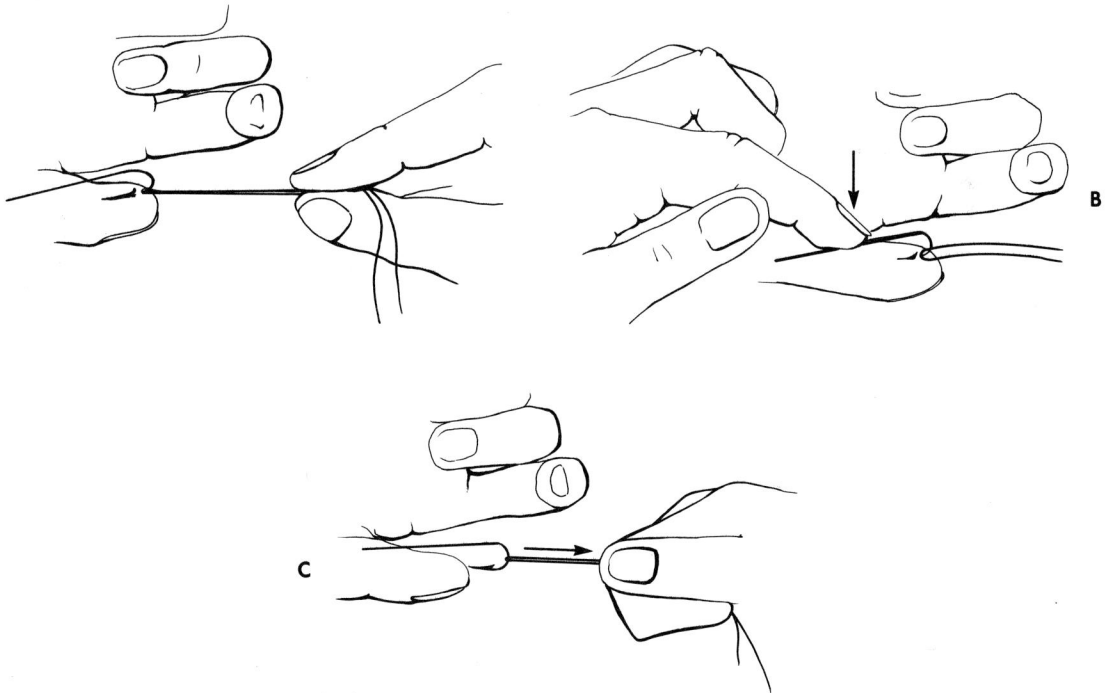

Fig. 6-12. Removal of fishhook using string mechanism.

against a firm surface. Disengage the barb by depressing the shank of the hook downward until it meets resistance (Fig. 6-12, *B*). Then pull the string out slowly until it is parallel with the shank of the hook. Finally, give a quick firm jerk to the taut string to expel the hook (Fig. 6-12, *C*).[15] NOTE: bystanders can be hooked themselves if they are in the line of the expelled hook. This method is practically painless and is now the preferred method of fishhook removal, but it does *not* work if there are two barbs or a double or triple hooking from a treble hook.

After removal of the fishhook the wound is treated as a puncture wound, and the tetanus immunization status is ascertained.

Ring removal

Whenever a ring, valuable or not, must be removed (finger swollen, cyanotic, or likely to swell due to injury or infection), a simple but most of the time effective maneuver may be applied.

Take a few feet of strong string or heavy silk suture and pass it under the ring either with a wood applicator stick, a toothpick, match, or small hemostat. Pull through a few inches of the string. Then begin tightly wrapping down the finger beginning at the ring and proceeding down the finger to the tip. The string wrap should be closely enough spaced to prevent any swollen tissue from bulging through (Fig. 6-13, *A*).

Then with the coil or wrap of string held firmly in place, begin pulling on the string on the proximal side of the ring and pull it slowly toward the tip of the fingers. As the string is pulled distally down the finger, the ring follows and finally drops off (Fig. 6-13, *B*).

This method is fairly painless because of the swelling and relative numbness of the digit already present.[16]

If this method does not work, then try the slipperiest substance one can find (soap, oil, grease), apply it all over and under the ring, and try easing the ring off slowly.

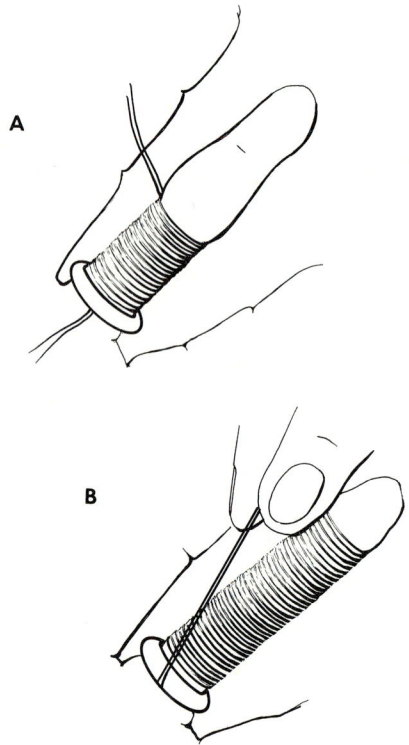

Fig. 6-13. Ring removal without cutting ring.

If the above methods do not work, a ring cutter is sure to work despite the ring owner's objection. Remember—a ring *can* be repaired by a qualified jeweler; a finger that becomes gangrenous usually *cannot* be fixed and must be amputated.

Subungual hematoma

Whenever a crushing injury occurs to any distal digit, there is the possibility of a subungual hematoma formation. These not only look terrible but are generally quite painful (due to pressure under the nail), even though the strongest narcotics may be given. This may last for several days until reabsorption of the blood takes place. An easy method to handle this problem is through the use of a hot paper clip. First, the area is lightly cleansed and the offended digit placed on a firm surface. Then a partially straightened paper clip

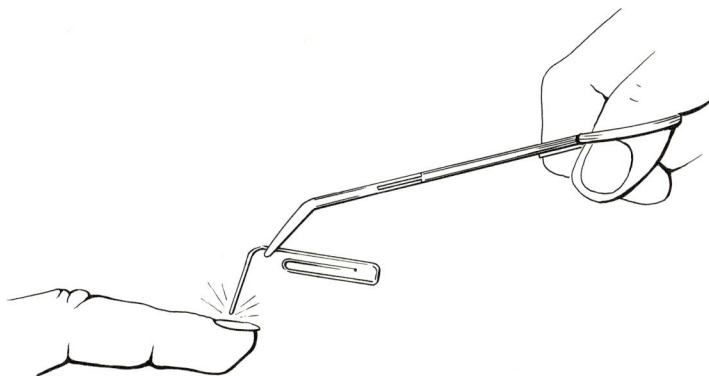

Fig. 6-14. Relieving a subungual hematoma using a red-hot paper clip.

held in a hemostat (Fig. 6-14) is heated to *red* hot with a lighter, alcohol lamp, bunsen burner, or the like. The red-hot clip is then gently but quickly thrust through the nail releasing the hematoma. There is a momentary sensation of pain, but this quickly subsides. Relief of the pressure pain is almost immediate. Other methods that have the same outcome are (1) using a no. 11 knife blade on a handle and drilling a hole in the nail until the blood is released, (2) drilling with a small hand-held drill and burr, or (3) using a red-hot electric hand-held cautery. All come to the same end— some a little slower and more painfully than others. After a hole has been formed, soaking of the wound to aid in draining the hematoma is in order.

HEMORRHAGE

Hemorrhage may be defined as any acute loss of blood. It can involve any amount of blood, being very small in some cases to life threatening in others. The causes of hemorrhage are as variable as the amount of blood lost. These can include lacerations, amputations, crushes, fractures, and internal conditions such as gastrointestinal bleeding or ruptured spleen.

There are three types of hemorrhage: arterial, venous, and capillary. These types are characterized as (1) arterial, spurting and bright red in color, (2) venous, continuous flow and dark, and (3) capillary, oozing and red. Of course, wounds are usually a mixture of at least two of these types.

The management of hemorrhage is twofold—stopping the bleeding and replacing the blood as needed. Probably the best and most basic way to stop external hemorrhage is direct pressure with or without subsequent ligation of the vessels involved. Tourniquets are restricted to life-saving measures only, and even then there are very few instances where they should be used. If major vessels are involved, repair or ligation should be carried out in an operating suite where all the necessary equipment and the best of lighting are available.

With severe hemorrhage of any kind the best volume expander is typed and cross matched with the blood. If this is not readily available, then plasma, plasmanate, fresh frozen plasma, Ringer's lactate, or normal saline may be given. As many intravenous infusions should be started as needed to cope with the blood loss. Intravenous needles should be the largest bore available (14 or 15 gauge). Central venous pressure (CVP) lines are frequently used. Vital signs are constantly monitored, and hematocrit determinations are a necessity in any emergency department. If shock is present, the patient should be in the shock position (head slightly down) or supine with the feet up, as many authorities now advocate. In addition, a Foley catheter is necessary to monitor urine output. If bleeding is internal, a nasogastric tube is quite useful and is a must in gastrointestinal hemorrhage; it facilitates removal of clots and collected blood and allows for lavage, which may be enough to stop the hemorrhage. Other laboratory studies frequently ordered (especially in gastrointestinal bleeding) are BUN, glucose, electrolytes, and a partial coagulogram (prothrombin time, partial thromboplastin time, platelets, fibrinogen level).

One test that can be done very simply to determine if there is significant acute blood loss is the tilt test. This consists of taking the patient's blood pressure and pulse after he has been lying and resting for a minimum of five to ten minutes. The patient is then asked to sit upright quickly, and again the pulse and blood pressure are taken. If there is a 20% rise in pulse rate or a 20% decrease in blood pressure, this is a positive reaction and indicates a definitive need for volume replacement in the patient. This test is done only if the patient's condition permits (i.e., he or she has no gross fractures, especially of the cervical spine, severe chest injuries, or certain extremity fractures and injuries).

Hemorrhage can be a life-threatening and panic-producing situation. It usually can be handled simply and most expeditiously if plain, simple common sense is applied to the situation with thoughts of immediate volume replacement and measures to stop the blood loss.[1-4,17]

REFERENCES

1. Ellis, M.: The casualty officers handbook, ed. 3, London, 1970, Butterworth (Publishers) Inc.
2. Davis, L.: Christopher's textbook of surgery, Philadelphia, 1972, W. B. Saunders Co.
3. Schwartz, S. I.: Principles of surgery, New York, 1969, McGraw-Hill Book Co.
4. Ferguson, L. M.: Surgery of the ambulatory patient, ed. 5, Philadelphia, 1974, J. B. Lippincott Co.
5. Hill, G. J.: Outpatient surgery, ed. 1, Philadelphia, 1973, W. B. Saunders Co.
6. Dushoff, I. M., Stitch in time, Emerg. Med., pp. 21-43, Jan. 1973.
7. Moore, D. C.: Regional blocks, ed. 4, Springfield, Ill., 1973, Charles C Thomas, Publisher.
8. Douglas, L. G.: Bite wounds, Am. Fam. Practice, p. 38, April, 1975.
9. Krupp, M. A., and Chatton, M. J.: Current diagnosis and treatment, Los Altos, Calif., 1976, Lange Medical Publications.
10. Faust, R. A., Vickers, O. R., and Cohn, I.: Tetanus: 2,449 cases in 68 years at Charity Hospital, J. Trauma 16(9):704-712, 1976.
11. Furste, W.: Prophylaxis against tetanus, Bull. Am. Coll. Surg., September 1972.
12. American Academy of Pediatrics: Report of the committee on infectious diseases, ed. 16, 1970.
13. Corey, L., and Hattwick, M. A. W.: Treatment of persons exposed to rabies, J.A.M.A. 232(3):272-275, 1975.
14. Hattwick, E.: When and how to treat rabies, Consultant, pp. 154-159, October 1976.
15. Friedenberg, S.: Removing an embedded fishhook, Hosp. Physician 8:71, 48-49, 1974.
16. Young, J. R.: A string to unring a finger, Emerg. Med. pp. 163-164, February 1971.
17. American Academy of Orthopaedic Surgeons: Emergency care and transportation of the sick and injured, Menasha, Wisc., 1976, George Banta Pub. Co.

CHAPTER 7

Assessment and therapy of the shock syndrome

R. W. Virgilio, M.D.
David E. Smith, M.D.

Although the first monograph on shock was written by Morris in 1867, it was not until World War I that physicians began to clinically investigate the pathophysiology of shock. In a review of the problem of shock following this war, Cannon stated: "The reader should understand from the beginning that the mystery of the onset of shock has not been definitely cleared away despite a considerable increase in our knowledge of it and that there still remains much work to be done before we shall have elucidated all the factors which play a role in its establishment."[1] Even though more than 50 years have since passed, this statement is still applicable.

The mortality of hemorrhagic shock has dropped dramatically with the use of blood and blood expanders. But in spite of our better understanding of the pathophysiology of shock, gram-negative bacteremic shock still carries a mortality rate between 60% and 70%, and cardiogenic shock has a mortality rate of over 80%. Shock is not a disease but rather a complex group of physiologic abnormalities that can be precipitated by various factors. Shock cannot, therefore, be thought of as a single clinical entity with a single remedy. Emergency personnel must first understand and treat the underlying cause precipitating the clinical state that is termed "shock" before they can reverse the physiologic derangements that are present. Prior to entering into the discussion of the shock syndrome, a clear definition of what is meant by the term "shock" must be stated.

DEFINITION

Shock is not a single entity with a specific causative agent and treatment; therefore, a simple, concise definition is not possible. In a recent monograph on shock, Thal stated: "Shock is in essence a story of survival, a struggle by the organism in an adverse environment to preserve the life of its most vital functions."[2] An understanding of this struggle requires knowledge of circulatory dynamics, adaptive mechanisms, and cellular physiology. Our survival in adverse environments is determined at the cellular level. The whole purpose of the cardiorespiratory system is to supply oxygen and other nutrients to the mitochondria within individual cells and individual organs. As cells die, so do major organs and ultimately the individual. Therefore, shock must be defined as *the condition in which the circulation or perfusion of blood is inadequate to meet tissue metabolic demands, thereby leading to cellular anoxia and death.* Unabated, this generalized breakdown of cellular function will eventually lead to the death of the organism.

We have not mentioned blood pressure in the above definition for a good reason. Shock should be thought of as a lack of adequate tissue perfusion regardless of the level of blood pressure. Following World War I, Archibald and McLean summarized their opinions regarding the value of blood pressure measurements in shock: "While a low blood pressure is one of the most consistent signs of shock, it is not the essential thing, let alone the cause of it; we have focused our attention far too much on blood pressure."[3]

THE SYSTEMIC RESPONSE TO SHOCK

Before examining the dynamics of the shock syndrome, a firm understanding of the body's normal physiologic response to stress must be established. This can be thought of as the body's ability to adapt or defend itself against an adverse environment, mainly a low flow state, or shock. When there is a sudden loss of intravascular volume from either blood loss or redistribution of large amounts of fluids as occurs in burns or sepsis, there is stimulation of the vasomotor center in the medulla of the brain to produce a marked sympathomimetic response, which increases peripheral resistance by stimulating the constriction of both the pre- and postcapillary sphincters in the microcirculation. This stimulation of the sympathetic nervous system also increases cardiac output by increasing the rate and force of contraction. In addition to this massive neural adrenergic vasoconstriction, there is a marked adrenal medullary response. This response can increase the circulating catecholamine (epinephrine and norepinephrine) titer from 10 to 50 times that of resting levels. These catecholamines are primarily alpha stimulants, which further increase the sympathetic vasoconstriction, thereby increasing the central pressure so that the heart and brain can be ensured prefusion. This response accomplishes two objectives:

1. It increases the central blood pressure, thereby ensuring perfusion of the brain and heart. The price that the body pays for this is diversion of blood flow from less vital areas such as muscle, skin, kidney, intestine, and liver.
2. It decreases capillary hydrostatic pressure, thereby causing a net movement of fluid from the interstitial space to the capillary space, helping to restore plasma volume (Fig. 7-1).

Thus a situation exists in which pressure has been preserved to ensure perfusion of the heart and brain at the expense of perfusion of the majority of body mass and less vital organs. If an individual is going to survive the immediate insult, this mechanism is absolutely necessary. However, prolonged diversion of perfusion from the bowel, kidney, liver, muscle, and so on will ultimately lead to the demise of the individual through progressive cellular anoxia and death in these organ systems. The early period of this adaptive response to cellular anoxia and death is a state of reversible shock (Fig. 7-1), and therapeutic intervention during this phase will usually be successful.

Other important adaptive mechanisms present to help restore plasma volume are the secretion of antidiuretic hormone by the anterior pituitary gland and aldosterone from the adrenal gland. These hormones cause retention of free water and sodium ion by the kidney, thereby helping to replenish plasma volume. Unlike the sympathetic response, these hormonal responses

Ischemia anoxia

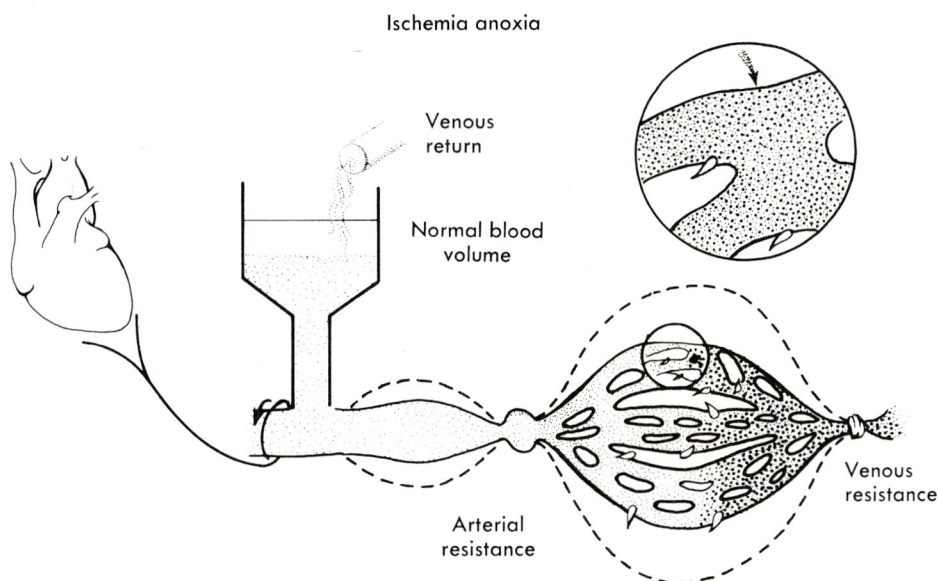

Fig. 7-1. Reversible shock. At this stage of the shock syndrome, both arterial and venous resistance are increased, resulting in a decrease in capillary pressure with a resultant net movement of fluid from the extravascular to the intravascular space. This process helps the individual maintain intravascular volume during the early shock phase. (From Dietzman, R. H., and Lillehei, W. C. In Schwartz, S. I.: Principles of surgery, New York, 1969, McGraw-Hill Book Co. Used with permission of McGraw-Hill Book Co.)

restore volume without being detrimental to cellular metabolism.

IRREVERSIBLE SHOCK

The systemic response to shock can be thought of as the compensated, or reversible, phase of the shock syndrome. Its purpose is to sustain the vital function of the heart and brain until the underlying pathology can be corrected, such as the restoration of blood volume following hemorrhagic shock. Sacrificing the perfusion of nonvital organs, however, sets the stage for progressive cellular anoxia and tissue death resulting in irreversibility of the shock state and ultimate death of the individual. The grace period afforded the individual prior to the development of irreversibility varies with the magnitude of the insult. In experimental hemorrhagic shock, however, it averages about two hours.[4]

The decreased perfusion present in the reversible stage of shock leads to cellular hypoxia, which forces metabolism into the anaerobic pathway (Fig. 7-2) producing higher lactate levels with resultant metabolic acidosis. Thus one of the earliest signs of shock is a metabolic acidosis at a time when the blood pressure may still be normal. As is seen in Fig. 7-1, during the phase of reversible shock the capillary hydrostatic pressure is decreased, thereby allowing the phenomenon of transcapillary refilling to take place with a resultant restoration of plasma volume. With continuous sympathetic stimulation, the venous tone will increase so that the influx of fluid from the tissues will cease. As tissue metabolites continue to accumulate, they

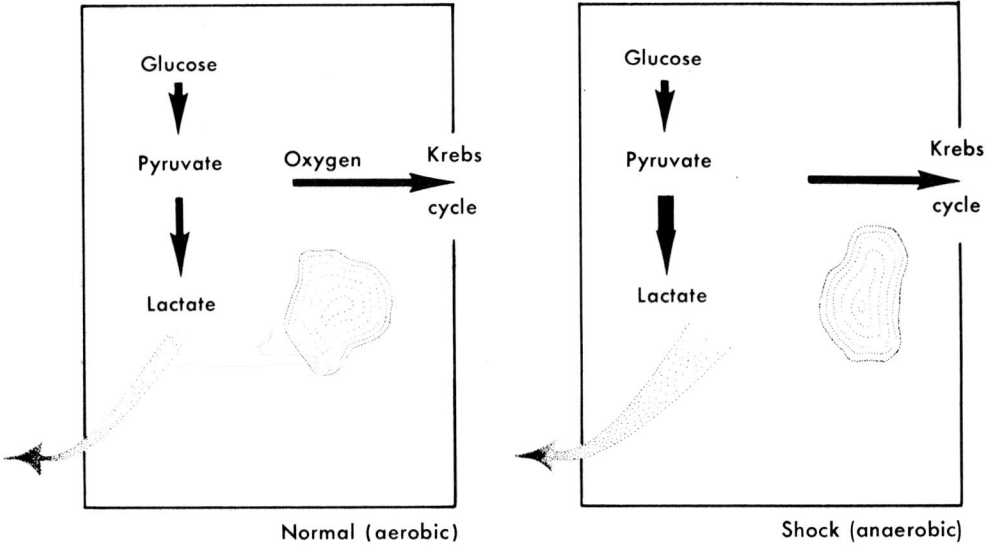

Fig. 7-2. The lack of oxygen at the cellular level during profound shock leads to anaerobic metabolism (right) with a resultant increase in lactate production and metabolic acidosis.[21]

Stagnant anoxia

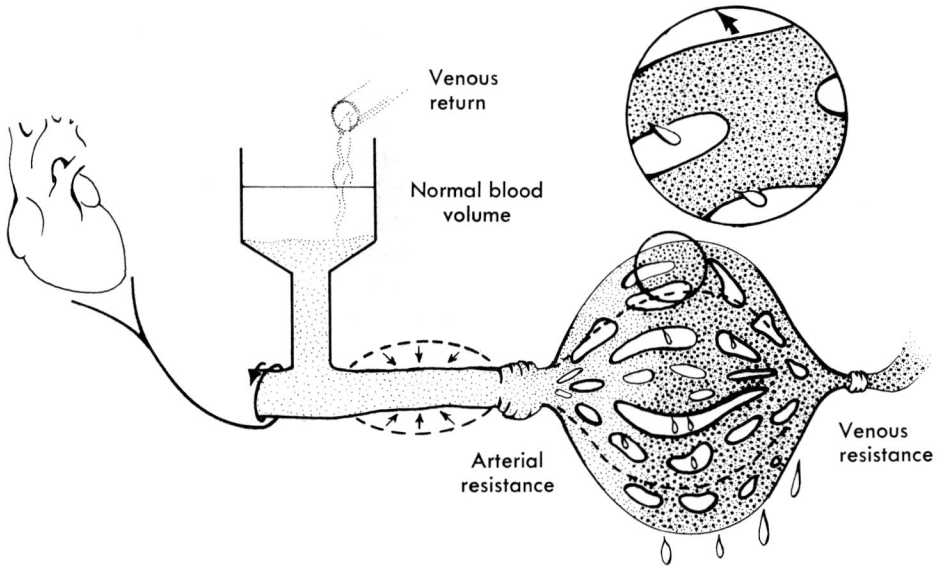

Fig. 7-3. Irreversible shock. At this stage of the shock syndrome, there is relaxation of the arterial sphincter; however, the venous resistance is maintained at a high level. This combination results in capillary hypertension with a resultant net movement of fluid out of the intravascular space into the extravascular space. This loss of intravascular volume further aggravates the shock state. (From Dietzman, R. H., and Lillehei, W. C. In Schwartz, S. I.: Principles of surgery, New York, 1969, McGraw-Hill Book Co. Used with permission of McGraw-Hill Book Co.)

act as a strong stimulus for vasodilatation that negates the constriction of the precapillary sphincter. The postcapillary sphincters, however, are more resistant to the vasodilatory effects of the acid metabolites, and they stay constricted long after the precapillary sphincters dilate (Fig. 7-3). This increases the capillary hydrostatic pressure, causing a net loss of fluid from the vascular space into the interstitial space. Thus the mechanism that originally ensured the maintenance of an adequate perfusion pressure for the heart and brain and the replenishment of the plasma volume ultimately works against

the individual by causing further loss of intravascular volume. With this decreasing volume there is a concomitant decrease in venous return to the right heart. This decrease in filling pressure causes further decrease in cardiac output with a concomitant decrease in the perfusion pressure of the heart and brain. When the perfusion of these two vital organs is no longer adequate for their metabolic demands, the organism dies.

The hemodynamic and tissue perfusion alterations seen in low flow states are depicted graphically in Fig. 7-4. The blood pressure responses in both reversible and

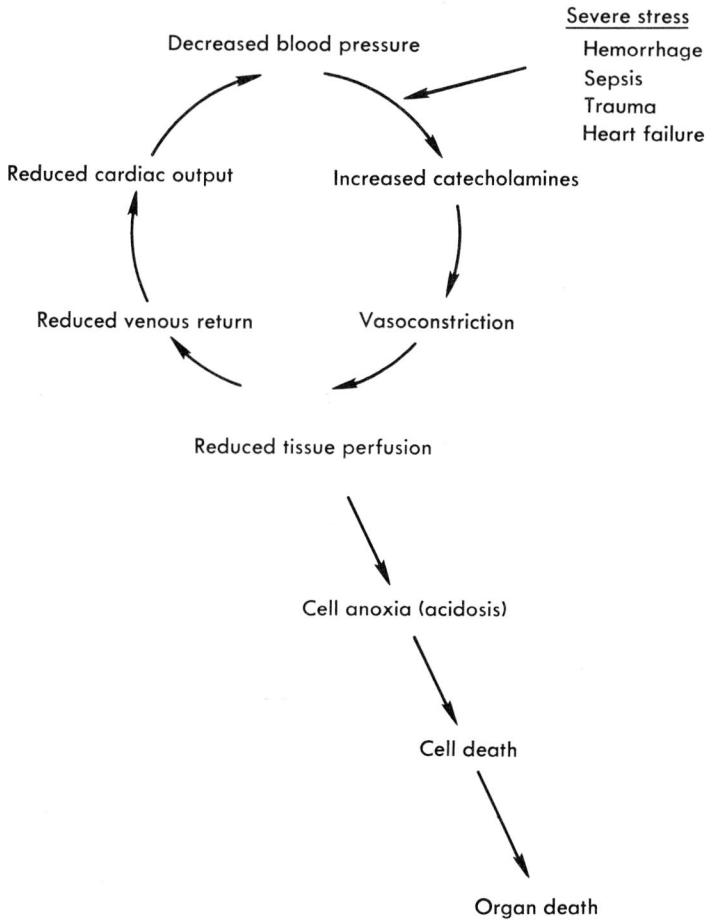

Fig. 7-4. Hemodynamic and tissue perfusion alterations in low flow states.

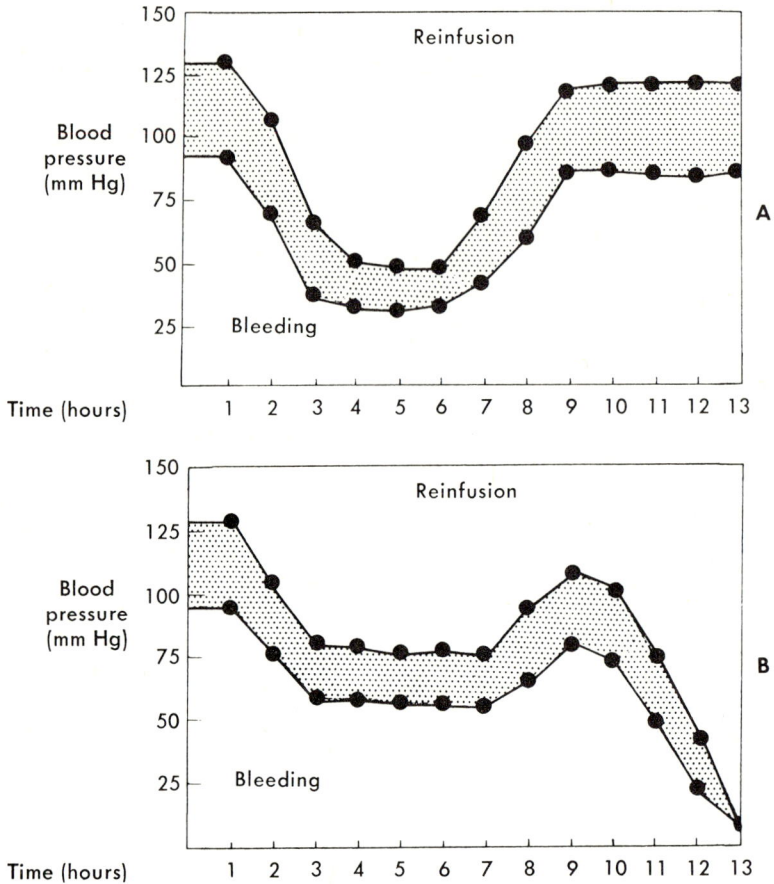

Fig. 7-5. Blood pressure response following reinfusion of shed blood in both the **A,** reversible, and **B,** irreversible, stages of shock. Note that initial favorable response in blood pressure during irreversible shock is only transiently sustained.

irreversible shock following the reinfusion of shed blood are illustrated in Fig. 7-5. Note that after the reinfusion of all the shed blood, there is an initial blood pressure response in the irreversible phase that is rather quickly replaced by the precipitous fall in blood pressure and ultimate death of the animal. This is in contrast to the favorable response after reinfusion of blood in the reversible shock phase in which there is a prompt return of the blood pressure to prehemorrhage levels, and this pressure is sustained.

DIAGNOSIS OF SHOCK

It is obvious from the above description of the pathophysiology of shock that the earlier one is able to diagnose the syndrome and institute appropriate therapy, the higher the salvage rate will be. Once there is cellular death, the restoration of blood flow to that tissue will not accomplish reversal of the anoxic changes. Emergency personnel must become astute at recognizing the early changes that occur in low flow states prior to the development of decompensated or irreversible shock. Consideration of the diagnosis of low flow states in clinical, hemodynamic, and biochemical terms is shown below.

Clinical changes

The early clinical changes in compensated shock are subtle, and unless one has a high index of suspicion, they will escape the notice of even the most experienced examiner. Common clinical situations that carry a high shock potential include not only postoperative and trauma patients, but all patients with chronic underlying disease processes in which septic complications are common. The early adaptive mechanisms in shock are increased sympathetic activity, which causes constriction of blood vessels in the skin resulting in a pale, cold, and clammy skin. There is ascending cooling of the extremities. The pulse is rapid and thready and the blood volume is marginal; it will decrease if the patient sits up, causing further tachycardia.

The metabolic acidosis caused by decreased perfusion and the resulting anaerobic metabolism is responsible for hyperventilation. This occurs in order to eliminate the carbon dioxide (H_2CO_3) and to maintain the blood pH in a normal physiologic range. With decreased perfusion in organs such as the kidney, a decline in the urinary output will be noted. In early stages, however, this change is usually not dramatic and goes unnoticed until the patient's course is evaluated retrospectively. The magnitude of these signs and symptoms in early compensated shock can be so inapparent that if they are noticed at all they are attributed to the patient's anxiety about the surroundings.

Once the blood pressure begins to fall, we are no longer talking about the early signs of compensated shock, but rather about a reflection of decompensation and late shock. The clinical signs of this stage are obvious, and there is little doubt even to the novice that an emergency exists.

In addition to the low systolic blood pressure (often 80 mm Hg or less), patient is usually hypothermic, diaphoretic, barely responsive, tachypneic, and either markedly oliguric or anuric. The declining arterial blood pressure reflects a decreasing venous return to the heart in spite of the previously described adrenergic compensatory mechanisms.

Since the early clinical signs of compensated shock are so subtle and can easily go unnoticed, attention must be given to other methods of diagnosis to help practitioners during this early phase. This becomes even more important considering the marked increase in the mortality when a patient slips from compensated shock to the phase of decompensation.

Hemodynamic changes

The unreliability of the physical examination in assessing early shock coupled with the value of aggressive early intervention has stimulated continuous monitoring of the major components of the cardiovascular system in patients at high risk of developing shock.

Arterial blood pressure. As was pointed out above, blood pressure is not a very helpful parameter in compensated shock because it is usually normal at the time perfusion is poor. Trends in blood pressure may be more helpful in showing the progression of low flow states, however. The marked peripheral vasoconstriction during compensated shock sometimes makes the use of a blood pressure cuff ineffectual. The present trend is to use intra-arterial lines in these high risk patients so that intra-arterial pressure can be continually monitored accurately. Femoral arterial lines placed percutaneously have a better longevity than similar lines placed in the upper extremity and are our personal preference. The point has been made that blood pressure is a poor indicator of compensated shock. It should be emphasized, however, that a systolic blood pressure below 80 mm Hg is always a sign of a low flow state which is now decompensated. According to Peterson:

1. A systolic blood pressure of 80 mm Hg, unless promptly reversed, is a warning of danger.
2. A systolic blood pressure of 70 mm Hg relates a serious degree of perfusion failure and must be corrected.
3. A systolic blood pressure of 60 mm Hg or less marks a critical reduction in perfusion. The most intensive resuscitative measures available must be introduced on an emergency basis. The mortality from shock in such cases is high. Thus, the monitoring of intra-arterial pressure by direct means is essential to follow the progression of low flow states and the adequacy of therapy.[5]

One cannot say what the optimal blood pressure should be following resuscitation. What is needed is a pressure great enough to supply adequate tissue perfusion. This may be a systolic pressure of 80 or 140 depending upon the individual circumstances. Some easily measurable parameters that indicate when the perfusion is adequate are discussed later in this chapter.

Cardiac output. When cardiac output is too low to supply adequate tissue perfusion, a state of shock exists. Measurement of this parameter, therefore, becomes an absolute necessity in evaluating the low flow state. In the phase of compensated shock when the arterial pressure may still be normal, the cardiac output will be low because of decreased intravascular volume (hemorrhagic shock) or pump failure (cardiogenic shock). A cardiac index of less than 3 liters/m²/minute (normal range is 3 to 4 liters/m²/minute) associated with an increased total peripheral resistance and reduced tissue perfusion is considered to represent a low output syndrome.[5] When it is less than 2 liters/m²/minute, a profound state of low flow exists and is usually associated with decompensation and hypotension.

Unfortunately, cardiac output by itself is not 100% reliable as an index of the degree of shock. There are clinical situations, which are usually associated with derangements of the microcirculation or primary cellular derangements, in which cardiac output is actually increased, and yet there is still biochemical and clinical evidence of inadequate perfusion. These situations are termed the "high output shock syndrome" of which certain cases of septic shock are classic examples.[6,7] The evidence now points to the fact that there is a primary cellular derangement in these patients with endotoxic shock that precludes the utilization of the delivered oxygen. The high cardiac output seen in these clinical situations is thought of as an attempted compensatory mechanism.[8] In all cases of hypovolemic or cardiogenic shock, however, and in some cases of septic shock, the use of the level of cardiac output as an index of the degree of shock is valid.

Total peripheral resistance. The calculation of total peripheral resistance (TPR) is based on measurements of the mean arterial pressure (MAP), central venous pressure (CVP), and cardiac output (C.O.):

$$TPR = \frac{MAP \text{ (mm Hg)} - CVP \text{ (mm Hg)}}{C.O. \text{ (liters/minute)}}$$

This number reflects the degree of peripheral vasoconstriction secondary to the sympathomimetic response seen in early shock. Normal values range from 1,000 to 1,500 dyne-sec.-cm⁻⁵. In the compensated phases of hypovolemic or cardiogenic shock this value may reach 3,000 to 3,500 dyne-sec.-cm⁻⁵. The clinical reflection of such high resistance is a marked degree of peripheral vasoconstriction with a resultant cool, clammy extremity, diminished or absent pulses, and the inability to get a good cuff blood pressure. Although the calculated total peripheral resistance does not in itself accurately reflect the degree of shock, when evaluated together with the cardiac output, central venous pressure, and degree of metabolic acidosis, it helps the physician make a reasonable estimation as to the underlying pathology responsible for the shock state. Its most important contribution in the care of the shock patient is in helping the physician decide if adrenergic drug therapy is needed and which drug to use. The results of this drug therapy will also be reflected by changes in the total peripheral resistance. These two considerations will be further elucidated in the discussion of the diagnosis and treatment of individual types of shock.

Central venous pressure. Attempting to diagnose and treat the shock patient without knowledge of the central venous pressure would be analogous to driving at night without the benefit of headlights. Arriving at the correct destination, that is, correct diagnosis and treatment plan, would surely be only by chance, and this is obviously not good enough when dealing with human life.

Central venous pressure is the pressure within the superior vena cava or right atrium. Techniques for insertion of this catheter are numerous and include using either the percutaneous or cut-down routes via an antecubital vein, jugular vein, or the subclavian vein. Our preference is the percutaneous infraclavicular subclavian route. Detailed descriptions of all the techniques can be found in the literature.[9-12]

In order for the monitoring of central venous pressure to be of value, one must first understand the various factors that directly affect this pressure. The level of the central venous pressure will be determined by the interaction of three factors:
1. Cardiac pump
2. Circulating blood volume
3. Degree of sympathetic venoconstriction in the veins that are responsive to adrenergic stimulation

The level of central venous pressure is directly proportional to the rate and volume of the venous return to the heart and inversely proportional to the degree of myocardial contractility. It is important to understand that the central venous pressure does not necessarily reflect the adequacy of circulating blood volume or the adequacy of cardiac output,[5,13] but rather it is only an index of right atrial filling pressure. Therefore, a patient may be relatively hypovolemic and have a normal or high central venous pressure because of compromised myocardial contractility or because of increased sympathetic stimulation of the peripheral venous system, which is increasing the venous return to the heart. As a result of the large venous capacitance, the central venous pressure may remain normal if there is normal cardiac function until there are far advanced volume deficits. A persistently low venous pressure— less than 5 cm of water (normal is 8 to 10 cm of water)—together with a low cardiac output is evidence that hypovolemia (relative or absolute) is responsible for the low flow state. Likewise, an elevated central venous pressure (over 25 cm of water) coupled with a low cardiac output is evidence that there is failure of the cardiac pump. This can either be a primary cause of the low flow state or a contributing factor in either hypovolemic or septic shock. In the latter cases further volume expansion is indicated but must be preceded with a drug that is going to increase myocardial function. It is apparent, therefore, that like the other hemodynamic measurements used in monitoring the patient in shock, the central venous pressure cannot be interpreted by itself but rather must be viewed as it relates to the arterial blood pressure, cardiac output, and total peripheral resistance.

Pulmonary artery pressure. There has been recent concern as to whether the central venous pressure adequately reflects changes that are taking place in the left ventricle in critically ill patients.[14-16] This is especially true in low flow states secondary to myocardial infarctions. Since the left ventricle is almost always involved in this disease, it becomes important to have an understanding of the dynamics of the left side of the heart, especially if it can be shown that the pathophysiology is not reflected in measurements of the right atrial filling pressure (CVP).

With the advent of the flow-directed pulmonary artery catheter,[17] direct measurements of the pulmonary capillary wedge pressure have become a reality in clinical medicine. The use of this catheter allows one to directly measure not only the pulmonary artery systolic and diastolic pressures, but also the pulmonary capillary wedge pressure (PCWP). Measurement of the pulmonary capillary wedge pressure is a much more accurate reflection of left atrial and left ventricular end diastolic pressure than is the central venous pressure. We can assume, therefore, that by measuring the pulmonary wedge pressure, a more direct assessment of the performance of the left ventricle is available. Over the past few years there has been convincing evidence that in low flow states, especially those associated with myocardial failure, there is no consistent relationship between central venous pressure and pulmonary capillary wedge pressure.[15] There can be rather far advanced heart failure reflected by elevated pulmonary diastolic and pulmonary capillary wedge pressures with the central venous pressure remaining normal.[15]

The procedure for insertion of the catheter is not difficult, and there are few significant complications associated either with its insertion or its presence in the pulmonary artery.[16,17] In our own trauma unit we have observed that even in the young trauma patient who is critically injured there is no consistent relationship between the central venous pressure and the pulmonary capillary wedge pressure. Therapeutic decisions as to fluid administration and drug therapy based on the use of central venous pressure rather than

pulmonary capillary wedge pressure would have been in error in well over one fourth of our patients. Our comments about the usefulness of central venous pressure should not be disregarded, however, because at present the use of the pulmonary artery catheter is a luxury restricted to specialized treatment and research units. Until the pulmonary artery catheter becomes as common place as the central venous catheter, particularly in the acute situation, physicians must utilize the central venous pressure while remaining aware of its limitations.

Biochemical changes

Earlier in this chapter shock was defined as a condition in which circulation or perfusion of blood is inadequate to meet tissue metabolic demands, thereby resulting in cellular anoxia and ultimately tissue death. Since blood pressure may be normal during the phase of compensated shock, a means of assessing cellular perfusion during this early phase becomes imperative. Laboratory evidence of poor perfusion with resulting cellular anoxia will allow diagnosis of a low flow state before the system decompensates, thereby increasing survival rates. A look at Fig. 7-2 will demonstrate what happens at the cellular level when cells are deprived of oxygen because of marked redistribution of blood flow from the nonessential organs to the heart and brain. Metabolism continues under anaerobic conditions with a resultant increase in the production of lactate. Compared to aerobic metabolism, anaerobic metabolism supplies only a small fraction of the body's energy requirements. It does allow for immediate cellular survival. The earlier the return to normal metabolism occurs, the better the chance for cellular survival.

The level of arterial lactate can be measured biochemically[18] and thus has been used in evaluating low flow states.[18-20] Carey and co-workers[21] demonstrated that arterial lactate levels were a good index

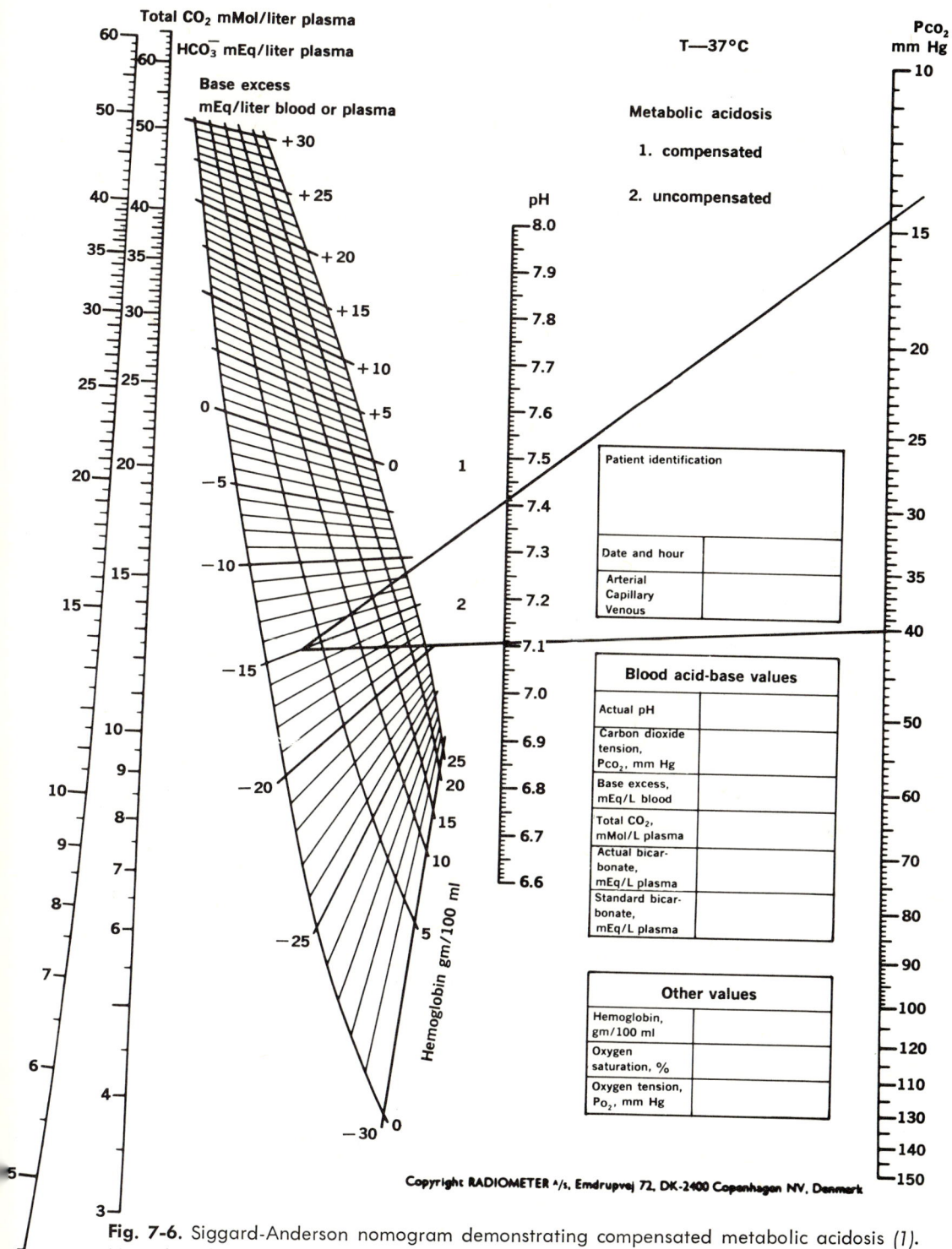

Fig. 7-6. Siggard-Anderson nomogram demonstrating compensated metabolic acidosis (1). Note that the pH is maintained in a normal range by the lowering of the Pco_2 through hyperventilation. In spite of the normal pH, however, there is a significant base deficit (-15 mEq HCO_3/liter) representing a marked degree of lactic acidemia. If the Pco_2 cannot be lowered (2), there would be a marked depression of the pH with the same degree of lactic acidemia.

of the presence and severity of shock from hemorrhage and trauma. Adequacy of therapy was reflected by decreasing serum lactate levels. There was a 100% mortality rate in patients whose arterial lactate levels continued to climb following initial resuscitation. Blood lactate levels are not immediately available to personnel caring for the acutely ill patient. Fortunately, however, there is a strong correlation between arterial lactate levels and the base deficit that is determined from the pH and the Pco_2 of arterial blood gas analyses. This latter test is available within minutes in most hospitals that have an emergency service.

With knowledge of the blood pH and Pco_2 and using the Siggard-Anderson nomogram[22] (Fig. 7-6) one can rapidly determine if there is any significant metabolic acidosis present. A significant degree of acidosis (base excess below –5 mEq of HCO_3 per liter) reflects poor perfusion, and if the blood pressure is normal, the patient is in a compensated low flow state. This is a frequent occurrence in the trauma patient who comes into the emergency department following injury. The patient who has had a significant volume loss may be in a state of compensated shock with a normal blood pressure because of the marked sympathomimetic response. Blood gas analysis may reveal a low or normal pH. If the pH is below 7.2, there is usually no question that the patient has a metabolic acidosis. One must not fall into the trap, however, of just looking at the blood pH, because most acutely traumatized patients will be hyperventilating and have a low Pco_2. If this is low enough to compensate for the metabolic acidosis, the pH will be normal in spite of a significant base deficit which represents inadequate tissue perfusion.

A case in point is that of a 22-year-old male motorcycle accident victim who arrived in the emergency department after his vehicle hit a telephone pole. His blood pressure was 110/80 with a pulse of 100, and he was fully alert and oriented. Initial blood gas analyses showed a Po_2 of 90, a Pco_2 of 15, and a pH of 7.4. By tracing the pH and Pco_2 values on the nomogram a severe metabolic acidosis with a base (Fig. 7-6), one can see that the patient had deficit of –15 mEq HCO_3/liter although his pH was normal at 7.4. The patient had an acute volume loss because of bilateral fractured femurs and a fractured pelvis. He was maintaining his central blood pressure at the expense of peripheral perfusion, and once his blood volume was replenished, the metabolic acidosis was rather rapidly corrected. If blood lactate levels had been obtained on this individual, they would have been markedly elevated.

The biochemical criteria for the diagnosis of shock, therefore, lies in our ability to measure the by-product of anaerobic metabolism. This anaerobic metabolism is occurring because of poor tissue perfusion and is reflected in elevated arterial lactate levels. A more practical measurement, which is much more universally available and can be obtained within minutes, is the base deficit, which is ascertained from arterial blood gases using a nomogram. It is imperative that this test be done on all acutely traumatized patients and that emergency personnel not be lulled into a sense of security because the patient has a normal blood pressure or because the pH is normal.

CLASSIFICATION

A simple means of classification of shock on the basis of the pathophysiology is outlined below:

I. Failure of venous return—hypovolemic
  A. Hemorrhage
  B. Fluid loss
    1. Gastrointestinal tract
      a. Cholera
    2. Third space
      a. Burns
      b. Peritonitis

II. Failure of cardiac pump—cardiogenic
   A. Ventricular ejection
      1. Myocardial infarction
   B. Ventricular filling
      1. Tamponade
      2. Pulmonary embolism
III. Primary cellular defect—septic
IV. Vasomotor collapse—neurogenic
   A. Spinal cord disruption

Failure of venous return (hypovolemic)

This is a classic hypovolemic state that is precipitated by blood loss or acute extracellular fluid loss as occurs in burns or severe peritonitis. During the compensated phase, the marked sympathomimetic response described earlier allows the individual to maintain an adequate pressure to perfuse the heart and brain, but perfusion to the nonvital organs is significantly depressed. This early phase will be detected by the presence of the metabolic acidosis that reflects the generalized anaerobic metabolism that is occurring. Hemodynamically, in pure volume loss the central venous pressure, pulmonary capillary wedge, and cardiac output will all be depressed, although the intra-arterial blood pressure may be normal because of the increase in total peripheral resistance. Fig. 7-7 illustrates the hemodynamic measurements present in decompensated pure hemorrhagic shock and how they differ from pure cardiogenic and septic shock. If there is a degree of myocardial failure complicating the hypovolemia, as can occur in an older patient with coronary artery disease who has an upper gastrointestinal hemorrhage, the central venous pressure may be normal or artificially elevated in spite of a critical volume deficit. Clinical evidence of the fluid loss is usually present and will help in differentiating this form of shock from that secondary to pure pump failure.

External blood loss and profound dehydration from heat prostration are clinically easily recognizable forms of hypovolemia. However, other clinical conditions with hypovolemia are subtle and often overlooked. Dehydration secondary to insidious external losses such as vomiting or diarrhea may be missed. Even more difficult to recognize is hypovolemia secondary to internal redistribution of fluids (third-space effect), which occurs in intestinal obstruction or peritonitis. In these conditions fluid is lost from the intravascular space into the bowel lumen or inflamed peritoneum. Similar occult losses occur in burns, crush injuries, pancreatitis, and effusions. The clinical findings that should point to this insidious hypovolemia are tachycardia, oliguria, decreased tissue turgor, and high urinary osmolality or specific gravity coupled with historical and physical evidence of intestinal obstruction, peritonitis, crush injury, and the like.

Electrolyte losses and redistribution occur concurrently and vary, depending on the underlying pathology. Decreased tissue perfusion may occur whenever these losses are rapid or exceed the organism's ability to restore plasma volume by aldosterone and antidiuretic hormone release. If effective plasma volume cannot be restored because of the rapid rate or large amount of fluid loss, the previously described sympathomimetic response occurs. Thus the hemodynamic and biochemical manifestation of compensated shock will be present. If this is allowed to progress, irreversible shock will occur, which will fail to respond to plasma volume replacement and correction of the electrolyte abnormalities.

Failure of cardiac pump (cardiogenic)

This form of shock is commonly termed cardiogenic shock and should be thought of as failure either of ventricular ejection or ventricular filling. Myocardial infarction is a classic example of the former and cardiac tamponade of the latter. As in hypovolemic shock, the cardiac output is depressed and the total peripheral resistance is markedly elevated. The main feature that helps differentiate this form of

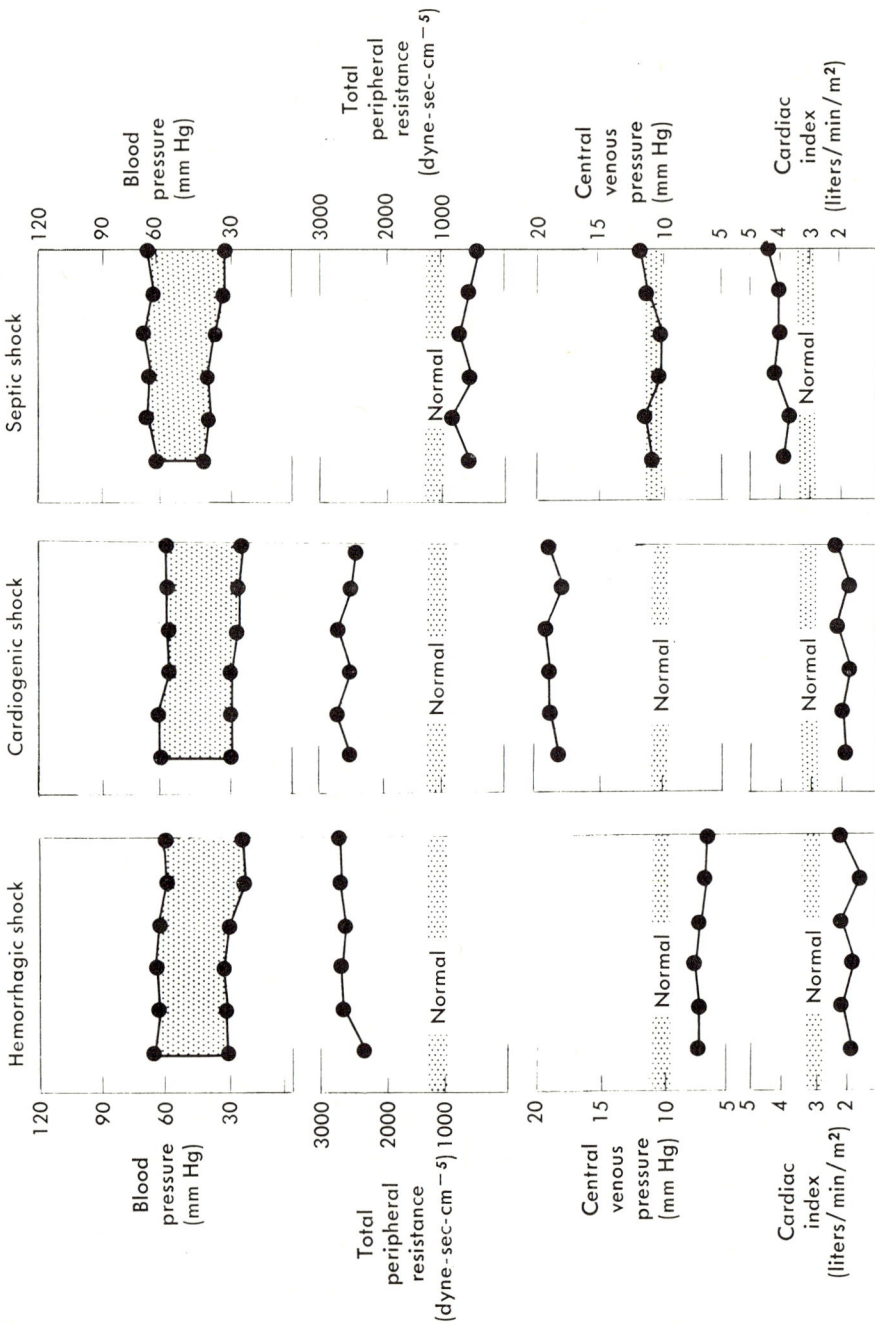

Fig. 7-7. Hemodynamic measurements in the three types of shock. Note that hemorrhagic shock can be differentiated from cardiogenic shock by elevation in central venous pressure while all other parameters are similar. Early septic shock is usually associated with elevated cardiac index and low peripheral resistance. This combination helps to differentiate pure septic shock from the other two types.

shock from hypovolemic shock is that the central venous pressure or, more specifically, the pulmonary capillary wedge pressure is significantly elevated (Fig. 7-7). Prior to a fall in blood pressure there is always an associated metabolic acidosis reflecting cellular anoxia. The elevated central venous pressure associated with a decreasing cardiac output in the case of cardiac tamponade becomes extremely helpful in evaluating the hypotension of the trauma patient. If personnel do not know that the central venous pressure is increased, they might mistakenly attribute the hypotension to blood loss from multiple injuries and begin to rapidly infuse blood or fluid. This would most certainly be detrimental and possibly fatal to this patient. Thus it is not enough to place a central venous catheter in a patient with acute trauma, but one must also determine the level of the central venous pressure.

Primary cellular defect (septic)

It is felt that a primary cellular defect is the underlying pathophysiologic factor in septic shock, and that the observed hemodynamic changes reflect a compensatory mechanism.[8] These cellular defects are precipitated by endotoxin released by gram-negative bacteria in the bloodstream. It is still not clear why only about 50% of patients with gram-negative bacteremia go into gram-negative shock, but host factors clearly are at play. The endotoxin can also be absorbed from the septic areas such as the peritoneal cavity or gastrointestinal tract without an associated bacteremia. The metabolic and physiologic effects of endotoxin are many and beyond the scope of this chapter. The reader is referred to a recent monograph on the subject for a comprehensive review.[23]

This form of shock usually occurs in the hospital population who are predisposed because of a chronic underlying condition such as diabetes, cirrhosis, leukemia, carcinoma, pyelonephritis, immunosuppressive

therapy, biliary tract obstruction, extensive surgical procedures, or burns. The offending organism is usually *Escherichia coli* or *Pseudomonas*. The clinical picture is characterized by marked elevations in temperature associated with shaking chills. The patient is alert and has a warm and flushed appearance. This is contrasted to the cold and clammy skin of the patient in hypovolemic or cardiogenic shock. The blood pressure is usually initially normal, but urine output is beginning to fall, and there is evidence of increasing acidosis.

Hemodynamically, in pure septic shock there is usually an elevation of the cardiac output with a normal or low central venous pressure and a low total peripheral resistance. This is the so-called high output, low resistance form of shock.[23,24] In spite of these consistently elevated cardiac outputs and low total peripheral resistances, the patient continues to have increasing anaerobic metabolism as is reflected by an increasing metabolic acidosis. Thus, although flow is high, it is still inadequate for the patient's tissue needs. This can be the result of a primary cellular defect that precludes the cell utilizing the oxygen, or there may be a defect in the oxygen delivery such that the hemoglobin cannot give up the oxygen at the cellular level.[25]

Prognosis in septic shock is directly related both to the severity of the underlying disease process and to the heart's ability to increase its output to meet the greatly increased metabolic demands. In one series the mortality rate for patients with an initial cardiac index of less than 2.5 liters/m²/minute was 75%, whereas the mortality rate for patients with an initial cardiac index of greater than 2.5 liters/m²/minute was only 15%.[2] There is now evidence that the endotoxin has a direct myocardial depressant action, which decreases myocardial performance in septic patients.[26,27] Also, there is usually a relative hypovolemic aspect of septic shock because of the sequestration of fluid into the area of inflammation. When both hypovolemia and myocardial failure complicate septic shock, it may become a low output, high resistance state similar to that seen in cardiogenic and hypovolemic shock. When this occurs, the prognosis is extremely poor. Fig. 7-7 demonstrates the classic hemodynamic abnormalities in pure septic shock as compared to those seen in pure hypovolemic and pure cardiogenic shock.

Vasomotor collapse

Either functional or actual transection of the spinal cord causes an interruption of vasomotor tone, marked vasodilatation, and hypotension from the loss of peripheral resistance. It is commonly seen with conduction anesthesia and its resulting sympathetic blockade. This hypotension can easily be treated by the use of an adrenergic drug and poses little or no problem for the personnel or patient.

THERAPY
Monitoring

All patients who have high shock potential or who have the clinical diagnosis of a low flow state should have the following catheters placed:

1. Central venous pressure catheter
2. A second large venous line
3. Intraarterial line
4. Foley catheter
5. Nasogastric tube

If facilities permit, a catheter should be floated into the pulmonary artery for monitoring of pulmonary capillary wedge pressure.

Surgical management

Before the medical treatment of shock is discussed, mention should be made of the role that surgery plays in its treatment. When the shock state is secondary to massive hemorrhage, one must obviously control this blood loss before any other therapy can be effective. The patient with acute cardiac tamponade will require initial pericardiocentesis followed by a formal thoracotomy. When septic shock is secondary to an intraabdominal abscess or peritonitis from a perforated viscus, surgery becomes an important part of the overall therapy. If the source of sepsis is not eliminated, other therapeutic modalities will surely fail. There has also been some recent interest in coronary artery bypass and infarctectomy for patients with cardiogenic shock secondary to massive myocardial infarction.[28] Except for these specific instances, the mainstay of shock therapy lies in the use of fluid replacement and drugs.

Drugs

For the most part, the drugs used in the treatment of the shock syndrome are powerful adrenergic substances. A brief look at the adrenergic receptor sites in the body reveals that the heart has only beta receptors and that stimulation of these receptors causes two basic responses:

1. Increase in the heart rate (chronotropic response)
2. Increase in the contractility of the myocardium (inotropic response)

The arteries perfusing the skin and mucosa have only alpha receptors, stimulation of which causes marked vasoconstriction. Arteries of the skeletal muscle and abdominal viscera have both alpha and beta receptors. Stimulation of the former causes vasoconstriction and of the latter vasodilatation. The peripheral veins that are sensitive to adrenergic stimulation have both alpha and beta receptors. Stimulation of both these receptors causes constriction of the veins. These responses to adrenergic stimuli are outlined in Table 7-1.

We have, therefore, two ways of manipulating the cardiovascular system with adrenergic drugs:

1. Stimulation of the beta receptors will increase the heart rate and myocardial contractility and also cause peripheral vasodilatation.

Table 7-1. Responses of effector organs to adrenergic stimuli

Effector organ	Receptor type	Response
Heart	Beta	Increase in rate; increase in myocardial contractility
Arteries, skin mucosa	Alpha	Constriction
Skeletal muscle; abdominal viscera	Alpha and beta	Constriction-dilatation
Systemic veins	Alpha and beta	Constriction

Table 7-2. Shock drugs

Generic name	Trade name	Site of action	
		Alpha	Beta
Isoproterenol	Isuprel	0	++++
Epinephrine	Adrenalin	++	+++
Metaraminol	Aramine	+++	+
Norepinephrine (levarterenol)	Levophed	++++	+
Phenylephrine	Neo-Synephrine	+++	+
Methoxamine	Vasoxyl	++++	0
Phentolamine	Regitine	Alpha blocker	
Phenoxyben-zamine	Dibenzyline	Alpha blocker	
Propranolol	Inderal	Beta blocker	

2. Stimulation of the alpha receptors will have no primary effect on the myocardium but will increase peripheral resistance.

This increase in peripheral resistance, while causing an increase in arterial blood pressure, will cause a reflex bradycardia and an actual decrease in the cardiac output. The alpha and beta receptors can also be blocked, causing a reversal of their basic pharmacologic response. Table 7-2 summarizes the commonly used adrenergic drugs in shock therapy together with their site of action. This brief review of the adrenergic drugs and the various receptor sites is limited and is intended only to help the reader better understand some basic principles of shock therapy. Refer to a recent monograph on the subject for a more comprehensive review.[29]

One additional agent that has to be mentioned before discussing specific treatment protocols is corticosteroids. Over the last several years there has been increasing interest in the effect of pharmacologic doses of steroids on both the cardiovascular system and the microcirculation in low flow states.[30-33] The effects can be summarized as follows:

1. Decreased peripheral resistance (acting as an alpha blocker)

2. Enhanced conversion of lactate to glucose
3. Preservation of cellular lysosomes
4. Positive inotropic effects

The most commonly used steroid preparation today is Solu-Medrol (methylprednisolone) in doses of 30 mg/kg in IV "push."

Therapeutic approach

As mentioned earlier, the patient who has a low central venous pressure (less than 5 cm of water) together with a low cardiac output and an increased total peripheral resistance is hypovolemic, and volume restoration is the treatment of choice. The increase in total peripheral resistance can be estimated clinically by the marked peripheral vasoconstriction. One easy method of getting a rough estimate of the cardiac output is to do a blood gas analysis on the blood obtained from the central venous pressure catheter. A normal central venous Po_2 is 40 mm Hg. In low flow states this is usually markedly depressed (less than 30 mm Hg). Rapid administration of 1,000 ml of a balanced salt solution while blood is being typed and crossmatched should cause some improvement as reflected by a rising CVP and blood pressure. One must remember that the drug of choice in hemorrhagic shock is blood. If the patient is still unstable after administration of 2,000 ml of balanced salt solution, typed specific blood should be given until crossmatched blood is available. If there is obvious continued blood loss, emergency surgery is indicated. Most patients in hypovolemic shock arrive at the treatment center still in a compensated phase with a normal blood pressure and metabolic acidosis. If the metabolic acidosis is not compensated for by hyperventilation and the pH is below 7.2, sodium bicarbonate should be given to help normalize the pH. This should be in association with, however, and not in place of adequate fluid resuscitation. If decompensation has occurred, there will be associated hypotension. Even if decompensated, the shock state is usually still reversible and will respond to adequate fluid replacement.

Probably less than 10% of all these cases become refractory to fluid therapy and will require drug intervention. As mentioned earlier, the primary factor in the pathophysiology of refractory shock is the marked increase in the pre- and postcapillarly sphincter tone in nonvital organs. Therefore, drug therapy must be directed at the capillary sphincter level. Isoproterenol (Isuprel) with its beta stimulation will dilate the arterioles in the skeletal muscle, kidneys, and abdominal viscera, thereby increasing flow to these organs. Because of its inotropic effect on the heart, it will also increase cardiac output. If the patient is still hypovolemic, there will be an initial drop in the blood pressure and also in the central venous pressure. This should signal the physician to give more fluid, not to stop the drug. When there is associated tachycardia, the use of this drug may lead to cardiac arrhythmias. If this should occur, small doses of epinephrine 0.1 to 0.5 μg/kg/minute should replace the isoproterenol. The epinephrine will act primarily as a beta stimulator without affecting the alpha receptors. Another approach is to block the alpha receptors with either phenoxybenzamine (Dibenzyline) or steroids and then use one of the adrenergic drugs that have alpha stimulating properties (Table 7-2).

One must always keep in mind that the goal of drug therapy is to increase tissue perfusion, not blood pressure. Therefore, the use of a pure alpha stimulator, such as Vasoxyl, is contraindicated without simultaneously blocking the alpha reactors. This will surely increase the blood pressure but will decrease perfusion and further aggravate the low flow state. If, after what is felt to be adequate replacement of blood volume, there is persistent hypotension associated with a low CVP and cardiac output, one must rule out continuing blood loss. Only after this has been done should the use of adrenergic drug therapy be entertained.

The relative hypovolemia and myocardial failure associated with septic shock require vigorous therapy. As a result of the myocardial failure, the central venous pressure may be high and preclude the giving of badly needed fluid. It has been demonstrated that the best inotropic drug to use in septic shock is digitalis.[27] (The onset of action of digoxin administered intravenously is 5 to 30 minutes with full development in one to five hours.) If this does not improve the myocardial performance, isoproterenol (Isuprel) may be tried. Unless myocardial function can be improved sufficiently to allow restoration of intravascular volume, the patient is surely going to die. Based upon the above described effects of steroids, their use in septic shock has rationale. Specific antibiotics and surgical drainage of sepsis are necessary adjuncts to therapy.

Shock associated with increase in central venous pressure (over 15 cm), decreased cardiac output, and increased total peripheral resistance is almost always the result of pump failure. Treatment of this type of shock is twofold:

1. To increase the filling pressure of the heart even above its already raised value in hopes of taking advantage of the Starling mechanism and increasing stroke volume and cardiac output
2. To augment cardiac output

The best drug to accomplish this is still controversial. Levophed is commonly used as is Dopamine. Cohn[34] has recently suggested that the myocardial failure is secondary to marked increase in afterload caused by the sympathomimetic response. He recommends that in certain cases of refractory shock a potent alpha blocker, which acts as a vasodilator, will improve cardiac function.

The objective of therapy in shock syndromes, whatever the underlying pathophysiology, is to restore tissue perfusion as early as possible. When fluid resuscitation alone cannot accomplish this, the use of appropriate drugs is indicated. Adequacy of therapy should be judged by the reversal of the metabolic acidosis that reflects poor tissue perfusion, the resumption of adequate urine output, and, lastly, the restoration of normal blood pressure.

SUMMARY

Shock is a condition in which the circulation is inadequate to meet tissue metabolic demands. It must be thought of as a lack of adequate tissue perfusion, not as a level of blood pressure.

The initial response to a sudden loss of intravascular volume is a marked vasoconstriction mediated by the autonomic nervous system and adrenal medulla. This ensures adequate perfusion of the heart and brain by diverting flow from less vital areas. This redistribution of perfusion is termed "reversible shock" and allows immediate survival. However, if this circulatory deficit is not corrected, progressive cellular anoxia leads to tissue death and irreversibility. Once there is cellular death, the restoration of blood flow to that tissue will not accomplish reversal of anoxic damage.

Early detection of compensated shock can be accomplished only by a combination of clinical, hemodynamic, and biochemical evaluations. This requires the use of a triple catheter technique, that is, the insertion of central venous, arterial, and Foley catheters. However, the most practical measurement of inadequate cellular perfusion is the base deficit, which represents the degree of metabolic acidosis. This can easily be determined from an arterial blood gas using the Siggard-Anderson nomogram.

The integration and interpretation of all the clinical, hemodynamic, and biochemical data allow the classification of low flow states into hypovolemic, cardiogenic, septic, and neurogenic shock. This pathophysiologic classification has considerable clinical import, since treatment varies for each. The mainstay of shock therapy lies in the appropriate use of fluid replacement and drugs. The objective of treatment is the restoration of tissue perfusion. When fluid resuscitation alone cannot accomplish this, the use of pharmacologic agents is indicated. However, the rational use of sympathomimetic drugs, adrenergic blockers, and corticosteroids depends on careful assessment of the individual hemodynamic profile and response to initial therapy. Beta-adrenergic stimulators (Isuprel) are useful for both inotropic and chronotropic cardiac effects as well as vasodilation of the microcirculation with improvement of tissue perfusion. This latter effect is also produced by alpha blockers (Dibenzyline). Alpha stimulants (Levophed) find considerable use in cardiogenic shock by increasing peripheral vasoconstriction and thereby increasing coronary flow. Corticosteroids have been useful because of their protective effect at the cellular level in septic shock. The response to any agent must be gauged by the reversal of anaerobic cellular metabolism as demonstrated by the correction of the metabolic acidosis. This indicates that adequate tissue circulation has been restored.

REFERENCES

1. Cannon, W. B.: Traumatic shock, New York, 1923, D. Appleton and Co.
2. Thal, A. P.: Shock: A physiologic basic for treatment, Chicago, 1971, Year Book Medical Publishers, Inc.
3. Archibald, E. W., and McLean, W. S.: Observations upon shock with particular reference to the condition as seen in war surgery, Ann. Surg. 66:281, 1917.
4. Mellander, S., and Lewis, D. H.: Effect of hemorrhagic shock on the reactivity of resistance and capacitance vessels and on capillary filtration transfer in cat skeletal muscle, Circ. Res. 13:105, 1963.
5. Peterson, C. C.: Perspectives in surgery, Philadelphia, 1972, Lea & Febiger.
6. Border, J. R., Gallo, E., and Worthington, G. S.: Systemic arteriovenous shunts in patients under severe stress: A common cause of high output cardiac failure, Surgery 10: 225, 1966.
7. Siegel, J. H., Greenspan, M., and Del Guercio, L. R. M.: Abnormal vascular tone, defective oxygen transport and myocardial failure in human septic shock, Ann. Surg. 165:504, 1967.
8. Wright, C. J., Huff, J. H., McLean, A. P. H., and MacLean, L. P.: Regional capillary blood flow and oxygen uptake in severe sepsis, Surg. Gynecol. Obstet. 132:637, April 1971.
9. Yoffa, D.: Supraclavicular subclavian venipuncture and catheterization, Lancet 2:614, 1965.
10. Borja, A. R., and Hinshaw, J. R.: A safe way to perform intraclavicular subclavian vein catheterization, Surg. Gynecol. Obstet. 130: 673, 1970.
11. Gallitano, A. L., Kondi, C. S., and Deckens, P. J.: A safe approach to the subclavian vein, Surg. Gynecol. Obstet. 135:96, 1972.
12. Parsa, M. H., Habif, D. V., and Ferrer, J. M.: Techniques for placement of long-term indwelling superior vena cava catheters, 56th Annual Clinical Congress of the American College of Surgeons, 1970.
13. Wilson, R. F., Sarver, E., and Bicks, B.: Central venous pressure and blood volume determinations in clinical shock, Surg. Gynecol. Obstet. 132:631, 1971.
14. Forrester, J. S., Diamond, G., McHugh, T. J., and Swan, H. J. C.: Filling pressures in the right-left sides of the heart in acute myocardial infarction: A reappraisal of central venous pressure monitoring, N. Engl. J. Med. 285:190, 1971.
15. Forrester, J., Diamond, G., and Ganz, V.: Right and left heart pressures in acutely ill patients, Clin. Res. 18:306, 1970.
16. Civetta, J. M., and Gabel, J. C.: Flow directed pulmonary artery catheterization in surgical patients, Ann. Surg. 176:753, 1972.
17. Swan, H. J. C., Ganz, V., Forrester, J., and others: Cardiac catheterization with a flow directed balloon type catheter, N. Engl. J. Med. 283:447, 1970.
18. Huckabee, W. E.: Relationships of pyruvate and lactate during anaerobic metabolism: Effects of infusion of pyruvate or glucose and of hyperventilation, J. Clin. Invest. 37:244, 1958.
19. Haller, J. A., Ward, M. J., and Cahill, J. L.: Metabolic alterations in shock: The effect of controlled reduction of blood flow on oxidative metabolism and catecholamine response, J. Trauma 7:727, 1967.
20. Rosenburg, J. C., and Rush, B. F.: Blood lactic acid levels in irreversible hemorrhagic and lethal endotoxin shock, Surg. Gynecol. Obstet. 126:1247, 1968.
21. Carey, L. C., Lowery, B. D., and Cloutier, C. T.: Hemorrhagic shock: Current problems in surgery, Chicago, 1971, Year Book Medical Publishers, Inc.
22. Siggard-Anderson, O.: Blood acid base alignment nomogram, Scand. J. Clin. Lab. Invest. 1963.
23. Hershey, S. G., Del Guercio, L. R. M., and McConn, R.: Septic shock in man, Boston, 1971, Little, Brown and Co.
24. Gilbert, R. P., Honing, K. P., Giffin, J. A., Becker, R. J., and Adelson, B. H.: Hemodynamics of shock due to infection, Stanford Med. Bull. 13:239, 1953.
25. Herman, C. D.: Advances and new concepts in shock. In Surgery annual, New York, 1972, Appleton-Century Crofts, pp. 1-49.
26. Hinshaw, L. B., Greenfield, L. D., Owen, S. E., and others: Precipitation of cardiac failure in endotoxin shock, Surg. Gynecol. Obstet. 135:39, 1972.
27. Hinshaw, L. B., Greenfield, L. J., Owen, S. E., and others: Cardiac response to circulation factors in endotoxin shock, Am. J. Physiol. 222:1047, 1972.
28. Gott, V. L., Brawley, R. K., Donahoo, J. S., and Griffith, L. S. C.: Current surgical approach to ischemic heart disease, Current problems in surgery, Chicago, 1973, Year Book Medical Publishers, Inc.
29. Hermreck, S. A., and Thal, A. P.: The adrenergic drugs and their use in shock therapy, Chicago, 1968, Year book Medical Publishers, Inc.

30. Dietzman, R. H., Castaneda, A. R., Lillehei, W. C., and others: Corticosteroids as effective vasodilators in treatment of low output syndrome, Chest **57**:440, 1970.

31. Sambhi, M. P., Weil, M. H., and Udhogi, U. N.: Acute pharamacodynamic effects of glucocorticoids on cardiac output and related hemodynamic changes in normal patients and patients in shock, Circulation **31**:523, 1965.

32. Rosenbaum, R. W., Hayes, M. F., and Matsumoto, T.: Efficacy of steroids in the treatment of septic and cardiogenic shock, Surg. Gynecol. Obstet. **136**:914, 1973.

33. Moses, M. L., Camishion, R. C., Tokunaga, K., and others: Effect of corticosteroid on the acidosis of prolonged cardiopulmonary bypass, J. Surg. Res. **6**:354, 1966.

34. Cohn, J. N.: Personal communication.

CHAPTER 8

Emergency management of diabetes mellitus and hypoglycemia

Richard C. Gross, M.D.

DIABETIC COMA

Ketoacidosis and hyperglycemic hyperosmolar nonketotic coma are the two most important acute complications of diabetes mellitus included in the term "diabetic coma."[1] Once associated with very high mortality, ketoacidosis is still fatal in 5% to 15% of cases. Mortality in the hyperosmolar syndrome is even higher, mainly because it is more common in older and debilitated patients. Because most instances of these complications have features of both entities and because the initial approach to treatment is similar, they will be considered together.

Pathophysiology

Insulin lack, either absolute or relative, is the underlying cause in every case of diabetic coma. This leads to a large number of abnormalities in carbohydrate, fat, and protein metabolism. The sequence of abnormalities in carbohydrate metabolism is outlined in Fig. 8-1. Inadequate insulin action leads to decreased transport of glucose from blood into tissues and to increased hepatic glucose output (secondary to accelerated glycogenolysis and gluconeogenesis), resulting in hyperglycemia. When blood glucose exceeds the renal threshold, glycosuria ensues. This causes an osmotic diuresis, with loss of water and electrolytes. If this continues, dehydration, decreased renal function, and vascular collapse (shock) occur.

Abnormalities in fat metabolism caused by insulin deficiency are outlined in Fig. 8-2. Free fatty acids are mobilized from adipose tissue triglycerides at an excessive rate. These are oxidized in the liver, leading to increased formation of ketone bodies (ketoacids). Ketone bodies are generated faster than the tissues can use them and faster than the kidneys can excrete them, which results in ketosis and metabolic acidosis. Compromised renal function caused by dehydration is also important in producing ketoacidosis.

Protein metabolism is also abnormal when insulin action is inadequate (Fig. 8-3). Muscle protein is broken down to amino acids at an increased rate, resulting in aminoacidemia and loss of potassium from tissues. Increased flux of amino acids to the liver promotes increased gluconeogenesis and thus hyperglycemia.

These derangements of carbohydrate, fat, and protein metabolism are generally all

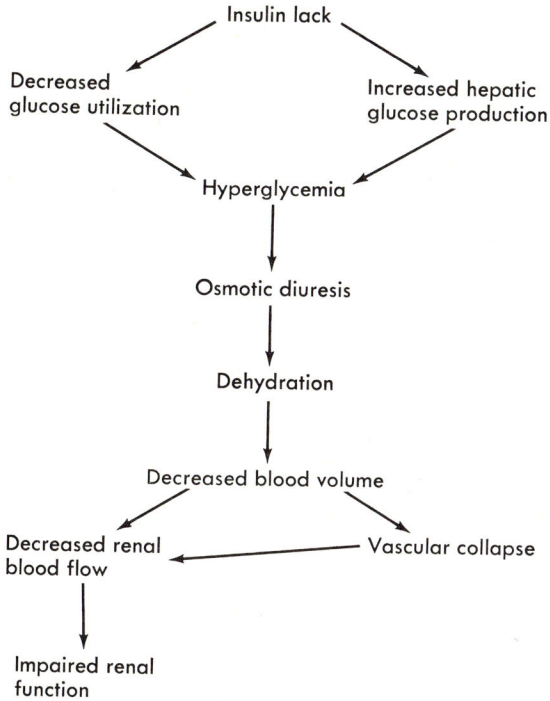

Fig. 8-1. Consequences of abnormal carbohydrate metabolism in uncontrolled diabetes.

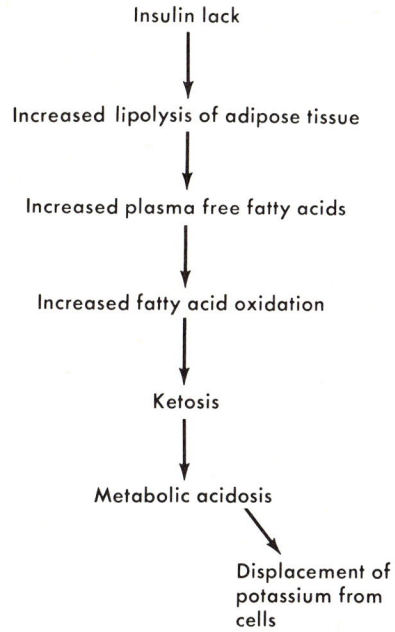

Fig. 8-2. Consequences of abnormal fat metabolism in uncontrolled diabetes.

present to some degree in most cases of diabetic coma. However, one abnormality may predominate, as in the hyperosmolar hyperglycemic syndrome. Here, hyperglycemia and dehydration are severe, ketosis is minimal, and acidosis is not seen. In some young diabetics hyperglycemia may be mild, but ketosis and acidosis are severe.

Causes

The most common precipitating cause of these complications is failure to take insulin or not taking sufficient insulin. Severe infections such as pneumonitis and pyelonephritis also commonly result in decompensation of diabetes and may precipitate coma in patients in whom diabetes was previously undiagnosed. In older patients or younger patients with diabetes of long duration, stresses such as myocardial infarction may provoke the episode. *An underlying cause*

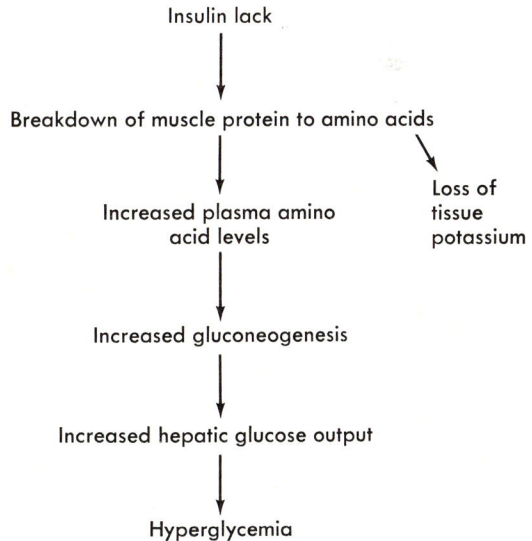

Fig. 8-3. Consequences of abnormal protein metabolism in uncontrolled diabetes.

for the diabetic coma should always be sought.

Clinical presentation and diagnosis

The patient may be only moderately ill, may be in a coma, or, in the hyperosmolar syndrome, may be having seizures. A history, if obtainable, will usually reveal polydipsia and polyuria for a few to several days. Only rarely do patients progress from good compensation to ketoacidosis in less than 48 hours, unless a severe precipitating stress is present; exceptions are brittle or unstable diabetics and pregnant women. Other frequent symptoms include abdominal pain, with nausea and vomiting as the syndrome progresses. When these occur, the condition of the patient can worsen rapidly because of additional loss of fluid and electrolytes and inability to maintain fluid intake. This is always an indication for hospitalization.

On physical examination the patient is usually febrile. The pulse is fast, and respiration is deep and rapid (Kussmaul or air-hunger breathing). Blood pressure may be low. Shock is a serious complication associated with a poor prognosis and requires prompt and vigorous treatment. Signs of dehydration are usually present—warm, dry skin with poor turgor and dry mucous membranes.

Usually the distinction between hyperglycemic and hypoglycemic coma is not difficult to make. Patients with hypoglycemia are generally pale and sweaty; Kussmaul respirations and signs of dehydration are not seen. If there is any question of hypoglycemia, 20 or 25 g of glucose (50% solution) can be given intravenously. This will revive the patient with hypoglycemia in most cases and will not worsen the condition of the patient with hyperglycemic coma.

A urine specimen should be obtained immediately. Unconscious patients should be catheterized. Very few conditions besides diabetes mellitus are associated with glycosuria and ketonuria, so urinalysis will usually confirm the diagnosis.

Venous blood should be obtained for determination of glucose, ketones, electrolytes, BUN, blood count, type and crossmatch, and blood culture. Arterial blood should be obtained for determination of gases and pH. Intravenous fluids should be started and insulin given without waiting for results of these tests.

Initial laboratory findings. Serum glucose may range from 300 to over 1000 mg/100 ml, with the higher values seen in the hyperosmolar syndrome. Presence of ketones in diluted serum always indicates severe ketosis. It must be remembered that serum and urine ketones measured by the nitroprusside reaction (Acetest or Ketostix) only reflect acetoacetic acid and free acetone levels.[1] This may be misleading, since beta-hydroxybutyric acid, which is not detected, is the predominant ketoacid present in blood and urine. If bicarbonate is less than 10 mEq/liter, acidosis is usually severe, but arterial blood pH is a better index. Serum levels of sodium and potassium may not reflect body content of these electrolytes. Sodium may be low if hyperglycemia is severe. If serum sodium is high in the presence of hyperglycemia, severe dehydration is indicated. Serum potassium is usually elevated due to metabolic acidosis in spite of marked losses of body potassium. Elevated BUN and hematocrit reflect dehydration. The white blood cell count may be as high as 12,000 to 18,000/mm³ even in the absence of infection.

Management

The following suggestions are only general guidelines for the management of diabetic coma in adults. It is impossible to give specific recommendations regarding dosages, fluids, and so forth, since these depend greatly on the individual situation. Very close monitoring of the patient's responses to initial therapy is required to provide data for direction of subsequent treatment.

Derangements in diabetic coma that most threaten the life of the patient are dehydration, insulin lack, and metabolic acidosis. These must be corrected rapidly and simultaneously.

Insulin. Only crystalline or "regular" insulin should be used. Until recently, relatively large doses given by intravenous push or subcutaneously, or by both routes, were recommended.[1] In the past few years much lower insulin doses, given by continuous intravenous infusion or by frequent intermuscular injection, have been used quite successfully.[2-6]

If *large doses* of insulin are used initially, the intravenous route may be preferable because of more certain delivery to tissues and less likelihood of hypoglycemia later in the course of treatment. With this approach the amount of insulin given depends on the severity of the patient's condition; there are schemes available for calculating initial insulin dosage based on such parameters as blood glucose and ketone levels. However, clinical research has shown that rapidity of recovery from ketoacidosis is not correlated with the amount of insulin given. The following schedule is reasonable: give 50 to 200 units initially depending on how seriously ill the patient seems. (The presence of coma or severe acidosis might be an indication for the higher dose.) This dose is repeated every two hours until there is evidence of insulin effect, such as a decrease in blood or urine glucose or ketones; these are checked approximately one hour after each dose. With this approach a response is usually apparent within six hours after beginning treatment. If no change has occurred by then, severe insulin resistance may be present. In that case the insulin dose should be doubled every two hours until a response is observed. When blood glucose has fallen to around 300 mg/100 ml, frequency of insulin administration should be decreased to every four hours, the dose may be decreased, and the subcutaneous route may be used. At this point 5% dextrose should also be added to the intravenous fluids. Some insulin should usually be given, even if only a small amount, every four hours during the remainder of the first 24 hours of treatment.

Patients with hyperglycemic hyperosmolar nonketotic coma may be more sensitive to insulin than those with ketoacidosis; therefore, smaller insulin doses are indicated after this diagnosis is apparent.

Continuous low-dose infusion of insulin by the intravenous route has recently been used successfully to treat diabetic ketoacidosis and the hyperosmolar syndrome.[2-4] Although not entirely new, the rationale for this approach was supported by findings that indicated a very short half-life of insulin injected intravenously—about three to five minutes—so that even very large doses will have essentially disappeared from the blood in 30 minutes. Other studies indicated that the maximal effect of insulin on blood glucose occurred at concentrations of 20 to 200 μU/ml, that concentrations in this range could be achieved by infusing insulin in a peripheral vein at rates of 2 to 12 units per hour, and that this procedure resulted in a fairly consistent, predictable fall of blood glucose in diabetic patients.

Crystalline insulin is diluted with physiologic saline to a volume allowing the desired infusion rate. (Example: 20 units in 100 ml, given at a rate of 10 ml or 4 units per hour.) Human serum albumin is usually added to a final concentration of 0.5 to 2.0 g/100 ml in order to minimize adherence of insulin to intravenous bottles and tubing, but has not been found to be essential by all investigators.[2] After an initial bolus of 2 to 8 units intravenously, the infusion is delivered by infusion pump or a pediatric drip set (such as that supplied by the Ivac Corporation) into the intravenous tubing or a separate vein at the rate of 2 to 8 units per hour. This results in a fall of blood glucose averaging 75 to 100 mg/100 ml per hour.[3,4] Insulin in dilute solution deteriorates fairly rapidly. Therefore, it may be advisable to prepare a fresh solution every four to six hours.

Infusion rate can be easily increased or decreased depending on the patient's response. Continuous infusion is maintained until the blood glucose has fallen to around 150 to 200 mg/100 ml, usually a matter of 6 to 12 hours. Blood glucose should be determined every two hours until it reaches 300 mg/100 ml; then it should be done hourly until the infusion is terminated.

Apparent advantages of this approach to insulin treatment are (1) less likelihood of hypoglycemia, (2) improved maintenance of serum potassium levels, (3) a beneficial fall in lactate levels during treatment, and (4) possibly more rapid recovery from ketoacidosis, since therapeutic levels of insulin in serum are constantly maintained, rather than widely fluctuating levels found after intermittent injection of intravenous boluses of insulin.

Small *intramuscular* doses of regular insulin have also been used to treat diabetic coma, with similar good results.[5,6] This regimen begins with a loading dose of 10 to 20 units followed by 5 to 10 units per hour.

Other aspects of management are the same as when large doses of insulin are used. Glucose must be added to intravenous solutions when the blood level falls to 300 mg/100 ml, and close observation of the patient's clinical condition remains essential. Administration of other intravenous fluids is similar with both types of insulin administration, so that the rate of infusion of insulin must be independent of that used for replacement fluids.

Fluids and electrolytes. It is essential that large amounts of intravenous fluid be given initially. Most patients receive from 5 to 10 liters during the first 24 hours with at least two thirds of that given during the first 12 hours. The tonicity of initial intravenous fluids is a point on which many disagree.

The composition of fluid losses estimated in clinical studies of diabetic coma most resembles 0.45% sodium chloride (half normal saline) solution with some potassium added. Hypotonic saline thus appears to be the most rational solution, at least for initial treatment. If the patient is severely volume depleted and hypotensive, 0.9% sodium chloride (normal saline) should be given. Some authorities feel that 0.9% sodium chloride should always be used, but this often results in excessive repletion of chloride and prolongation of acidemia and may initially worsen hyperosmolality.

Alkali. Alkali should be given if arterial pH is less than 7.15 to 7.20. Although some feel that rehydration will normalize renal function sufficiently to allow for quick return of pH to safe levels, severe acidemia (pH less than 7.0) can affect cardiovascular function adversely and should be corrected to approximately pH 7.20. Alkali should always be given as sodium bicarbonate. Depending on the initial pH, from 1 to 3 ampules (44 to 132 mEq) are added to the first 2 liters of intravenous fluid, and response of arterial blood pH is followed closely. Attempting to completely replace estimated bicarbonate deficits usually results in metabolic alkalosis.

Potassium. If the initial serum potassium level is elevated, potassium replacement is not begun for three to four hours, at which time serum levels will usually have fallen. Patients in ketoacidosis with normal or low serum potassium levels initially should have replacement started immediately, since this indicates severe body potassium depletion. Everything given for treatment of ketoacidosis (insulin, alkali, fluids) drives potassium back into cells and may lower serum potassium to dangerous levels. Potassium should always be given when bicarbonate is used. Ordinarily potassium chloride, 100 to 200 mEq over the first six to eight hours, is used to partially replace the potassium deficit. Neutral potassium phosphate, if available, may be preferable to potassium chloride, since most patients are also phosphate depleted. Phosphate depletion causes decreased levels of red blood cell 2,3-diphosphoglycerate, which may adversely affect oxygen delivery to tissues as acidemia is corrected.

General considerations. General support of the patient should not be neglected during treatment of diabetic coma. Vital signs should be followed closely. Whole blood, plasma, or other plasma expanders should be given if initial rehydration with normal saline does not reverse hypotension. A nasogastric tube should be placed, since gastric dilatation is frequently present due to electrolyte disturbances. Central venous pressure should be monitored if shock is present or if the patient's cardiac compensation is questionable. Treatment of any infection present should be initiated. If myocardial infarction is suspected, the patient must be monitored carefully for cardiac arrhythmias. Other causes of shock, such as sepsis, renal papillary necrosis, hemorrhagic pancreatitis, or gastrointestinal hemorrhage, must also be considered if the patient does not respond to initial volume replacement.

Potential hazards. The approach outlined above represents vigorous treatment of diabetic coma. This is recommended purposely so that even the most severely ill patient will be adequately treated. The treatment is not without some risk, which can be largely avoided if the hazards are anticipated.

Hypokalemia occurs frequently during the treatment of ketoacidosis and, if severe, can result in cardiac arrhythmias, paralysis, and death. Frequent monitoring of the electrocardiogram can alert one to potential danger of hypokalemia, but serum potassium levels must be checked frequently. As noted above, if initial serum potassium levels are low or even normal, replacement should begin immediately. Some patients may require very large amounts of intravenous potassium, far in excess of those recommended above.[7]

Cerebral edema occurs rarely during the course of treatment of diabetic coma but is often fatal. It is suspected if the patient seems to respond initially but then lapses into a deeper coma. If this occurs, immediate treatment with dexamethasone may be helpful. The complication is probably the result of movement of water into the central nervous system, which maintains elevated osmolality even after extracellular fluid osmolality has been lowered by treatment. Recent experiments in animals suggest this problem can be minimized by avoiding reduction of blood glucose below 300 mg/100 ml in the first several hours of treatment. Therefore, intravenous glucose should be given to maintain that level for sufficient time to allow central nervous system osmolality to equilibrate with that of extracellular fluid, perhaps 12 to 18 hours.

Hypoglycemia may also occur during treatment but will be averted if the above guidelines for glucose administration are followed.

Lactic acidosis

Lactic acidosis is a rarer cause of diabetic coma, although elevated lactate levels can also be present in ketoacidosis. Infection, infarction, shock, administration of phenformin, and ethanol ingestion are among the precipitating causes. The patient may be either hyper- or hypoglycemic. Initial emergency treatment includes vigorous bicarbonate therapy, hydration, and administration of glucose and insulin. Major efforts must be devoted to finding and treating the cause of the elevated lactic acid levels.

HYPOGLYCEMIA

It is well established that the brain is dependent upon glucose for normal metabolism. In the absence of glucose, intracellular metabolites are diverted for energy use by the neural cells, and important changes occur in membrane transport functions, lipid and protein biosynthesis, concentration of high energy phosphate compounds, and secretion of neurotransmitters. Sensitivity to glucose deprivation of various areas of the brain appears to be correlated with their oxygen consumption.[8] The cortex is the area most sensitive to hypoglycemia, followed by the subcortical, diencephalic, and more primitive areas. Although hypoglycemia is often arbitrarily defined as a concentration of plasma glucose less than 50 mg/100 ml, hypoglycemic symptoms also relate to the rate of fall of plasma glucose levels. The glucose and oxygen requirements of the brain at the time, the state of cerebral circulation, the presence of any agent interfering with glucose oxidation, and the presence of previous brain damage will also influence the appearance of symptoms.

To defend against hypoglycemia, plasma glucose concentration is closely regulated. Hormones involved in glucose homeostasis include growth hormone, insulin, glucagon, cortisol, and epinephrine. When hypoglycemia occurs, the normal response includes the increased secretion of these hormones, accompanied by suppression of insulin secretion.

Signs and symptoms

The adrenergic or epinephrine-like features of hypoglycemia relate to the rate of fall of plasma glucose as well as to the level of plasma glucose. These, therefore, may occur before any abnormality in cerebral function is apparent. Manifestations of adrenergic stimulation include tachycardia, anxiety, diaphoresis, nervousness, tremor, weakness, pallor and increase in blood pressure. These signs and symptoms may be blunted or absent in patients receiving sympathetic antagonists, such as propranolol, in patients with neuropathy of the autonomic nervous system (as may occur in diabetes mellitus), in older patients, or in patients with chronic hypoglycemia.

Neurologic manifestations of hypoglycemia are varied and often subtle; hence the diagnosis of hypoglycemia must be considered in any patient showing neurologic abnormalities. The initial symptoms and signs relate to cortical glucose deprivation and include headaches, faintness, hunger or nausea, increased irritability, mild to severe confusion, somnolence, hallucinations, aimless hyperactivity, hypotonia, and visual disturbances. Other manifestations of hypoglycemia are protean but are frequently similar in a given patient with recurrent episodes of hypoglycemia. In addition, previous areas of brain injury or focal restriction of cerebral blood flow may produce focal signs, either paralytic or convulsive, during hypoglycemia. Additional signs and symptoms secondary to neuroglucopenia include somnolence, hypotonia, hypothermia, tremor, loss of consciousness, primitive movements such as sucking, grasping, and grimacing, tonic spasms, hyperesthesia, ophthalmoplegia, Babinski signs, extensor spasms, seizures, status epilepticus, and ultimately deep coma with bradycardia, miosis, atonia, and slowed respirations. Even the most severe of these symptoms, which reflect glucose insufficiency in the more primitive areas of the brain, can usually be entirely reversed; however, every minute that hypoglycemia is prolonged results in further damage. Therefore, once the diagnosis is made or even suspected, it is imperative to begin rapid treatment of the hypoglycemia. Although reversal of signs may occur within minutes following glucose administration, hours or days may be required for recovery from prolonged hypoglycemia. For this reason, lack of immediate response to administration of glucose does not exclude the diagnosis of hypoglycemia.

Etiology

There are many causes of hypoglycemia; some of the more common are considered below[9]:
A. Drugs
    1. Insulin
    2. Oral hypoglycemics
    3. Ethanol
    4. Miscellaneous (salicylates, propranolol, pentamidine)

B. Hepatic disorders
  1. Hepatocellular destruction
  2. Inborn errors of metabolism (glycogen storage disease, galactosemia, hereditary fructose intolerance)
  3. Passive congestion secondary to congestive heart failure.
C. Hormone deficiencies
  1. Cortisol
  2. Growth hormone
  3. Glucagon
  4. Epinephrine
D. Tumors
  1. Insulinoma
  2. Massive extrapancreatic tumors
    a. Mesotheliomas
    b. Fibrosarcomas
    c. Liposarcomas
E. Reactive disorders
  1. Leucine sensitivity
  2. Early adult-onset diabetes mellitus
  3. Post gastric surgery
  4. Functional hypoglycemia

Drug induced. Most important in this category is excess exogenous insulin taken either accidentally or intentionally by diabetic patients (insulin reaction or insulin shock). Other commonly used drugs that can cause profound hypoglycemia include ethanol and oral hypoglycemic agents. The metabolism of ethanol by the liver causes a decreased NAD/NADH ratio, the result of which is a marked decrease in glucose production by the liver. The combination of ethanol ingestion with other hypoglycemic drugs or with fasting can lead to profound hypoglycemia. The sulfonylureas are the oral hypoglycemic agents most often associated with hypoglycemia, and of these, chlorpropamide (Diabinese) is by far the most common offender. This drug is excreted mostly unmetabolized by the kidney and persists in the blood over 24 hours, exhibiting a half-life of 36 hours. Hence, blood levels of this drug can increase insidiously, particularly in the presence of renal insufficiency. The most susceptible patients are the elderly, in whom the complication of hypoglycemia is not uncommon. Other sulfonylureas less frequently cause hypoglycemia.

Beta adrenergic blocking agents such as propranolol can produce severe hypoglycemia because of their inhibitory effects on hepatic glycogenolysis. Hypoglycemia must be considered in any patient receiving beta blocking agents, especially in those also taking insulin. In the latter, adrenergic response to hypoglycemia may be masked. Other drugs occasionally associated with hypoglycemia include biguanides such as phenformin, salicylates, haloperidol, propoxyphene, prochlorperazine, para-aminobenzoic acid, pentamidine, phenylbutazone, and antihistamines. In most instances, hypoglycemia associated with these drugs occurs in patients with concurrent hepatic or renal disease.

Hepatic disorders. Several conditions including severe hepatocellular damage and various congenital metabolic abnormalities such as glycogen storage diseases, galactosemia, and hereditary fructose intolerance can be associated with hypoglycemia. Right-sided heart failure with passive congestion of the liver may also cause hypoglycemia, especially in children with congenital cardiac disease.

Hormone deficiencies. Deficiencies of those hormones that tend to raise plasma glucose through stimulation of glycogenolysis or gluconeogenesis or through peripheral antagonism to insulin may cause hypoglycemia. Cortisol deficiency (due to primary hypoadrenalism or hypopituitarism), growth hormone deficiency in children, and rarely catecholamine or glucagon deficiency can all present with hypoglycemia.

Tumor hypoglycemia. One category of tumors causing hypoglycemia is those tumors of the pancreatic islet cells that produce insulin, or insulinomas. Hypoglycemia under these circumstances can be profound and refractory to therapy. A second category of tumor hypoglycemia includes tumors that produce substances, not insulin, that promote hypoglycemia or tumors that cause hypoglycemia by yet unknown mechanisms, possibly through excessive utilization of glucose. These tumors are usually of mesothelial or epithelial origin, are generally very large and easily detected, and include fibrosarcomas, lymphosarcomas, mesotheliomas, liposarcomas, adrenocortical carcinomas, hepatomas, cholangiocarcinomas, and gastric and cecal carcinomas.

Reactive or nonfasting hypoglycemia. Most causes of hypoglycemia mentioned above operate during the fasting state. There is another category of hypoglycemia: that which occurs at variable times following ingestion of a meal. Reactive hypoglycemia has several etiologies. These include leucine sensitivity, functional hypoglycemia, early adult-onset diabetes mellitus, post gastric surgery, and several rare hereditary disorders, such as fructose intolerance, listed at the beginning of this discussion.

Diagnosis and treatment

Diagnosis of hypoglycemia should be considered in any patient who manifests unusual behavior, neurologic signs, seizures, or coma, especially if the patient has diabetes mellitus, takes drugs, has a history of ethanol intake, or a history of recurrent episodes suggestive of hypoglycemia. The initial approach to the patient should include a rapid history, if available, and physical examination; blood should be drawn for glucose and ethanol, and enough serum should be frozen and saved to permit measurement at a later time of immunoreactive insulin, growth hormone, cortisol, or toxicology screening, if indicated. In addition, an estimate of blood glucose, by use of Dextrostix should be made to help support or discard the diagnosis; however, absolute reliance on this test is unwise. It is preferable to err in the direction of making the diagnosis, as the danger of not treating hypoglycemia when it is present is always greater than the danger of treating nonexistent hypoglycemia.

If the diagnosis of hypoglycemia is suspected, an intravenous infusion should be started, and 25 g of glucose (50 ml of D50/W) should be given slowly by intravenous push; thereafter, administration of D5/W can be started and the rate of infusion adjusted, based on frequent plasma glucose determinations. Large amounts of glucose, even in a concentration of 10%, may be required if massive doses of insulin or oral hypoglycemics have been taken, or if the cause is an insulinoma, or non-insulin-producing tumor. Since glucose provides the major stimulus for secretion of endogenous insulin, it is preferable to maintain a constant rate of glucose infusion rather than giving intermittent large boluses that could stimulate the pancreas to produce more insulin. For the vast majority of patients this therapy will be adequate.

Other procedures that should be performed in the emergency department include an accurate determination of core body temperatures to ascertain the presence of profound hypothermia; pulse and blood pressure should be measured carefully. An ECG should be obtained since hypoglycemia represents a major stress on the myocardium. On occasion, despite the glucose administered, the hypoglycemia may persist. This may not be clear until after the patient has been admitted to the hospital. Although this is generally not a problem for emergency care personnel, it will be discussed briefly.

At this point, the critical problem is to diagnose the cause of the hypoglycemia. For example, in patients taking long-acting insulin preparations or chlorpropamide, the stimulus producing hypoglycemia can be expected to persist for many hours to several days; therefore the patient will clearly require admission to the hospital and treatment until the cause of the hypoglycemia is resolved. *Premature discharge of the patient is hazardous.* Explanation of the symptoms of hypoglycemia and admonitions to take glucose-containing food at the first sign of hypoglycemia may not prevent a fatal episode, especially if it occurs when the patient is sleeping or becomes confused and somnolent. If the patient has been taking insulin regularly, he may require admission for adjustment of dosage.

Supplemental treatment

Administration of drugs is rarely required to control hypoglycemia. Glucagon, 1 mg IM, can be given to stimulate hepatic glucose release[9,10]; however, one should keep in mind that glucogen in pharmacologic amounts is a potent stimulus to insulin secretion. Nevertheless, there is an occasional use for this drug in the emergency treatment of hypoglycemia. Similarly, epinephrine, 1 mg SC, may be given, although it is rarely required. Administration of glucocorticoid is justified in any patient with resistant hypoglycemia or suspicion of adrenal or pituitary insufficiency (see below). Hydrocortisone succinate (Solu-Cortef), 100 mg by IV continuous drip, may be given as initial treatment. An effective drug for recalcitrant hypoglycemia, particularly in those patients with nonresectable insulinomas, is the benzothiadiazine diazoxide, a nonnatriuretic and nonkaliuretic thiazide that acts primarily by blocking release of insulin from the beta cell. From 200 to 600 mg of diazoxide may be given intravenously over several hours or taken orally in doses of 100 to 200 mg every six hours. The drug should be given in association with a diuretic to prevent salt retention. Patients must be carefully followed for weight gain, fluid retention, and blood pressure. Patients not responding to initial treatment with intravenous glucose and glucagon after one hour, even though normo- or hyperglycemia had been achieved, may be given corticosteroids and 200 ml of 20% mannitol over 20 minutes on the assumption that cerebral edema may be present.[10]

Prevention

Obviously, explanation of the symptoms of hypoglycemia to the patient and appropriate instructions to take glucose-containing food (e.g., orange juice with added sugar) are indicated. All patients with diabetes mellitus and anyone who has had an episode of hypoglycemia should obtain an appropriate Medic-Alert bracelet. Some patients on insulin should have glucagon available at home to be administered by a relative should the patient become unconscious or too obtunded to take oral fluids. A dose of 1 mg can be administered subcutaneously or intramuscularly and may be repeated in 20 minutes.

REFERENCES

1. Hockaday, T. D. R., and Alberti, K. G. M. M.: Diabetic coma, Clin. Endocrinol. Metabol. 1:751-788, 1972.
2. Page, M. M., Alberti, K. G. M. M., Greenwood, R., et al.: Treatment of diabetic coma with continuous low-dose infusion of insulin, Br. Med. J. 2:687-690, 1974.
3. Kidson, W., Casey, J., Kraegen, E., and Lazarus, L.: Treatment of severe diabetes mellitus by insulin infusion, Br. Med. J. 2:691-694, 1974.
4. Semple, P. F., White, C., and Manderson, W. G.: Continuous intravenous infusion of small doses of insulin in treatment of diabetic ketoacidosis, Br. Med. J. 2:694-698, 1974.
5. Alberti, K. G. M. M., Hockaday, T. D. R., and Turner, R. C.: Small doses of intramuscular insulin in the treatment of diabetic "coma," Lancet 2:515-522, 1973.
6. Kitabchi, A. E., Ayyagari, V., Guerra, S. M. D., and Medical House Staff: The efficacy of low-dose versus conventional therapy of insulin for treatment of diabetic ketoacidosis, Ann. Intern. Med. 84:633-638, 1976.
7. Abrahamson, E., and Arby, R.: Diabetic acidosis with initial hypokalemia, J.A.M.A. 196:401-403, 1966.
8. Ensinck, J. W., and Williams, R. H.: Disorders causing hypoglycemia. In Williams, R. H., editor: Textbook of endocrinology, Philadelphia, 1974, W. B. Saunders Co., pp. 627-659.
9. Baruh, S., Sherman, L., Kolodny, H. D., and Singh, A. J.: Fasting hypoglycemia, Med. Clin. North Am. 57:1441-1462, 1973.
10. MacCuish, A. C., Munro, J. F., and Duncan, L. J. P.: Treatment of hypoglycemic coma with glucagon, intravenous dextrose, and mannitol infusion in a hundred diabetics, Lancet 2:946-949, 1970.

CHAPTER **9**

Endocrine emergencies

Jeffrey A. Sandler, M.D.

ACUTE ADRENAL CRISIS[1,2]
Precipitating factors

Patients with Addison's disease, hypopituitarism, or illnesses being treated with therapeutic doses of glucocorticoids may develop an acute adrenal crisis under a variety of circumstances. Abrupt cessation of steroid medications by the patient or physician, failure to increase glucocorticoid dosage during situations of stress, removal of an adrenal adenoma with contralateral glandular suppression, or adrenal hemorrhage secondary to sepsis, anticoagulants, or metastatic carcinoma may all predispose the patient to the development of acute adrenal insufficiency. Glucocorticoid requirement may increase up to tenfold during stress in patients with adrenal insufficiency or limited adrenal reserve. Stressful situations such as infection, fever, or surgery should be met with increased glucocorticoid replacement. Certain concurrent illnesses such as hyperthyroidism may increase requirements for glucocorticoids via increased metabolism of the steroid. Similarly, drugs such as phenytoin (Dilantin) increase the rate of metabolic inactivation of adrenocortical steroid, although this is rarely of clinical significance. Another unusual circumstance in which adrenal insufficiency may be expected is in the acute development of an adrenal arterial or venous thrombosis. Addison's disease should be considered strongly in patients with tuberculosis or with certain autoimmune diseases, such as pernicious anemia or Hashimoto's thyroiditis.

Signs and symptoms

Since adrenal crisis is often precipitated by an intercurrent illness, signs and symptoms are referable to both the adrenal insufficiency and the precipitating condition. Generally the patient will give a history of progressive anorexia, weakness, and irritability, followed by nausea and vomiting, headaches, cramping abdominal pain, diarrhea, arthralgias, and hyperpyrexia, often marked, over an 8- to 12-hour period. If untreated, the patient may progress to shock and coma.

On physical examination the patient may have hyperpigmentation, particularly noticeable in recent scars, intertriginous regions, palmar creases, as vertical dark bands in the nails, or on buccal, rectal, or vaginal mucosa. Hyperpigmentation is only seen in patients with primary adrenal failure, and it is thought to be due to the excessive secretion of melanocyte-stimulating activity from the unsuppressed pituitary. Evidence of auricular calcification and signs of other endocrine deficiencies, such as hypogonadism or hypothyroidism, should be sought.

In adrenal crisis associated with the Waterhouse-Friderichsen syndrome (adrenal hemorrhage of septicemia), high fever and purpura with meningeal signs and coma are characteristic.

Laboratory data

Hyponatremia and hyperkalemia, occasionally marked, with evidence of hemoconcentration and an increase in BUN, may be seen in primary adrenal insufficiency with loss of mineralocorticoid activity. This rarely occurs with hypopituitarism or hypothalamic-pituitary suppression from long-term glucocorticoid therapy. Eosinophilia may be striking. Acidosis may also be present. Occasionally, with severe volume depletion, hypercalcemia is seen. Hypoglycemia may occur and may be marked; therefore a plasma glucose level should be determined in any patient in whom the diagnosis is considered. When hypoglycemia or severe hypotension occurs, hypothermia may be seen. The hypotension may be the result of hypovolemia as well as of loss of glucocorticoid activity needed for maintenance of vascular tone. An ECG should be obtained to evaluate possible arrhythmias, looking for signs of hyperkalemia. Blood for determination of arterial pH, plasma cortisol, electrolytes, BUN, creatinine, and a complete blood count with differential should be obtained. Therapy is begun on the basis of the clinical diagnosis.

Treatment

Therapy is directed at correction of the glucocorticoid deficiency, fluid and electrolyte abnormalities, and any accompanying hypoglycemia or infection. The most important aspect of therapy is the administration of glucocorticoids in substantial doses.[1] Once the diagnosis is suspected and blood for appropriate laboratory studies is obtained, a secure intravenous infusion should be started and appropriate drugs and fluids administered.

Glucocorticoids. One commonly used replacement regimen is to administer 100 mg hydrocortisone succinate (Solu-Cortef) or hydrocortisone phosphate slowly by intravenous infusion over five to ten minutes; then an infusion is begun of 100 mg of hydrocortisone succinate in 1,000 ml of 5% dextrose in normal saline (D5/NS) at the rate of about 100 ml per hour or as needed to maintain blood pressure and urine output.[2] An additional 50 to 100 mg of hydrocortisone may be given intramuscularly in divided doses at several sites to ensure adequate absorption. Over the initial 12 hours of treatment no more than 200 mg of hydrocortisone or its equivalent is generally required, and no more than 300 mg is needed over the first 24 hours. Analogues of cortisol with relative lack of mineralocorticoid activity, such as prednisolone or dexamethasone, should not be used to treat adrenal crisis.

Mineralocorticoid replacement. Because of the salt-retaining properties of high doses of hydrocortisone, mineralocorticoids are generally not required and particularly in the elderly should be avoided to obviate the development of fluid overload and pulmonary edema. However, if the patient is severely ill with profound hypotension or has marked hyponatremia and hyperkalemia, desoxycorticosterone acetate, 5 to 10 mg IM, may be given daily; fludrocortisone (Florinef), 0.1 to 0.2 mg, may be given daily when the patient is able to take medications by mouth.

Fluids and electrolytes. Generally, administration of 2,000 to 3,000 ml of D5/NS intravenously during the first 24 hours will correct salt and water depletion as well as hypoglycemia. Initially one should administer fluids rapidly enough to maintain blood pressure; for example, in a dehydrated, hypotensive patient in crisis, giving 1,000 ml of D5/NS intravenously over the first one to two hours would be reasonable. If the patient is massively dehydrated (e.g., a patient with panhypopituitarism who has both adrenal insufficiency and diabetes insipidus) or has questionable cardiac reserve, fluid replacement may be required using evaluation of central venous pressure (CVP) as a guide. Even if severe hyponatremia is present, hypertonic saline should not be given because of the attendant exacerbation of intracellular dehydration. In those patients with profound acidosis as evidenced by arterial pH less than 7.2 or with total bicarbonate less than 10 mEq/liter, sodium bicarbonate can be given intravenously. The mild hypercalcemia seen in some patients requires no specific therapy and is corrected with administration of fluids and glucocorticoid.

Other measures. The patient in addisonian crisis should be adequately treated for this life-threatening problem before unnecessary procedures or examinations are done. The hypothermia or hyperthermia requires no specific corrective measures other than those for suspected sepsis. The administration of fluids and adequate steroid replacement will generally be sufficient to correct hyperthermia due to adrenal insufficiency. Since a rapid drop in temperature may precipitate hypotension, aspirin, in the rare instance in which it is given for hyperpyrexia, should be administered in low doses (begin with 60 to 120 mg). Hypotension usually responds to the steroid and fluid therapy outlined above; if severe circulatory collapse is present, colloids and vasopressors may be necessary. If this is required, however, other causes such as bacteremic shock should be suspected.

Appropriate cultures including cerebrospinal fluid should be obtained, and administration of broad-spectrum antibiotics should be started routinely in most patients who suddenly develop acute adrenal crisis without apparent precipitating cause. In these cases infection clinically inapparent because of dehydration or hypothermia is commonly responsible.

Since total body potassium may actually be depleted in patients with adrenal insufficiency, despite hyperkalemia, the potassium should be monitored very carefully;

later in treatment, supplemental potassium may be required. Overhydration and water intoxication should be avoided.

Following emergency treatment the patient should be admitted to the hospital for further evaluation and therapy. Hydrocortisone succinate (Solu-Cortef), 25 mg IM, every six to eight hours, or an equivalent dose of cortisone acetate given orally every 12 hours, will generally be adequate to maintain the patient; the dose should be tapered and maintenance with oral steroid medication continued. Search for other hormonal deficiencies is indicated for two reasons: (1) the patient may have secondary adrenal insufficiency from hypopituitarism, and (2) other primary "autoimmune" endocrine dysfunction has been seen in patients with primary adrenal insufficiency.

THYROID STORM
Precipitating factors

Thyroid storm is a loosely defined clinical diagnosis in which there is an exaggerated expression of the hyperthyroid state, generally with increased hypermetabolism accompanied by hyperpyrexia ($> 40°$ C), marked tachycardia, and exaggerated central nervous system, hepatic, and gastrointestinal features of hyperthyroidism. In patients with hyperthyroidism the stress of infection, anesthesia, surgery, diabetic ketoacidosis, preeclampsia, and parturition may precipitate uncontrolled hypermetabolism. Treatment of an overtly thyrotoxic patient with a large goiter by surgery or, rarely, by radioactive iodine has been reported to cause thyroid storm. The syndrome may progress rapidly to shock, cardiovascular collapse, coma, and death. Since the syndrome cannot be precisely defined, estimates of mortality vary but may exceed 20%. Therefore, the clinical diagnosis impels immediate therapy before laboratory confirmation of the diagnosis.

Signs and symptoms

Characteristically, the patient gives a history compatible with hyperthyroidism, including heat intolerance, weight loss, voracious appetite, hyperdefecation, muscle weakness, nervousness, hyperhidrosis, and palpitations.[3,4] Symptoms and signs of frank congestive heart failure or ischemic heart disease may be present. On physical examination the patient may be febrile (38° to 41° C) and may have shaking chills in addition to the usual signs of hyperthyroidism, which often include marked asthenia, smooth, flushed, and moist skin, significant sinus tachycardia (often more than 140 beats per minute) or cardiac arrhythmia, a tremor, muscle weakness, exophthalmos, lid lag, alopecia, vitiligo or hyperpigmentation, pretibial myxedema, and onycholysis. The patient may have hepatosplenomegaly and lymphadenopathy and on occasion may even be jaundiced. Blood pressure is usually well maintained. The patient is restless, confused, emotionally labile and may display psychotic behavior. Convulsions and stupor may ultimately occur. Generally the thyroid gland is quite enlarged and firmer than usual in Graves' disease; it may be uninodular or multinodular in the less common forms of thyrotoxicosis. Rarely the gland may be impalpable or normal sized. Thyroid storm may be seen with factitious thyrotoxicosis caused by ingestion of thyroid hormone. In elderly patients with severe thyrotoxicosis usually due to toxic multinodular goiter, the patient may express few of the symptoms of hyperthyroidism, although tachycardia is almost always present; the patient may be somnolent and drift into coma. This syndrome is referred to as apathetic hyperthyroidism but is equally life threatening. In untreated thyroid storm, hyperpyrexia progressively increases and ultimately reaches lethal levels, with shock and coma occurring within 24 to 48 hours.

Evaluation and treatment[5,6]

The patient should have a full blood chemistry profile and blood count. Blood should be sent for determination of cholesterol and total thyroxine (T_4) and an as-

sessment of thyroid-binding globulin (T_3 resin uptake), and T_3 by radioimmunoassay. An ECG should be obtained and all vital signs recorded.

Therapy is begun immediately and is directed at three major objectives: (1) prevention of thyroid *hormonogenesis* (PTU, methimazole), (2) prevention of thyroid *hormone release* (iodides), (3) treatment of some of the peripheral effects of thyrotoxicosis (propranolol).

Prevention of further synthesis of thyroid hormone. Propylthiouracil, 300 mg, or methimazole, 30 mg, should be given orally or by nasogastric tube immediately and every eight hours to prevent further thyroid hormone synthesis. This is achieved by immediate blockage of organic binding and coupling of thyroid hormone.

Prevention of thyroid hormone release. Thirty minutes following institution of propylthiouracil or methimazole, 10 drops of a saturated solution of potassium iodide (SSKI), should be given orally to prevent release of stored thyroid hormone; this dose may be repeated every eight hours, although as little as ⅛ of 1 drop of SSKI is sufficient to inhibit thyroid hormone release. If the patient cannot take oral medication, sodium iodide can be given in an intravenous drip (1 to 2 g/24 hours).

Treatment of some of the peripheral manifestations of thyrotoxicosis. On the basis of some indirect evidence it has long been felt that many of the features of hyperthyroidism are the result of enhanced sensitivity to catecholamines produced by thyroid hormone. Although this proposed synergism may exist, a significant portion of the cardiovascular and metabolic effects of thyroid hormone are direct and not mediated by enhanced catecholamine sensitivity. Unfortunately, at the time of this writing no antagonists of thyroid hormone are clinically available. However, on the basis of postulated thyroid-catecholamine interrelationships, various sympatholytic agents have been used to treat hyperthyroidism with improvement of the tachycardia, hyperhidrosis, tremor, and nervousness. Beta blocking agents such as propranolol act immediately to compete with catecholamines at the membrane receptors and do not cause acute release of stored catecholamines. Propranolol can probably be recommended as the drug of choice in thyroid storm despite the lack of a large controlled study regarding its usage and optimal dose. Although generally contraindicated in congestive heart failure, propranolol appears beneficial in the treatment of heart failure of thyrotoxicosis due to tachyarrhythmias or high cardiac output. Nevertheless, to be cautious, an initial test dose of propranolol, 0.5 mg IV, should be given, and if it is tolerated, an additional 1 mg may be given. If no worsening or failure occurs, the patient can then be started on oral propranolol at a dose of 20 mg every six hours, increasing the next dose based on the pulse rate and clinical signs. Propranolol is contraindicated in patients with bronchial asthma or with congestive heart failure secondary to factors other than high cardiac output or tachyarrhythmia.

Treatment of complicating factors

Although extremely unlikely, there is a possibility of coexistent adrenal insufficiency in some patients. There is no data to support a decrease in adrenocortical reserve in patients with thyrotoxicosis. However, standard practice recommends the short-term use of glucocorticoid therapy in patients suspected of having thyroid storm. Hydrocortisone succinate (Solu-Cortef), 200 mg, should be given intravenously, and a total dose of 300 mg should be given over the first 24 hours.

Dehydration and electrolyte abnormalities should be treated with appropriate fluid replacement. Occasionally significant hyponatremia may be present. D5/NS is an intravenous solution of proven benefit during the initial treatment of these patients. Vasopressor agents are used only with extreme reluctance.

Since thyrotoxicosis is associated with increased utilization and subclinical deficiencies of B vitamins, large doses of B vitamins should be included in the intravenous infusion, particularly thiamine (100 to 200 mg), since an exacerbation of high output heart failure by thiamine deficiency in thyrotoxicosis is a serious complication.

Congestive heart failure, if unresponsive to control of the heart rate, can be treated by administration of digitalis, oxygen, and diuretics.

Treatment of hyperthermia should be restricted to the use of a cooling blanket for high fevers, being careful to remove the blanket as the temperature reaches 38° C. Only with extremely high fevers should one consider the use of salicylates or phenothiazines in large doses, since hypotension may be precipitated by the use of these drugs.

Treatment of coexistent or precipitating illnesses

A vigorous search should be made for a precipitating illness, particularly infection. Cultures of blood, urine, and sputum should be obtained, and a thorough evaluation for a source of infection should be done. Because these patients frequently present with neurologic signs, examination and culture of the cerebrospinal fluid may also be indicated. Strong clinical suspicion of infection is justification for administration of broad-spectrum antibiotics, pending bacteriologic results. Cardiac arrhythmias, if unresponsive to propranolol, should be treated with the appropriate antiarrhythmic agent.

MYXEDEMA COMA[7]

Myxedema coma is the extreme expression of untreated hypothyroidism and is a serious medical emergency. As with many medical emergencies, treatment must be initiated on the basis of history and physical examination since confirmatory laboratory data are not immediately available.

In plasma there are two active thyroid hormones—thyroxine (T_4) and triiodothyronine (T_3). These hormones are secreted directly by the thyroid gland, but the major contribution to serum T_3 is from peripheral deiodination of T_4. It is currently debated whether T_3 or T_4 is the primary hormone, with much recent evidence favoring T_3. Thyroid hormone exerts numerous effects on growth, differentiation, and expression of differentiated function in a large number of tissues, and deficiency of thyroid hormone produces a severe clinical syndrome with manifestations in several organ systems.

Signs and symptoms

Myxedema coma occurs in patients with long-standing untreated hypothyroidism. Suspicion should be high in anyone with a history of neck surgery, known thyroidectomy, radioactive iodine therapy, previous hyperthyroidism, and any signs suggestive of panhypopituitarism. Myxedema coma is more common in the elderly, particularly females who have significant arteriosclerotic disease. Common precipitants of this acute illness include cold winter weather, infection, or ingestion of a large variety of drugs, especially narcotics, sedatives, and tranquilizers.

The syndrome is characterized by stupor, progressing to a comatose state, with hypothermia, often profound, and hypoventilation. The patient has a pale, sallow complexion, often with a yellowish orange tint due to carotenemia; dry, cool skin; large tongue; scant and coarse scalp or eyebrow hair; and usually puffiness of the face (particularly in the periorbital area) and extremities. The patient generally has a deep, hoarse voice and slow movements. There is a bradycardia, often profound; the reflexes are hypoactive and demonstrate a marked delay in the relaxation phase. A critical finding is that of hypothermia, and survival is roughly correlated with the degree of hypothermia, being extremely poor with temperatures below 32° C. Therefore, to accurately assess the core body temperature, the thermometer must be shaken to below 27° C. Additional features include bizarre behavior and slow mentation if the patient is awake. Because of central nervous system depression and occasional cerebellar ataxia and muscle weakness, patients with severe myxedema may fall, and evidence of subdural hematomas and rib fractures should be sought.

Myxedema coma may be due to disordered cerebral metabolism caused by the hypothyroidism itself, or it may be related to complicating features. Since these complications must be treated, evidence of the following conditions should be sought in every patient.

Hypoventilation and CO_2 narcosis. Hypoventilation and CO_2 narcosis are the most common and most serious treatable complications of myxedema. Respiratory insufficiency and CO_2 retention to some degree occur in more than 50% of patients. Severe decrease in ventilation may occur. Obesity, congestive heart failure, pleural and pericardial effusions, central nervous system depression, macroglossia, muscle weakness, ingestion of any sedatives or narcotics, and aspiration are all possible contributing mechanisms. In addition, the large tongue and myxedema of the trachea may make intubation quite difficult. Death from CO_2 narcosis is a well-reported, and avoidable, cause of death in this syndrome.

Hypoglycemia. Hypoglycemia is uncommon but felt to be responsible for the death of several patients with myxedema coma. It may be due to concomitant pituitary or adrenal insufficiency. Therefore, plasma glucose should be determined for each patient.

Hypothermia. Hypothermia, often severe, is present in 80% of patients. It is generally agreed that active warming is detrimental and may divert blood supply from vital organs; at most a blanket or sheet can be placed on the patient, and allowance should be made for thyroid hormone replacement to restore hormonal balance and body temperature.

Hyponatremia and inappropriate secretion of ADH. Almost half the patients reported have hyponatremia, often marked, and generally felt to be due to inappropriate secretion of ADH (antidiuretic hormone) and diminished renal perfusion with impaired ability to excrete free water.[7]

Adrenal insufficiency. In the past it was often suggested that adrenal insufficiency occurred commonly in severe myxedema. It now appears that only a few examples of actual adrenal insufficiency in myxedema coma have been documented. Nevertheless, it is customary to assume a relative adrenal insufficiency in these patients because (1) hypothyroidism occasionally is the result of pituitary insufficiency; (2) hemorrhage into the adrenal glands in myxedema coma has been reported; (3) administration of thyroid hormone may increase metabolic inactivation of steroid hormones and unmask a limited adrenal reserve; and (4) Hashimoto's thyroiditis, a common cause of hypothyroidism, frequently coexists with other "autoimmune" diseases such as adrenal insufficiency.

Other complicating factors. Other complicating factors include paralytic adynamic ileus, bladder, atony, anemia with a wide spectrum of red blood cell morphology, aspiration, bleeding tendency, and seizures. Pleural and pericardial effusions generally require no immediate therapy but should be aspirated if extremely large and contributing to cardiac or pulmonary decompensation.

Evaluation and therapy

The initial laboratory data should include arterial blood gases and pH, electrolytes, BUN, and calcium. Other laboratory tests performed are liver function; toxicology screen, especially for sedatives; cortisol; cholesterol; T_4; T_3 resin uptake; free T_4; and TSH. Some serum should be frozen and saved for determinations of other hormones at a later date. Obviously the results of thyroid function tests will be unknown when therapy is begun. The ECG may show marked low voltage, sinus bradycardia, T wave depression, and increased QT and PR intervals. A chest film should be obtained to look for pleural and pericardial effusions, and an echocardiogram, if available, will be helpful in the diagnosis of pericardial effusion. Therapy should be initiated as soon as the blood for initial tests is obtained. Evidence of infection should be sought, and blood, urine, and sputum cultures taken.

Once the diagnosis is suspected, the two major aspects of therapy are (1) to evaluate the possible presence of secondary complicating factors and (2) to decide the dose of thyroid hormone that should be given. The gravity of this illness is such that even with optimal treatment, mortality rates of up to 40% have been reported.

Thyroid replacement. There is a vast amount of literature which has suggested that large doses of thyroid hormone given to myxedematous patients may be associated with myocardial insufficiency or infarction, arrhythmias, cardiac decompensation, and even death. For this reason, cautious replacement doses were initially used in the treatment of myxedema coma. Even though there is no carefully controlled study that can be cited, it would appear that survival in myxedema coma is greatly improved with administration of large doses of thyroid hormone, apparently because the dangers of thyroid hormone lack outweigh the cardiovascular risks of treatment. A patient with myxedema coma has a severe deficit of thyroxine in the extrathyroidal pool; in addition, turnover of thyroxine is much decreased in hypothyroidism and is not immediately corrected by administration of thyroid hormone. Although the entire calculated deficit has been replaced by some authors, most series have used initial replacement doses of one third to one half the calculated deficit. Since oral and intramuscular administration of thyroxine produce uncertain or variable absorption, intravenous administration is the mode of choice. A single initial dose of T_4, 500 μg, may be given followed by 50 μg each day thereafter.

T_3 has theoretical advantages over T_4: (1) it may represent the active form of the hormone; (2) it has a more rapid onset of action; and (3) should toxicity occur, it has a far shorter half-life (about three days versus seven days for T_4 in euthyroid patients). However, since T_4 is peripherally converted to T_3 and metabolically active within hours and is readily available in a parenteral form (T_3 is not), it is considered the treatment of choice.

Clinical judgment is required to decide the dose of thyroid hormone to be used. If coma is secondary to other factors and easily corrected or if severe myocardial ischemia or arrhythmias are present, a lower dose might be used.

Treatment of complicating factors

1. Hypoglycemia and hyponatremia are treated by water restriction and beginning a D5/NS infusion. If required, additional glucose can be given. Care must be taken not to overhydrate the patient who may already have congestive heart failure.
2. Ventilatory insufficiency is probably the most life-threatening aspect of myxedema coma. If severe hypoventilation with elevated P_{CO_2} exists, intubation should be considered to permit mechanical ventilatory assistance. Care must be taken to avoid hypoxia and to minimize use of local anesthetics, since they may accumulate in toxic amounts.
3. Evidence of infection should be carefully sought since clinical manifestations will be blunted; infection is treated with appropriate antibiotics.
4. As discussed, hydrocortisone, 200 to 300 mg, should be given over the first 24 hours of treatment to preclude adrenal

insufficiency, giving the initial dose prior to administration of thyroid hormone.
5. Active warming of the patient should be avoided. Pressor agents to elevate blood pressure should also be avoided unless absolutely required.

HYPERCALCEMIA

Calcium plays a role in a variety of metabolic activities, including blood coagulation, enzyme activation, peptide hormone secretion, and function of cellular membranes and organelles. The most dramatic consequences of abnormalities in blood calcium involve neural function and the contractility of cardiac and skeletal muscle.

In blood and extracellular fluids almost one half the total calcium is protein bound, mostly to albumin. Hormonal regulation of calcium homeostasis is controlled by the level of ionized calcium, and it is the ionized fraction, comprising most of the non-protein-bound calcium, which mediates the physiologic effects of calcium. The remaining calcium is complexed to phosphate, citrate, and other ions. Blood, extracellular fluids, and soft tissues contain only about 1% of total body calcium; bone contains the remaining 99%, deposited in the form of hydroxyapatite (calcium and phosphate in the ratio of 1.5:1).

Blood calcium homeostasis is maintained primarily through the use of bone calcium reserves. This is not a process of simple diffusion but is under elaborate hormonal control. The kidney is the principal route of elimination of calcium, and urinary calcium excretion rises rapidly in the presence of hypercalcemia. However, even in patients with hypercalcemia, from 95% to 99% of filtered calcium is reabsorbed.

The blood calcium level is regulated primarily by parathyroid hormone, calcitonin, and vitamin D. The rate of parathyroid hormone secretion is inversely related to the blood level of ionized calcium; calcitonin secretion increases as the blood calcium level rises. Parathyroid hormone, when vitamin D levels are adequate, stimulates release of calcium from bone. It also increases intestinal absorption and renal reabsorption of calcium, although this action is of lesser importance in calcium homeostasis. The major actions of calcitonin are to inhibit bone resorption and increase urinary calcium and phosphate excretion. Vitamin D, converted by hepatic and renal hydroxylation steps to the active form (1,25 dihydroxycholecalciferol), increases calcium absorption in the intestine. Other agents exerting effects upon calcium metabolism include blood phosphate, glucocorticoids, growth hormone, thyroid hormone, and estrogen.

A high serum calcium (15 mg/100 ml or greater) or rapid development of hypercalcemia of lesser degree must be considered a medical emergency. The normal range for serum calcium is usually from 8.8 to 10.5 mg/100 ml.

Spurious abnormalities in serum calcium are noted under a variety of circumstances. A 1 g/100 ml elevation or depression of albumin or globulin is associated with a parallel serum calcium alteration of roughly 0.8 mg/100 ml. Venous stasis during sample collection may result in an overestimation of calcium concentration because of the resultant hemoconcentration.

Etiology

A list of causes of hypercalcemia are included in Table 9-1. The most common and most clinically significant are the hypercalcemias associated with malignancy and hyperparathyroidism, which together account for more than 80% of cases. Malignant tumors usually produce hypercalcemia as a result of bony metastases. Many carcinomas produce parathyroid hormone or a parathyroid hormone–like substance; this is most frequently reported in pulmonary, renal, ovarian, and cervical tumors, the so-called syndrome of ectopic hyperparathyroidism. Other humoral substances implicated in malignant hypercalcemia include

prostaglandins (hypernephroma) and osteoclast-activating factor (multiple myeloma and other lymphoreticular malignancies). Initiation of estrogen therapy in metastatic breast cancer can be associated with a severe hypercalcemia, usually occurring within the first week, but occasionally as late as two to three weeks. Excess vitamin D or large quantities of absorbable antacids associated with increased dietary calcium may result in hypercalcemia. Certain conditions thought to cause hypersensitivity to vitamin D, presumably by an increased conversion to 1,25-dihydroxycholecalciferol, also result in similar toxicity. These include sarcoidosis and tuberculosis, as well as some of the idiopathic hypercalcemias of childhood.

Signs and symptoms

The manifestations of hypercalcemia stem from effects on multiple organ systems. Distressing polyuria, nocturia, and accompanying polydipsia are early signs. Other symptoms include weakness, fatigue, general malaise, abdominal pain, nausea, vomiting, anorexia, constipation, and dehydra-

Table 9-1. Causes of hypercalcemia

Common causes or those associated with severe hypercalcemia	Uncommon causes or those associated with minor Ca^{++} elevations
Malignancy with or without osteolytic metastases	Sarcoidosis
	Leukemia; lymphoma
Hyperparathyroidism	Hyperthyroidism
Primary	Myxedema
"Ectopic"	Addisonian crisis
Multiple myeloma	Diuretic phase of acute
Hypervitaminosis D	tubular necrosis
Thiazide therapy	Post-renal transplant
Immobilization	Acromegaly
Estrogen therapy for	"Idiopathic" hyper-
metastatic breast	calcemia of infancy
carcinoma	Hypervitaminosis A
"Milk-alkali syndrome"	Syndrome of watery
	diarrhea, hypokale-
	mia, and achlorhy-
	dria (WDHA)

tion. Mental symptoms may include drowsiness, inability to concentrate, forgetfulness, and anxiety or depression. Severe hypercalcemia inhibits neuromuscular and myocardial depolarization and impairs renal responsiveness to vasopressin, resulting in nephrogenic diabetes insipidus, which may lead to severe dehydration. Psychosis, metabolic coma, and cardiac arrest can occur in untreated patients.

Other pathologic complications of hypercalcemia include peptic ulceration, pancreatitis, hypertension, and nephrocalcinosis with nephrolithiasis, occasionally producing acute renal failure.

On physical examination evidence of subcutaneous calcification (particularly over joints), band keratopathy (deposition of calcium phosphate crystals as a thin, granular aggregation in the medial and lateral aspects of the cornea close to the corneoscleral junction), and conjunctival calcification may be present. Muscular weakness and hypotonia are often profound.

Blood must be analyzed immediately for electrolytes, BUN, calcium, magnesium, osmolality, and a complete blood count. A chemistry profile, including the concentrations of total protein, albumin, phosphorus, and creatinine, should also be obtained. An ECG is advisable, including a rhythm strip, and the presence of a shortened QT interval should be looked for. Chest and abdominal roentgenograms may reveal pulmonary, gastric, vascular, and renal calcifications. Urinary osmolality, sodium, and calcium should be determined. The patient should be weighed and placed on a cardiac monitor. Frequent measurement of vital signs is indicated. Accurate records of fluid input and urine output are crucial. Failure to maintain an adequate urine output should be noted.

Treatment[8]

In considering therapy directed toward correction of hypercalcemia, it is important to take into account the magnitude and rapidity of development of the disorder. Most hypercalcemias are mild, appearing as constipation, polyuria and nocturia, lassitude, and nausea. This condition requires less vigorous treatment. Serum calcium levels less than 13 mg/100 ml are usually associated with mild symptoms and are well tolerated. Almost no treatment of hypercalcemia is without disadvantages, and these must be balanced against the need for rapid lowering of the serum calcium. In general, relatively mild hypercalcemia is treated by hydration with sodium chloride. The level of dehydration can be considered marked if there is dryness of the mouth, reduced skin turgor, postural hypotension, hemoconcentration, and subnormal central venous pressure. Because of the possibility of renal damage from hypercalcemia per se, azotemia is not necessarily a reflection of the magnitude of dehydration. Florid hypercalcemia, with vomiting, abdominal pain, obstipation, severe dehydration, cardiac arrhythmias, or psychosis, requires more vigorous therapy.

The various therapeutic modalities will be individually discussed; an overall plan for treatment will then be presented.

Saline diuresis and diuretics. The hypercalcemic patient is generally severely dehydrated. The goal is to replace the extracellular fluid volume and then to initiate a sodium diuresis, which produces a facilitation of calcium excretion because of the linear relationship between calcium and sodium excretion. The major initial clinical improvement relates to relief of the dehydration.

If congestive heart failure is not present, diuresis is initiated with isotonic (0.9%) or half isotonic (0.45%) saline infusion until the central venous pressure reaches 10 cm of water, followed by infusion of either 0.9% or 0.45% saline, 1 liter every three hours. During diuresis approximately one third of hypercalcemic patients will experience a lowering of serum calcium. When this treatment alone is not effective, a calciuretic diuretic is given in conjunction with intravenous saline after the initial rapid infusion has restored the central venous pressure to normal.

The diuretic of choice for initiation of a sodium diuresis is furosemide, 40 mg IV; repeat doses are given, if required, when the drug-induced diuresis is terminated. Because of the attendant potassium and magnesium losses, one must follow blood levels closely; it is generally wise to add both to the intravenous solutions (e.g., 10 to 20 mEq K^+, 2 mEq Mg^{++} per liter). Thiazide diuretics, which uncouple sodium and calcium excretion, are definitely contraindicated, since their use alone may produce hypercalcemia. The prodigious fluid loss necessitates that the patient be carefully monitored, with accurate serial weights (preferably using a bed scale), frequent vital sign checks, and monitoring of cardiac rhythm and central venous pressure. If the patient is on a digitalis preparation, the situation becomes doubly dangerous, since the increased sensitivity to digitalis in the face of hypercalcemia may be exaggerated with the development of hypokalemia.

In patients with serious renal disease or cardiovascular disease and in the presence of congestive heart failure, vigorous infusion of saline may be quite dangerous. All patients should be carefully followed for the development of congestive heart failure and pulmonary edema.

Sodium sulfate. Intravenous isotonic sodium sulfate (0.12 M sodium sulfate [38.9 g of sodium sulfate decahydrate per liter] with 10 to 20 mEq potassium phosphate and 2 g magnesium sulfate to replace losses) is often used with beneficial results. Sodium sulfate may be substituted for saline and diuretics since less fluid administration is required and the procedure seems to have no side effects other than nausea at infusion rates greater than 10 ml/min. It is speculative as to whether sodium sulfate is really more effective than sodium infusion alone. Other modes of action include the formation of a urinary complex of calcium and sulfate and diminution of calcium binding to plasma protein. These two putative effects are small in comparison to the effect of natriuresis, however. Magnesium and potassium losses are also promoted.

The total dose and rate of administration are limited only by the positive fluid balance (not over 1% to 3% of the body weight, depending on the cardiac reserve) and by the nausea that occurs at higher infusion rates. Since the mechanism of action depends on renal excretion, sodium sulfate is not useful in patients with renal insufficiency. Generally, 1 liter is infused over three hours, and up to 5 liters may be given.

Urinary calcium losses of several grams have been noted with the use of sodium sulfate. As discussed in the previous section, careful monitoring is required, and frequent determinations of serum sodium, potassium, chloride, magnesium and calcium should be obtained. Some hypernatremia is to be expected, since each liter infused contains 240 mEq of sodium but only 122 mEq of sulfate.

Phosphates. Soluble oral phosphates are quite effective in the therapy of hypercalcemia. The mechanism of action is to promote deposition of calcium and phosphate in skeletal and extraskeletal sites. A typical dose is 5 ml of Fleet's Phospho-Soda (3.3 g of sodium phosphate) or two tablets of Neutra-Phos (500 mg of phosphorus) every six to eight hours. If oral medication cannot be taken, the phosphates may be given as a rectal enema; they are well absorbed from the sigmoid colon. Diarrhea may be a complication of the oral therapy. Since intravenous phosphate has been felt by some to cause death from extensive extraskeletal calcification, its use is no longer recommended. The use of insoluble phosphates, such as cellulose phosphate, has not been proven to increase fecal calcium sufficiently to be considered of value in this situation.

Corticosteroids. Glucocorticoids are not helpful in lowering serum calcium levels acutely, but their administration is generally begun during the acute period in order to help control hypercalcemia during the subsequent course. Prednisone (30 to 100 mg/day) or hydrocortisone (up to 250 to 400 mg every eight hours) will lower serum calcium over a period of several days. Glucocorticoids produce substantial benefits in the hypercalcemias associated with vitamin D intoxication, sarcoidosis, "milk-alkali syndrome," and most importantly with the hypercalcemias of certain malignancies (multiple myeloma, lymphoproliferative disorders, and tumors responsive to steroids). There is no response in the overwhelming majority of patients with hyperparathyroidism. Glucocorticoids are felt to decrease abnormally elevated intestinal absorption of calcium by antagonizing the effect of vitamin D and to decrease both bone turnover and renal tubular calcium reabsorption.

Dialysis. Hemodialysis or peritoneal dialysis against a calcium-free dialysate has the advantages of (1) speed, (2) efficacy in the absence of renal function, (3) not requiring deposition of calcium into extraskeletal tissues for its effect, and (4) minimizing the need for toxic or dangerous medications. Grams of calcium can be removed from the body within hours of hemodialysis. One should attempt to lower blood calcium at a moderate rate since too rapid a reduction is hazardous. Determination of blood levels is the guide to therapy.

EDTA. For completeness, the use of a calcium-chelating agent must be mentioned. Disodium EDTA chelates free ionized calcium, reducing very swiftly the level of the active fraction of plasma calcium, independent of urinary excretion. However, it can cause severe renal damage and is used only in cases of life-threatening cardiac arrhythmias. The usual dose is 50 mg/kg of body weight given over four to six hours. Its use should not be continued any longer than necessary to control the cardiac arrhythmias. One gram of disodium EDTA will complex about 120 mg of calcium ion,[9] but the complex continues to circulate in the bloodstream until cleared by the kidney. The measurement of changes in the total serum calcium, therefore, will not reflect fluctuations of the biologically active ionized fraction when EDTA is present. Therefore, calcium monitoring depends on determination of free calcium by the calcium activity electrode or total non-EDTA-bound calcium by EDTA titration. This methodology is cumbersome and not readily available.

Mithramycin. Mithramycin, available as Mithracin, is a cytotoxic drug related to actinomycin D, which was being given as cancer chemotherapy (particularly for testicular tumors) when its hypocalcemic properties were first noted. The drug diminishes bone resorption in addition to its antitumor effects. The doses now given to control hypercalcemia are significantly lower than those used in cancer chemotherapy, but a debate over the safety of the drug continues. It is clear that in many cases it can safely reduce serum calcium and maintain it within the normal range with intermittent infusions of 25 μg/kg of body weight. One effective regimen is to add the mithramycin to 1,000 ml of 5% dextrose and water and infuse it slowly over three hours; direct slow injection of the full dose may increase the nausea but is also frequently used. Intermittent administration when serum calcium rises again above the normal range (within 7 to 14 days) usually reduces the serum calcium within 36 hours. Because of the long duration of action, more frequent administration carries the potential risk of inducing hypocalcemia. A lowering of serum calcium by several milligrams per 100 ml is usually seen in one to four days.

Nausea and vomiting are frequent side effects of mithramycin therapy; this can occur anytime up to six hours after the infusion and last for several hours thereafter. Prochlorperazine helps to reduce these effects. More seriously, however, mithramycin can cause reversible thrombocytopenia, and renal and hepatocellular damage.

At present, mithramycin is used only in the hypercalcemia of steroid-resistant malignancy because of its dangerous side effects. In addition, its slow onset of action makes it of no value in emergency situations. Sodium infusion, diuretics, oral phosphates, steroids, and sulfates should all be used before the decision is made to administer mithramycin.

Calcitonin. Calcitonin is not currently available for general use in the treatment of hypercalcemia. Theoretically it appears to be indicated in every patient with hypercalcemia associated with increased bone resorption. In the few studies currently available a moderate decrease in serum calcium is usually noted following the infusion of calcitonin; the drug is particularly efficacious in severely hypercalcemic patients. The optimal dose and a clear formulation of its efficacy are as yet unknown. Salmon calcitonin, which is even more potent than human calcitonin, has been used in most studies. As little as 0.1 μg has been reported to have significant effects in humans.

Treatment plan. The primary decisions to be made when confronted with a patient with hypercalcemia are to determine the severity of the calcium elevation and to estimate the immediate danger to the patient's life. Only if the patient is in immediate danger of death due to cardiovascular complications of hypercalcemia should one consider the administration of EDTA. It is almost never used because of its renal complications. If a critically ill patient has impaired renal function, arrangements for hemodialysis should be made immediately while proceeding with initial hydration and administration of oral phosphates as described below.

In any but the above situations the therapy outlined below should initially be considered. The doses and special considerations of each treatment have been previously discussed.

1. Hydrate the patient with half normal (0.45%) or normal (0.9%) saline until the CVP is 10 cm of water; then continue 0.9% saline to initiate enhanced calciuresis.
2. If the hypercalcemia is severe and not dropping with saline diuresis alone, one might consider furosemide with prompt replacement of urinary fluid and electrolyte losses as previously described.
3. Administer oral phosphates every six hours. If the patient cannot take oral medication, administer phosphates via rectal enema.
4. Initiate corticosteroid therapy if the cause of hypercalcemia is one of those thought to be steroid responsive.
5. If hypercalcemia persists and renal function is good, consider a trial of sodium sulfate therapy.
6. In patients with malignancies in which the hypercalcemia is refractory to all other therapeutic modalities, mithramycin may be considered.

During the management of hypercalcemia it is important to keep the patient in meticulous fluid and electrolyte balance during the manipulations. The patient should be followed with cardiac monitoring. Digoxin should not be given because of its increased cardiac toxicity in the face of hypercalcemia; if the patient is already taking digoxin, further drugs should be withheld. The patient should be placed on a low-calcium diet prophylactically.

Another important consideration is that too rapid a decrease in serum calcium itself may produce hypotension, cardiac failure, and renal failure. Therefore, the goal of therapy is not to decrease serum calcium to the low normal range (e.g., to drop from 16 mg/100 ml to 9 mg/100 ml) over 24 hours, but rather to slowly lower the serum calcium concentration. Since the onset of action of most modes of therapy requires more than 24 hours, this is usually not a problem.

The patient will subsequently require therapy directed at maintaining a normal serum calcium level, which generally involves oral phosphates, loop diuretics, and definitive treatment of the underlying disease.

HYPOCALCEMIA

Hypocalcemia is an uncommon endocrine emergency and has multiple etiologies. A partial list of some of the diseases that can be present with hypocalcemia includes hypoparathyroidism and pseudo-hypoparathyroidism; vitamin D deficiency, "vitamin D resistance"; hyperphosphatemia; malabsorption; acute pancreatitis; hypomagnesemia; renal tubular acidosis; Fanconi syndrome; and renal failure. A decrease in the ionized calcium with normal serum calcium concentrations is seen in alkalosis (e.g., with hyperventilation, loss of gastric acid as with excessive vomiting, or administration of large amounts of alkali) and may, therefore, produce symptoms of hypocalcemia.

Signs and symptoms

A major clinical finding in patients with hypocalcemia is tetany, due to increased neuromuscular irritability. This is generally seen when serum calcium approaches 7 mg/100 ml or less. The patient may complain of numbness and tingling in the perioral and acral regions. Latent tetany can be elicited by tapping over the facial nerve to elicit a positive Chvostek's sign in which twitching of the mouth, nasolabial fold, and eyelids may be seen. A more specific and reliable finding is Trousseau's sign in which flexion of metacarpophalangeal and carpometacarpal joints, interphalangeal extension, and thumb adduction become evident within three to four minutes after occlusion of the brachial artery using a blood pressure cuff inflated to above systolic pressure; the test may be made more sensitive by concomitant hyperventilation (von Bonsdorff's phenomenon). Bizarre mentation or other manifestations of increased neuromuscular irritability should further suggest the presence of hypocalcemia. Hypotension and renal failure may result from hypocalcemia, making the treatment of acute symptomatic hypocalcemia a medical emergency.

Hypocalcemia should be particularly suspected following parathyroid surgery, thyroidectomy, or any other surgical procedures in the neck. Laboratory data obtained immediately should include BUN, creatinine, sodium, potassium, chloride, CO_2, calcium (with ionized calcium, if available), phosphorus, and magnesium. An ECG should be obtained and prolongation of the QT interval specifically looked for. Tetany has been reported with hypokalemia, which may also promote alkalosis, and with hypomagnesemia, which can promote hypocalcemia by inhibition of parathyroid hormone release and effect.

Treatment

Therapy is based upon clinical judgment of the severity of the hypocalcemia. If hyperventilation alone is suspected as a cause of symptomatic tetany, the patient is asked to rebreathe from a paper bag, and evidence of symptomatic improvement is sought. However, if more serious hypocalcemia is present, administration of 10 to 30 ml of 10% calcium gluconate intravenously over 10 to 15 minutes is indicated. Further titration can be achieved by adjustment of an intravenous infusion containing 10 to 30 ml of 10% calcium gluconate in 500 ml normal saline. The total calcium required may be quite high. For example, in patients undergoing parathyroid surgery for hyperparathyroidism, the postoperative course may be complicated by severe and protracted hypocalcemia, secondary to avid calcium deposition in diseased bone in conjunction with suppressed parathyroid function. Under these circumstances, as much as 15 mg/kg of body weight of calcium may be required over a period of several hours. In the presence of hypomagnesemia, frequently seen in patients with hypocalcemia, magnesium sulfate replacement may also be required. This can be accomplished by administration of 50% magnesium sulfate (4 mEq/ml) in a dose of 2 to 4 ml intramuscularly every 12 hours. Calcium replacement can be guided by frequent determinations of serum calcium.

The patient is hospitalized for continued control, diagnosis, and institution of adequate oral calcium supplementation, vitamin D therapy if indicated, and treatment of any underlying disorder.

HYPERTENSIVE CRISIS

Emergency treatment for hypertension is required when the diastolic blood pressure exceeds 150 mm Hg (even in the absence of symptoms), or when pulmonary edema, cerebral hemorrhage, or encephalopathy develops in a patient with moderate elevations in blood pressure (diastolic pressure > 120 mm Hg).

Signs and symptoms

Approximately 5% of patients with either essential or secondary hypertension develop a malignant phase requiring emergency therapy.[10] Symptoms are frequently neurologic (severe headache, vomiting, visual disturbances, transient blindness, paralysis, convulsions, stupor, and coma) and cardiorenal with full-blown pulmonary edema and oliguria.

Physical examination is remarkable for marked elevation in blood pressure, papilledema, hyperreflexia, and signs attributed to the magnitude of neurologic or cardiac decompensation.

Laboratory data should include electrolytes, BUN, creatinine, calcium, and complete blood count (with examination of the peripheral smear to look for evidence of microangiopathic hemolytic anemia).

Treatment

The aim of therapy should be to gently lower the blood pressure *toward* normal, but not below. A diastolic pressure of 90 to 95 mm Hg should be low enough to alleviate the acute emergency situation.

Drugs with immediate onset of action (minutes)

Nitroprusside. Nitroprusside is a potent peripheral vasodilator (arterial and venous) and highly effective in allowing instantaneous control over the blood pressure. Aside from its relief of systolic afterload, it has the added benefit of promoting venous pooling, which will be helpful in the treatment of the patient in pulmonary edema. Nitroprusside is given by an intravenous infusion of 0.5 to 8 μg/kg/min and carefully monitored based on repeated blood pressure determinations.

Diazoxide (Hyperstat). Diazoxide (Hyperstat) is another vasodilator whose advantage lies in its ease of administration. A dose of 300 mg is administered rapidly intravenously; an effect is seen within minutes and lasts for several hours. The dose can then be repeated. Because of its sodium-retaining properties, a diuretic should be administered simultaneously (e.g., furosemide, 40 mg orally). Rare complications include significant hyperglycemia and profound hypotension.[11]

Trimethaphan (Arfonad). Trimethaphan (Arfonad) is a ganglionic blocker with a rapid onset of action. An intravenous solution of 500 mg in 500 ml D5/W (1 mg/ml) can be administered at an initial rate of 3 to 4 mg/min and adjusted based on the blood pressure response.

Drugs with a delayed onset of action (> 30 minutes). Several drugs in this category have the advantage of effectiveness upon oral as well as parenteral administration and can be used for long-term management of hypertension.

Methyldopa. Methyldopa, 500 to 1,000 mg IV, is given over 30 minutes and every six hours until the blood pressure is stabilized. Oral administration is frequently as effective and may be substituted as soon as blood pressure control is obtained.

Hydralazine. Hydralazine, 10 mg IV or IM, is given every 10 to 15 minutes as needed up to 50 mg; then the total dose may be repeated every six hours or substituted orally. To lessen the reflex tachycardia, propranolol, 20 mg orally, may be given before initiation of hydralazine therapy. Caution is advised in the use of hydralazine in patients with ischemic heart disease, and propranolol in patients with congestive heart failure.

Adjuncts to therapy. Adjuncts to therapy include intravenous diuretics and digitalis if congestive heart failure is present. If pheochromocytoma is suspected (an uncommon form of hypertension, and an even more unusual cause of hypertensive crisis), drugs that may release stored catecholamines (methyldopa, reserpine, guanethidine) should be avoided.

REFERENCES

1. Lipsett, M. B., and Pearson, O.H.: Pathophysiology and treatment of adrenal crisis, N. Engl. J. Med. **254:**511-514, 1956.
2. Thorn, G. W., and Lauler, D. P.: Clinical therapeutics of adrenal disorders, Am. J. Med. **53:**673-684, 1972.
3. McArthur, J. W., Rawson, R. W., Means, J. H., and Cope, O.: Thyrotoxic crisis, J.A.M.A. **134:**868-874, 1947.
4. Waldstein, S. S., Slodki, S. J., Kaganiec, G. I., and Bronsky, D.: A clinical study of thyroid storm, Ann. Intern. Med. **52:**626-642, 1960.
5. Ingbar, S. H.: Management of emergencies. IX. Thyrotoxic storm, N. Engl. J. Med. **274:**1252-1254, 1966.
6. Mackin, J. F., Canary, J. J., and Pittman, C. S.: Thyroid storm and its management, N. Engl. J. Med. **291:**1396-1398, 1974.
7. Blum, M.: Myxedema coma, Am. J. Med. Sci. **264:**432-443, 1972.
8. Goldsmith, R. S.: Treatment of hypercalcemia, Med. Clin. North Am. **56:**951-960, 1972.
9. American Hospital Formulay Service. American Society of Hospital Pharmacists, Washington, D.C., 1977.
10. Jagger, P. I., and Braunwald, E.: Hypertensive vascular disease. In Thorn, G. W., Adams, R. D., Braunwald, E., Isselbacher, K. J., and Petersdorf, R. G., editors: Harrison's principles of internal medicine, New York, 1977, McGraw-Hill Book Co., pp. 1307-1318.
11. Nies, A. S.: Adverse reactions and interactions limiting the use of antihypertensive drugs, Am. J. Med. **58:**495-503, 1975.

CHAPTER **10**

Transfusion practices

Stewart E. Dadmun, M.D.

Emergency departments across the country are giving more transfusions of blood and blood products and rightly so. Transfusion of severe trauma cases while awaiting definitive treatment elsewhere in the hospital is a well-established procedure. More emergency departments are becoming established as transfusion centers where patients with chronic, intermittent blood needs can be served on a come-and-go basis, thereby avoiding hospitalization. This increasing role in the use of blood and blood products makes it important for personnel to be familiar with transfusion techniques.

HARVEST AND STORAGE

Blood is a tissue that is transplanted from the donor to a needy recipient. Approximately 450 ml of blood is drawn from a donor, mixed with a preservative anticoagulant mixture (usually acid citric dextrose [ACD] solution) and put in containers. Plastic bags have replaced glass bottles in most areas, decreasing the chance of pyogenic reactions and air embolism. Up to 70% of the red cells can be kept viable for three weeks in a blood bank refrigerator at 1° to 5° C.[1,2] After 21 days blood is considered outdated and is not used for transfusion. Frozen blood has the advantage of longer bank life. It is available in some areas on a limited basis but is not yet available for general use because of technical and cost problems.

TYPE AND CROSSMATCH

To avoid serious reactions blood must be matched to each patient. Everyone's blood carries several membrane antigen systems which determine that person's blood type. The plasma carries natural antibodies to some of these antigens. A person may develop acquired antibodies to the antigens of other peoples' blood.[3]

The best known antigen system is the ABO system. Most people have either A or B antigen or neither (type O) on their red cells. These same people will have antibodies against the antigens of this system that they do not carry on their own red cells (Table 10-1).

The Rh system is made up of several

Table 10-1. ABO system of red blood cell antigens

Red cell antigen	Serum antibody	Patient type
A	Anti B	A
B	Anti A	B
A and B	None	AB
O	Anti A and B	O

red cell antigens: C, D, E, c, and e. An individual may inherit one of the upper or lower case antigens of each letter from either parent. "Rh positive" refers to the presence of the highly antigenic D antigen. Anti-Rh antigens do not occur naturally but develop after previous transfusions with nonmatched blood or during pregnancy with a fetus of a different Rh type. Several other antigen systems of lesser importance are known but will not be discussed here.

Red cell typing is carried out with commercial antibody preparations, which clump the red cells containing type-specific antigens. Serum from a type A patient will clump with donor type B cells, because A patient's serum has antibodies against the B antigens on the donor's cells. This fact forms the basis for the standard crossmatch. This procedure requires that the donor cells be incubated with the patient's serum (major crossmatch) and that the patient's cells be incubated with the donor's serum (minor crossmatch). By varying the conditions of these mixtures, potentially dangerous incompatability can be detected by observing clumping of either the patient's or donor's cells. Once the unit has been successfully crossmatched, it should be safe to give to the patient.

It is often important to give blood in a hurry and the 30 to 45 minute delay required for the crossmatch is frustrating. In such instances it is tempting to give type O negative blood. This type blood presumably carries no antigens to which the patient might react. This would satisfy the needs of the major crossmatch mentioned above. However, this seemingly safe procedure is not totally without a hazard. Remember that all type O blood contains anti-A and anti-B antibodies. Emergency type O, Rh-negative transfusions can have commercially available A and B antigen added to neutralize these antibodies. Nonetheless, one of the other lesser antibody systems might cause a problem in such an un-

crossmatched transfusion. Obviously, the risk of delay must be weighed against the risk of a transfusion reaction in such situations.

ADVERSE REACTIONS

Even when the crossmatching procedures show compatibility between donor and patient, several things can go wrong when blood is transfused. People who take responsibility for monitoring transfusions must be aware of the potential problems and what to do about them.[4] The following section outlines some of these potential problems. How these difficulties can occur is discussed in a later section.

Immediate reaction

The immediate hemolytic reaction is the most dreaded side effect of transfusion. Hemolytic reactions may be either immediate or delayed. An immediate reaction usually occurs in the first 30 minutes or during administration of the first 50 ml of the transfusion. It is heralded by fever, back or chest pain, nausea, and vomiting. Hypotension and dyspnea may be noted. If the transfusion is not discontinued immediately, profound signs of hemolysis such as hemoglobulinuria, jaundice, and renal shutdown may supervene. The patient may also develop generalized signs of bleeding as clotting factors are consumed by the hemolytic reaction.[5] The most common cause of such reactions is donor-patient ABO incompatibility, although patients previously strongly sensitized to Rh or other antigens may experience this reaction without incompatibility of the ABO system. In such a serious reaction the major crossmatch would be expected to be positive (donor's cells–patient's serum). Minor crossmatching incompatibilities may cause this reaction as well if the patient's red cells become coated with enough antibody to cause lysis in circulation.

The presence of the hemolytic type reaction is confirmed by demonstrating free hemoglobin in the patient's plasma. A gently spun sample of the patient's blood may show pink plasma or serum. Hemoglobin in the urine is an ominous diagnostic sign. Treatment consists of immediate discontinuation of the transfusion, followed by blood pressure support with agents that do not impede renal blood flow. A urine output of 60 ml per hour minimum is encouraged by the use of such diuretics as Mannitol and Lasix.[6] A repeat of the crossmatch will usually demonstrate the incompatibility. Most fatalities reported from transfusions occur with this reaction.

Delayed reaction

The delayed hemolytic transfusion reaction may occur from hours to weeks after the blood is given. The patient may develop anemia, malaise, and mild to moderate jaundice. This reaction occurs when red cells are coated only with enough antibody to sensitize them to phagocytosis in the reticuloendothelial system of the liver, spleen, and marrow. The lysis of red cells occurs outside the vascular space with this type of reaction. This condition may be difficult to differentiate from autoimmune hemolytic anemia. If the reaction occurs late enough, hepatitis may be suspected. Careful evaluation of the patient should lead to the correct diagnosis. Usually no specific treatment is required for delayed hemolysis.

Allergic reactions

Fortunately, hemolytic reactions are rare. Allergic reactions are much more common. These reactions usually start with fever. Patients with the allergic reaction should not have a shaking chill. Usually such a chill indicates a more serious problem (i.e., hemolytic reaction or sepsis). Bothersome pruritus or urticarial rashes are common. Nausea and chest and back pain may occur. Rarely, there may be dyspnea from bronchospasm or an angioedema-like reaction, which may compromise the airway by causing swelling of oropharyngeal tissues.

Allergic reactions may occur by one of three mechanisms. (1) Occasionally patients who have been transfused several times develop allergies to serum proteins foreign to their own. (2) The donor's white cells and platelets may contain different antigen systems from the red cells. Typing white cells and platelets is not practical in routine transfusion practice, and occasionally allergies to these cellular elements develop and cause reactions. (3) Finally, it is possible for the donor to have circulating allergic antibodies that will react to a substance recently eaten by the recipient and vice versa.[7] These reactions usually can be managed effectively with antipyretics and antihistamines. Occasionally, epinephrine is needed. Transfusions with buffy-coat-poor blood or packed or washed red blood cells may prevent or diminish allergic reactions. Such precautions may be necessary in patients who have previously had a more serious allergic transfusion reaction.

Transmission of infected material

One dreaded complication of transfusions is the transmission of infected material.[8] Blood is an excellent culture medium; bacteria may be picked up from the skin of the donor at the time the needle is inserted into the vein. Organisms that grow well at low temperatures, such as *Pseudomonas*, can grow in great numbers in the bank blood. A transfusion of such a contaminated unit causes rapid signs of sepsis, such as chills, fever, hypotension, and shock. Vigorous resuscitative methods with antibiotics, corticosteroids, and antihypotensive agents are usually not successful in saving these unfortunate patients. Units of blood that show cloudy plasma, extensive hemolysis, or a brown or unusual purple color should be suspected as harboring infection.

Hepatitis

A common hazard of transfusion is the transmission of hepatitis, either the serum or infectious type.[9] Development of testing methods that can demonstrate the hepatitis-associated antigen (Australia antigen) has eliminated many units of blood which otherwise would have caused hepatitis.[10] Unfortunately, this test has not been refined to the point that it will pick up all units transmitting serum hepatitis (hepatitis B). This test is of no value for finding units that might transmit the infectious hepatitis virus (hepatitis A). Until a more perfect means of checking blood for hepatitis is available, this disease must be confined by a combination of using currently available testing methods and careful selection of donors. It is well known that volunteer donors are much less likely to harbor hepatitis than paid donors.

Other reactions

All transfused blood is checked for signs of syphilis with routine serologic studies. Nonetheless, it is possible for syphilis to be transmitted by transfusion if infection is so recent that blood studies are negative. Fortunately, the pesky spirochete cannot survive at low temperatures for more than 72 hours. Transfusion must be a very uncommon way to contract this disease. Another infection rarely transmitted in transfusions is malaria.[11]

BLOOD COMPONENT TRANSFUSION

The term "blood transfusion" usually conveys the idea of giving a patient whole blood. Whole blood is actually made up of several separable components, which may be given individually as needed, saving the rest of the whole blood unit for other purposes.[12] The capacity to separate whole blood into components has drastically limited the indications for whole blood transfusions.[13] However, whole blood must be given when transfusion is indicated for the patient who is losing whole blood.

Risks of multiunit blood transfusion

Bleeding tendencies. Occasionally, massive bleeding will require the transfusion of several times the patient's blood volume in whole blood. Massive transfusions of stored whole blood do not replace those blood components which become inactivated during storage. The most notable examples of these labile factors are the components of blood necessary for clotting. Low levels of viable platelets and certain clotting factors (notably factors V and VIII) in bank blood can lead to a generalized bleeding tendency during or following multiunit transfusions.

Potassium in plasma. Another potential problem can arise from the fact that red cells which normally lyse during storage release large quantities of potassium into the unit's plasma. Tranfusions of this potassium-laden plasma in large quantity may lead to serious hyperkalemia. This is a particular problem in patients who have impaired renal function or who have other reasons for a high serum potassium, such as a crush injury of a major extremity.

Lack of calcium. The citrate in ACD solution is added to units of blood in greater quantity than is needed to complex the calcium to prevent clotting of donor blood. The lack of calcium available to the patient in transfused blood, as well as the calcium-complexing capacity of this excess citrate, may lead to tetany.

2,3-DPG depletion. Stored whole blood develops depletion of 2,3-diphosphoglycerate (2,3-DPG), a moleclule closely linked to the red cell's capacity to give its oxygen to the tissues. Many units of 2,3-DPG-deficient transfused blood may deprive the patient's tissue of oxygen desperately needed in a state of massive bleeding, shock, sepsis, and so forth. Fortunately, 2,3-DPG will increase in these transfused red cells after they have had a chance to circulate for several hours in their new host.

Other risks. The complications of serious

hypothermia may result from the rapid transfusion of large volumes of blood taken directly from the refrigerator. Also, large volume transfusions carry the risk of overloading the recipient's cardiovascular system; congestive heart failure and pulmonary edema are dangers in older patients and in patients with heart disease who must undergo transfusion.[4]

Rapid transfusions

When rapid transfusion of more than six units of whole blood is indicated, the following guidelines should be observed:

1. Give two units of fresh blood as the seventh and eighth pints transfused, and give two units of fresh blood for every six units thereafter. This precaution helps to replace the platelets and clotting factors lost in bank blood.

2. Patients undergoing massive transfusions should have ECG monitoring. A prolonged ST segment and falling T wave may point to calcium complexing by citrate. The serum calcium level available from laboratory studies is of no help here because it is a measure of both bound and unbound calcium. Signs of tetany, such as muscular twitching and carpopedal spasm, may be followed rapidly by seizures because adequate calcium is not available to the central nervous system. Giving 1 ampule of 10% calcium gluconate intravenously with the two units of blood given after six units should compensate for the rapidly infused citrate.

3. Peaking of T waves on the ECG and a rising serum potassium level indicate that any additional rapidly given units of blood should be fresh whole blood, packed red cells, or washed red cells in order to prevent a further and possibly dangerous rise in the serum potassium level. (Incidentally, the circumstances mentioned in this section and in No. 1 are about the only times fresh blood is ever needed.)[14]

4. By the time six units have been rapidly transfused, central temperature monitoring should begin, and arrangements should be made to warm future blood units if the patient's temperature begins to fall.

5. The need for further rapid transfusion should be reassessed if there is a normal or high central venous pressure. Should further blood transfusion be required, one should seriously consider decreasing the rate of infusion to 0.5 ml/kg/hour.

6. Oxygen transport impairment caused by low levels of red cell 2,3-DPG may be helped slightly by administering nasal oxygen. Maneuvers that might cause systemic alkalosis (hyperventilation, bicarbonate administration, etc.) tend to accentuate the low 2,3-DPG oxygen transport problems and should be avoided when possible.

PACKED CELLS

A patient who is not rapidly losing whole blood generally need not be transfused with whole blood. Some form of packed red cells is better therapy for the patient with a slowly progressive anemia. Most patients with such anemia need not be transfused at all until they begin to show signs of cardiovascular compromise.[15] Packed cells lessen the volume overload risk, which might put such patients into congestive failure. Another advantage of packed red cells is a decrease in the risk of hepatitis transmission. In addition, elimination of donor plasma essentially eliminates the possibility of a donor plasma vs. patient red cells type hemolytic reaction. Furthermore, the patient is exposed to fewer plasma antigens which might induce an allergic reaction.

Giving buffy-coat-poor blood further decreases the risk of white cell and platelet allergic reactions. Buffy-coat-poor blood should be the transfusion of choice to patients who may require organ transplantation in the future. White cells contain antigens that overlap with tissue antigens and may cause patient sensitization, which could decrease the chance of a successful transplantation "take." Transfusing one of the forms of packed cells allows the blood bank to use the donor's plasma and platelets for other purposes.

Washed red cells are rarely necessary. They are used in patients suffering from hemolytic reactions that might be accelerated by the donor's complement (i.e., cold agglutinin hemolysis, paroxysmal nocturnal hemoglobinuria, etc.). In order to wash red cells, the unit must be opened and washing solution added, which increases the risk of bacterial contamination.

PLATELETS

Patients with thrombocytopenia caused by marrow failure (i.e., aplastic anemia, leukemia, and aplasia from marrow-toxic drugs) may need platelet transfusions.[16] From 40% to 50% of a blood unit's platelets can be expected to be viable up to 24 hours after donation. Platelets removed from such blood as platelet-rich plasma or platelet concentrates have better viability at room temperature than at low temperatures.[17] Platelet packs kept at 22° C can be of value up to 72 hours following preparation. One must bear in mind the fact that there is an increased risk of transmitting bacterial infection with platelet packs kept at room temperature.

The decision to transfuse thrombocytopenic patients with platelets often cannot safely wait until life-threatening bleeding occurs. Nonetheless, predicting such bleeding danger from the platelet count can be a chancy business. Generally, a platelet count above 25,000 will prevent spontaneous bleeding. Counts in excess of 50,000 should protect against bleeding from surgical or accidental trauma. These figures naturally assume normal platelet function. Patients with a rapid platelet turnover, as in idiopathic thrombocytopenia, generally do not bleed so readily at the same level of thrombocytopenia as do patients with impaired platelet production, as in aplastic anemia. The fact that platelet transfusions are virtually ineffective in the rapid-turnover thrombocytopenias makes their use in these disorders unusual. Infections and exceedingly high leukemic white counts increase the risk of thrombocytopenic bleeding. Platelets have a normal life span of 8 to 10 days; frequently repeated transfusions are often necessary. Repeated platelet transfusions from random donors sooner or later lead to platelet isoantibodies in the recipient, which limit the effectiveness of subsequent transfusions.

Platelet typing is possible but because of the many platelet antigen systems different from red cells, platelet crossmatches are not routinely used. Tissue typing of donor and recipient by the HL-A lymphocyte tissue matching method tends to avoid isoantibody induction. Unfortunately, a random donor has only about one chance in a thousand of matching a given patient's HL-A type. A sibling has about one chance in four. Repeated platelet phoresis of as much as one half of the circulating platelets of an HL-A–matched sibling is an increasingly practical way to transfuse this blood component without risk of isoantibody induction. Because of the high risk of isoantibody production, non–HL-A matched platelets should be used only for severe need. As a rule, platelet transfusions are indicated in the marrow failure type of thrombocytopenia at a platelet count of about 10,000 in noninfected patients, and at a platelet count of 20,000 in the presence of sepsis. The platelets from eight donated blood units will raise an adult's platelet count about 50,000 in the absence of isoantibodies. Four units can be expected to do about the same in a child.

WHITE BLOOD CELLS

To date, there is no generally available way to transfuse these fragile and skittish cellular blood elements. So far, white blood cell transfusions are limited to centers with specialized cell separating equipment.[18]

WHOLE PLASMA OR SERUM ALBUMIN

Plasma or albumin supplementations may be needed when the infusion of colloid is indicated for expansion of the plasma volume, as in treatment of septic shock, burns, and the like.[19] Units of pooled plasma that have been obtained from many donors carry a high risk of transmitted hepatitis. Freshly frozen plasma from individual donors decreases this risk. Plasma should either be matched for ABO type or supplemented with A and B antigen substance in order to avoid hemolytic reactions of the minor crossmatched type. Human albumin can be separated from plasma, lyophilized, and treated so as to essentially eliminate the hepatitis danger. Its main drawback is relatively high cost. One should consider other safe and readily available volume replacement agents such as electrolyte and dextran solutions before deciding to use human plasma or albumin for replacement therapy.[20]

CLOTTING SUBSTANCES

Fresh plasma or fresh frozen plasma contains close to the original donor levels of the usual clotting factors. Fresh plasma has been used for years to treat the bleeding problems of hemophiliacs and other patients with nonthrombocytopenic bleeding disorders.[21] A major drawback of plasma in such treatment situations is the high volume of this substance needed to raise the patient's deficient clotting factor to a level that will stanch bleeding. In recent years it has been possible to separate several clotting factors from native plasma and to concentrate these fractions into small volumes.

The most commonly used clotting factors in transfusion practice are preparations containing factors VIII and IX and fibrinogen (Fig. 10-1).

Hemophilia

Patients with severe hemophilia may have less than 1% of the normal amount of factor VIII in their plasma. These low levels are often responsible for spontaneous bleeding problems. The most common sites of such bleeding are the major joints. Repeated, uncontrolled, joint bleeding may lead to crippling joint deformities. Elevation of a hemophiliac's factor VIII level to as low as 5% to 10% of normal may

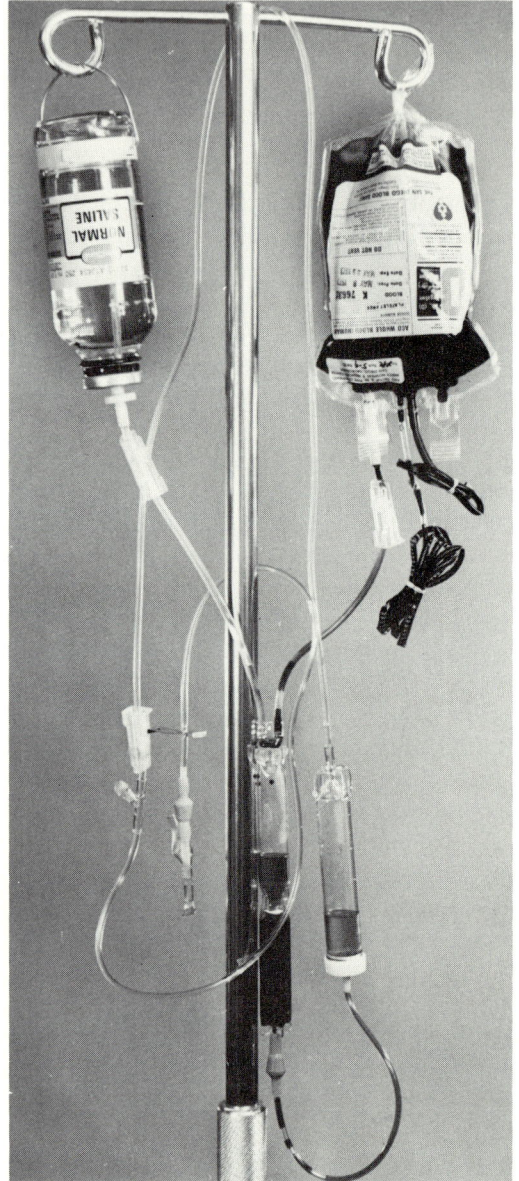

Fig. 10-1. Blood infusion setup with filter.

stop this bleeding. Elevations to 25% can even permit minor surgery, such as tooth extractions, without excessive bleeding. From 25% to 50% levels of factor VIII should prove sufficiently hemostatic for even major injuries or surgery. One may calculate the number of factor VIII units needed to raise a patient's antihemophiliac factor to a desired level in the following way: One unit is considered to be the amount of clotting factor present in 1 ml of normal plasma.[21] Commercial factor VIII concentrates are assayed and then labeled with the number of units they contain. Cryoprecipitate concentrates of factor VIII prepared at local blood banks usually have between 70 and 100 units of factor VIII per bag.[22] Commercially prepared antihemophilic factor concentrate now contains approximately 1,000 AHF units per 30 ml (Hemofil). This supplies large doses without excessively overloading the patient's circulatory system. A useful formula for calculating the number of units of factor VIII required is:

$$\text{Units factor VIII} = (\text{Desired factor VIII level} - \text{Initial factor VIII level}) \times \text{Plasma volume} \\ (\text{about 41 ml/kg})$$

The above figure should be increased by 25% to account for the factor VIII lost in the extravascular space. If one plans to give factor VIII every 12 hours, the initial postinfusion level of this factor should be about twice the desired level in anticipation of its 12-hour half-life.

A condition called von Willebrand's disease is a fairly common complex inherited clotting disorder, which is associated with low levels of factor VIII. Transfusion therapy in this condition is similar to classic hemophilia with the important exception that fresh plasma or factor VIII concentrates contain an "anti–von Willebrand's factor," which tends to induce these patients to make their own factor VIII after a 12 to 24 hour delay.[23] Therefore, patients with von Willebrand's disease should receive less than the calculated dose of factor VIII.

Christmas disease (hemophilia B)

This is a less common type of hemophilia, which is caused by an inherited deficiency of factor IX. Like classic hemophilia, it is transmitted as an X-linked recessive trait and is, therefore, a disorder essentially limited to males. Its clinical presentation is identical to hemophilia A. Hemophilia B is only about one-eighth as common as classic hemophilia. Factor IX concentrates or plasma are given in much the same way as previously described for factor VIII.[24] Factor IX has a longer half-life (approximately 24 hours) than factor VIII, but more (50% or more) of this clotting substance seems to leave the vascular space and is, therefore, unavailable for general distribution following infusion. The factor VIII formula already presented is modified to add 50% more units than calculated based on plasma volume. This increased requirement for factor IX is offset by the fact that these infusions can be stretched out to every 24 hours if the desired level is the same as in the formula given for factor VIII deficiency.

Several other inherited clotting disorders have been described but are so rare that they will not be discussed here.[21]

Oral anticoagulants

Factor IX concentrates are rich in the clotting factors depleted by oral anticoagulants such as Dicumarol and Warfarin. These same clotting factors (i.e., prothrombin and factors VII, IX, and X) are also depleted in severe liver disease. Severe bleeding associated with prolonged prothrombin times in patients on oral anticoagulants or suffering from severe liver disease can be stopped more rapidly with factor IX concentrates than with vitamin K.[25] Furthermore, vitamin K has an effect on the prothrombin time for up to three weeks. The delayed effectiveness of vitamin K makes it less desirable in the acute situation, and its prolonged effect may be undesirable if one plans to return the patient to oral anticoagulant therapy. Transfused factor IX concentrate clotting factors have the advantage of providing an immediate improvement of the prothrombin time which lasts only a few hours.

Fibrinogen

Fibrinogen can be extracted and concentrated from many units of plasma. However, there is high risk of hepatitis transmission with this substance. A high incidence of serum hepatitis is noted following infusions of factor IX concentrate

as well. Improved methods of treating fibrinogenopenic states have markedly decreased the need for direct infusions of this clotting factor.

TRANSFUSION TECHNIQUE

It is usually best to start a blood transfusion into an infusion of normal saline which is already running freely. It is not wise to use 5% dextrose solutions for this purpose, because they cause lysis of red cells, which makes a gummy mass in the tubing. Transfusion intravenous equipment should be used exclusively. This type of intravenous set-up has a filter that catches any small clots of cells or fibrin that may have formed in the unit of blood (Fig. 10-2). Blood transfusion intravenous

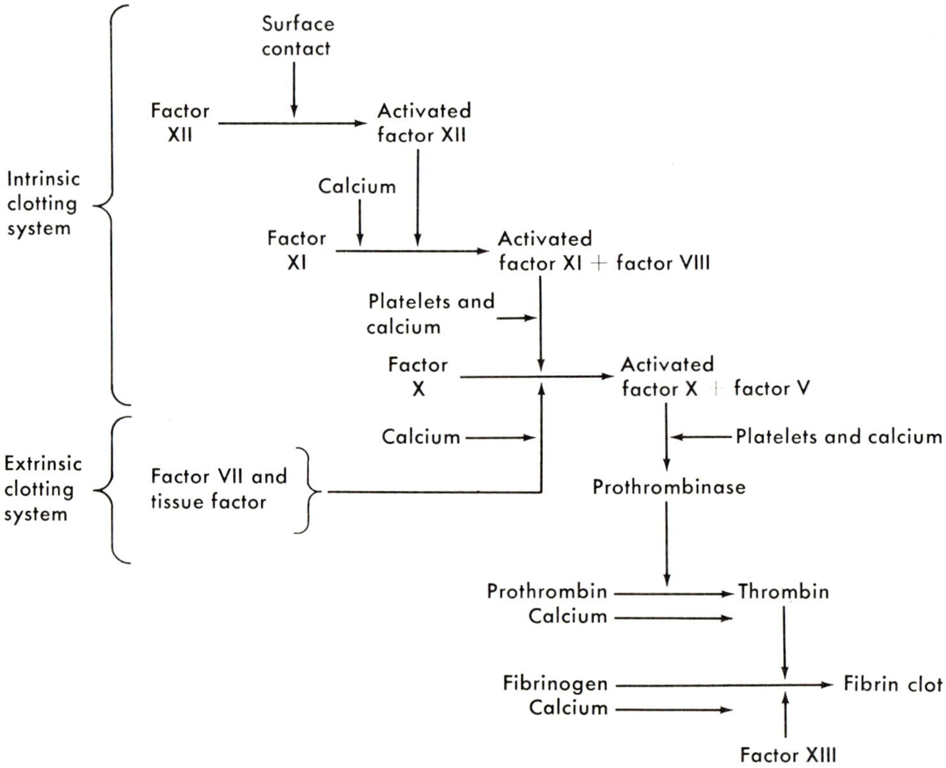

Fig. 10-2. Clotting sequence. Classical hemophilia (hemophilia A) and von Willebrand's pseudohemophilia have defects in factor VIII. Christmas disease (hemophilia B) has a defect in factor IX. Oral anticoagulants such as Warfarin and Dicumarol deplete factors VII, IX, X, and prothrombin. (These latter factors are all found in commercial preparations of factor IX.) The other factors listed here may be depleted in rare inherited bleeding disorders.

tubing should be changed at least every eight hours because of the danger of infection developing in the small clots trapped on the intravenous filter. If blood is to be given rapidly, a large needle should be used. However, small gauge needles can be used safely for slower infusions. One must keep in mind the danger of bacterial growth in a unit of blood kept at room temperature for a long period of time. For this reason blood should not be outside the blood bank refrigerator more than four hours before it is transfused into the patient.

The need for careful identification of the patient cannot be overemphasized. This identification must be clear, both at the time the blood is drawn for crossmatch and at the time the unit of blood is started for transfusion. Require the conscious patient to speak his or her name. Check the wristband to identify the comatose patient. When a patient has a fairly common name, it is wise to check to be sure that there is only one patient with that name in the treatment area. Always check the unit's blood type and serial number against the corresponding identification on the requisition. Another wise precaution is to have all the above information checked by two people. *The overwhelming majority of transfusion accidents and deaths are the direct result of inadequate patient identification, not laboratory error.*[4] Check the unit of blood for any signs of infection as already described. Never put any kind of medication into a unit of blood. It is always wise to monitor a patient closely as to temperature, blood pressure, and sense of well being during the first 30 minutes or the first 50 ml of each unit of blood. Most serious reactions will be preceded by some symptoms during that period. The patient should be checked every 30 minutes during the remainder of the transfusion. The transfusion should be stopped immediately if the signs or symptoms of a serious reaction occur.

As mentioned earlier, it is not always possible to determine the severity of a transfusion reaction from the early signs, because the signs of a dangerous or mild reaction may overlap. The patient's physician should decide whether a given reaction is mild enough to warrant continuing transfusion. If a serious reaction is suspected, the laboratory should be notified. All the remaining transfusion tubing and equipment should be returned to the laboratory with a freshly drawn sample of the patient's blood. The laboratory will use this material to recheck its crossmatch. Treatment and monitoring methods for transfusion reactions are described in an earlier section.

Blood transfusion, although potentially life saving, is also potentially dangerous. The dangers can be diminished by careful patient identification and monitoring, combined with restraint and care in the use of blood and blood products.

INTRAVENOUS AND INTRAARTERIAL TECHNIQUES

Proper placement of a needle into a vessel is both an art and a science. The science can be taught, but the art can only be gained through practice. The following section is an introduction to some of the techniques that you will need for the proper placement of intravascular needles.

Venipuncture

Generally, it is safest to limit venipuncture sites to the antecubital space and forearm, although other sites could be used by physicians and other trained personnel familiar with them. For venipuncture in the antecubital space one begins by placing a tourniquet around the midbiceps area so that it is tight enough to stop venous return from the forearm but does not diminish or cut off the palpable radial pulse. Look for distended peripheral veins. Check carefully over the antecubital space, lateral wrist, and dorsum of the hand. Sometimes veins that are poorly visible will become more dilated by patting the area sharply with the hand (Fig. 10-3). Occasionally, a blood pressure cuff tourniquet pumped up to two-thirds systolic pressure will be of help. When veins are particularly hard to find, it may be necessary to have the patient lie down so that the arm will be dependent. Wrapping the arm in a warm, moist towel will sometimes bring out small, shallow veins. Some claim that the red goggles that radiologists used to wear prior to fluoroscopy make indistinct blue veins more visible. Often good veins can be felt more easily than they can be seen.

As a rule, veins in the mid- or lateral antecubital areas are best for drawing blood. Veins in the medial antecubital area often are larger but are more likely to rupture and form hematomas when punctured. The medial antecubital skin is also more sensitive to pain.

Intravenous infusions are best started in the lateral wrist or the dorsum of the hand because of the likelihood of infiltration when the arm is bent around an antecubital needle. Splints to prevent such bending at the elbow are usually quite uncomfortable.

Once an appropriate vein has been found, sterilize the area and pull the skin tight around the forearm with the thumb and fingers of your left hand. (Do not pull so tight as to collapse the vein). This action helps to prevent the vein from rolling away from the needle tip. Puncture the skin above or near the vein with the needle pointing proximally at an acute angle to the arm and near parallel to the vein. Keep the needle bevel down. This decreases the chance of puncturing the other side of the vein upon insertion. Advance the needle into the vein until blood can be drawn into the syringe or Vacutainer attached (Fig. 10-4).

Starting an intravenous solution utilizes much the same techniques. Attach the tubing to the intravenous bottle and fill the tubing and needle with fluid. It is helpful to keep the IV bottle below the level

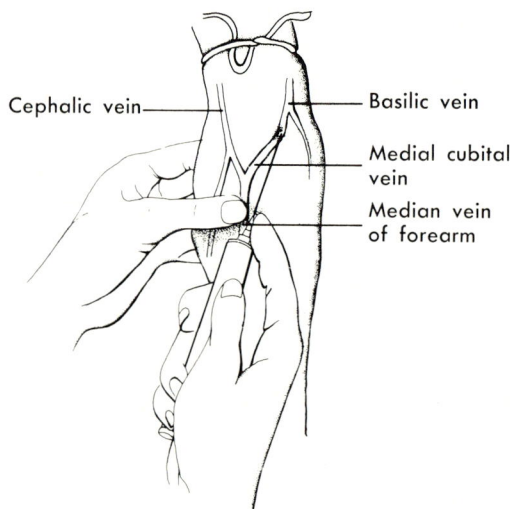

Fig. 10-3. Arm positioning for proper venipuncture. If available, the antecubital (medial cubital) vein or the cephalic vein should be attempted first since these veins pose less of a problem than others.

Cephalic vein

Basilic vein

Medial cubital vein

Median vein of forearm

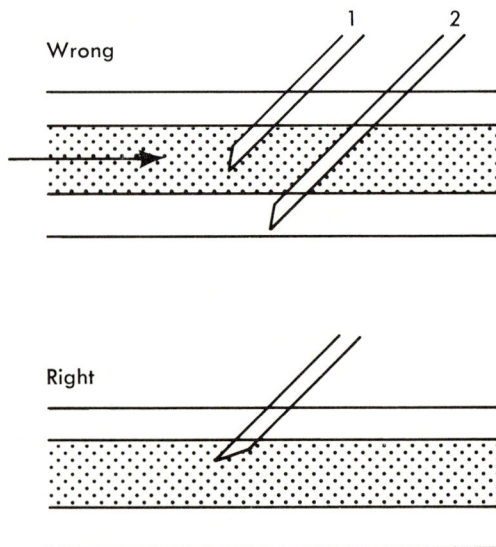

Fig. 10-4. Correct and incorrect methods of venipuncture.

Wrong

Right

of the vein. When the skin is punctured, open the IV valve. The return of blood into the tubing indicates that the needle has entered the vein. At this point release the tourniquet and raise the bottle without dislodging the needle. The needle can be advanced into the vein carefully while the intravenous solution is running rapidly. Fluid running out of the needle tip will help keep the vein distended and away from the sharp point as it is advanced. Tape the needle and tubing securely to the arm so that movement will not dislodge the needle and cause the vein to rupture.

Additional consideration should be taken with the use of intracatheters. If the stylets are saved and taped to the patient's chart, they can be measured against the plastic catheter upon removal. This assures that a piece of loose plastic is not free floating in the circulation.

Use of an antibiotic ointment at the puncture site will reduce the possibility of infection. This can be routinely applied when the catheter is being secured.

The right antecubital space should not be used in a cardiac patient. Should heart block occur, this space could be used to start a temporary pacemaker.

Arterial puncture technique

Many arteries in the body are accessible for needle puncture. For safety's sake this technique is best limited to the radial artery at the wrist. The hand is normally supplied by both the radial and ulnar arteries through an interconnecting arching arterial system in the palm. Therefore, in the rare event of an intra-arterial thrombosis of the radial artery following arterial puncture, the ulnar artery would supply blood to the entire hand.

Suggested equipment for arterial puncture includes (1) a 3 ml glass syringe, (2) a 22-gauge needle, (3) sterile heparin for injection, (4) small cork or rubber stopper, and (5) a basin with crushed ice, large enough to hold syringe and needle. Draw heparin into the needle and syringe so that the entire barrel of the syringe is coated, then expel the heparin and any air bubbles. Feel the radial pulse and mark its location with a fingernail indentation into the skin. A small amount of local anesthetic may be put in the skin at this site after sterilizing the area with alcohol. Grasp the patient's supinated hand with your left hand and forcibly hyperextend the patient's wrist. Hold the body of the syringe like a pencil or dart in your right hand so that the needle bevel is up and the angle of the needle to the patient's forearm is from 100 to 120 degrees (Fig. 10-5). Slowly push the needle into the skin at the point where the radial pulse is marked. As the needle enters the radial artery, arterial blood should enter the syringe, pushing the plunger up. Occasionally, a needle tip will collapse the artery and puncture both walls at once so that the tip of the needle comes to rest against the radial bone. In this case the needle should be slowly withdrawn until the bevel is within the radial artery and blood enters the syringe. It may be necessary to advance and withdraw the needle two or three times before a small rolling radial artery is entered. Once the syringe is full, the needle is withdrawn and a cotton ball is immediately and forcibly squeezed down against the puncture site. This pressure should not be released for a minimum of ten minutes in order to prevent extravasation of arterial blood. *Do not leave application of this pressure up to the patient!* After pressure has been maintained for ten minutes, an elastic pressure bandage should be applied to the puncture site. This should stay in place for at least 12 hours. As soon as the needle is removed from the skin, the tip should be plunged into the rubber or cork stopper. Be sure no bubbles are present. Put the syringe, needle, and stopper into the bowl of cracked ice (Fig.

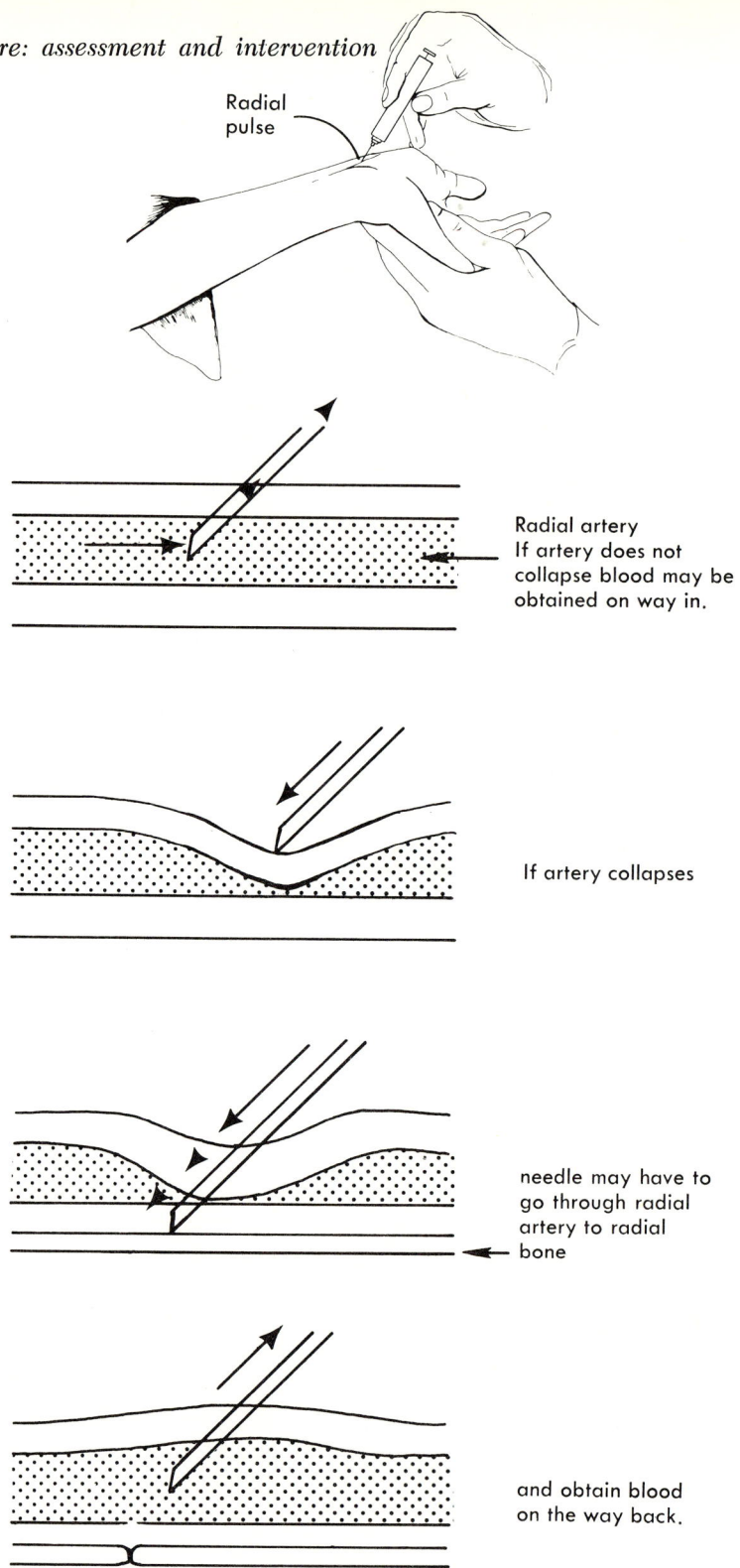

Radial pulse

Radial artery
If artery does not collapse blood may be obtained on way in.

If artery collapses

needle may have to go through radial artery to radial bone

and obtain blood on the way back.

Fig. 10-5. Arterial puncture technique.

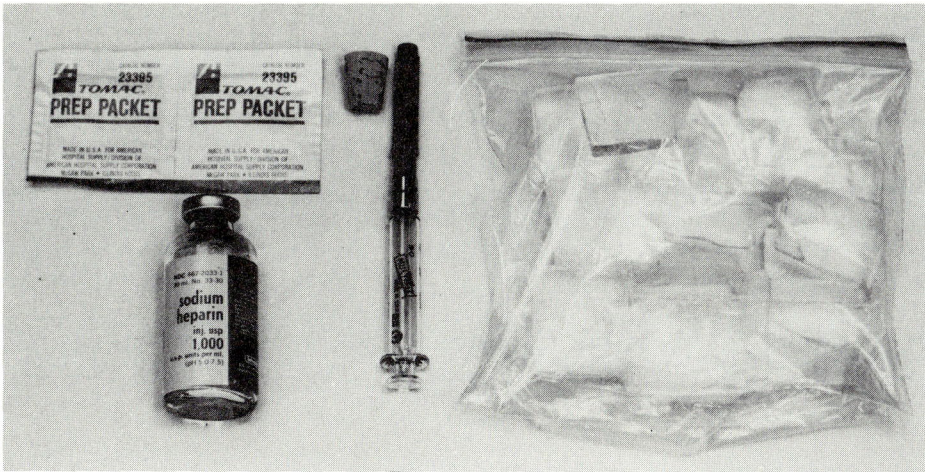

Fig. 10-6. Arterial puncture tray.

10-6). This should be transported to the laboratory so that the blood gas determinations may be done as soon as possible.

Careful adherence to the techniques mentioned, combined with plenty of practice, should make you an expert at finding veins and puncturing the radial artery. Nevertheless, it is usually best to observe these techniques as performed by skilled individuals before trying them yourself.

REFERENCES

1. Mollison, P. L.: Blood transfusion in clinical medicine, ed. 4, Philadelphia, 1967, F. A. Davis Co.
2. American Association of Blood Banks: Standards for a blood transfusion service, ed. 4, Chicago, 1966, The Association.
3. Race, R. R., and Sanger, R.: Blood groups in man, ed. 5, Philadelphia, 1968, F. A. Davis Co.
4. Merritt, J. A., and Maloney, W. C.: Management of emergencies. XII. Untoward reactions to blood transfusions, N. Engl. J. Med. **274**:1426, 1966.
5. Ingram, G. I. C.: Editorial review: The bleeding complications of blood transfusion, Transfusion **5**:1, 1965.
6. Barry, K. G., and Crosby, W. H.: The prevention and treatment of renal failure following transfusion reactions, Transfusion **3**:34, 1963.
7. Dameshek, W., and Nober, J.: Transfusion reaction to a plasma constituent of whole blood, Blood **5**:129, 1950.
8. Braude, A. I.: Transfusion reactions from contaminated blood: Their recognition and treatment, N. Engl. J. Med. **258**:1289, 1958.
9. Allen, J. G.: Post-transfusion hepatitis: A serious clinical problem, Calif. Med. **104**:293, 1966.
10. Prince, A. M., and Burke, K.: Serum hepatitis antigen (SH): Rapid detection by high voltage immunoelectrophoresis, Science **169**:593, 1970.
11. Chojnack, R. E., Brazinsky, J. H., and Barrett, O.: Transfusion-introduced falciparum malaria, N. Engl. J. Med. **279**:984, 1968.
12. Vogel, J. M., and Vogel, P.: Transfusion of blood components, Anesthesiology **27**:363, 1966.
13. Blackburn, E. K.: Indications for blood transfusion, Practitioner **195**:174, 1965.
14. Oberman, H. A.: The indications for transfusion of freshly drawn blood, J.A.M.A. **199**:96, 1967.
15. Chaplin, H., Jr.: Packed red blood cells, N. Engl. J. Med. **281**:364, 1969.
16. Becker, G. A., and Aster, R. H.: Platelet transfusion therapy, Med. Clin. North Am. **56**:81, 1972.
17. Murphy, S., and Gardner, F. H.: Platelet preservation: Effect of storage temperature on maintenance of platelet viability and deleterious effects of refrigerated storage, N. Engl. J. Med. **280**:1094, 1969.
18. Graw, R. G., Jr., Eisel, R., Bockner, C. D., and Perry, S.: Granulocyte procurement from normal donors for transfusion into leukopenic patients, Clin. Res. **17**:401, 1969.

19. Moyer, C. A., and Butcher, H. R.: Burns, shock and plasma volume regulation, St. Louis, 1967, The C. V. Mosby Co.
20. Golub, S., and Bailey, C. P.: Management of major surgical blood uses without transfusion, J.A.M.A. **198:**1171, 1966.
21. Biggs, R., and MacFarlane, R. G., editors: Treatment of hemophilia and other coagulation disorders, Philadelphia, 1966, F. A. Davis Co.
22. Pool, J. G., and Shannon, A. E.: Production of high potency concentrates of antihemophiliac globulin in a closed bag system; assay in vitro and in vivo, N. Engl. J. Med. **273:**1443, 1965.
23. Biggs, R., and Matthews, J. M.: The treatment of hemorrhage in von Willebrand's disease and the blood levels of factor VIII (AHG), Brit. J. Haemat. **9:**203, 1963.
24. Bidwell, E., Booth, J. M., Dike, G. W. R., and Denson, K. W. E.: The preparation for therapeutic use of a concentrate of factor IX containing also factors II, VII and X, Brit. J. Haemat. **13:**568, 1967.
25. Tullis, J. L., Melin, M., and Jurigiam, P.: Clinical use of human prothrombin complexes, N. Engl. J. Med. **273:**667, 1965.

CHAPTER 11

The unconscious patient, seizures, and headache

Randall W. Smith, M.D.
Jack C. Sipe, M.D.

Initially, a definition of unconsciousness must be reached if personnel are to know which patients fall into this diagnostic category. Unconsciousness can be considered to be synonymous with coma or semi-coma. Patients demonstrating such states cannot be aroused sufficiently to speak or follow commands. Such patients may move purposefully in response to pain or may posture their extremities but they will do little else (see Chapter 20, p. 320).

THE UNCONSCIOUS PATIENT

Unconscious patients all have a common abnormality—depression of brain function. This depression has many causes as shown in the following outline.

- I. Shock (cardiogenic)*
  - A. Cardiac arrest
  - B. Myocardial infarction
  - C. Pericardial tamponade
- II. Shock (hypovolemic)*
  - A. Dehydration
  - B. Hemorrhage
- III. Metabolic
  - A. Renal (uremic)
  - B. Hepatic (ammonia)
  - C. Diabetic (glucose)*
- IV. Metabolic (chemical)
  - A. Sodium—hypernatremia, hyponatremia
  - B. Potassium—hyperkalemia, hypokalemia
- V. Metabolic (toxic)
  - A. Drug overdose
  - B. Sedatives
  - C. Narcotics
  - D. Poisons
- VI. Seizures*
- VII. Infection
  - A. Meningitis*
- VIII. Respiratory insufficiency* (hypoxia, hypercapnia)
  - A. Airway obstruction
  - B. Pneumothorax
  - C. Lung disease (pneumonia)
- IX. Intracranial hematoma*
- X. Stroke (brain stem)

Neurologic depression may occur because the entire brain is subjected to the effects of excessive or insufficient amounts of chemicals or drugs. The chemicals may

---

*These disease categories need emergency department diagnosis and treatment.

be those normally present in the body but altered in their concentration by an underlying disease process. Certain chemicals may be accidentally or purposefully ingested. Drugs, prescribed or otherwise, can seriously depress the brain when present in excessive amounts.

All chemical and drug-induced unconsciousness is called *metabolic, or toxic, encephalopathy.* The goal in these patients is to identify the chemical or drug by history, physical examination, or laboratory tests.

Unconsciousness may be caused by compression of the brain stem and resulting dysfunction of the reticular activating system (see Chapter 20, p. 318). This occurs as a result of cerebral hemorrhage or a tumor inside the head. A cerebral thrombosis (stroke) that involves the brain stem itself can cause unconsciousness. A patient with unrecognized trauma (brain injury without obvious scalp injury) can be unconscious because of either brain stem contusion or brain stem compression from hematoma (see Chapter 20, pp. 323-336).

The above patients all are unconscious as a result of primary intracranial pathology. The goal of emergency department care is to decide which of the intracranial lesions is present and, particularly, to recognize brain stem compression and its immediate threat to life.

Certain patients, particularly the elderly, may become semicomatose in the presence of infection or abnormally low blood pressure. Patients who sustain a generalized seizure will be comatose, then semicomatose for an hour or so.

The outline of causes of unconsciousness given above is lengthy. By taking a careful history, performing a reasonable examination, and making judicious use of the laboratory, many of these causes can be ascertained in the emergency department.

A reasonable question to be asked in the care of the unconscious patient is, What should be the emergency department's role in the evaluation of these patients? Although the answer to this question may vary from hospital to hospital, the following might be a fair response: The ability to diagnose and treat disease that can be rapidly and simply substantiated and that can lead to death or permanent damage if not immediately recognized. Once it has been established that the patient does not have immediate life-threatening disease, further evaluation and care should take place on the ward or in the intensive care unit. There is little justification for a stable patient to undergo a prolonged stay in the emergency department while awaiting results of laboratory tests. Observation and waiting can occur elsewhere.

Assessment

No matter how long an unconscious patient remains in the emergency department and no matter how stable the patient, emergency department personnel must be responsible for (1) as detailed a history as possible, (2) a physical examination plus a baseline neurologic examination, and (3) ongoing measurement of vital signs (Fig. 11-1).

History. No aspect of the emergency department evaluation of the unconscious patient is more crucial than obtaining a history. Nothing can narrow down the diagnostic possibilities more quickly than a good history of how the unconsciousness occurred. Find out as much as possible from whomever is available. Whoever accompanies the patient may have invaluable information. Contact relatives or friends; it is crucial to know the usual state of the patient's health. When was the patient last seen awake? What diseases does the patient have? What drugs are usually taken? Any history of previous drug abuse or suicide attempts? Any history of seizures? Heart disease? Stroke? High blood pressure? Recent headaches? Diabetes? Insulin reactions?

Any identification the patient may have

The unconscious patient

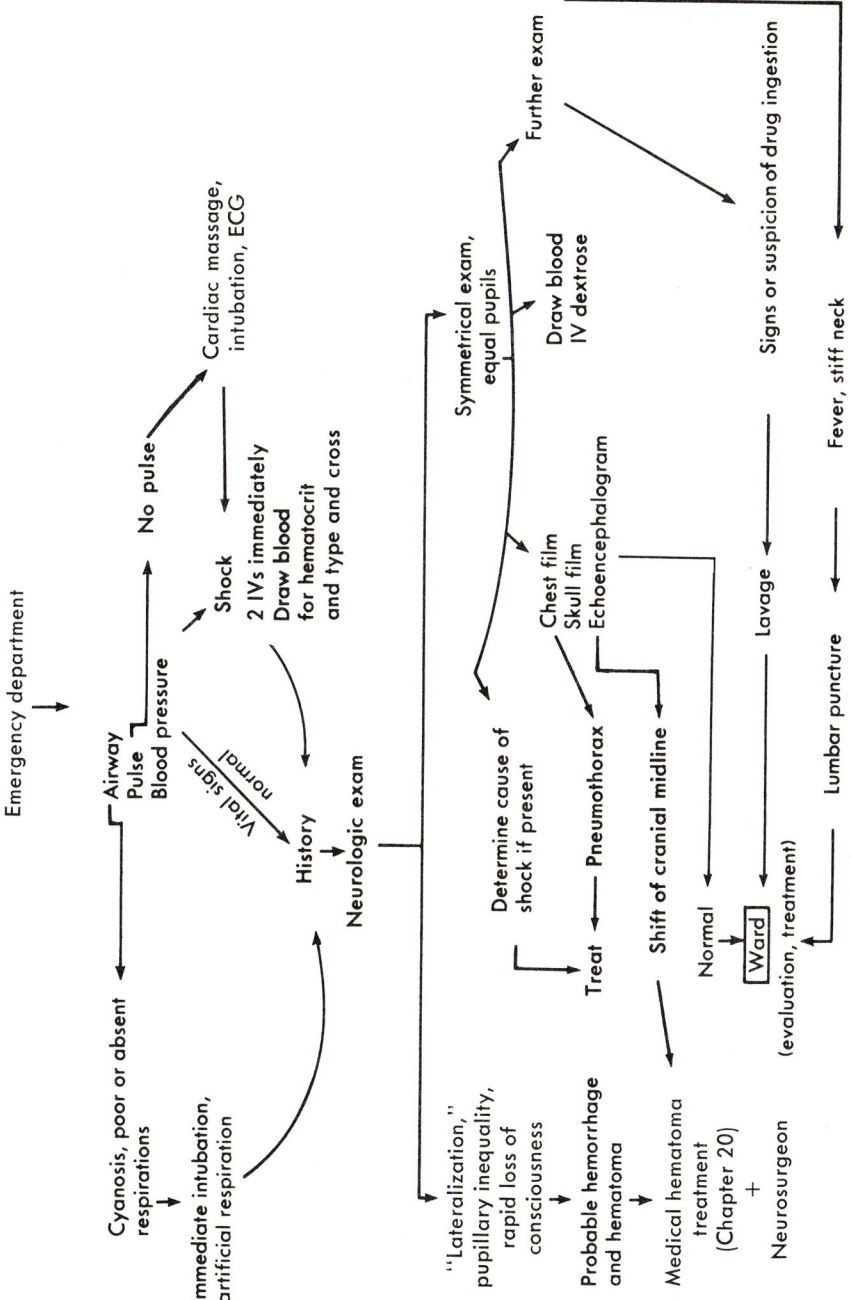

Fig. 11-1. Management outline for unconscious patients.

can be useful. The family physician should be contacted if possible. Look for medical bracelets that may indicate diseases.

Of course, some patients arrive with no history whatsoever. They are found unconscious in the street or in their homes, and no one knows how they became so afflicted. When there is no history, assume that the onset of unconsciousness was acute and that an intracranial hemorrhage is likely. This will increase the intensity of search for a life-threatening intracranial hematoma, which is one of the most lethal and disabling causes of unconsciousness.

Physical examination. The physical examination can be most informative. Vital signs should be rapidly checked. Respirations that are shallow, very irregular, or slow should be immediately assisted. The patient in shock requires immediate intravenous fluid therapy, while treatment of elevated blood pressure can usually wait until the rest of the evaluation has been completed. Dentures should be removed, and contact lenses, if present, should be removed or their presence called to the attention of the physician.

Absence of visible blood vessels on the white (scleral) portion of the eye suggests significant anemia. Dusky or cyanotic lips, tongue, or nail beds suggests low oxygen levels and imply shock or respiratory embarrassment necessitating *immediate breathing assistance.* Needle marks on the abdomen or thighs identify the diabetic, while those found on the arms suggest a hard drug user. The patient's breath may reveal the heavy pall of alcohol, or the distinctive odor of acetone in the diabetic. It should be emphasized that the odor of alcohol cannot be presumed to explain unconsciousness. Alcohol alone rarely causes coma or semicoma; an additional diagnosis must be considered.

Yellow discoloration of the sclera or the skin is noteworthy as it may suggest liver failure with unconsciousness due to abnormal amounts of blood ammonia. Look at the tongue for lacerations (a seizure) and check the moistness of the mucous membranes of the mouth. A very dry mouth suggests dehydration which, coupled with renal failure, can cause unconsciousness in the elderly.

Check for pressure marks on the skin. These suggest that the patient has lain immobile for some time (hours) and is useful information when history is lacking.

Note any evidence of incontinence of bowel or bladder. Incontinence suggests seizure, intracranial hemorrhage, or a considerable duration (hours) of unconsciousness.

A careful search must be made for signs of trauma. Contusions, abrasions, and lacerations discovered anywhere must alert one to the possibility of head injury.

Neurologic examination. The neurologic examination (see Chapter 20, p. 319) must be performed as soon after admission as possible. The purpose of the examination is to detect the signs of mass and herniation. This examination takes less than two minutes and cannot be neglected. If nothing else, it forms the baseline against which to compare the future course of the patient.

The examiner should check for neck stiffness (nuchal rigidity) because of its importance in indicating intracranial disease. Normally, the head can be easily bent forward by the examiner until the patient's chin rests on the chest. If the unconscious patient's neck offers resistance to this maneuver and the chin cannot be brought to the chest, then nuchal rigidity is present. This means one of the following: intracranial mass with herniation, intracranial hemorrhage, or meningitis.

Diagnostic tests. Diagnostic tests that are rapidly and simply performed can be helpful. An electrocardiogram in patients over 40 may indicate myocardial infarction and explain cyanosis and shock. Chest and skull x-rays are easily obtained and may offer significant help. No patient with undiagnosed unconsciousness should leave the emergency department without skull films and an echoencephalogram to hopefully detect an occult mass lesion. Echoencephalography (see Chapter 20, p. 325) is rapidly performed and can indicate the presence of brain shift and thus an intracranial mass. Unfortunately, this test is anything but infallible, and even if results are negative, it cannot be relied upon to rule out a mass lesion. If definitely positive, then a mass must be presumed and further investigation undertaken (angiogram, computerized cranial tomogram).

Lumbar puncture is a diagnostic test of considerable assistance in the presence of meningitis. It should not be performed in the unconscious patient unless meningitis is considered likely (fever, nuchal rigidity) and the following criteria are met: (1) no neurologic lateralization (see p. 320), (2) equal, reactive pupils, and (3) no brain shift (midline calcified pineal gland on skull film; echoencephalogram with 2 mm or less of shift).

Finally, two diagnostic maneuvers related to diabetes mellitus should be performed. As the intravenous line is started, but before fluids are administered, a small blood sample should be saved and immediately tested for blood glucose with a Dextrostix. A value greater than 250 suggests the possibility of *hyper*glycemic coma, whereas a value of less than 100 raises the possibility of insulin reaction. In the latter instance, 50 g of dextrose should be immediately injected into the intravenous line (not the bottle). If *hypo*glycemic coma is present, the patient should begin to awaken within minutes.

Remember that electrocardiographic abnormalities will never explain unconsciousness unless the patient is in shock or has sustained a cardiac arrest.

Diagnoses

As already mentioned, a certain group of diagnoses are worthy of being made because of their immediate threat to life or their simplicity of discovery. These diagnoses will be dealt with in some detail while the rest will not be covered (see outline on p. 137). The detailed evaluation and therapy of the latter group should occur on the ward and skills related to these diagnoses gleaned from other volumes.

Following the above criteria pares the emergency department list of causes of unconsciousness down to eight: cardiac arrest, shock, respiratory insufficiency, diabetes, intracranial hematoma, drug overdose, meningitis, and seizures.

Cardiac arrest. Cardiac arrest is detected by ambulance attendants, police, or by the first set of vital signs. For its further evaluation, see Chapter 30.

Shock. Refer to Chapter 7.

Respiratory insufficiency. Respiratory insufficiency causes unconsciousness by supplying insufficient oxygen to or by removing too little carbon dioxide from the brain. The patient who is unconscious for this reason is close to death. The situation must be rapidly corrected (see Intervention section).

The usual hallmark of insufficient respiration is cyanosis. The patient's lips, tongue, or nail beds are some shade of blue. Any patient with pink skin and red lips and tongue probably does not have respiratory insufficiency, and certainly this is not the cause of unconsciousness. The rare exception to this is the patient with severe emphysema who can be pink but have a very high carbon dioxide level and be in a coma from the hypercapnia.

Insufficient respirations are caused by obstruction of the airway, collapse of a lung, consolidation of the lung by pneumonia, or dysfunction of respiratory drive from the brain.

The diagnosis of these various forms of respiratory insufficiency is discussed in detail in the chapter on acute respiratory emergencies (Chapter 27).

Diabetes. Diabetic coma is detected by immediate blood sugar determination. It must be pointed out that high blood sugar does not necessarily explain a patient's coma. The rest of the evaluation must be performed, and if no other life-threatening diseases are detected, then hyperglycemia is presumed to be the problem.

Intracranial hematoma. Intracranial hematoma is one of the diagnoses most often missed. This is extremely unfortunate, because intracranial hemorrhage with a resultant hematoma and herniation is a common cause of unconsciousness. The diagnosis must be made in the emergency department and *immediate* therapy undertaken if death or significant neurologic disability is to be avoided.

The hematoma may be the result of one of a number of underlying disease processes (hypertension, aneurysm, arteriovenous malformation, unknown or unrecognized head injury), but the problem is always the same: hemorrhage → hematoma → brain shift → brain stem compression → unconsciousness.

The history is crucial and often indicates sudden, catastrophic onset of unconsciousness. The patient is literaly felled like a tree. There is frequently an antecedent history of hypertension. Patients who are not rendered totally unconscious will have complained of a severe headache followed by rapid neurologic deterioration to coma or semicoma. This particular history always means intracranial hemorrhage and hematoma.

Not infrequently, the patient will be found some hours to days after having last been seen awake and well. This kind of limited history is often obtained in unconsciousness due to a variety of causes and does not necessarily mean hematoma. Thus, the physical examination becomes all important.

Blood pressure is almost always normal or elevated in the presence of hematoma. Indeed, a patient in shock is quite unlikely to have a hematoma, and if the neurologic examination is symmetrical, then attention should be directed toward another diagnosis.

Respirations vary from hyperventilation to eupnea to very irregular breathing with periods of apnea. Therefore respiratory pattern is not a good guide to the diagnosis of intracranial hematoma.

The neurologic examination usually reveals lateralization, that is, movement of only one side of the body in response to pain. Usually the larger pupil reacts sluggishly to light, and nuchal rigidity is frequently found. Lateralization is rarely seen in metabolic encephalopathy and is not found in cardiac arrest, respiratory insufficiency, diabetes, shock, or meningitis.

Deeply unconscious patients (coma) may posture their extremities (see Chapter 20). Decerebrate or decorticate posturing is not usually seen in unconsciousness due to metabolic or toxic causes and must be presumed to mean a hematoma.

The echoencephalogram will usually show a significant (greater than 2 mm) shift, and if the pineal gland is calcified, its position will be shifted on the skull x-ray films.

If the diagnosis of hematoma is made, immediate therapy must follow plus neurosurgical consultation and further diagnostic tests.

Just as important as making the diagnosis of hematoma is deciding that hematoma is not present. This will allow diagnostic and therapeutic efforts to be concentrated in other areas. An unconscious patient who fulfills the following criteria is unlikely to have a hematoma:

1. No history or history of gradual (days) lapse into unconsciousness without headache complaints
2. Normal or low blood pressure
3. Symmetrical response to pain
4. Equal pupils that react to light (very small pupils are always reactive)
5. Absence of decerebrate or decorticate posturing
6. Supple neck

7. Normal echoencephalogram

8. Normal skull films; no pineal shift

About the only form of hematoma that meets the above criteria is bilateral chronic subdural hematoma. The diagnosis of this disease will not be forthcoming until other causes of unconsciousness are ruled out on the ward and subsequent diagnostic tests are performed.

Drug overdose. The sooner gastric lavage occurs in drug overdose cases, the better the chances of retarding the depth of central nervous system depression. If a history of oral overdose is obtained, a lavage tube is immediately passed. If there is no history available, visual examination of the gastric contents for tablet or capsule fragments may be enlightening. A 0.4 mg injection of naloxone (Narcan) may prove lifesaving if physical examination reveals pinpoint pupils and there is suspicion of narcotic use. Naloxone will not alter bodily function and, therefore, is a useful diagnostic as well as therapeutic agent. If the diagnosis is established only by blood tests, treatment will occur on the ward, where the patient should be located awaiting results of toxicologic tests.

Meningitis. Meningitis is mentioned only to point out that the nuchal rigidity, hallmark of meningitis, *does not by itself mean meningitis*. It may mean hematoma. A "meningitis" patient should not undergo a lumbar puncture until the criteria for absence of hematoma are met (see p. 141).

Intervention

Comments regarding therapy will be limited to therapeutic maneuvers common to all unconscious patients and those absolutely necessary to treat the previously listed life-threatening diseases in the emergency department.

Initially, all unconscious patients need their life safeguarded to allow time for history, physical examination, and diagnostic tests. This means assuring adequacy of respirations, blood pressure, and kidney function.

An endotracheal tube should be placed in every comatose patient. This will usually solve airway obstruction and improve lung consolidation or collapse. It will also allow artificial respiration in those with poor respiratory drive.

The only exception to intubation is a clear diagnosis of postseizure depression or hypoglycemic coma. In the former, recovery is expected to occur rapidly and spontaneously; the diabetic patient should awaken within minutes after 50 ml of 50% dextrose is injected intravenously.

An intravenous line is rapidly placed after multiple blood samples are drawn; one sample is immediately tested for glucose with a rapid indicator (Dextrostix), and the rest is set aside or sent to the laboratory. If the Dextrostix indicates a blood sugar less than 50 mg/100 ml or if hypoglycemia is suspected, an infusion of 50 ml of 50% dextrose is given into the intravenous line. A bladder catheter should be placed to monitor the adequacy of urine production and thus renal perfusion. A nasogastric tube should be placed to empty the stomach, detect pill residue, and prevent vomiting.

Once the above steps have been accomplished, further history is taken and the examination is performed. As soon as a diagnosis is felt to be probable and it falls within the group of diseases needing actual treatment, the therapy must begin.

Management of cardiac arrest is detailed in Chapter 30, intervention for respiratory failure is covered in Chapter 27, and shock therapy is outlined in Chapter 7. Therapy for meningitis, which involves administration of antibiotics, occurs on the ward and should not be an emergency department concern.

Drug overdose. Treatment of oral drug overdose beyond the initial gastric lavage should occur on the ward. However, when suspicion of this problem is high (needle marks, history, shallow respirations), a narcotic antagonist, such as naloxone (Narcan), 0.4 mg, can be injected intravenously and in cases of overdose will acutely reverse the narcosis and result in rapid awakening of the patient. If successful, the drug may be repeated as necessary to sustain consciousness.

Intracranial hematoma. Treatment of intracranial hematoma and the reasons for it are considered in some detail in Chapter 20 and need not be repeated here. Once medical treatment has begun, the exact location of the hematoma and its cause must be ascertained by angiography or computerized cranial tomography with a neurosurgeon in attendance ready to act upon the findings.

SEIZURES

A generalized (includes both arms and legs) seizure has been likened to an "electrical storm" in which the brain cells fire in great volleys, resulting in the generalized jerking muscular activity and clenched teeth. The diaphragm is jerking in the same manner, respirations are ineffective, and cyanosis develops. Autonomic nerve impulses result in urination and excessive salivation. The tightly clenched teeth, saliva, poor respiration, and cyanosis present an alarming picture and have given rise to the misconception that these patients have "swallowed" their tongue. (It is impossible to swallow the tongue, and any attempt by medical personnel to insert a finger and pull up the tongue is usually rewarded with failure if not digital trauma.)

As the seizure continues, the patient tends to injure the flailing extremities, lacerate the tongue between clenched teeth, and become more and more cyanotic. It is this increasing cyanosis that finally makes the brain hypoxic, and because of a lack of adequate oxygen, the brain cells stop firing. This explains why most generalized seizures cease spontaneously after a few minutes; only occasionally does a seizure continue for more than five minutes, that is, status epilepticus.

Status epilepticus constitutes a major threat to the patient for two reasons. First, although the hypoxia is not quite severe enough to force the discharging nerve cells to cease firing, it can be severe enough for irreparable damage to occur to other more normal nerve cells as well as other organs (heart, kidney). Second, extreme amounts of energy are required, and heat is created by the muscular system to keep up the repetitive jerking movements. The heart may be taxed so much to supply blood to these muscles that cardiovascular collapse can occur.

Seizures become an emergency department concern under two circumstances:

1. When a patient is brought to the emergency department because of a generalized seizure and is still having the seizure upon arrival (i.e., status epilepticus)
2. When a patient undergoing evaluation (of any problem) has a generalized seizure while in the emergency department

Assessment

The assessment here is usually obvious since the patient has regular jerking motions of all extremities, is salivating excessively, has clenched teeth (often with the tongue trapped between them), irregular respirations, and cyanosis. This clinical picture generates quite a bit of excitement and frenzied activity and frequently results in a good deal of inappropriate therapy.

Intervention

The convulsing patient should be protected (pillows, blankets) so that the extremities and head are not repeatedly beaten against metal side rails or hard flooring. Try to wedge a bite block (tongue blade wrapped at one end with a few turns of adhesive tape) between the teeth *only* if the tongue is trapped. Prying open the mouth by itself does not assist respirations, which are inadequate because of the diaphragmatic spasm, not airway obstruction. Remain calm; seizures that begin in the emergency department will likely stop spontaneously in a very few minutes. Medication should be prepared for possible use.

Most drugs used to abruptly stop seizures do so by their depressant effect on the brain. Since a patient's postictal (following a seizure) state of consciousness is one of temporary coma, the use of depressive drugs to stop a seizure deepens and prolongs the usual postictal coma. This additional sedation can effect the following:

1. Retard the expected resumption of respirations
2. Leave the patient heavily sedated
3. Interfere with subsequent neurologic evaluation, particularly important when the cause of the seizure is unknown

Use depressants *sparingly* in treatment of seizures that begin in the emergency department. Give the seizure a few minutes to stop by itself while medications are readied and an appropriate vein is identified for injection. If the seizure persists longer than five minutes, medication should be carefully employed as indicated below.

In the emergency treatment of *generalized status epilepticus,* there are two chief concerns:

1. Prompt institution of general care measures (including respiratory and cardiovascular supportive measures) to maintain patient's rapidly dissipating strength
2. Intervention with anticonvulsive drugs in an effort to abort the continuing seizures

Drug reservations do not apply in this situation. Continuous seizures may lead to prolonged cerebral hypoxia, hyperpyrexia, and eventual cardiovascular collapse. General care measures are instituted at once

(IV, ECG monitor, mask O_2), and at the same time, anticonvulsant drugs are prepared for intravenous administration. Slow intravenous infusion is begun when anticonvulsant drugs are available. Preparations are made for endotracheal intubation if respiratory function is significantly depressed postictally.

Intravenous phenytoin (Dilantin) is considered by many to be the anticonvulsant drug of choice in the treatment of generalized status epilepticus. The use of intramuscular Dilantin is not recommended because of the drug's poor water solubility and consequent unpredictable absorption from muscle. Intravenous Dilantin should not be mixed with intravenous fluids since microprecipitation occurs. Dilantin is supplied in 100 mg/2 cc vials predissolved in propylene glycol and should be administered by direct intravenous infusion using a small scalp vein set. The Dilantin solution should be infused slowly at a rate not to exceed 50 mg/min together with monitoring of blood pressure and ECG during infusion. Hypotension and arrhythmias usually disappear upon cessation or slower administration of the drug. For children below the age of 3 years the use of Dilantin is controversial and there is evidence that the drug may not be an effective anticonvulsant in this age group. In children between the ages of 3 and 5 years the intravenous dose is 100 to 200 mg. For children up to 10 years the Dilantin dose range is 200 to 500 mg IV. In teenagers and adults an initial dose of 1,000 mg of intravenous Dilantin is recommended.

Often hypnotic or sedative anticonvulsant drugs are used instead of, or in conjunction with, intravenous Dilantin. The most commonly used drugs include phenobarbital sodium, diazepam (Valium), and sodium amobarbital (Amytal). Of the barbiturates, phenobarbital appears to have the widest margin of safety for parenteral use. The usual dose is 4 to 6 mg/kg given intramuscularly or by slow intravenous infusion. About two hours after the initial dose is given, parenteral administration of phenobarbital in divided doses according to the age of the patient is begun.

Some consider intravenous diazepam (Valium) to be the drug of choice because of its swift action and relatively good margin of safety, if administered properly *as the initial sedative anticonvulsant drug*. The margin of safety is greatly reduced when Valium is given together with barbiturates since each drug potentiates the respiratory depression and muscle relaxation of the other. The usual dose is administered by slow intravenous infusion at the rate of 1 mg every one to five minutes up to 10 mg in children 5 years or older. In adults the usual dose range is 20 to 30 mg by slow intravenous infusion. Diazepam is infused through a large peripheral vein undiluted (if possible), since microprecipitation occurs upon mixing with aqueous solutions.

Sodium amobarbital (Amytal) has the advantage of rapid anticonvulsive action, but its use is limited by respiratory depression and by the fact that the drug solution must be prepared just prior to injection. The dose range is 150 to 200 mg in adults by slow intravenous infusion.

The chief pitfalls to avoid are the following:

1. Rapid intravenous infusion of anticonvulsant drugs
2. Concurrent use of intravenous Valium and barbiturates thereby reducing the safety margin of both
3. Lack of preparation for endotracheal intubation

It may be necessary to use large amounts of anticonvulsant drugs to abort convulsive status, but if injection is performed slowly, this route of administration is preferred as long as respiratory assistance is available when the seizure stops. Aggressive anticonvulsant drug therapy is recommended only for *generalized status epilepticus* and not for other types of continuous seizures involving only one or two limbs or the face.

HEADACHE

Headache is said to be the most common symptom about which patients consult their doctors, and it is certainly a common symptom in the emergency department. Although most physicians realize that 85% to 90% of all headaches are not due to serious causes, it must also be recognized that those due to serious intracranial disease may have disastrous consequences for the patient if treatment is delayed. Every patient suffering from headache requires careful consideration and sometimes thorough investigation. In this section, primary consideration will be given to headaches due to serious nervous system disease.

The great majority of patients who have headaches from serious intracranial disease fall into the following categories: meningitis, intracranial hemorrhage, intracranial tumors (including abscesses), hydrocephalus, chronic subdural hematoma, and temporal arteritis (Table 11-1).

Assessment

History. History is crucial in patients with headache because the mode of onset, location, accompanying symptoms, and past history of headache may well suggest the diagnosis prior to the examination. One must inquire about a history of *sudden* headache; when present, this suggests intracranial hemorrhage and *must be investigated*. Generally, the location of headache is not very helpful, but temporal (in front of the ear) headache in the elderly must bring to mind temporal arteritis (see below). Headache that awakens the patient from sleep or is most severe upon arising in the morning, accompanied by nausea, vomiting, lethargy, or dullness of affect, suggests increased intracranial pressure (tumor, hydrocephalus). A patient with a

Table 11-1. Characteristics of serious headache

Symptom	Meningitis	Intracranial hemorrhage	Tumors	Abscess	Hydrocephalus	Chronic subdural hematoma	Temporal arteritis	Migraine
Headache								
Severity	Severe	Severe	Moderate to severe	Moderate to severe	Moderate to severe	Absent to moderate	Moderate	Moderate to severe
Duration	Days	Hours	Weeks	Days	Days	Weeks	Weeks	Hours
Onset	Gradual	Sudden	Gradual	Gradual	Gradual	Gradual	Gradual	Gradual
Miscellaneous	Generalized	Emesis common	± Emesis	± Emesis	Emesis common	Confusion	Temporal tenderness; visual disturbance	Long history; usually unilateral; usually nausea without emesis
Neck stiffness	Yes	Yes	No	Maybe	No	No	No	No
Fever	Yes	No or slight (38° C, 101° F)	No	Yes	No	No	No	No
Unilateral weakness	No	Frequent	Common	Common	No	Common	No	Rare
Unequal pupils	No	Frequent	Occasionally	Frequent	No	Uncommon	No	Rare
Stupor or coma	Uncommon	Frequent	Uncommon	Sometimes	Unusual	Sometimes	No	No

long series (years) of similar headaches is no particular cause for concern, whereas a first severe headache or a short history of such complaints is of greater importance. A history of head injury within the recent past may suggest chronic subdural hematoma in the patient with gradually increasing headache and confusion.

Physical examination. Elevated blood pressure and bradycardia with headache should raise the suspicion of increased intracranial pressure. Fever (greater than 38° C [101° F]) with headache, particularly when nuchal rigidity is present (neck cannot be flexed so that chin touches sternum), means that meningitis, encephalitis, brain abscess, or intracranial hemorrhage must be considered. Palpably tender temporal arteries suggest temporal arteritis. Any abnormality in the level of consciousness or lateralization of the neurologic examination is cause for further evaluation of the patient with headache.

Diagnosis

Meningitis. Meningitis is marked by the gradual (hours/days) onset of generalized headache, stiff neck, and fever. These patients are *not* unconscious (except the very elderly) and are *not* lateralized.

Intracranial hemorrhage. Intracranial hemorrhage is heralded by the *sudden* onset of severe headache and is usually followed by the rapid onset of neck stiffness. Fever is not prominent, but emesis is common. The level of consciousness can vary from alert or lethargic to deeply comatose. Lateralization on the neurologic examination is common. If the patient is comatose with unequal pupils, this constitutes an emergency situation requiring immediate medical treatment for herniation (p. 328) followed by angiography or computerized cranial tomography. When awake and talking, these patients will need to undergo angiography but require immediate admission to the ward or ICU for further evaluation.

Intracranial tumors. Patients with intra-

cranial neoplasm usually have a long history (weeks, months) of increasingly severe headache that is usually most noticeable upon awakening in the morning. One-sided weakness may be seen, but unconsciousness and pupillary inequality are not often present. Fever is absent.

Brain abscess. Brain abscess is usually indicated by a short (days) history of increasing headache and somnolence plus unilateral weakness. Neck stiffness may be absent, but fever is common. Unequal pupils are unusual unless stupor or coma is present.

Hydrocephalus. Patients are usually known to have this disease and come to the emergency department because of malfunction of the subcutaneously implanted shunting device utilized to control the problem. In the main, any patient who complains of headache and is known to have hydrocephalus or a shunt warrants at least a telephone call to the neurosurgeon. Somnolence or vomiting is cause for even greater concern. These patients should not have lateralizing neurologic findings or have unequal pupils; neck stiffness is uncommon. Fever is not seen with malfunction of the shunt, but a recent operation to repair the system followed within a few weeks by fever with or without headache suggests infection of the shunt system.

Chronic subdural hematoma. Chronic subdural hematoma is one of the most difficult problems to delineate at any time, certainly during an emergency department visit. Although headache can be absent in the disease, when present it has no striking characteristics to identify it as such. Somnolence is common, as are focal neurologic signs, although unequal pupils are rare short of accompanying coma.

Temporal arteritis. Extracranial vascular inflammation due to temporal arteritis is an infrequent but important cause of headache in patients over the age of 55, and it is considered a medical emergency because permanent unilateral or bilateral loss of vision may occur if treatment is delayed. When the complaint is of pain in the temples and the superficial temporal arteries are observed to be prominent, tender, and pulseless, the diagnosis should never be in doubt. The pain, however, may be occipital, nuchal, or even in the jaw. Tenderness may be slight and arterial pulsations normal. If there is any suspicion of temporal arteritis, an erythrocyte sedimentation rate (ESR) should be obtained and the results ascertained immediately (usually greater than 60 mm/hour in this disease; more than 30 mm/hour is suspicious).

Other headaches. As implied in the introduction of this section, most headaches are not a cause for alarm, although they may be quite uncomfortable. Migraine is the easiest nonserious headache to identify, since the usual long history, the one-sided location, the typical prodrome that the patient experiences prior to onset of the actual head pain, the nausea, and photophobia all mark this type of headache rather clearly. These patients, as well as others whose headaches do not fall into the serious categories, can be given analgesics and safely discharged from the emergency department to see their private physician in the office. In essence, any patient less than 50 years old with a headache that came on gradually and who has a supple neck, no fever, and a normal neurologic examination including level of consciousness requires only limited emergency department attention.

Intervention

Meningitis. When meningitis is felt to be the problem, an immediate lumbar puncture (LP) and intravenous antibiotics are in order. The LP may be done in the emergency department, and the results should be ascertained as quickly as possible. Remember that this procedure should *not* be performed on any patient with suspected meningitis when the patient demonstrates lateralizing neurologic findings or has unequal pupils. In such circumstances

an intracranial contrast study (brain scan, computerized cranial tomogram, angiogram) must be done first to rule out brain abscess.

Intracranial hemorrhage. In the presence of a poor history, possible sudden onset of headache, and equivocal examination (slight stiff neck, otherwise normal), a lumbar puncture will clearly establish or rule out hemorrhage and may be safely performed in the emergency department. When the history and examination are definite, angiography is warranted. The lumbar puncture is performed subsequently. When hemorrhage is suspected and the patient has lateralized neurologic findings, the LP is contraindicated until after angiography.

Intracranial tumor. Patients suspected of harboring tumors should be admitted, given a detailed neurologic examination and diagnostic studies (brain scan, EEG, computerized cranial tomogram, angiogram) within 24 hours of admission. When the patient is stuporous or comatose, immediate neurologic consultation or contrast study or both should be obtained.

Brain abscess. Brain abscess, when suspected, necessitates immediate intracranial contrast study, which, if positive, should result in rapid surgical drainage of the abscess.

Hydrocephalus. Patients with hydrocephalus vary from mildly to severely ill. Any patient with known hydrocephalus who has an abnormal level of consciousness should be seen by the neurosurgeon. Since this disease is most common in children, the patient's mother will be an excellent source of information. If the mother thinks the patient's cerebrospinal fluid shunting system is malfunctioning, she is almost always correct since she probably has extensive experience with her child's behavior when ill from inadequate function of the shunt.

Chronic subdural hematoma. If chronic subdural hematoma is suspected, the patient should be admitted and closely observed and a brain scan, computerized cranial tomogram, or an angiogram performed within 24 hours. If the patient is semicomatose or comatose, one of these procedures should be done immediately.

Temporal arteritis. Temporal arteritis can be documented in the emergency department by history, physical examination, and a sedimentation rate. Treatment should be started immediately and consists of prednisone, 100 mg orally, followed by chronic oral therapy at doses of 80 to 100 mg per day while the patient undergoes further evaluation in the hospital.

SUMMARY

Every unconscious patient arriving in the emergency department brings to mind the same pertinent question: Why is this patient in coma? Although initial and emergency treatment should occur simultaneously with the history and physical examination, a probable diagnosis must rapidly be established if ongoing therapy is to be effective. This chapter offers a guideline for initial evaluation of these patients and for the rapid recognition of immediately life-threatening diseases. It is suggested that stable patients who are likely to have less severe causes of coma be

rapidly admitted to the ward or intensive care unit for further investigation and treatment. If personnel are well attuned to separating these two groups, then there will be efficient use of the emergency department and efficient preservation of life and function.

Continuous major generalized seizures can result in permanent brain damage, and aggressive therapy must be given to such patients.

Headaches are infrequently a cause for alarm, but certain types need early recognition and treatment to prevent brain damage.

REFERENCES

1. Hinterbuchner, L. P.: Evaluation of the unconscious patient, Med. Clin. North Am. **57:** 1363-1372, 1973.
2. Plum, F., and Posner, J. D.: Diagnosis of stupor and coma, ed. 2, Philadelphia, 1972, F. A. Davis Co.
3. Headaches and cranial neuralgia. In Vinken, P. J., and Bruyn, G. W., editors: Handbook of clinical neurology, Amsterdam, 1968, North-Holland Publishing Co., vol. 5.
4. Dalessio, D. J.: Wolff's headache and other head pain, New York, 1972, Oxford University Press.
5. Lombroso, C. T.: The treatment of status epilepticus, Pediatrics **53:**536-540, 1974.

CHAPTER 12

Psychiatric emergencies

Thomas N. Rusk, M.D.
Barbara J. Edwards, R.N.

When need satisfaction is threatened, people are in crisis. The severity of the crisis depends on the person's ability to handle individual feelings and needs. When needs are unfulfilled in fact (as when one loses a loved one) or threatened (as in a job promotion in which one fears reprisal from competitive peers or fears failure in new responsibilities) then two major alternatives emerge: (1) crisis resolution through creative problem-solving by behaving so as to change the life situation so that needs are satisfied or (2) failure to cope and increasing distress, with escape maneuvers to reduce the discomfort of frustrated needs by drinking, drug abuse, suicide attempts, psychiatric illness, or running away.

In this chapter the concept of a crisis or emergency is discussed first, followed by the general approach to psychiatric emergency care; finally, approaches to specific emergency situations are presented.

CRISIS CONCEPT

Whitehorn[1] describes four human needs shared by everyone that are critical for optimal life functioning.

1. Love—to love and be loved by another (parents in the case of a young child; someone outside the original family from adolescence on)

2. Security and control—security that biologic needs for food, air, shelter, and so forth, are provided for and that the world is reasonably consistent and predictable; the need for some control over day-to-day life changes.

3. Significance—the feeling that one is worthwhile, valued by self and others

4. Fun

Many illnesses can be viewed as resulting from coping inadequately when one of these needs is threatened. Many patients would rather take large doses of various medications, be hospitalized, labeled medically ill, have numerous surgeries, or be charged large amounts of money for diagnostic tests and expensive treatments than honestly face their current life situation. They cannot admit to the harsh reality that they feel unloved, insecure, and insignificant and that in order to alter that reality they must change how they live and interact with others, an extraordinarily difficult task.

The rule of thumb for the clinician remains to look beyond the chief complaint. Theodore Reik speaks of "listening with the third ear," and with time, practice, and determined detective work, the effective clinician can expose the underlying problem that has been too painful for the patient to encounter directly.

Consider the following example:

A 28-year-old woman, single, bright, and employed as a teacher, presented with insomnia and fear of staying alone at night, all of recent onset. She wanted medication for relief of these symptoms and could think of no reason why they had occurred. Everything was going "well." Confident, intrusive, empathic exploration into her current life situation revealed that the man she had lived with for a month had returned to his wife just before the onset of symptoms. She curiously experienced no anger at him, probably for several reasons. Open anger of any sort was never displayed by her family, and if she did get openly angered at him, she feared he might never return to her. Also, if she became angry and told him to decide in her favor or forget her, he might decide to leave his wife and marry her. This consequence contradicted her self-fulfilling prophesy that she was born to be rejected and hurt by men and to live a lonely life. This "script," although painful, was less anxiety-provoking than risking a life-style that allowed intimacy and mutual respect, a life-style foreign to her.[2]

How can emergency personnel be of more direct help to patients needing psychiatric care? What should you do if there is a significant discrepancy between a patient's complaint and its organic basis, or if you are convinced that tension, depression, or other emotional distress is significant? Although further exploration is indicated, you may be inclined to avoid this step: If you open up Pandora's box, what might it take to close it again and what dire consequences might ensue? Is there any possibility of more severe anxiety, depression, suicide attempt, or other catastrophic occurrences? The following discussion should help emergency personnel handle some of the more common psychiatric emergencies.

GENERAL PRINCIPLES OF MANAGEMENT
Assessment

Bridges[3] recommends that information be elicited in five significant areas: (1) the patient's behavior, (2) the patient's complaint (the patient's own account, told as freely as possible), (3) physical examination, (4) history from others (e.g., relatives and psychiatric hospitals), and (5) observation of the patient over a period of time, if necessary. Pertinent laboratory tests should be done if an organic brain syndrome is suspected, for example, blood tests for determination of bromides, barbituates, alcohol, or amphetamines when indicated. On one occasion a simple blood smear on a confused man referred to psychiatry revealed that he had a lymphocytic leukemia; a simple urinalysis on another occasion showed that the patient's confused state was caused by diabetes.

The presence of signs of an organic brain syndrome, acute (delirium) or chronic (dementia), with or without the psychotic manifestations of grossly disorganized behavior (hallucinations, delusions, etc.), is a medical, not psychiatric, diagnostic emergency. Vagueness, hesitancy, and errors or difficulties in smooth flow of thought and recall of recent events are the subtle indicators of cerebral insufficiency. Once loss of recent memory and disorientation to day and date are present, significant impairment exists. An EEG would indeed be useful, for example, to differentiate the withdrawal of a schizophrenic or the lethargy of depression from impending coma.

Personnel should increase their diagnostic acumen so as to recognize early cerebral impairment. It is their urgent duty to uncover its organic origins. Too often the florid psychologic manifestations in delirium sidetrack clinicians into spending too much time and effort suppressing the symptomatology with medication or referring these patients to psychiatrists. In so doing, they abrogate their medical responsibility for the patient.

Expansion of each of Bridges' five areas is important:

1. Patient's behavior: If the patient is totally disorganized or totally mute and stuporous, little other than this observation can be made. Otherwise,

the symptomatic behavior of the patient can often be translated by applying the question, "What is the patient saying and asking by this behavior?" The cowering, shaking figure in the corner is saying, "I am helpless, harmless, and frightened; please don't hurt me." The angry, destructive, threatening patient is saying, "You all want to hurt me; I can trust no one, which scares me so much I'll fight and destroy anyone to protect myself."

2. Patient's complaint: Let the patient relate complaints in his or her own words, but lead the exploration by focusing on the question, "Why now?" The current life situation has precipitated the emergency. The interaction between the patient and the principal people in his or her life has created dissatisfaction in regard to the three essential needs of every human being: affection, significance, and security. The clinician's job: discover what happened and how and why this has happened.

3. Physical examination: This is a crucial aspect of care, but it hardly needs emphasis to this book's audience.

4. History: A psychiatric emergency is a psychosocial emergency. The better the information and cooperation from those important to the patient, the better the prognosis.

5. Observation of patient: This might involve overnight hospitalization when the diagnosis is unclear. In our experience most emergencies occur in the late afternoon or evening, as well as on special days like holidays or at particular times of the year such as spring. Astrologers' conceptions to the contrary, the presence of a full moon does not increase the incidence of psychiatric emergencies. Many crises seem less significant to a patient in the morning, especially after a good night's sleep has restored the ego.

Therapeutic approach

A useful therapeutic approach in crisis involves five components: explicit empathy, confidence, warmth, hope, and intrusiveness.

Explicit empathy. Explicitly conveyed empathy for the patient's discomfort enhances the crucial therapeutic alliance. This can be relied on to effect changes necessary to alleviate the emergency. The feelings that threaten to overwhelm a patient in a crisis provide an excellent opportunity to be empathic. The tailspin of increasing anxiety and depression followed by progressively more primitive coping behavior (regression) tends to isolate the patient from family and friends. Empathic involvement reverses the isolation, relieving the loneliness and providing a primitive comfort akin to early mothering. Make explicit observations as to how the patient actually looks: "You look really depressed (sad, angry, lonely, etc.) to me." Explain that in your experience, people with similar complaints are not presently having their needs for love, security, significance, and fun satisfied. Ask if that applies to the incurrent life.

Confidence. A calm, confident approach reduces anxiety and increases the likelihood that the patient will identify with your competent approach to crisis situations. Explore the present life situations, especially in regard to home and work. Side with the patient's needs. "You have the right to be loved, secure, and feel important. Anyone would be tense, upset, and depressed if he had as unsatisfactory a life as you seem to have." Make the patient aware of your confidence in yourself and your concern for his or her needs. There is no place here for a passive, permissive approach. You must take the firm lead to get the patient back on course before returning control to his or her hands. Explain that there are times when people have to be helped when unable to help themselves. *Only do for patients what they cannot do for themselves—no more!*

Warmth. A truly warm individual is especially sensitive to anxiety levels. One can love another without being explicitly loving toward another. Sharing one's understanding with words and feelings is more likely to elicit some reciprocal behavior. Warmth can be silently experienced, too, but is useful therapeutically only when put into explicit action: a hand gently placed on an arm, shoulder, or knee will say a thousand unspoken words. To take another's hand in yours wihle speaking will rapidly erect the solid bridge over which all therapeutic effects pass. This does not deny that even silent warmth is useful in increasing understanding, but in the therapeutic process, understanding helps only when shared.

Hope. Hope, like confidence, is contagious. If honestly experienced and effectively conveyed, it is a prime motivator for therapeutic change. Your willingness and eagerness to explore the patient's alien emotions and to allow their expression demonstrate a desire to truly become involved, to understand, and to help. Support and hope of this type is desperately desired and yet so rare in the lives of most people by the time they are in crisis. By providing hope you will discover that you have all the leverage needed to accomplish short-term goals.

Intrusiveness. The person in crisis, unable to competently survey all aspects of the siutation, experiences tunnel perception instead. In an abortive attempt to cope, the patient often chooses a single inappropriate focus or jumps in a disorganized manner from one to another. As the therapist, you must be established as a crucial variable in the patient's life, demanding some of the limited available attention if you are to have influence. At times this demands that a dramatic quality be introduced. Very often you must do the unexpected in a very human, personal manner to yield dividends. You may have to grasp the patient's hands or shout to gain attention. You can display your anger or pain when ignored by withdrawn patients. In all of these actions the message is, "I count, and I refuse to be ignored or to accept your hopeless view of the situation." Explore what the patients would like their lives to be. Ask how they intend to get there. How do they intend to change their behavior in life so they can get their needs satisfied. Emphasize that you expect the patient to "risk" new behaviors. Put the emphasis on changing to more productive behaviors rather than on insight as to why things are currently so unrewarding. Now you can clearly place responsibility where it belongs. If a patient has a terrible current life situation, is miserable and symptomatic, yet is unwilling to risk change, then you have no magic potion that will relieve the situation. You can confront this patient warmly and reasonably, yet firmly, and with self-respect, knowing you can do only so much with emergency care. These patients must change the reality of their lives if their complaints are to be relieved.

Goals

Aim for the last best level of adjustment. The more acute the onset, the more severe the external stress, the more reliable and available are relatives and friends, the less the emotional and behavioral regression, the better the prognosis.

Accurate estimation of the patient's potential and residual capacity to cope requires a careful mental status (thought processes, affect [feelings or emotions], orientation, etc.), along with the usual historical data, such as current life adjustment, educational, marital, and military background, and previous illnesses, especially duration and response to treatment. The sole ally you have in therapy is the healthy part of the individual. The crucial test is the empirical one, the critical trial. All the enthusiasm, hope, and confidence you can muster should be employed in order to involve the patient in creative intervention. If emergency intervention fails, you can always resort to hospitalization; but never hospitalize without giving emergency intervention a trial.

TACTICS IN CRISIS INTERVENTION
Affectual release

The release of pent up feelings induces appreciation. Second, it provides an opportunity for empathy. Labeling, as in, "You must feel very uncomfortable (confused, upset) inside," may help to open the affectual floodgates. Most people attempt to minimize and suppress strong negative feelings in others, for example, grief, anger, or jealousy. Your willingness and eagerness to explore these alien emotions and to allow their abreaction demonstrates a desire to truly get involved, to understand, and to help.

Fostering maturity

Ultimately, the therapist works toward having patients assume as much responsibility for their life as their potential will allow. At first, meet the patient where he or she is in regard to individual coping capacity. You cannot afford the luxury of professional appropriate distance, and often the patient's ego is not healthy enough for an independent, introspective growth experience. Therefore, you should supply whatever nurturing is needed at the onset of the crisis regardless of degree and then proceed with the expectation of growth to at least the previous best adaptive capacity. Many therapists are concerned that they may foster regression, which would deprive the patient of the required support needed during this crisis phase. In this way they lose the chance to diminish anxiety and establish an alliance. Others, discouraged or frightened by an infantile state, do not attempt crisis intervention and hospitalize immediately. In so doing, they demean both the patient and themselves.

Current life focus

Focus on the events that led to the crisis in the first place, as well as the reasons for seeking help that day. The current situation should constitute the nodal point of the entire intervention. You can do nothing about past situations. Memory remains fresher for current data and is less contaminated by intrapsychic distortions. This focus on the patient encourages patient responsibility for the adaptive task at hand and discourages unrealistic expectations that early traumatic sources can be found that will "solve everything." A person in crisis is frequently unable to address the current stress or conflict directly. This inability to deal effectively with a current situation is the crisis. To face it directly would rekindle the anxiety. The therapist must gently lead the patient back to face the crisis. The unwary therapist who pursues material from the past (over one year) unwittingly encourages a defense flight into pseudocrisis:

A 47-year-old truck driver who had been driving and teaching novices for the same firm for 20 years came to us in 1969 with nightmares, insomnia, tremulousness, and inability to work for six weeks due to concerns for, and memories of, a subordinate who had died while on patrol with the patient in Korea in 1952! Under persistent exploration we found that the patient had failed in his attempts to train a psychopathic student driver who was infuriating him. Six weeks prior to coming to the emergency department, while driving with this young man who was sleeping inappropriately through his driving time, the patient fantasized stalling his truck at a particularly dangerous crossing and leaping out himself prior to a train's demolishing the truck and his young nemesis. This would satisfy his anger and eliminate the shame of his first failure as an instructor.

Pseudocrisis represents but one of a group of techniques employed by patients to avoid reexperiencing the events that precipitated the current crisis. These maneuvers include preoccupation with physical symptoms, depression, suicide attempts (a cry for help in themselves), drug overdose, and other bizarre behavior. Search for the most recent reasonably adequate life adjustment. Use this as a starting point rather than belaboring the details of the vicious decompensation cycle.

Unsatisfied needs

Explore patiently the current life situation that has transpired in which the patient's needs are frustrated or threatened. Gentle but persistent exploration into all life areas, such as home, work, and school, will reward you with success. The patient's needs for affection, security, and significance are imperiled. Which one or combination is primarily threatened? Just as important, *who* is disappointing the patient? What coping methods has the patient generally used? Why are these no longer effective? This focusing will lead you to the significant problem area or focal conflict.

Affectual cues

Verbal or nonverbal cues, or affectual inappropriateness, indicate problem areas worthy of exploration. Anxiety reflects that one's ability to cope is being severely tested. Handle it gently, leaving existing defenses intact unless others can be substituted. Note wringing of hands, sweating, facial expressions, and leg and arm movements.[4] If the patient states, "I just need something to calm my nerves," and you note restlessness, tear-brimmed eyes, and head-hanging, it is your clue to reflect back this nonverbal evidence. The statement, "You look terribly upset and anxious," may literally open the flood gates. Depression, on the other hand, represents resignation to defeat of coping efforts. Explore depression relentlessly lest the anger and hopelessness beneath the defensive front erupt at another time when therapist support is not as readily available.

Fostering feedback

As a therapist you should actively foster feedback to and from the patient. There may be no true crisis; the patient may not be in significant distress and may simply want to manipulate you to intercede in the current situation. Examples include seeking increases in compensation benefits, hospitalization to punish a spouse, letters to convince authorities of some disability, or to avoid imprisonment. In these situations the visit is not due to crisis; rather you are being used as an agent for well-established chronic defenses. Practicing clear feedback will help you arrive at a "clean," explicit, mutually agreeable therapeutic contract. Repeated feedback of what the patient states will elucidate a clear-cut picture of why the patient is there and will emphasize your partnership efforts to solve problems with the patient.

Emphasis on the positive

Emphasizing the positive follows an overall principle of working with and from strength. What was the previous optimal level of performance? What are the available strengths in the patient and family? These are frequently difficult facts to elicit. By acknowledging them, the patient contradicts the state of regressive behavior selected to convince the therapist to take over. Having failed, no one is motivated to try again. For this very reason, every possible strength should be thoroughly explored.

At this point, environmental manipulation may be necessary. It is of immense importance to discuss the problem with the relatives or friends of the patient, preferably after the patient's version has been presented, then again at the time future plans are worked out. This provides a more objective history, while encouraging the family's support of the patient. Inviting the family in with the patient to summarize your total understanding helps to establish the positive encounter as a mutual foundation on which to build constructively, rather than as a weapon to punish one another. At times, you can actually work out a focal family conflict. A therapist can supportively "tell it like it is" and clear the air. The emphasis again is on the positive. Which needs of each have not been satisfied? How can each person in the family help the other? Ask them! Has one member had to devalue another in order to have needs satisfied? An attempt should be made to reverse destructive negative feedbacks and encourage positive ones.

Sequence of intervention

Although there can be no simple formula applicable to the wide variety of individuals in crisis, you can plan an overall approach to the intervention. Early in the session work to release dammed-up emotions, using focal probes into potentially significant life areas until results begin to flow. Then, or at the onset, if the patient seems overwhelmed by feelings, explicitly empathize with his or her distress, laying the foundation for the therapeutic alliance. This stage involves information-gathering for a formulation of the current life crisis. In the third phase, become an active, creative problem-solver enlisting help from the patient concerning possible alternative ways of dealing with the present life situation. Included in this phase is building the patient's hope, self-esteem, and independence by emphasis on the positive. Proceed as rapidly as the patient permits from the role of trust-inducing parent to one that encourages initiative. At times only diminished anxiety and halted regression can be accomplished, but time is gained until more definite care is possible.

In brief, then, the intervention plan includes the following: (1) presentation of the therapist as an empathetic, calm, warm, hopeful, intrusive leader; (2) focusing on affect release; (3) fostering of maturity; (4) searching for current focal life situation with the patient; (5) delving into unsatisfied needs; (6) consensual summary and feedback; (7) structured planning, with shifting of responsibility and confidence to the patient while encouraging him or her to select from appropriate alternatives; and (8) reviewing future possibilities of stress, methods of resolution, and sources of further help.

Termination

The following hints are useful in determining whether efforts at intervention have been adequate, or if further immediate steps are necessary:

1. Has the manifest anxiety level decreased significantly?
2. Can the patient independently describe a plan of future action?
3. Is the patient explicitly and genuinely hopeful regarding the immediate future?
4. Is the patient spontaneously appreciative of your attempts to help?
5. Is there a realistic expectation that unmet needs now have a better chance of satisfaction?

In general, the more adequate the current available interpersonal relationships, the less concern we have in releasing patients rather than hospitalizing them, regardless of their coping capacity.

Environmental manipulation

Manipulation of the patient's environmental situation includes physical force, hospitalization, job change, changes at work, alterations in living arrangements, commitment, and so forth. Be cautious of simplistic notions, such as the idea that vacations are always beneficial for persons who overwork. Overwork exists but should be regarded as symptomatic rather causal in almost all situations. Precluding this defensive behavior can release a serious depression, perhaps even leading to suicide.

Physical force deserves more detailed consideration. The violent or disorganized patients who are out of control and not responsive to talk must be restrained for their own sake, as well as others'. Frequently, the root of the outburst is overwhelming anxiety born of the incapacity to control and protect the self. The solution is to muster an overwhelming number of calm, competent, firm but nonpunitive, able-bodied individuals—at least "one for each limb, plus one." Confront such patients with the "show of force" and a humane determination to protect them from harming themselves or others. If calm does not ensue, do not hesitate to put force into action. A well-trained crew of mental health assistants, rather than untrained police, relatives, or friends, will ensure success. The violence may reflect a desire to save face or displace anger. Considerable skill is then necessary to avoid actual fighting and injury. Once the patient is subdued, temporary sedation is indicated rather than prolonged physical restraint.

Chemotherapy

Drugs should be used with caution in the emergency situation. Three categories of drugs are of use in psychiatric emergencies. They all serve as sedative tranquilizers. Chlorpromazine (Thorazine), orally in doses of 50 to 100 mg repeated every 45 minutes to 4 hours, may be necessary. Hypotension is a danger with intramuscular use. Blood pressure should be checked after each dose, recumbency encouraged, and shock position employed if hypotension occurs. Thorazine is the drug of choice with schizophrenic and manic excitements.

In organic disorders, especially when seizures are a concern as in alcoholic withdrawal, diazepam (Valium) is the drug of choice for initial and continuing care. Oral doses of 10 mg three to four times daily for the first day and 5 mg three to four times daily thereafter should be employed. The adult intramuscular or intravenous dose for initial treatment of muscle spasm, status epilepticus, or recurrent convulsive seizures is 5 to 10 mg. A second dose may be given

in one to four hours. For agitation due to alcohol withdrawal the initial intravenous dose is 10 mg followed by 5 mg every five minutes until control is achieved. As little as 15 mg or as much as 250 mg may be required for initial calming.[5] Intramuscular injections should be made deep into the muscle. The rate of intravenous administration of diazepam should not exceed 5 mg/min. Caution is warranted, however, since diazepam has a prolonged (20 to 50 hour) half-life and, therefore, is capable of inducing cumulative central nervous system depression. High doses should be avoided in patients with liver insufficiency.

Some clinicians still prefer rapid-acting, parenterally administered barbiturates such as thiopental (Pentothal), intramuscularly or injected slowly intravenously in a dose of 150 to 250 mg initially over 30 seconds with additional drug injected after one minute as necessary. Anesthesia is rapidly produced. Drawbacks include the potential for laryngospasm and cardiac arrest. If agitation persists, as the sedation wears off, one still faces the necessity of either reanesthetizing the patient or using the major or minor tranquilizer that could have been used in the first place. Severe liver damage is a contraindication to the use of rapid-acting barbiturates and chlorpromazine (Thorazine).

Great care should be taken and generally much lower doses employed in elderly or debilitated individuals when utilizing any of the drugs mentioned. In any patient already sedated, omit the next scheduled dose.

As with force, do not use homeopathic doses of medication. If, for the sake of safety and humaneness, the patient needs tranquilization, give adequate doses repeated frequently until calm ensues. Small doses diminish the patient's control further and thus can paradoxically increase anxiety.

Severe suicidal depressions of emergency nature do not respond to these agents, although the frequently associated agitation might. In those rare cases of malignant depression with self-multilation behavior, emergency electroconvulsive therapy dramatically alleviates the problem. Antidepressant therapy (e.g., Tofranil, Elavil) in emergency situations is inappropriate, since these drugs are toxic in relatively low overdose (10-day supply), are nondialyzable, and do not begin to work therapeutically for ten days to two weeks. An exception is the use of amitriptyline (Elavil) or imipramine (Tofranil), 50 mg, at night to improve sleep in anxious-depressed patients. Tolerance usually develops to the sedative side effects of tricyclic antidepressants in one to two weeks, though beneficial effects on sleep persist.

Major tranquilizers, such as the phenothiazines (chlorpromazine—Thorazine; trifluoperazine—Stelazine; perphenazine—Trilafon; fluphenazine—Prolixin; thioridazine Mellaril) and minor tranquilizers in the benzodiazepine group (chlordiazepoxide—Librium; diazepam—Valium; oxazepam—Serax) have a potentially fatal massive dose (MD) to daily dose (DD) ratio of at least 30 to 1. This allows the patient to have up to a month's supply with safety.

Antidepressants of the tricyclic (imipramine—Tofranil; amitriptyline—Elavil) or the monoamine oxidase (MAO) groups (phenelzine—Nardil; tranylcypromine—Parnate) and minor tranquilizers of the substituted diol group (meprobamate, tybamate—Solacen) have a MD/DD of only 10 to 1. Dialysis is useful only with the small-molecule MAO inhibitor antidepressants and substituted diols. Note that tricyclic antidepressants, the drugs of choice in severe depressions, are the most lethal in overdose and not effectively dialyzable.[6] Since patients in crisis require a minimum of once or twice weekly visits, 30-day supplies are rarely indicated.

Management of emergencies calls for a calm, deliberate, yet creative use of environmental manipulation and chemotherapy.

Often the most useful benefit the patient derives from the crisis intervention is the feeling of genuine interest from a confident professional person. Further, the assurance that the therapist and colleagues remain available demonstrates continuing interest, concern, and support during the days and weeks of precarious balance that follow the initial crisis visit.

MANAGEMENT OF SPECIFIC EMERGENCY SITUATIONS
Social emergencies

On social emergencies there is threat of actual loss of behavioral control with resultant destructive behavior toward self, others, or property. In preparing this section we have freely drawn from a number of sources[7-10] to supplement our own experiences.

Suicidal behavior. Officially the tenth leading cause of death with more than 20,000 deaths recorded per year, suicide probably accounts for ten times this figure, as well as for a large number of accidental deaths that are naively assumed to be unintentional rather than intentional or "subintentional."[11] The number of attempts has been estimated at seven to ten times this rate.

Women attempt suicide at least twice as often as men, especially in the second and third decade. Men complete suicide two to four times as frequently as women, the incidence increasing with age.

Suicide occurs less among the married (x), especially those with children, than among the single ($2x$), widowed ($4x$), or divorced ($4x$). In the United States suicide predominates among the poor, the foreign born, and the white, although the rate for urban blacks is rising rapidly.

Data on women indicate that the menstrual period is a time of increased suicidal and accidental behaviors.[12] Spring brings increased suicidal behaviors, while in midwinter self-destruction is at a low ebb.[13]

Alcoholics, patients with chronic debilitating or terminal diseases, and those recently informed of a serious pathology comprise the high risk groups in routine practice, especially if they also display the dependent, dissatisfied personality pattern.[14-16]

Sixty percent of completed suicides have histories of previous attempts. Ten percent of attempted suicides will eventually kill themselves. Seventy-five percent of completed suicides have given rather clear warning.[10] Repeated attempts often increase in seriousness.[17]

Among those primarily psychiatrically ill, the depressive constitute the highest suicide risk. This occurs particularly if a person is significantly depressed while retaining high energy levels, as in agitated depressions.

Suicide occurs in other psychiatric diagnostic groups as well. The most unpredictable is the schizophrenic, especially if the patient suffers depression or threatening hallucinations.

Persons who attempt suicide present some diagnostic difficulty. Is it a gesture or a real attempt? This is a dangerous and artificial dichotomy. Shneidman[16] proposes that every suicidal patient be evaluated on two bases: Evaluate how upset or disturbed the patient is and then evaluate the patient's lethality. For example, an adolescent girl might be very upset with her parents but have no intention of killing herself, while an elderly man who is slowly dying and alone in the world might be very lethal but not particularly disturbed. In addition, evaluate the following:

1. The method employed: is it rapidly fatal or slow and not likely to succeed?
2. To what extent is the behavior giving a message designed to manipulate others rather than simply to effect death?
3. How socially isolated from significant others is the patient? Has the patient become significantly alienated from or suffered what appears to be an irretrievable loss of a person? This would increase the risk significantly. In a recent article Fawcett and co-workers[18] found that the relationships to significant others constitute the crucial ingredients in determining the seriousness of suicidal intent. These relationships serve as "shock absorbers" in times of crisis.
4. After the attempt, has the constellation of events altered sufficiently to diminish the chance of a repeat performance?
5. Have close relatives suicided? This increases the risk.
6. Can the patient talk hopefully and spontaneously about the future?
7. A history of previous attempts, associated with significant depression requiring hospitalization, including drug or electroconvulsive treatment, increases the lethality rating.*

Suicidal behavior demands referral to a psychiatrist for evaluation of the preceding factors. Utilize the therapeutic approach recommended earlier to establish a therapeutic alliance. Obtain the information recommended in this section and evaluate the psychosocial constellation. After this has been done, the decision regarding admission should be clear. Admission to hospital does not preclude a successful suicide attempt, which can occur anywhere. The best preventive is an alteration of circumstances, clearing the path for hope while diminishing the current distress. This may ensue as a result of the attempt itself or efforts at intervention. Until it has, the patient is not safe anywhere.

Anxiety and panic. The reverberating circuit of anxiety and its physiologic con-

---

*Two excellent articles on the evaluation of suicidal risks by Havens[19] and Litman and Farberow[20] are worth reading.

comitants, such as palpitations, dyspnea, tremor, sweating, and restlessness evoke the fear of death and loss of control. The therapist should first attempt to talk to the patient, as recommended earlier. As an adjunct or substitute, if talk is impossible, drugs may be employed and discussion postponed.

Anxiety must be differentiated from more serious conditions. Schizophrenics suffer great anxiety and need a more careful approach because of their great difficulty in trusting others. Phenothiazines are required, generally in high doses (from 400 to 1,000 mg of chlorpromazine [Thorazine] per day) or haloperidol (Haldol), 10 to 30 mg or more, in the acutely excited state. There will be comparable difficulty in calming hypomanics with talk. Often they respond only to massive doses of chlorpromazine while lithium therapy is initiated.

Patients with organically caused confusions can demonstrate marked anxiety and restlessness that can mask early signs of intellectual impairment. Specific treatment is required over and above symptomatic care. Agitated depressives, as noted earlier, are very serious suicide risks. These patients must be differentiated from those in simple acute anxiety states.

Aggressive or bizarre behavior. This is among the most common major psychiatric emergencies. Aggression and bizarre behavior are common in schizophrenics, manics, the intoxicated, the organically confused, epileptics during seizures or in postical confusion, and psychopaths.

An attempt should be made in a kind, confident, nonthreatening manner to clarify the reality of the situation and to reassure these patients that no harm will come to them, nor will they be allowed to harm anyone. Never deceive them by giving false promises or going along with a delusion in order to gain control. If an honest discussion fails, resort to overwhelming (and thus humane) doses of drugs or manpower.

Delusional or paranoid patients. To be paranoid is not necessarily to be schizophrenic. Many paranoid patients have localized and guarded delusional beliefs, ideas of reference or persecution. Often they are of above average intelligence and are very sensitive to criticism. In fact, their paranoia can be explained as the necessity to protect their self-esteem, which in men is intricately involved with masculinity. A common past history includes mental hospitalization, frequent lawsuits, frequent marriages, and job changes with blame always ascribed to others or circumstances. Overintellectualization or extraordinarily detailed knowledge, especially in the area of law, rules, or regulations, is common.

These are risky, unpredictable people who make unreasonable demands and misinterpret communications of all sorts. If they feel slighted by authorities, such as physicians or nurses, they become extremely angry and may then make direct or indirect attacks through police, courts, or other channels. These patients are notoriously bad risks for elective surgery, yet they frequently seek treatment, especially for chronic back and rectal difficulties. (Worthy of note is the clinical clue that incipient schizophrenics often complain of vague or bizarre physical complaints of recent onset.)

Be firm, matter-of-fact, calm, passively friendly, avoiding a conciliatory or aggressive approach. Never deceive. Agree to disagree openly and *without anger* if, in fact, you do disagree. Have witnesses present if possible. Make it clear that you are available as an ally, but only if the patient desires it. Avoid even the slightest hint that you have a vested interest in dealing with the patient. Phenothiazines are useful only in patients with an underlying schizophrenic thought disorder or in acute paranoid states. Chronic paranoid personalities defeat any and all efforts at treatment.

Organic brain syndromes. In this category we refer to the organic brain syndromes mentioned in the section on assessment. These syndromes must be differentiated from psychiatric conditions such as hysterical fugues or amnesias and catatonic or manic stupors. Expert consultation and observation over time may be necessary to differentiate the "functional" stupors from organic disturbances. Treatment, as noted earlier, requires attention to the specific underlying disorder, as well as symptomatic treatment with sufficient medication to avoid restraints. A well-lit room, friendly, competent, consistent attendants (or responsible family members) around the clock, and frequent efforts to orient and reassure the patient are crucial.

Alcohol and drugs. Although the disorders produced by these agents fall into the previous category, the tremendous incidence of alcohol-related problems, the ever increasing problem of drug abuse, and the special problems related to these kinds of intoxications merit a separate discussion.

One tends to be irritated by those who misuse alcohol and drugs and to minimize the inebriated state as the simple, reversible overindulgence it often is. But keep in mind that in 50% of all fatal automobile accidents at least one intoxicated driver is involved.[21] In a similar percentage of all major crimes in this country the perpetrators were intoxicated. Many suicidal people take drugs in addition to alcohol, and the effects are often additive. Occult head injuries are frequent in the intoxicated. Alcohol is the most common sedative used for self-treatment even by severely ill schizophrenics. If there is any doubt, the following is indicated: hospitalization, observation with careful neurologic examinations, skull films, EEG, and only enough sedation to prevent injury or exhaustion of the patient and to allow evaluation and management. Recent studies show the superiority of diazepam (Valium) over all other sedatives for these patients as well as

for those suffering from delirium tremens.[5,22]

Emergencies caused by overdose or withdrawal from other sedatives, such as barbiturates and hypnotics of other types, pose similar problems. Wikler[23] describes in detail the management of those withdrawing from these drugs.

In brief, alcoholics in withdrawal require adequate doses of Librium or Valium to avoid restraints, 4 to 8 liters of nutritive juices by mouth (if cardiac and renal functions are adequate), and high doses of B vitamins intramuscularly for several days.

Sedative addicts in a withdrawal emergency should be replaced on their medication, or liquid pentobarbital substituted after a 200 mg test dose is administered while the patient is in the neutral state between intoxication and withdrawal. If no effect occurs, including the absence of nystagmus on lateral gaze, then the equivalent of 1,200 mg or more of liquid pentobarbital per day may be required to prevent the almost inevitable seizures and delirium that ensue in those who have been taking the equivalent of over 800 mg of pentobarbital per day.

Patients showing some indication of intoxication two hours subsequent to the test dose require intermediate maintenance doses. Once maintenance is established, initiate slow withdrawal of no more than 100 mg of pentobarbital per day. If withdrawal symptoms reappear, the dose should be maintained or raised slightly until such symptoms disappear. Severely dependent patients may be withdrawn from barbiturates in 14 to 21 days.

Narcotic addicts in withdrawal can be stabilized with 5 to 20 mg of methadone four times a day orally followed by slow withdrawal. Those suffering overdoses of narcotics can be cautiously treated with regular doses of naloxone, 400 μg intravenously every two to three minutes, until vital signs remain at acceptable levels. If there is no significant improvement after two to three doses, the depressive condition may not be due to a drug or disease state responsive to naloxone. Since the duration of the narcotic is often longer than that of naloxone, the depressant effects of the narcotic may return, requiring additional doses of naloxone. Naxolone is the drug of choice when the identity of the depressant drug is unknown because it does not cause further respiratory depression. Another danger is the violent abstinence syndrome that antagonistic agents can precipitate.

The hallucinogens or psychotomimetics constitute a different problem. Although these emergencies are rare in relation to their total use, "bad trips," "flashbacks" (recurrence of phenomena induced by drug without new ingestion of it), confused behavior while on a poorly guided experience, and prolonged psychotic episodes constitute bona fide emergencies. Marijuana rarely produces these kinds of problems, although panic attacks and paranoid reactions do occur. Patients intoxicated with drugs of the LSD or mescaline type should be hospitalized. The same supportive measures that are indicated for patients with organic disease are necessary, along with chlorpromazine in sufficient doses to calm the patient. Rarer, but more complicated, is a combined hallucinogen overdosage, especially if one drug is an antichlolinergic, such as stramonium, scopolamine, atropine, or the more potent newer analogues Serynl or Ditran.[24] Care for overdosages of the latter with phenothiazines may aggravate parasympathetic blockade. Valium has been recommended for the treatment of all types of hallucinogenic drug crises,[25] since it is effective and does not aggravate the parasympathetic blockade.

Other problems. Other "urgencies" encountered in practice are touched on by Shurley and Pokorny.[26] They include the following.

The self-mutilating patient. Deluded, hallucinating schizophrenics, patients with organic disease, or suicidal patients may mutilate themselves directly or by sabotaging the treatment devices used on them, such as casts, stitches, catheters, and the like. Constant care, adequate sedation, and treatment of the underlying disorder are indicated.

The uncooperative patient. The "ounce of prevention" proverb is applicable. Those clinicians who develop adult therapeutic partnerships with their patients will be plagued much less by lack of cooperation and loss of patients. These productive therapeutic partnerships stand in contrast to those clinician-patient relationships characterized by minimal involvement or paternalistic omnipotent-omniscient attitudes. The latter evoke magical expectations and unrealistic demands, with disappointment the inevitable result.

Most uncooperative patients are responding to anxiety, anger, and diminished trust in the therapist. Rather than arguing, a calm, reassuring exploration of the basis of these feelings ameliorates the majority of these situations. The largest stumbling block remains the therapist's threatened self-esteem when his or her care is questioned. The competent secure individual will weather the abuse, explore the concerns, and in so doing, give tremendous reassurance.

If the situation is emergent and the patient is psychotic and dangerous to self or others, commitment may be indicated. If so, calmly and firmly inform the patient and family while carefully justifying your recommendation to them and in your records.

The patient who feels hopeless. There is increasing evidence that the "giving up, given up"[27] attitude complex contributes to the development of disease states, as clinicians have suspected for generations. In addition, suicide potential is great, and cooperation in care and convalescence is poor or perfunctory. The best solution remains the well-cultivated relationship between the clinician and the patient, coupled with active, concerned, direct exploration of the patient's concerns.

The patient about to receive bad news. How much one tells a patient should depend on how much the patient indicates he or she desires to know. In the case of impending death, a responsible adult family member must, of course, be informed (a private, explicitly empathic, unhurried discussion). The personal physician, privy to all the medical details and having the advantage of an established relationship and the patient's trust, should handle this most difficult of all medical responsibilities. This approach would apply as well to family members about to be told of a patient's death.

Personal crises

An extensive discussion of the multitude of potential crises throughout the life cycle is beyond the scope of this chapter. Some excellent references in this area are noted at the end of the chapter.[28,29] Several important life crises with emergency potential are outlined below to exemplify this group of problems.

School phobias. Almost invariably this is a separation anxiety stemming from difficulties in the relationship between the child and parents.[30] Generally less serious in the young child, it nonetheless requires that the child immediately return to school while, not after, counseling is provided as necessary to child and parents. School authorities should be included in the diagnostic evaluation and treatment planning. Onset of school aversion in adolescence may herald an incipient psychosis. Referral to a psychiatrist is generally indicated.

Death of a loved one. The prolonged and destructive effects of unresolved grief are excellently described by Lindemann.[31] Survivors deserve an opportunity to thoroughly "work through" the grief. Bowlby[32] has described the three stages of

normal grief as protest, despair, and detachment. Those who express little grief and who discuss their relationship with the deceased very little are prime candidates for unresolved grief and prolonged life-crippling symptomatology. Marked grief persisting longer than three to six months also indicates a pathologic process worthy of psychiatric referral. Emergency personnel should encourage the survivors to openly express to them and to teach other thoughts, feelings, and memories of the deceased.

A special case involves suicide. Those who survive the suicided person must be helped to cast off the legacy of guilt that the common anger-motivated suicide leaves in its wake.

Often just as painful and far more common in routine emergency department practice is rejection by a lover or spouse. The stages of grief are analogous but messier since the inevitability of the rejection is far less certain.

Menopause. The shibboleths of eternal youth and drug panaceas for any and all symptomatology prevail in our culture. Growing pains afflict the muscles of many youngsters. Many adolescents experience breast tenderness. In a similar way, most menopausal women experience the discomforts of flushing, irregular menses, and cramping. Although careful, regular examinations are necessary, much psychologic and physical distress can result from overenthusiastic therapeutic zeal. Especially in women, the "change of life" involves physiologic endocrine readjustment and psychologic life inventory reassessment, which can lead to significant depression masking as physical symptomatology. Parasuicidal encouragements to physicians to recommend surgery with the inevitable physical and psychologic sequelae may constitute an irresistible seduction for "cure-oriented" physicians. A thorough work-up is indicated. If significant definite pathology is not found and exploration of the patient's life situation indicates significant life disappointments, then earnest discussion of these problems should ensue. Psychiatric referral should be considered in addition to appropriate hormonal treatment.

Middle and late middle age impotence is the male equivalent to menopause and is commonly precipitated by retirement, job change, or even a transurethral resection of the prostate. Management is similar to that indicated for menopause. In the absence of definite hormonal imbalance, however, hormonal therapy is *specifically contraindicated*. The overwhelming majority of men with late onset impotence suffer an underlying depression.

SUMMARY

Emotional crises constitute a rather severe test of a therapist's own coping capacities. Multiple systems and variables must be considered in a very brief time in order that very significant and, at times, even life-and-death decisions be made. The emergency department is no place for the passive, permissive, blank screen approach. Good therapy should be judged solely on the basis of its results. The greater the well-being of the individual and the more personally satisfying the life adjustment emanating from crisis therapy, the better the psychotherapy. Further, the more quickly this is accomplished, as in all medical care, the better. In crisis intervention one does what one can as rapidly as possible.

REFERENCES

1. Whitehorn, J. C.: A working concept of maturity of personality, Am. J. Psychiatry **119**:197-202, 1962.
2. Berne, E.: The relationship between transactional analysis and other forms of treatment. In Berne, E., editor: Principles of group treatment, New York, 1966, Grove Press, pp. 292-319.
3. Bridges, P. K.: Psychiatric emergencies, Postgrad. Med. J. **43**:599-604, 1967.
4. Nierenberg, S. I., and Colero, H. H.: How to read a person like a book, New York, 1971, Hawthorn Books, Inc.
5. Thompson, W. L., Johnson, A. D., and Maddrey, W. L.: Diazepam and paraldehyde for treatment of severe delirium tremens: a controlled trial, Ann. Intern. Med. **82**:175, 1975.
6. Brophy, J. J.: Suicide attempts with psychotherapeutic drugs, Arch. Gen. Psychiatry **17**:652-657, 1967.
7. Ewalt, J. R.: Other psychiatric emergencies. In Freedman, A. M., and Kaplan, H. I., editors: Comprehensive textbook of psychiatry, Baltimore, 1967, Williams & Wilkins Co., pp. 1179-1187.
8. Shneidman, E. S., and Farberow, N. L.: Clues to suicide, New York, 1957, McGraw-Hill Book Co.
9. Farberow, N. L., and Shneidman, E. S., editors: The cry for help, New York, 1961, McGraw-Hill Book Co.
10. Hendin, H.: Suicide. In Freedman, A. M., and Kaplan, H. I., editors: Comprehensive textbook of psychiatry, Baltimore, 1967, Williams & Wilkins Co., pp. 1170-1179.
11. Shneidman, E. S.: Suicidal phenomena: Their definition and classification, Los Angeles Suicide Prevention Center.
12. Mandell, A. J., and Mandell, M. P.: Suicide and the menstrual cycle, JAMA **200**:792-793, May, 1967.
13. Henderson, D., and Batchelor, I. R.: Gillespie's textbook of psychiatry, London, 1962, Oxford University Press, p. 71.
14. Farberow, N. L., McKelligott, J. W., Cohen, S., and Darbonne, A.: Suicide among patients with cardiorespiratory illnesses, JAMA **195**:422-428, Feb., 1966.
15. Farberow, N. L., Shneidman, E. S., and Leonard, C. V.: Suicide among general medical and surgical hospital patients with malignant neoplasms, Medical Bulletin 9, Veterans Administration, Department of Medicine and Surgery, Feb., 1963.
16. Shneidman, E. S., Farberow, N. L., and Leonard, C. V.: Suicide evaluation and treatment of suicidal risk among schizophrenic patients in psychiatric hospitals, Medical Bulletin 8, Veterans Administration, Department of Medicine and Surgery, Feb., 1962.
17. Sneddon, J.: Casualties in the casualty department, Practitioner **195**:785, 1965.
18. Fawcett, J., Neff, M., and Bunney, W. E.: Suicide: Clues from interpersonal communication, Arch. Gen. Psychiatry **21**:129-137, Aug., 1969.
19. Havens, L. L.: Recognition of suicidal risks

through the psychologic examinations, N. Engl. J. Med. **276**:210-215, Jan., 1967.

20. Litman, R. E., and Farberow, N. L.: Emergency evaluation of self-destructive potentiality. In Farberow, N. L., and Schneidman, E. S., editors: The cry for help, New York, 1961, McGraw-Hill Book Co.

21. Litman, R. E., and Tabachnick, N. O.: Fatal traffic accidents, Los Angeles Suicide Prevention Center. Unpublished.

22. Brown, J. H., Moggey, D. E., and Shane, F. H.: Delirium tremens: A comparison of intravenous treatment with diazepam and chlordiazepoxide, Scott Med. J. **17**:9, 1972.

23. Wikler, A.: Diagnosis and treatment of drug dependent of the barbiturate type, Am. J. Psychiatry **125**:758-765, Dec., 1968.

24. Mandell, A. J., and West, L. J.: Hallucinogens. In Freedman, A. M., and Kaplan, H. I., editors: Comprehensive textbook of psychiatry, Baltimore, 1967, Williams & Wilkins Co., pp. 247-253.

25. Solursh, L. P., and Clement, W. R.: Use of diazepam in halucinogenic drug crises, JAMA **205**:644-645, Aug., 1968.

26. Shurley, J. T., and Pokorny, A. D.: Handling the psychiatric emergency, Med. Clin. North Am. **46**:417-426, 1962.

27. Schmale, A. H., Jr., and Engel, G. L.: The giving up—given up complex illustrated on film, Arch. Gen. Psychiatry **17**:135-145, 1967.

28. Parad, H. J., editor: Crises intervention: Selected readings, New York, 1965, Family Service Association of America.

29. Berlin, I. N.: Secondary prevention. In Freedman, A. M., and Kaplan, H. I., editors: Comprehensive textbook of psychiatry, Baltimore, 1967, Williams & Wilkins Co., pp. 1541-1548.

30. Work, H. H.: Psychiatric emergencies in childhood. In Wayne, C. J., and Koegler, R. R., editors: Emergency psychiatry and brief therapy, Intern. Psychiatry Clin. **3**:27-37, Nov. 4, 1966.

31. Lindemann, E.: Symptomatology and management of acute grief, Am. J. Psychiatry **101**:141-148, 1944.

32. Bowlby, J., The Adolf Meyer lecture: Childhood mourning and its implications for psychiatry, Am. J. Psychiatry **118**:481-498, 1961.

CHAPTER 13

Substance abuse*

Randolph A. Read, M.D.

WHAT IS SUBSTANCE ABUSE?

Substance abuse is drug abuse . . . but drugs are not just heroin, barbiturates, LSD, or marijuana. Almost any chemical substance can be used as a drug, that is, for the ways its use affects the body and mind. Alcohol is a drug. Tobacco is a drug. Even sugar can be used as a drug.

In the late 1960's, various authors evolved the label "substance" in an effort to overcome our society's blind spot regarding alcoholism and the abuse of prescription medications. People often use the term "drug abuse" to refer only to the narcotic junkie, the glue-sniffing adolescent, or the marijuana-smoking college student. "Substance abuse" emphasizes the inclusion of the executive alcoholic, the housewife sedative addict, and for that matter, the obese person, for they all abuse chemical substances. "Substance abuse" will probably never supplant the phrase "drug abuse" since the latter is so firmly entrenched, but it may help broaden the social definition of drugs. Educational programs in the schools have started spreading the word: "Booze is a drug too."

But such a broad definition of drugs points up the vagueness of our concept of abuse. What *is* abuse? Generally, it has been defined as use at odds with social norms. Jerome Jaffe succinctly summarized this standard in 1969 as "the use, usually by self-administration of any drug in a manner that deviates from approved medical and social patterns within a given culture."[1] Unfortunately, those "approved medical and social patterns" are rarely explicit or consistent. How much use is OK? How much use is too much? Are some drugs acceptable for recreation? Should other drugs never be self-administered? Social values in this area are vague and often contradictory. The "double standard" for alcohol is a good example. On the one hand there are frequent social encouragements to "have a drink" as part of having a good time. Yet, a person who regularly responds to these drinking cues may soon step over that almost invisible line of acceptable use and become ostracized as an "alcoholic."

Part of the problem is that as a society we are "in love" with chemicals. We use them so regularly in our everyday lives that

*Copyright R. A. Read 1977. The author wishes to thank J. Schibanoff, M.D., for his helpful comments on this chapter, and J. Brophy, M.D., for his years of superb teaching.

we can not seem to agree on what constitutes abuse. Consuming chemicals and other material goods is seen as a way to achieve status, pleasure, and satisfaction. Commercial advertising goads us, "Here, take this!" and we are offered automobiles, appliances, foods, and, of course, drugs—remedies for headaches, nervous tension, and every conceivable bowel irregularity.

We live in a society that believes in material solutions to every problem. It expects a "drug for every ailment," as though it were a constitutionally guaranteed right. People take drugs more often than not for that evasive "relief," as if it is inconceivable that one should ever feel anything even slightly unpleasant. It is hardly surprising that substance abuse problems are one of the most common classes of emergencies. Like vehicular accidents, they are simply a by-product of the way we live.

Discussions regarding drug abuse often begin with this sort of handwringing. Obviously this chapter is no exception. The point needs to be made, however, for as health care professionals we have all too often become the high priests of drugs. Treatment of substance abuse problems often focuses on "medications" and "antidotes"—treating with even more drugs—and thereby reinforcing the myth that chemicals solve all problems. Humanity can get lost when material approaches become enshrined as fixed rituals. Ipecac and emesis can become an assembly line routine or, even worse, administered as punishment to teach the patient a lesson.

Our attitudes and beliefs have profound effects. Mechanical, perfunctory care may get the patient through the intial emergency but interfere with what comes next. If the emergency department experience is dehumanizing, the patient might not bother going to the counseling center he had been referred to for follow-up care. If he does not go, he may be back next week with another substance abuse emergency. Staff attitudes affect patients. As much as

blood pressure cuffs or ECG machines, we also are instruments of care.

This chapter will focus on substance abuse emergencies, ways to optimize acute care and to increase chances for successful follow-up treatment. Substance abuse problems come in almost endless varieties, but here we will consider only the most *common, serious* threats to health that appear in *emergency situations*. This usually means an emergency department at a general hospital, but these problem areas are also regularly seen on the fire department rescue call, at the walk-in clinic, and even at home. Since this text is intended for a mixed audience of physicians, nurses, and paramedics a basic review of pharmacologic principles and drug reactions is included. Approaches to assessment and management vary widely, and local problems may demand unique interventions. Overall, an effort has been made to present the most widely accepted approaches to the most common substance abuse emergencies.

SOME BASIC PHARMACOLOGY

The mechanisms of action of most drugs are poorly understood. What *is* known is often complex and confusing. Research may reveal that a drug interacts with a particular enzyme or nucleotide, but the clinical significance of the new finding may be obscure. Part of the problem is that we know relatively few details about the "normal" physiologic processes, let alone how these processes are influenced by drugs.

Fortunately, our ignorance regarding events at the biochemical level does not preclude our determining which drugs can be useful in medicine. If the substance seems to produce an effect with some therapeutic benefit, it becomes labeled a "medication." If, on the other hand, it regularly produces toxic or lethal effects, it is called "poison." Through gross observation of the patient, drug classifications have been developed based on the most striking or useful effect, such as stimulant, narcotic, or anesthetic.

Such categories can be misleading, however, since they suggest that drugs always show the same actions. For example, amphetamines are usually referred to as stimulant drugs, since in most people they produce increases in alertness, rate of speech, or general motor activity. Exactly how they act upon the body to produce these effects is unclear so that we are left with the general term "stimulant" without any good idea of what it is that is being stimulated. Our confusion may be increased by their calming and sedating effects observed in hyperactive children; how can a stimulant act like a tranquilizer? Only partial answers are possible at this time. Drug effects are rarely simple and straightforward so that not too much should be expected from our limited knowledge. Ultimately, each drug and patient is a unique case.

A useful approach is to break down the total drug effect into various subeffects that may add, cancel, or even multiply (Fig. 13-1). In the emergency setting a working understanding of these principles is extremely helpful since clinical signs in the patient that initially don't make sense may be understood when the contribution of the separate effects is taken into consideration.

Drug-specific effects. Drug-specific effects reflect the primary pharmacologic actions of a drug on its *receptor sites* in the body. Drugs are thought to exert their effects by interacting with these receptors in a fashion similar to enzyme lock-and-key reactions. A drug's molecular configuration (the key) allows contact with the receptor site (the lock), which then leads to changes in biochemical processes that produce the drug-specific effects (Fig. 13-2).

These effects may be unique to that substance or shared by other members of its drug class. Substances have been grouped

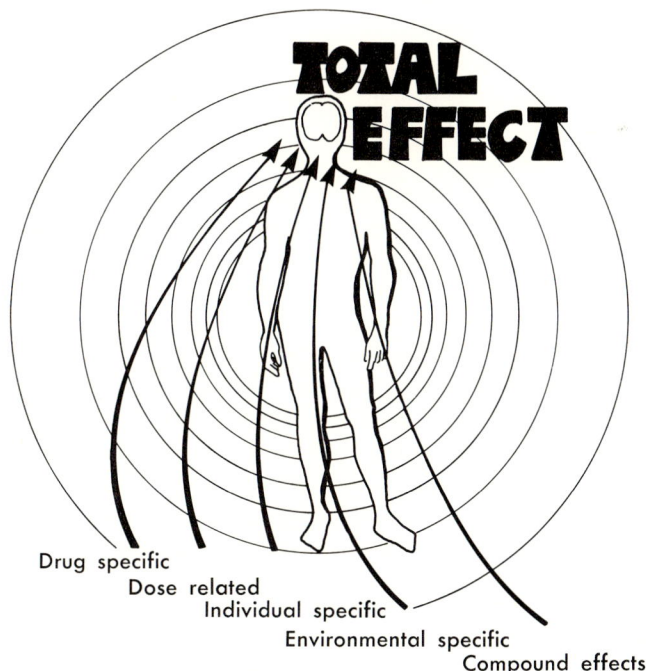

Drug specific
Dose related
Individual specific
Environmental specific
Compound effects

Fig. 13-1. A drug's overall effect can be understood as interacting subeffects.

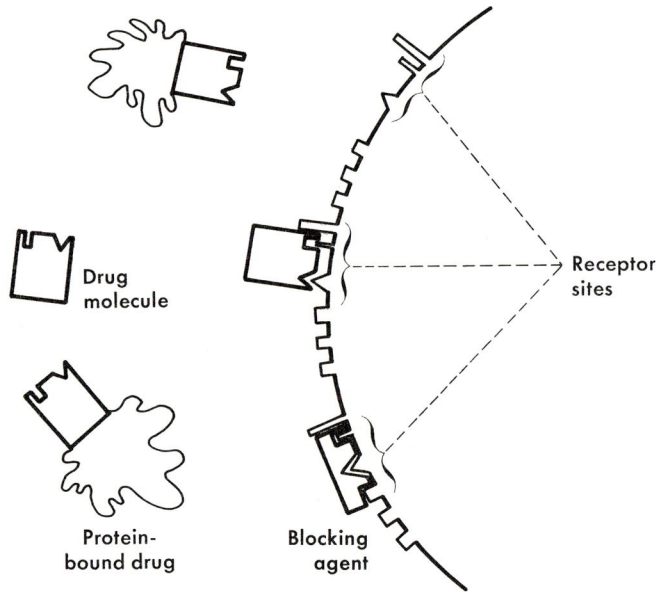

Fig. 13-2. Drug-specific effects are initiated by drug to receptor interaction ("lock and key" combination).

in categories based on one particular drug-specific effect, such as analgesics, sedatives, or stimulants. Broader categories are also possible, for example, drugs that influence thinking, feeling, or behavior are often referred to as psychotropic or psychoactive. Abused substances invariably have some psychotropic drug-specific effect; indeed, that is why they are used in the first place. Heroin, amphetamine, diazepam, and secobarbitol, for example, get abused because respectively they can make a person feel either euphoric, energetic, relaxed, or half asleep. In other words, they produce drug-specific effects that can be interpreted as a "high."

Psychotropic effects do not necessarily mean a drug *will* be abused. Chlorpromazine (Thorazine) rarely tempts anyone since few people interpret its action as a high. Widely used substances usually produce feelings of well-being and euphoria, but almost any strong psychotropic action will make a drug attractive to someone. Drugs that are essentially without psycho-tropic properties, such as digitalis, almost never get abused.

From the user's perspective drug-specific effects can be divided into two general areas: desired and undesired effects. In medicine, desired effects are often referred to as *therapeutic actions* and reflect why a particular drug was administered. Undesired or *side effects* are the unwanted or harmful actions that are part of how that drug interacts with the body. Morphine is usually used for the desired effect of pain relief, yet it also produces the undesired effect of respiratory depression.

Ultimately, what constitutes a side effect depends on the observer's point of view. The street drug phencyclidine (known as PCP, angel dust, or THC) typically produces numbness, paresthesias, feelings of lightheadedness, and kinesthetic halucinations of physical movement. One individual may interpret these effects as nausea, vertigo, and disorientation, yet another person may label the same effects as "rushing, flying through space, and being incredibly high." Thus the adage "one man's side effect is another man's remedy." For most psychotropic drugs the essential drug-specific effects can never be disentangled from one's *perception* of those effects; objective descriptions become impossible. To answer questions regarding a psychotropic drug's actions, one must first ask who is taking it and in what setting.

Individual-specific effects. Individual-specific effects are those attributable to the individual and his expectations. They are the "who is taking the drug?" part of the equation. The person's mental set is most important: his beliefs and desires regarding the drug's effect, history of previous use, and internally experienced stress or psychological pain. Age, sex, body mass, and other physiologic factors affect drug metabolism. Also significant is the person's general state of health including preexisting medical diseases, drug allergies, and idiosyncrasies.

In some situations, individual effects can account for most of the observed total drug effects. Psychedelic drugs produce increased suggestibility (probably a drug-specific effect), which in turn lets a person's fears and desires shape the "trip." At the extreme of individual-specific effects are placebo reactions, responses not attributable to a chemical substance. Thus, when an individual ingests a capsule of talcum powder or smokes a banana peel and gets a high, the reaction is largely the product of his expectations—the individual-specific effect—since both of these substances are almost inert pharmacologically. Flashback reactions, the reexperiencings of psychedelic drug intoxications, have not been shown to have a biochemical basis and probably are placebo reactions that occur without even the "prop" of taking a pill.

Environmental-specific effects. Environmental-specific effects are those attributable to the environment surrounding the use of the drug. They are the "in what setting is the drug taken?" part of the

equation. The immediate environment—people, buildings, time of day—dramatically influences the perception of the effects of many psychoactive drugs. Indeed, in the case of marijuana, consumption by first-time users in the sterility of a laboratory environment may hardly produce any effects at all.[2]

In many ways, individual-specific effects are the products of environmental-specific effects. An individual's reaction to the environment, along with his internalized social values, can strongly alter his perception of drug effects. In the case of bad trips, treatment can exploit these effects by placing the patient in a relatively quiet, nonstimulating, supportive environment.

Various drugs come in and out of vogue, like clothing and cars, and these fads contribute to environment-specific effects. In the United States opiate use enjoyed a boom following the Civil War, but by the 1920's accumulating legal and social pressures led to its replacement by alcohol. In the 1960's, psychedelic drugs enjoyed a surge in popularity, but today only marijuana remains a widely popular survivor. Cocaine, the "in drug" of the idle rich in the 1920's, fell out of favor but seems to have made a recent comeback as the drug for the socially clever. Nevertheless, alcohol continues to be our country's most popular drug, with hypnotic sedatives and tranquilizers probably a poor second.[3] Drug fads will no doubt continue to evolve, and as technology makes other manipulations possible, new highs will be born.

Dose-related effects. Dose-related effects are the changes in drug-specific effects attributable to the quantity of drug used. Generally, but not always, this means "more drug, more effect." In the case of alcohol ingestion an average individual, for example, drinking screwdriver cocktails at a weekend party, would show changes in drug effects as more alcohol is consumed. After one drink a slight to moderate feeling of relaxation might be noted. After two or three drinks this effect may become more pronounced and may be accompanied by feelings of well-being and a sense of increased social ease. If more alcohol is consumed in a one-hour period, by six or seven drinks, signs of impaired motor coordination may become prominent: slurring of speech, unsteady gait, and double vision. By nine or ten drinks, extreme ataxia, lethargy, and somnolence may appear, particularly if the alcohol comsumption has occurred rather rapidly. Sleep usually intervenes before gross poisoning occurs, but ingestion of alcohol can cause coma or death.

This relationship between increasing dosage and changing effects can be plotted graphically and is known as a dose-response curve (Fig. 13-3). As the number of drinks is steadily increased, the total effect changes from little or no observable response through signs of moderate intoxication to the extremes of unconsciousness and eventually death. With increasing dosage the intensity of some drug-specific

effects may level off. Thus, euphoria or feelings of well-being may increase initially and later diminish as nausea or vertigo appears (Fig. 13-4, *A*). Other effects, such as alcohol-induced respiratory depression, may not appear at all until extreme dosage levels are reached (Fig. 13-4, *B*). These dangerous or lethal responses are referred to as toxic effects and usually occur at higher dosages.

The expression "overdose" is commonly used to describe almost any acute drug reaction but properly refers to toxic effects from excess drug. Some overtly poisonous substances, such as organophosphate insecticides, produce toxic effects with even slight exposure. On the other hand, even the most benign materials can produce toxicity at very high dosages (such as occurs in the syndrome of water intoxication). The notion that too much of anything is bad is borne out by the fact that a sufficient quantity of almost any substance will produce toxic effects. The rapidity of the transition from desirable therapeutic

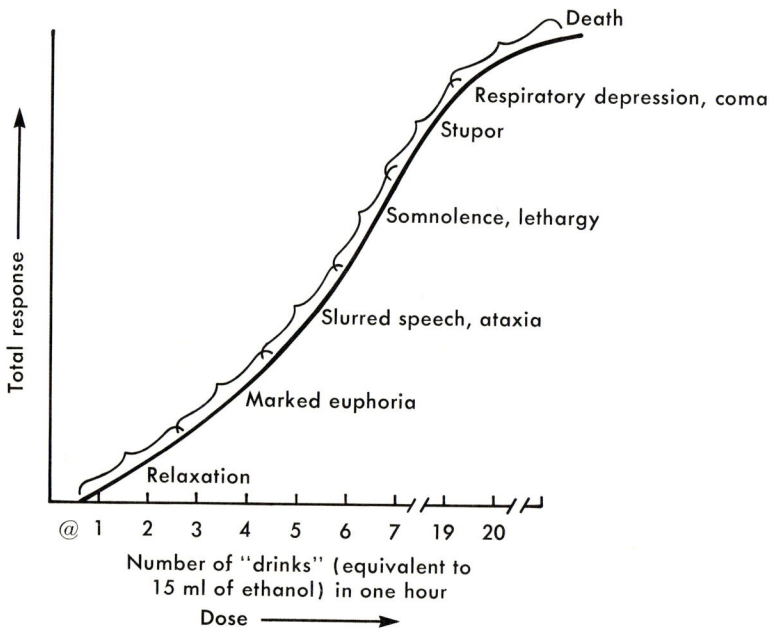

Fig. 13-3. Hypothetical dose/response curve for an "average individual."

effects to unwanted toxic effects as dosage is increased is reflected by the *therapeutic index*. Drugs with low therapeutic indices, such as lithium carbonate, have steep dose-response curves and can produce extreme toxicity following small errors in dosage. Other drugs, such as diazepam, have large margins of safety so that ingestion of even 200 times more than therapeutic amounts has not been lethal.

Dose-related effects are complicated by the various dynamic equilibria of the body's biochemistry; that is, consumed drug does not just go to the receptor sites. A drug is admitted or excluded from physiologic compartments depending on its fat solubility, protein-binding capacity, ionic charge, and other properties. When a capsule of secobarbital is ingested, some stays in the bowel and is never absorbed. What is absorbed is exchanged through various areas. Some dissolves into body fat stores, some is metabolized by the liver, some is excreted by the kidneys, and finally a small portion enters the central nervous system to exert its action. The im-

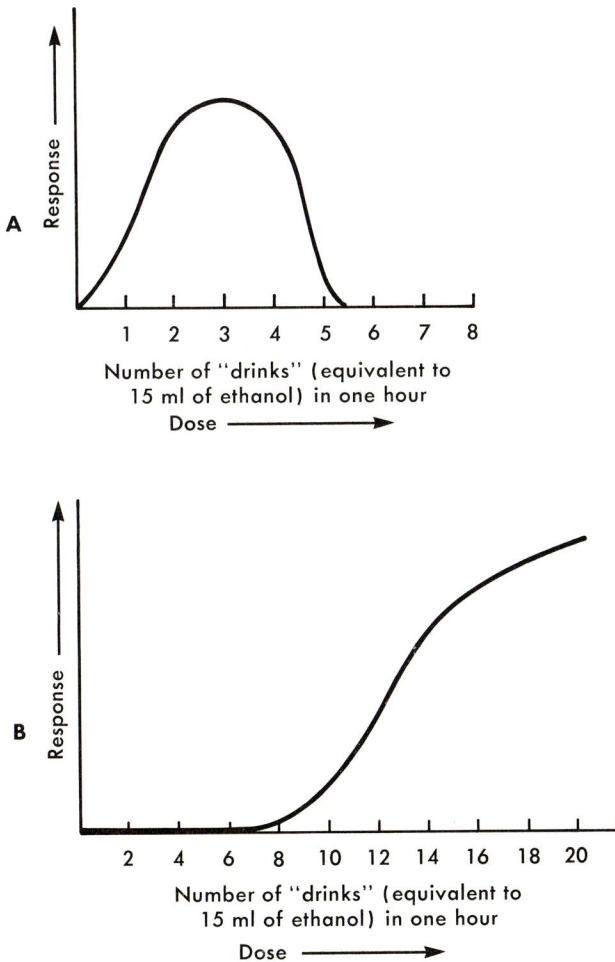

Fig. 13-4. Hypothetical dose/response curves for alcohol induced euphoria **(A)** and respiratory depression **(B)**.

portant point is that what goes into the mouth does not necessarily get to the brain. Putting drugs into the body is like pouring water into a leaky bucket: the amount of filling is dependent not only on the quantity going in but also on the relative rate at which it leaks out. Clinically this is important since for the vast majority of drugs there is little that can be done to reverse drug-specific effects once the substances have reached their receptor sites. Most treatments, therefore, depend on slowing absorption, increasing excretion, and other means of diverting the passage of drugs through the body.

Compound effects. Compound effects are attributable to interactions between drug-specific, individual, environmental, and dose-related effects. Complicated interactions are possible. An opiate addict (individual effects) who has shallow respirations and coma following a shot of heroin (drug and individual effects) may recover only to lapse into coma again. A contributing cause of coma is revealed when gastric lavage produces fragments of secobarbital capsules (drug and individual effects) that were still present in the stomach, as opiates increase antral tone and decrease gastrointestinal motility (drug effect). Typical interactions may not always be this complex, but when unexpected signs appear, compound effects should be considered.

Drug-drug interactions. Drug-drug interactions are the combinations of effects between two or more different drugs. Although diminution or cancellation can occur, with abused drugs multiplication of effect or *synergism* is the general rule. Typically this occurs when an individual who is using sedative hypnotic drugs also ingests alcohol, inadvertently producing more sedation than had been expected. Drug-drug interactions may be deliberately produced as a therapeutic maneuver. For example, many antihypertensive drugs potentiate each other's actions and so provide a way to manage cases refractory to milder treatments. Drug oppositions are also useful, as when an antagonist antidote is used to block another drug's effects. In the case of narcotic analgesics, their primary or "agonistic" actions of respiratory depression and decreased level of consciousness can be dramatically reversed by narcotic-antagonist drugs. These antagonists probably compete with the opiate receptors of the brain and thus produce a drug-drug interaction of nearly complete cancellation.

Tolerance. Tolerance or tachyphlaxis occurs when dosage must be increased in order to produce the same total effect. Although tolerance is mostly a drug-specific effect, individual effects are present in the altered physiology of the user. A chronic user of barbiturates or opiates, drugs that rapidly produce tolerance, may show minimal effects from a dose that in a nontolerant individual would be promptly lethal. Yet tolerance actually increases the likelihood of overdose since with increased tolerance the therapeutic index usually decreases and the difference between effective and toxic doses becomes smaller (Fig. 13-5). To maintain the desired euphoria, a chronic user of tolerance-producing drugs must not only increase the dosage but also tread ever more near a deadly overdose.

Even more dangerous than this increased risk of toxicity is the personal, moral, and physical decay that seems to invariably accompany chronic consumption of tolerance-producing drugs. Multiple factors are involved in this deterioration, such as the rat race of keeping up with one's habit, the gradual replacement by drug use of other sources of pleasure in one's life, and the alienation of a life based on getting and using drugs. Labels like "alcoholic deterioration," "drug casualty," and "burned-out addict" have been used for these various end-stage disorders. The causes remain obscure; all that is clear is how much damage the person has suffered.

Withdrawal. Withdrawal or abstinence

syndromes are the reactions to decreasing use of a drug. They represent the rebound of the body's homeostatic mechanisms that have become "used to" having that drug present. Thus, where euphoria, miosis, and constipation are produced by opiates, an abstinence syndrome of dysphoria, mydriasis, and diarrhea is produced on withdrawal after chronic use. Tolerance and withdrawal go hand in hand so that the more extreme the tolerance, the more likely the withdrawal will be severe. Although some drugs such as narcotics produce classic withdrawal syndromes, many abused drugs have been assumed not to produce abstinence phenomenon. Amphetamines, for example, had been assumed not to produce withdrawal since obvious clinical signs consistent with an abstinence syndrome had not been observed. This concept has been changed by laboratory studies that showed rebound disturbances in the EEG and REM sleep following amphetamine withdrawal.[4] Physical and psychological addiction can not be as neatly distinguished as was once thought. Probably almost any substance, if used long enough, leads to disruption of physiologic mechanisms that may produce some withdrawal findings. Substances in general could accordingly be arranged on a spectrum ranging from those that regularly produce severe abstinence syndromes to those that produce mild or minimal symptoms. Coffee is an excellent example of a drug that produces withdrawal at the milder end of the spectrum, since even a three-cup a day user may notice a decrease in energy and enthusiasm if that drug is withdrawn. As the street wisdom says, "You can get a habit behind anything."

CLASSES OF DRUG REACTIONS

Emergency department care has more than its share of monotony, both from nightly repetitions of the "current overdose drug of choice" and slack periods of trivia and boredom. It is the odd case that challenges us; the occult head trauma, the atropine poisoning, or multiple-drug overdose can make us use all we know. Drug-abuse reactions are often treated as stereotypes, and most of the time this assembly line approach "gets by." Here and there the unusual sneaks in. The best clinical care demands receptivity to the unusual, a readiness to modify working hypotheses as new data evolve. Rigid protocols never work as well as the rough mental outlines or checklists that prod one to remain alert. Questions to keep in mind should be based on *common* problems likely to occur and *uncommon* problems likely to be overlooked. Such a list will consistently evolve, depending on the geographic area, prevailing drugs fads, and current medical knowledge. Specific approaches generally outlive their usefulness in a few years so that continuous updating is necessary.

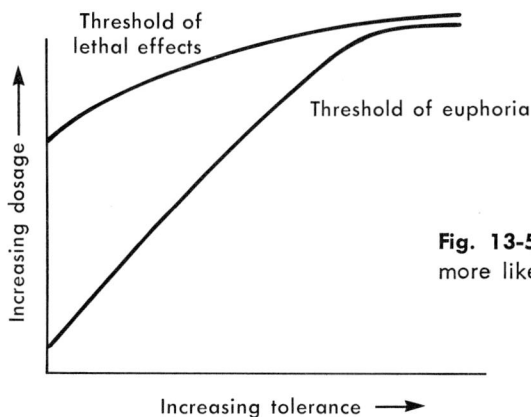

Fig. 13-5. Increasing tolerance makes accidental overdose more likely.

A useful general approach to substance abuse emergencies is to form an initial hypothesis based on a brief history and examination of the patient: type of drug reaction and the relative contributions of drug-specific, individual, environmental, and dose-related effects. Further evaluation can guide treatment based on specific problems, such as respiratory failure or arrhythmias, while the working diagnosis is tested against all new data. Various classifications of adverse drug reactions are possible, but the following outline seems to be most generally applicable.

Drug intoxications. Drug intoxications are attributable to the biochemical actions of a substance. Included are reactions caused mostly by drug-specific and dose-specific effects (such as poisonings and overdose) and also the untoward reactions to otherwise moderate doses of a drug (such as pathologic intoxication or "bad trips"), where individual and environmental effects may be significant. The class is quite broad so that both mild inebriation with alcohol and frank poisoning with lead are called intoxication. In a sense, drunkenness is the prototype state so that "intoxication" is used to refer to any reaction where drug effects produce noticeable impairment of function. Although "intoxication" is often used to emphasize the appearance of toxic effects, the "one man's side effect is another man's remedy" principle applies here since an individual may interpret the toxic effects to be the reason for taking the drug. For example, barbiturates are actually mild CNS poisons: their depressant actions can easily cause death. Habitues use these drugs to get a high of euphoria, disinhibition, and temporary amnesia. In medicine a similar name game is played; the same drugs are given to induce a coma that passes for sleep.

Severe intoxications are often labeled "overdoses," but the term is also used to refer to the patients themselves and also the constellation of lifestyles and environmental effects that lead to their emergency presentation. Overdoses tend to come in two general varieties: the planned overdose of the suicide attempt and the less-intentional variety of the narcotic addict who misestimates his requirement. Chronic users often seek extreme rather than mild or moderate degree of intoxication and thus increase their risk of an overdose. Their attitude is expressed in the street argot for intoxication—"loaded," "wasted," "destroyed"—and in the junkie maxim, "It's better to go out from a shot (i.e., become unconscious) than not get high at all!"

Drug-specific effects can increase the likelihood of overdose. Barbiturates commonly produce "automatic behaviors" where the individual, in a semistuporous state, forgets how much has been consumed and mechanically swallows more pills. Drug-drug interactions through synergism can also produce extreme intoxications. Typically this occurs when alcohol potentiates the action of a sedative drug.

Many abused drugs are distributed illicitly and lack controls on their purity or strengths. These street drugs frequently contain adulterants and contaminants that may produce intoxications of their own.[5] Some frankly poisonous compounds, such as strychnine, are frequently used to bring back the kick in drugs that have been diluted with maltose or other substances. That such a process would be widespread may seem surprising unless one considers that many users of street drugs require only some strong effect to make their purchase worthwhile. A few adulterants have become almost traditional, such as the use of quinine in the heroin distributed in New York City. Some say its use followed an outbreak of malaria among New York junkies in the 1940's, but most users claim that it is added to accentuate the initial rush of the heroin euphoria, as a sort of intravenous cocktail.

A syndrome of sudden death, associated

with opiate use, has often been considered to be the result of heroin overdose, but considerable question exists as to whether these reactions can be attributed solely to excess drug.[6] The reaction is often so swift that the individual is found with a needle still in a vein so that a true pharmacologic overdose, a much slower process, seems unlikely. The cardiotoxic effects of quinine have been proposed as a cause of this syndrome, but in areas where that adulterant is not used, the reaction may still be common.[7,8] Proposed causes for this acute toxicity syndrome have included anaphylactic reactions to contaminants, acute disturbances of respiratory or cardiovascular regulatory centers, and drug-drug interactions between opiates and alcohol, but the cause of sudden heroin death remains obscure.[9]

Drug withdrawals. Drug withdrawals are a common class of drug reactions and are produced by abstinence or reduction in dosage after tolerance has been established. The most serious reaction in this class is the sedative hypnotic withdrawal where life-threatening seizures may occur. Alcohol withdrawal may produce varying degrees of incapacitation, up to the full blown clinical syndrome of delirum tremens (the DT's). Stimulant drugs, such as amphetamines, can also produce serious withdrawal syndromes since profound depressions often occur and probably increase suicide risk. Complaints of withdrawal reactions are also used by malingering addicts who hope to obtain drugs during their emergency visit.

Allergic and hypersensitive reactions. Allergic and hypersensitive reactions are uncommon but may be quite dramatic. Skin reactions are probably the most frequent and range from rashes to exfoliative dermatitis. Anaphylaxis, asthma, urticaria, Stevens-Johnson syndrome, and various fixed drug eruptions are occasionally seen. Of this last category, an impressive bullous eruption following barbiturate overdose is one of the most frequent forms. Drug

fever, a serum sickness–like syndrome with fever, leukocytosis, arthralgia, and dermatitis also occurs.

Drug reactions with concomitant illness, injury, or psychiatric disorders. Concomitant disorders are not infrequent, so that often an overdose is not just an overdose. Trauma is probably most common, particularly in association with sedative hypnotics and alcohol, and often takes the form of vehicular-accident injuries. Subtle varieties of trauma also occur, such as peripheral nerve compressions produced by body weight on a limb during the immobility of drug-induced stupor. Head trauma is occasionally overlooked and must be considered in the examination of every unconscious patient.

Infections, such as pneumonia or meningitis, are far from rare, especially among street-drug users and chronic alcoholics whose general health may be poor. Aspiration pneumonia is a frequent complication of drug-induced coma. Usually vomitus is aspirated, resulting in a chemical burn of the lung. Since a sprinkling of mouth anaerobes and other organisms accompanies the vomitus, severe infections are common. The risk of aspiration pneumonia can be reduced during resuscitation if the patient is not left supine. Intubation may be necessary to protect the airway when vomiting persists.

Intravenous drug use drastically increases the risk of medical complications. The usual routine for parenteral administration of street drugs includes cooking the drug in a small quantity of water to enhance its solubility, then drawing it into a syringe through a wisp of cotton before injection. Not only is the cotton "strainer" ineffective at removing inert particulate matter, such as the talc and cornstarch adulterants in street drugs, it also adds bits of cotton to the drug solution in the process. These insoluble materials can produce foreign body granulomas, thrombotic and embolic lesions in various organs, including the lungs, brain, and eyes.[10-12] Parenteral drug use also carries increased risk of a long list of infectious disorders, including pneumonias, lung and brain abscesses, hepatitis, endocarditis, osteomyelitis, tetanus, malaria, and septicemia.[13]

Bacterial endocarditis associated with intravenous drug use often takes a rapid and devastating course. It most commonly affects the aortic or mitral valve and is caused by *Staphylococcus aureus* in more than half the cases. *Pseudomonas* and *Klebsiella* are probably the next most common groups, with *Streptococcus viridans* infections relatively rare. Infections with unusual or exotic organisms, such as *Candida albicans, Hemophilus vaginicola,* or *Serratia marcescens,* may represent sporadic outbreaks but probably overall do not account for more than 10% of the cases.[14-16]

Drug reactions may also be complicated by concomitant illnesses not related to the substance abuse. Preexisting medical disorders such as diabetes and preexisting psychiatric disorders such as schizophrenia do not preclude drug abuse and, at the very least, make treatment more complicated.

ASSESSMENT AND MANAGEMENT

Precise treatment depends on precise diagnosis. In the management of substance abuse emergencies, however, such luxuries must often be foregone. A diagnosis can rarely be made with complete certainty since hidden problems may exist. A patient who responds to narcotic antagonists following opiate overdose may later slip into coma from orally ingested barbiturates. "Best guess" impressions, based on presenting signs and local patterns of abuse, must usually suffice. Diagnoses must often be revised as new data accumulate. Indeed, the clinician is confronted with a threefold pattern: reliable history is often unavailable; pathognomonic signs are rare; laboratory testing to identify suspected agents takes too long.

History is the biggest problem. Usually little is available, and what there is may be inaccurate or misleading. What exactly a patient took, when, and why may be unanswerable: the patient may not remember or be so obtunded or combative that meaningful conversation, let alone reliable history, is impossible. Friends or family members may be confused, unsure, or unable to agree on just what did happen. Even worse, when the patient can talk, he may be misinformed as to the identity of the drug or know it only by its street name. Chronic users, in an effort to obtain more drugs, may exaggerate the facts or simply lie.

Physical signs are of more reliable help in setting priorities of treatment and gauging the course of therapy, but they rarely guarantee diagnoses. Even the classic sign of opiate intoxication, pinpoint pupils, may not be present if the heroin was used along with amphetamine or cocaine. Yet, it would be folly to withhold a narcotic antagonist in an apneic patient with fresh needle marks on his arm because he did not have pinpoint pupils. Physical signs should raise questions and suggest directions for therapy, but since changes in condition are frequent, close observation provides the most reliable data.

Most of the difficulties could be neatly circumvented if rapid and accurate quantitative laboratory methods were available for emergency use. Unfortunately, at the time of this writing such is not the case; blood and urine levels require a minimum of an hour and often more than half a day to provide needed answers. It is perhaps this lack of precise information that makes drug abuse problems one of the most challenging areas of medicine. In spite of the complexities, it can also be one of the most rewarding, since with prompt and aggressive care, lethally ill patients can routinely be saved.

The outline below contains some approaches for the management of substance abuse emergencies. It is worth reemphasizing that it is intended as a general guide so that some warnings are in order. This outline is limited to reactions to commonly abused drugs; reactions to overtly poisonous substances, such as insecticides and heavy metals, will not be included. Such poisonings may be produced by the "substance abuse" of industrial carelessness, but their treatment is detailed elsewhere in several specialized texts.[17] Substance abuse emergencies are often far too complex to be "cookbooked," so this outline *does not* represent a protocol or formula. Concurrent medical illnesses or trauma frequently complicate the patient's status so that therapy must be tailored to each individual case. Most importantly, this outline represents approaches that are considered useful at the time of this writing. Medicine is very much a "state of art" endeavor; treatments that are prudent today may be embarrassingly obsolete tomorrow. Continuing education is the only safeguard.

Overall, the basic principles of intervention will remain, for they are fundamental to sound management. First, treat what most urgently requires care (support of vital functions, first aid, etc.); second, while treating the urgent conditions, make an effort to identify the underlying causes and evolve a treatment plan suitable for that individual; third, take measures to restore optimal health and minimize the risk of further illnesses.

Preparation: know what to expect

Before treating any patients, have a general idea of what kind of problems might be seen in your geographic area. Although the specific agents involved can not always be identified while the patient is still in the emergency department, local fads in drug use may be recognized. For example, in a given emergency department, Friday night may bring overdoses of methaqualone or heroin. Each holiday weekend may guarantee one or two com-

bative alcoholics. Comatose, middle-aged individuals brought by their families may have tricyclic antidepressant overdoses that demand careful monitoring for cardiac arrhythmias.

Knowing the local trends can be quite useful, especially when a new drug makes its appearance. Nurses, aides, and even clerks often possess almost uncanny knowledge regarding drug-problem frequencies, yet may be reluctant to share their observations since they are based on "intuition" or "hunches." It is the involved staff who looks for the unusual and follows up hunches with laboratory testing of street samples who will recognize changes in trends of drug use early and be prepared with adequate treatment.

Across the United States the general trend over the last ten years has been away from the mid-1960's psychedelics with their attendant bad-trip epidemics to a peak of opiate overdoses and a return to hypnotic sedative comas as the most frequent severe drug problems. Alcohol, hypnotic sedatives, tricyclic antidepressants, and recently phencyclidine (PCP) seem to account for most substance-related emergencies. Street or illicit drug use, if not actually decreasing, seems to be producing far fewer adverse reactions, perhaps because users have become more sophisticated in avoiding unwanted reactions.

Information regarding trends of emergency department cases is often available from local drug-abuse treatment agencies, and a useful summary of national patterns is published by the National Institute of Drug Abuse in the Drug Abuse Warning Network (DAWN) bulletin. Analyses of drug samples can be performed by various laboratories, probably the most well-known of which is PharmChem Research Foundation.

Local trends can be assessed by keeping a drug problem register in the emergency department that can be augmented by the periodic analyses of samples of street drugs. Such assays are useful also for tablets and capsules that appear to be of legitimate manufacture but may be bootlegged and adulterated (a practice common with barbiturates, hypnotic sedatives, and the amphetamines). Even at a very informal level a knowledge of likely patterns of drug abuse helps to raise questions regarding treatment, such as, "Given this patient's age and appearance, what drugs are likely to be involved?"

Always back up guesses with careful examination to avoid falling into the trap of treating the stereotype rather than the patient. The middle-aged housewife with a meperidine (Demerol) overdose or the junkie with early signs of meningitis can be confusing surprises. The best rule of thumb seems to be to know what's common in your area but to be alert for the exceptions.

First-priority problems

Priorities cannot be rigidly defined, but a useful checklist includes first ruling out conditions that pose the greatest threat to life. Drugs usually kill by disrupting homeostatic mechanisms; respiratory failure from depression of CNS centers is most common, although cardiac arrest, massive hypotension, and status epilepticus also occur. Examine comatose patients immediately, rapidly assessing pulse, respirations, and evidence of bleeding or trauma. Adequate cardiopulmonary function allows a more leisurely approach to the patient, but if signs of arrest are present, treat promptly.

Cardiopulmonary arrest. Cardiopulmonary arrest is somewhat uncommon in drug abuse emergencies but may occur abruptly in an otherwise stable patient as he slips into deeper coma. Signs are *coma, absent pulse and respirations,* and *cyanosis.* The usual cardiopulmonary resuscitation measures are appropriate.[18] A team approach works best since there are often several things to do at once. All health

care personnel should have basic training in CPR techniques since the patient with cardiopulmonary arrest needs *immediate* attention. A delay here can be fatal.

1. *Deliver a sharp blow to the precordium* with the side of a closed fist. This simple maneuver works often enough to make it a worthwhile first step.

2. *Begin external cardiac massage* over lower half of sternum using a rocking motion. Monitor effectiveness by checking for carotid pulse. Check pupil size for return to normal as the marked dilation, produced by severe CNS hypoxia, should recede as cerebral blood flow is improved. Pupillary signs may be obscured by drug actions, however, so that the carotid pulse is the most reliable indicator. Arrhythmias usually convert spontaneously with correction of hypoxia and acidosis, but further measures may be necessary (see below).

3. *Support ventilation.* Rapidly clear the oropharynx of vomitus, dentures, and the like. The patient should be lying supine with his head tilted back, but avoid hyperextension of the neck. Tilt the tongue forward to clear the airway and begin ventilatory support. Start with 100% O_2 by Ambu bag or cuffed endotracheal tube. If these are not available, use mouth-to-mouth resuscitation. Endotracheal intubation should only be attempted by those skilled in its use. *Do not waste time* waiting for specialized personnel or specialized equipment since an Ambu bag or even mouth-to-mouth resuscitation can keep the patient alive.

4. *Maintain a pulse of 60/min and respiratory rate of 12/min.* With a team of two individuals, one can provide cardiac massage and the other respiratory support by five cardiac compressions, followed by one respiratory inflation. If a second person is not available, a single rescuer can maintain this rate by alternating 15 external cardiac-massage compressions and two respiratory inflations. Patients with drug-induced cardiopulmonary arrest are usu-

ally in otherwise good health and will survive if adequate care is given. Continue cardiopulmonary support until other care is feasible.

Respiratory failure. Respiratory failure is quite common with substance-related coma since commonly abused drugs often have significant respiratory depressant effects. Also, it may precede the development of anoxia-induced arrhythmias and cardiopulmonary arrest. Signs are *slow, shallow, irregular, Cheyne-Stokes respirations to total apnea.* Cyanosis is usually present in severe respiratory depression but may be reduced by shock, carbon monoxide poisoning, or anemia.

1. *Support ventilation* as with cardiopulmonary arrest, always clearing oropharynx first, then administering 100% O_2 by cuffed endotracheal tube or Ambu bag. Since many drugs depress cough and gag reflexes, a cuffed endotracheal tube is the best insurance against aspiration. When these reflexes are not depressed, as often occurs in phencyclindine poisoning, the patient may fight intubation or extubate himself. In these cases, restraints are prudent, and intubation should be done smoothly to avoid inducing emesis through undue pharyngeal stimulation. Since external cardiac massage is not required for simple respiratory failure, mechanical respirators can be used immediately.

2. *Administer antagonist* whenever narcotic-induced respiratory depression is suspected. Naloxone (Narcan) is essentially without agonistic actions of its own (such as respiratory depression) and has replaced nalorphine (Nalline) as the drug of choice. It is effective against opiates, synthetic analgesics, including pentazocine (Talwin), propoxyphene (Darvon), and diphenoxylate. Naloxone, 0.4 to 0.8 mg (0.01 mg/kg), should be given intravenously and repeated within five minutes if the patient fails to respond. If the patient responds slightly to the second dose, a third dose should be given, but complete failure to respond suggests nonanalgesic respiratory depression. Naloxone should *not* be given to comatose patients who are breathing adequately.[19]

Shock syndromes. Shock syndromes can be produced by various drug effects that lead to peripheral vasodilation, relative hypovolemia, or rarely directly cardiotoxic actions. Shock may occur alone or with cardiopulmonary arrest or respiratory failure. Signs are *hypotension, tachycardia, cold, clammy skin, and decreased level of consciousness.*

1. *Rapidly check vital signs.* In addition to pulse and respiration, check blood pressure, temperature, and reflexes. Extreme fever (greater than 40° C [104° F]) or hyperreflexia may warn of impending seizures.

2. *Start reliable intravenous route.* Indwelling intravenous catheters are best, and jugular or subclavian sites may be necessary in chronic intravenous users with heavy vein scarring. Intravenous routes can easily become avulsed in the furor of resuscitation or by patients who become combative as they emerge from coma. A well-taped intravenous catheter will usually do the job, but butterfly needles and other devices of doubtful security should be avoided.

3. *Correct hypotension.* If systolic blood pressure is less than 100 mm Hg, treat first with cautious fluid replacement. In drug-induced coma, relative hypovolemia from venous pooling is common, and the resultant hypotension usually responds well to moderate fluid replacement and correction of hypoxia. Lower than normal systolic pressure should be expected, however, especially with barbiturates. Adequate tissue perfusion can usually be expected if systolic blood pressure is above 100 mm Hg and urinary output by Foley catheter is maintained at 20 ml per hour. Warming of core body temperature in hypothermic patients also suggests improved perfusion. Overvigorous fluid re-

placement should be avoided, as it can lead to pulmonary edema. In the rare case, pressor drugs may be required (see below). Where intravenous equipment is not available, the effects of hypotension can be reduced by keeping the patient warm, laying him on his side, and elevating his feet slightly. Frequent rotation is useful, but avoid the supine position as it encourages aspiration.

4. *Correct blood chemistry irregularities.* Where metabolic acidosis is present or strongly suspected, such as after cardiopulmonary arrest, administer sodium bicarbonate ($NaHCO_3$), 43 mEq IV bolus, repeated every five minutes as necessary. Iatrogenic alkalosis is a frequent result of overvigorous bicarbonate therapy. Determine necessity of further replacement by following arterial blood gases. ("Ideal" values: Po_2 100 mm Hg, Pco_2 40 mm Hg; HCO_3 25 mEq/liter; pH 7.4). The femoral artery is the site of choice when pulse is faint or absent. Use anatomic landmarks; red blood confirms arterial puncture. Keep in mind other causes of coma, such as diabetic ketoacidosis, which require less vigorous replacement of bicarbonate.

5. *Administer glucose* (glucose 50%, 50 ml IV bolus) to any comatose patient in order to correct any possible hypoglycemic effects. *This step should never be overlooked.*

Seizures. Seizures may occur during intoxication or withdrawal from drugs. Idiopathic epilepsy or cerebral trauma may also be present. Signs are *generalized major motor or clonic-tonic movements, lateralized or focal fits.*

1. *Treat conservatively.* Correction of hypoxia is the best single maneuver. Medications should be used judiciously. Seizures produced by withdrawal from alcohol or hypnotic sedative drugs are best managed by slow detoxification. Drugs that are more likely to cause seizures during intoxication or overdose include codeine, propoxyphene, methaqualone, amphetamine, cocaine, phencyclidine, and strychnine. The lithium ion is a relatively toxic drug whose poisoning syndrome may develop insidiously. Thirst, nausea, obtundation, hyperreflexia, and seizures may be produced by accidental overdose or even electrolyte disturbances from a bout of diarrhea. Lithium is increasingly widely prescribed, but fortunately its toxic syndrome is easy to recognize and it responds well to electrolyte replacement or forced diuresis.

2. *Recurrent seizures* may require chemotherapy. Diazepam, 15 mg IV, is both effective and avoids the respiratory depressant effect of phenobarbital. In patients with preexisting seizure disorders, phenytoin (Dilantin), 1 g slowly IV q 2 h to achieve adequate drug levels, will provide good control but can further depress consciousness. Since intravenous phenytoin can cause arrhythmias, always give it slowly, preferably with ECG monitor. When seizures persist, after hypoxia and acidosis have been corrected, other causes should be sought, including fever, increased intracranial pressure, intracranial hemorrhage, electrolyte disturbances, or drug toxicity.

3. *Neurologic/neurosurgical consultation* is indicated for any patient with focal seizures, lateralizing signs, and recurring seizures resistant to chemotherapy (status epilepticus). Curariform drugs, intubation, and mechanical ventilation may be necessary in rare instances.

Autonomic crises. Autonomic crises are rare but often lethal syndromes produced by substances that disrupt neurotransmitter physiology. Although usually caused by ingestion of overtly poisonous substances, autonomic crises may be produced by overdoses of psychotropic drugs.[20,21] Treatment is prompt drug treatment so that early recognition of these symptoms is vital.

1. *Adrenergic crises* are produced by the sympathomimetic actions of CNS stimulants. Tachycardia, fever, profuse perspiration, delirium, seizures, extreme hypertension, and intracerebral hemorrhage may

follow overdose of amphetamines, monoamine oxidase (MAO) inhibitors, or related drugs. Adrenergic crises may be precipitated by the interactions between MAO inhibitors and tricyclic antidepressants or foods rich in the amino acid tyramine (eggs, some wines, and cheese). Blocking agents may be required for the extreme hypertension, but no single drug seems useful to oppose the entire hyperadrenergic syndrome. Problems are best treated as they appear, the most serious being seizures, hypertension, and extreme fever.

2. *Anticholinergic crises* can be produced by a large variety of drugs that exert atropinelike effects. Belladonna alkaloids (atropine, scopolamine, hyoscyamine, and stramonium extract) cause a classic syndrome of delirium, dilated and nonreactive pupils, fever, flushed dry skin, tachycardia, atrioventricular conduction defects, and seizures. Overdoses with over-the-counter sleep agents containing scopolamine are a common cause of this syndrome. Synthetic anticholinergic agents may be present in street psychedelic drugs, and occasionally stramonium-based asthma remedies (Asthmador) are smoked along with marijuana. Some drugs with marked anticholinergic side effects, such as tricyclic antidepressants and some phenothiazines, may precipitate or exacerbate anticholinergic delirium. Treatment consists of care for delirium and fever and titration with the specific antidote physostigmine (1 to 2 mg IM or IV q 30 min PRN). Occasionally physostigmine has been used as a general stimulant in comatose patients, but such use is unjustified and dangerous. Rather, it should only be administered to oppose clear signs of anticholinergic toxicity.

3. *Cholinergic crisis* is an unusual syndrome caused by drugs with muscarinic or cholinergic effects. The hypercholinergic syndrome is characterized by pinpoint pupils, salivation, hyperactive bowel sounds, muscle fasciculations, paralysis, and coma.

Cholinergic crises are most often caused by organophosphate insecticides or poisonous mushrooms (*Amanita muscaria*, "fly agaric"). In the past, mushroom poisonings were usually the result of misidentification by gourmet mycophiles, but recently seekers of drug highs have deliberately used these extremely toxic plants. In addition to cholinergic crises, *Amanita* species can also produce anticholinergic and directly hepatotoxic effects. Atropine (0.4 to 0.8 mg IV or IM q 30 min PRN) is the drug of choice, with intravenous titration producing the fastest results. Overvigorous titration with either atropine or physostigmine can lead to iatrogenic anticholinergic or hypercholinergic syndromes, but with back titration, symptoms usually readily abate.

Second-priority problems

As the name implies, second-priority problems involve milder degrees of impairment of vital functions than first-priority problems do. Where cardiopulmonary arrest demands maneuvers within seconds, problems such as respiratory failure or severe hypertension allow slightly more time—treatments required in a space of minutes. Prompt and effective management with careful observation is necessary since many of these problems may persist for hours, with sudden transition back to first-priority problems of cardiac or respiratory arrest. Once again, several things often need to be done at once so that a team approach is extremely useful.

Lighter grades of coma. The unconscious patient with stable vital signs is a common drug abuse emergency. Depth of coma is an important clinical sign, and the patient's status should be frequently recorded. To this end the various systems of classification have been proposed, probably the most popular being Reed's system[22]:

Grade I: response to painful stimuli present; deep tendon reflexes intact; vital signs stable

Grade II: pain response absent; deep

tendon reflexes present; vital signs stable

Grade III: pain response absent; deep tendon reflexes absent; vital signs remain stable

Grade IV: pain response absent; deep tendon reflexes absent; vital signs require external support

Although these levels also represent the various stages of anesthesia, such an abbreviated classification system is adequate since signs such as pupillary dilation and spontaneity of respirations may be complicated by variations in drug effects. In addition to the treatment of specific problems, general measures should include the following:

1. *Obtain relevant history.* Although history regarding substance abuse problems is notoriously inaccurate, data should still be sought and considered. Friends, family, rescue personnel, and police may be able to provide information. Questions should include the following:

a. How was the patient found (after phone call, note, suicide threat? unconscious with needle still in vein?)

b. Is patient known to have consumed any specific drugs? (new batch of street drugs? psychotropic medications from physician?)

c. Was alcohol consumed with or near the time of drug ingestion? (quantity? time of ingestion?)

d. Is patient a habitual user of alcohol or other drugs? (what drugs? previous overdoses?)

e. Was patient under psychiatric care? (receiving psychotropic medications? previous hospitalizations? previous suicide attempts?)

f. Does patient have concurrent medical problems (diabetes, hypertension, epilepsy, renal disease, or other medical problems? on medications, such as phenobarbital, digitalis, thyroid? any allergies, especially to antibiotics?)

Additional historical information can often be obtained by searching the patient's personal effects (purse, wallet, Medi-Alert bracelet) and examination of any drugs found (pills, tablets, packets of powdered substances). Bottles with prescription labels should have their contents checked since it is not uncommon for old containers to be used for illicit drugs.

2. *Perform a rapid physical examination.* Record observations *legibly,* along with the *time of each examination.* A complete physical examination should be performed with particular attention to the following:

a. *Vital signs:* pulse, respirations, blood pressure, temperature measured and recorded accurately.

b. *General appearance:* age, sex, ethnic group, apparent socioeconomic level may suggest drug used—alcohol, barbiturates, opiates, or others. Strong body odor may be caused by uncleanliness, but extremely acrid perspiration suggests chronic amphetamine use. Also check odor of breath for alcohol, ethchlorvynol (Placidyl), gasoline, acetaldehyde (from disulfran/alcohol reaction) or ketoacids (from diabetic ketoacidosis).

c. *Skin:* evidence of injections, abscesses, or trauma. Assess skin temperature, color, and degree of hydration. Dusky erythematous plaques or tense vesicles or bullae ("barb burns") may occur over areas of pressure in comatose patients. Sweat gland necrosis, presumably the effect of skin hypoxia and trauma, seems to be the common finding in these dramatic lesions.[22a]

d. *Head:* Evidence of trauma, blood, or CSF in ears or nose.

e. *Eyes:* Eye signs are a rich source of information regarding drug effects. Check pupil reactivity and eye movements. Pupil size is useful for following clinical course but is rarely pathognomonic. Miosis is classic with opiates but may be obscured by amphetamines or cocaine. Barbiturates usually produce near-normal pupillary size and reactivity, but some sedative hypnotics, such as glutethimide, can produce marked mydriasis. Atropine and strongly anticholinergic agents produce dilated, unreactive pupils, whereas amphetamines, cocaine, and psychedelic drugs usually produce dilated but reactive pupils. Glutethimide and other hypnotic sedatives may produce the worrisome finding of unequal pupils that resolves as the coma lightens.[22b] Nystagmus on lateral gaze is frequent with barbiturates but can occur with other hypnotic sedatives and occasionally marijuana. Spontaneous nystagmus with vertical components can occur with phencyclidine intoxication.[23] Conjunctival injection classically occurs with marijuana intoxication. Lacrimation, particularly with rhinorrhea, is frequent in early heroin withdrawal. Fundi should be inspected for evidence of emboli, hypertension, diabetes, or increased intracranial pressure.

f. *Chest:* rate and depth of respiration should be recorded. Presence or absence of rales or other adventitious sounds should be noted.

g. *Heart:* rate and rhythm, presence or absence of murmurs or gallops should be noted.

h. *Abdomen:* examine for bowel sounds, organomegaly, and stool occult blood.

i. *Neurologic signs:* as with any comatose patient, carefully recorded neurologic examinations are essential. Pathologic signs, such as doll's eyes and decerebrate or decorticate postures, should be noted as they occur. Closely follow eye signs, deep tendon reflexes, Babinski sign, and response to pain. Various painful stimuli have been used, but quadriceps withdrawal following Achilles tendon pinch is quite

sensitive and produces minimal trauma. Repeated sternal pressure or pinprick may produce needless iatrogenic injury.

3. *Promptly obtain relevant laboratory studies.* If outside facilities involve a significant delay, testing should be performed within the emergency department. Hematocrit and leukocyte and differential counts are more essential than other CBC indices and may be quickly performed. Serum values for glucose, electrolytes, BUN, and creatinine, along with a urinalysis, should be obtained as rapidly as possible. Other studies may include arterial blood gases, serum or urine toxicology, and analysis of gastric aspirate or other drug samples. Chest roentgenograms and electrocardiograms should be performed routinely; lumbar puncture is indicated if CNS infection is suspected. The EMI scan has replaced the lumbar puncture, skull films, and echo studies as the procedure of choice for suspected head trauma. Unfortunately, although it is reliable and relatively noninvasive, the equipment is expensive and not always available.

4. *Suspect salycilate poisoning* in younger patients with hyperventilation or marked blood gas aberrations. (Most poisoning texts contain management approaches for the complex disruptions aspirin overdose can produce.) In such cases arterial blood gases and serum K^+ must be observed closely. Salicylates often lead to bleeding disorders; prothrombin time should be checked and vitamin K_1 (10 mg IM) given. Whole blood is occasionally necessary.

5. *Rule out other causes of coma,* including the common (hypoglycemia, ketoacidotic coma, head trauma, postictal coma) and the uncommon (intracranial hemorrhage, hepatic coma, encephalitis, myxedema, addisonian crisis).

6. *Continue to observe the patient* at a frequency determined by depth of coma and stability of condition. Examinations of vital signs at 15-minute intervals may be

appropriate, particularly when there is a chance of recurring respiratory depression. If focal neurologic signs appear or patient remains in severe coma, neurologic or neurosurgical consultation is indicated.

7. *Avoid the use of analeptic drugs.* Stimulants (amphetamines, methylphenidate, pentylenetetrazol) are worthless for comatose patients. At best they produce a diffuse agitation, but morbidity and mortality are clearly increased.[24]

Continuing drug exposure. Within the body, significant pools of drug may lead to increasing toxicity. Patients with such problems require measures to terminate exposure by removing or inactivating remaining drugs. The most frequent pattern occurs with ingested substances that may be only partially absorbed when the patient is first seen. For example, after a suicide attempt with 50 secobarbitol capsules, a patient may initially manifest only mild coma, since most of the drug remains in the stomach. Procedures to remove unabsorbed drugs are useful maneuvers to prevent the development of more serious toxicity later.

The patient's exposure to the substance can also be decreased by blocking absorption to reduce bioavailability or by enhancing rates of excretion. This wide variety of approaches reflects the lack of methods to *directly* block drug actions at the level of the receptor sites. Were complete, direct antagonism possible, normal rates of excretion would be adequate since the drug, although present, would exert no pharmacologic effects. Unfortunately, blocking is usually only partial and antagonists can produce toxic effects of their own.

Once cardiopulmonary functions are stabilized, measures to decrease drug exposure can be utilized. The choice of approach depends on when and how (PO, IV, SC) the drug was taken and the patient's condition (level of consciousness, presence of trauma, etc.). Studies are lacking regarding the relative effectiveness of these various maneuvers for decontamination of the patient, but accumulated clinical studies have shown that they are generally effective. As in any case where data is scarce, opinion rules, so that champions of lavage over emesis will argue interminably with those who see it the other way. Which measures are truly the most effective remains to be proven, but many earlier maneuvers, such as the use of tannic acid, which clearly had toxic side effects, have been abandoned.

Removal of ingested drugs. Massive quantities of drugs can easily be taken orally. It is quite possible to ingest 10 g of a sedative hypnotic, but intravenous self-administration of a tenth of that amount may be quite difficult. Administration of drugs *per rectum* (usually opiates or cocaine) is used as the preferred route by some individuals. Drug smugglers frequently hide drug-filled balloons in their bowels. Accidental leaks and subsequent overdose are hazards of this method of carrying contraband. The usual overdose route is oral, however, and therapeutic maneuvers are directed at removing the substances through either end of the gastrointestinal tract.

Emesis. Recently ingested drugs are probably best removed by emesis. The utility of emesis decreases with time, and after three hours, emesis is unlikely to recover significant amounts of drug. Concomitant use of other drugs, such as opiates, which markedly decrease gastric emptying, may make emesis a practical option several hours after ingestion.[25] Since it is a well-tolerated and relatively safe procedure, it should be performed whenever significant quantities of drug may be in the stomach. To reduce the possibility of aspiration, emesis should only be induced in a fully conscious and cooperative patient. It should not be attempted after signs of frank poisoning have developed. Likewise, emesis should not be used following ingestion of corrosives (lye, other caustic acids, or alkalis), which may produce esophageal stricture, or liquid hydrocarbons (kerosene, dry cleaning fluid), which increase the risk of aspiration pneumonia.

Syrup of ipecac, 30 ml given with 100 ml of water, is usually effective. Successful induction of emesis requires fluid in the stomach, but larger volumes of water should be avoided since they may stimulate gastric emptying and thus increase absorption. Emesis is usually produced within 15 minutes, but a repeat dose of ipecac may be necessary. No more than 60 ml of ipecac should be given to avoid producing cardiac arrhythmias.

Apomorphine, 3 to 4 mg IV or SC, has often been advocated as an emetic. Although it can produce respiratory depression, it is quite effective, and its action can be rapidly terminated by naloxone. It has not been as widely used as ipecac, and since questions regarding its safety do exist, apomorphine should probably be considered the second choice.[26] Other emetics, such as fluid extract of ipecac, copper sulfate, powdered mustard, and sodium chloride, may lead to serious toxicity and should be avoided.

Gastric lavage. Gastric lavage is probably less effective than emesis since it produces less thorough emptying and it cannot recover tablets or capsules larger than the stomach tube aperature. Nevertheless, it is the procedure of choice in unconscious patients. Lavage is also useful when emetics fail, as may happen when phenothiazines or other strongly antiemtic drugs have been ingested. Gastric lavage, followed by intermittent low suction, has been advocated for overdoses of glutethimide, tricyclic antidepressants, and other substances with marked enterohepatic circulation.[27]

Gastric intubation. Gastric intubation can be achieved with a well-lubricated Levin tube of the largest size that will comfortably pass through the nose to the pharynx. In the conscious patient, passage is facilitated by having the patient sit upright and swallow once the tube reaches the posterior pharynx. The tube should be advanced smoothly and briskly to avoid provoking emesis through undue pharyngeal stimulation. In the comatose patient, endotracheal intubation is necessary to prevent aspiration. After the tube is in place, its position can be confirmed by auscultation over the stomach. Injection of 30 ml of room air through the tube should produce clearly heard tympanic sounds. Repeated injection and withdrawal of 50 ml of normal saline will flush most of the gastric contents. Care should be taken not to introduce large quantities of water, which may stimulate gastric motility and thus enhance absorption.

Reduction of bioavailability. Even when procedures to empty the stomach are successful, significant amounts of drugs can remain in the gastrointestinal tract. From time to time various means have been employed to reduce bioavailability, such as demulcents and ion exchange resins, but in the overwhelming majority of drug poisonings, absorption with activated charcoal is the preferred method.[28] Although the murky suspension of activated charcoal powder in water may appear distasteful to the staff, it is flavorless and enjoys fair patient acceptance. Other adsorbent materials, although more appealing in color, such as mineral clays, are clearly inferior at decontamination.

Activated charcoal powder. The average adult dose of activated charcoal powder is 50 to 100 g in 75 ml of distilled water. Activated charcoal powder is safe and effective for adsorption of most psychotropic drugs. It is ineffective for poisonings with mineral acids, bases, electrolytes (lithium, HCL, NaOH, KOH, NaCL, etc.), or cyanide compounds. Activated charcoal should not be given immediately after ipecac since it readily absorbs that drug and can prevent the induction of emesis. In the unconscious patient the activated charcoal suspension can be administered by nasogastric tube after lavage. Suction should not be resumed for at least two hours to allow dispersion of the adsorbent. In the occasional patient who has ingested several hundred tablets or capsules, drug concretions may be produced and may be visible on plain films of the abdomen. Protracted coma often results, and the administration of activated charcoal every 12 hours should be continued as long as the patient is unconscious.

Lipid cathartics. Lipid cathartics are potentially toxic and should be used with care. Mineral oil and castor oil, 75 ml, are most widely used. In addition to their cathartic effect, they also form a nonabsorbable lipid phase within the gastrointestinal tract into which some drugs such as diazepam and glutethimide are readily dissolved. This partitioning into a lipid phase slows absorption, thus further reducing bioavailability. Hazards associated with lipid cathartics include lipid pneumonia following aspiration, and prolonged bowel irritation when used after drugs that decrease gastrointestinal motility. Some authorities prefer activated charcoal over cathartics, but since the risk/benefit ratios of the two approaches are not established, many physicians use them together.

Facilitation of excretion. Clinically significant routes of drug excretion include routes through gastrointestinal, respiratory, and urinary systems. Maneuvers depend largely on predominant metabolic pathways of the drug in question.

Gastrointestinal excretion. Many drugs are excreted through the bile or directly into the gut. Unfortunately, this often occurs without complete detoxification steps through the liver, so that active drug may be resorbed. This enterohepatic or enteroenteric circulation is particularly important with glutethimide and tricyclic antidepressants. The resultant secretion and resorption often produce gross fluctuations in the clinical picture. Interruption of enterohepatic and enteroenteric circulation can be best achieved with activated charcoal

suspensions and possibly gastric suction. Nonabsorbable lipid cathartics may also help by increasing gastrointestinal motility and interfering with reabsorption.

Respiratory excretion. Inhaled substances such as hydrocarbon solvents or fluoroalkane gases are primarily excreted through expired air. Adequate excretion is ensured through normal respiration, but carbon monoxide is a notable exception. Its high affinity for hemoglobin requires that 100% oxygen should be used until oxygen transport functions have returned to acceptable levels.

Urinary excretion. Since many drugs are excreted in part through the urine, an extra 500 ml per day output is useful. Adequate hydration should be maintained with replacement of fluid losses (both measured and insensible) and correction of electrolytes in all comatose patients.

Forced diuresis. Forced diuresis is indicated only for markedly water-soluble drugs that are poorly protein bound (bromide, lithium, and other electrolytes, amphetamines, and long-acting barbiturates) and then only in patients with grade II coma or deeper. Forced diuresis is not a conservative procedure. When it is indicated, an output of 250 ml per hour should be maintained, monitored by indwelling catheterization. Intravenous fluids should contain adequate amounts of sugar and electrolytes; serum values should be regularly checked. In the rare patient, diuretics may be required.[29]

Acidification. Acidification of urine will enhance excretion of amphetamines and some monoamine oxidase inhibitors. Urinary pH of 4 should be maintained by ammonium chloride (NH_4Cl), 500 mg q 3 h, with adjustments as necessary. *Alkalinization* of urine enhances excretion of salicylates, long-acting barbiturates, and meprobamate. A urinary pH of 8 should be maintained with sodium bicarbonate ($NaCHO_3$), 43 mEq IV q 2 h, adjusted as needed.

Dialysis. Dialysis and the even more heroic procedure of exchange transfusion were once used more frequently for drug overdoses than they are now. When dialysis is indicated for drug poisoning, hemodialysis is the procedure of choice since it is several times as effective as the peritoneal route and avoids interference with diaphragmatic excursions and tidal volume. Criteria for dialysis in cases of drug poisoning have been proposed by Schreiner[30] and include severe coma following potentially lethal overdose of dialyzable drug, impairment of normal routes of excretion (e.g., kidney disease), concomitant medical illnesses that increase hazards of prolonged coma (e.g., cardiac or pulmonary disease), and progressive deterioration despite careful medical management. Many centers have discontinued use of dialysis altogether, even for extreme poisonings with poorly water-soluble drugs such as glutethimide. It is probably only necessary in a rare instance, and since it is a procedure with considerable risk, dialysis should be employed only when all else fails.

Persistent respiratory failure. Emergency measures to support respiration often produce immediate and gratifying results, yet relapses may occur since many drugs can produce protracted respiratory depression. Various degrees of respiratory assistance can be provided depending on the degree of failure.

1. *Check blood gases regularly.* Although cyanosis and clinical signs are useful, arterial blood gases are the most reliable indicator of respiratory failure. $Po_2 < 60$ mm Hg or a $Pco_2 > 50$ mm Hg suggests the need for external ventilatory support.

2. *Assist ventilation* with a pressure or volume-controlled mechanical respirator through a cuffed endotracheal tube. In some cases, protracted coma or concomitant trauma may make tracheostomy necessary. After emergency resuscitation with 100% O_2, lower oxygen tension should be employed. Many drugs depress the sensitivity of the Pco_2 receptors so that breathing becomes dependent on the stimulus of hypoxia. A patient who might be breathing spontaneously can become apneic or respirator dependent when the Po_2 of inspired air is excessive. In cases of carbon monoxide poisoning, 100% O_2 must be used to overcome that substance's affinity for hemoglobin.

3. *Monitor respirations every 15 minutes* for at least two hours on all unassisted patients with respiratory depression. When narcotic antagonists are used, repeat doses may be necessary since initial clearing may be followed by the sudden reappearance of coma. Titrate with the smallest effective dose to avoid antagonist-induced withdrawal since it is resistant to treatment and unnecessarily stresses the patient. Antagonists should not be given to comatose patients who are breathing adequately.

4. *Observe closely* when long-acting narcotics are suspected. Multiple-drug overdoses are not uncommon, including such combinations as intravenous heroin with orally ingested methadone and alcohol. Patients with such combinations may breathe adequately following naloxone, only to later become apneic when the antagonist wears off. Naloxone, along with the shorter-acting narcotics such as heroin and Dilaudid, has a duration of action of two to three hours. Methadone, a drug used in narcotic maintenance for its long duration of action, can produce respiratory depression for up to 48 hours. For patients who lapse in and out of coma but respond well to antagonists, a naloxone drip of 4 mg/liter has been proposed.[31]

Since an even longer-acting narcotic, L-methadyl acetate (LAAM or long-acting methadone), is soon to be available, antagonist infusion may be necessary to treat the respiratory depression of up to three days that this drug may produce.

5. *Regularly attempt respirator weaning.* Ensure that respirator sensitivity is appropriate to the patient's efforts, or weaning

may be made more difficult. "Low pressure cuff" endotracheal tubes are superior, especially for protracted coma as they reduce the likelihood of tracheal injury and make periodic inflation unnecessary.

Cardiac arrhythmias. Most drug-induced arrhythmias improve after correction of hypoxia and acidosis. Some drugs, however, especially tricyclic antidepressants and phenothiazines, may produce arrhythmias that are especially difficult to manage. In overdose with tricyclic antidepressants a 2RS interval longer than 100 msec suggests severe toxicity.[31a] Since these drugs have long half-lives, unexpected deaths several days after the overdose may be the result of recurring arrhythmias.[31b] Fortunately, physostigmine seems to be effective in controlling these problems.[31c] Management should include the following:

1. *Correct hypoxia and acidosis* first since this may be adequate to restore normal rhythm. Never use chemotherapeutic agents first as their effectiveness is reduced by these blood chemistry aberrations. Monitor effectiveness of treatment with ECG and blood gases.

2. *Ventricular tachyarrythmias* respond best to DC cardioversion repeated as necessary, with antiarrhythmic drugs such as lidocaine (50 to 75 mg IV bolus, then IV drip, 2 to 4 mg/min). Procaine amide is a second choice, but phenytoin (Dilantin) should be avoided since it may contribute to CNS depression.

3. *Atrial tachyarrhythmias* usually convert spontaneously, but carotid sinus massage followed by edrophonium, 10 mg IV push, may be necessary. In cases of anticholinergic crisis (tachycardia conduction defects, dry, flushed skin, fever), physostigmine, 1 to 2 mg IV repeated as necessary, is useful. Tricyclic antidepressant poisoning may require frequent titration over a period of days.

4. *Bradyarrhythmia* should be treated only if cardiac output is markedly compromised. Atropine and adrenergic drugs should be avoided if poisoning with tricyclic antidepressants or phenothiazines is suspected. Transvenous ventricular pacing is probably safest in severe conduction problems since it avoids pharmacologic complications.

Hypotension. Systolic blood pressures below 100 mm Hg that do not respond to correction of hypoxia and moderate fluid replacement may require further measures. Treatment should be aggressive as hypoperfusion may produce acute renal failure (16% of all barbiturate overdose fatalities in one large series).[32]

1. *Foley catheterization* is useful in any comatose patient as it permits continuous monitoring of urinary output. Unless forced diuresis is indicated, an output of at least 40 ml per hour should be maintained. Since urinary output reflects renal perfusion, it is a sensitive measure and may drop before the development of obvious hypotension.

2. *Periodic urinalysis* can warn of renal damage. Oliguria produced by volume depletion and mild hypotension alone reflects near-normal excretory functions. Oliguria from acute renal failure typically shows salt-wasting (urine $Na^+ > 10$ mEq/liter) and urea retention (urine/plasma urea ratio < 10). Correction of hypotension, administration of diuretics, and other treatment maneuvers for acute renal failure may be necessary.

3. *Central venous pressure monitoring* is also quite useful. Pressures below 15 cm H_2O are usually adequate. Swan-Ganz catheterization is useful, especially in patients with preexisting heart or lung disease.

4. *Plasma expanders*—saline, plasma, Ringer's lactate, dextran, serum albumin, or even whole blood—help increase intravascular volume, but observe central venous pressure to warn of overreplacement.

5. *Vasopressor drugs* should only be used if the above measures fail to keep systolic blood pressure at least 100 mm Hg. Dopamine, 400 mg in 250 ml D5W (5 to

10 μg/kg/min), can be used, but epinephrine should be avoided, especially in phenothiazine intoxication where selective alpha adrenergic blockade may produce paradoxical hypotension.

Pulmonary edema. Decreased arterial Po_2 and acidosis along with rales suggests the presence of pulmonary edema. Classic signs, such as frothy pink sputum, may be present, although more subtle forms, with little findings other than positive chest roentgenograms, may follow drug overdoses. Two varieties probably exist: a cardiogenic form that is the result of acute bacterial endocarditis or direct cardiotoxic effects of drugs such as barbiturates; and a more variable form associated with intravenous opiate abuse. The cardiogenic form is similar to classic pulmonary edema and is easily exacerbated by overvigorous fluid replacement. The opiate-associated or heroin-induced pulmonary edema may be quite common (up to 50% of some heroin overdoses) and is associated with significantly higher morbidity and mortality.[33] Pulmonary edema following opiate use usually clears within 48 hours if treated with oxygen and ventilatory support. Although various conjectures regarding its cause have been advanced, none have been completely supported by research. Treatment should remain conservative. Since pulmonary edema makes its appearance several hours after exposure to the drug, it is easy to overlook. Although risk of pulmonary infections is high, prophylactic antibiotics are not indicated. Close observation with appropriate laboratory tests is the best course. In both cardiogenic- and opiate-associated forms treatment should include:

1. *Positive pressure ventilation* with 100% O_2 along with frequent blood gas monitoring. Positive end expiratory pressure systems are especially helpful. Swan-Ganz catheterization is also useful.

2. *If clearly cardiogenic*, employ cautious use of tourniquets, phlebotomy, and diuretics. In any case, avoid opiates and use digoxin only if more conservative measures fail.

Hypertension. Elevated diastolic blood pressure greater than 120 mm Hg may occur following severe stimulant overdoses. Additional signs include decreased urinary output, congestive heart failure, and signs of increased intracranial pressure (papilledema, bradycardia, seizures, focal signs, etc.). Severe drug-induced hypertension usually follows overdoses of amphetamines, monoamine oxidase inhibitors, or tricyclic antidepressants. Hypertensive crises can also occur when patients taking MAO inhibitors consume food or beverages that contain high levels of the amino acid tyramine (eggs, some cheese, sausage, beer, and wine). Hypertension can be caused by or cause increased intracranial pressure.

1. *Adrenergic blocking or vasodilating drugs* are two general approaches. For amphetamine or other stimulant drug overdoses producing systolic elevations greater than 210 mm Hg, phentolamine (Regitine), 2 to 5 mg by IV drip, has been advocated to reduce pressure to 160 to 170 mm Hg.[34] For diastolic elevations over 120 mm Hg, the vasodilating drug diazoxide, 300 mg IV bolus, can be used, followed by a diuretic such as furosemide, 40 mg IV.

2. *Suspect increased intracranial pressure* as a cause of hypertension if above measures are ineffective. Mannitol, 50 g IV, with dexamethasone, 10 mg IV, can be given to reduce intracranial pressure. Excessive replacement of fluids may produce cerebral edema, but intracranial hemorrhage from trauma or overdose of stimulant drugs should not be overlooked as possible causes.[35]

Thermoregulatory disorders. Thermoregulatory disorders may occur as signs of disordered physiology and can become life-threatening problems on their own.

1. *Hypothermia* is quite common, especially after overdoses with sedative-hypnotic drugs and major tranquilizers. Treatment is supportive, but one should keep

in mind that attempts to warm a patient in a cold room are usually ineffective.

2. *Hyperthermia* is most often caused by drug poisoning, infection, or both. Infection must be ruled out, particularly in users of intraveneous drugs, since nonsterile techniques bring an endless array of microorganisms. It is not at all uncommon for addicts to inject drugs through peri-venous abscesses, which then disgorge their contents into the bloodstream. Pneumonias, infections, endocarditis, thrombophlebitis, and other frequent complications of intravenous drug use should be ruled out whenever fever is present. Tuberculosis, urinary tract infections, and meningitis should also be considered.

3. *Extreme fevers* with core body temperatures greater than 40° C (104° F) suggest gram-negative septicemia or drug poisoning. Direct interference with hypothalamic thermoregulatory centers may occur with some drugs, such as atropine amphetamines, MAO inhibitors, tricyclic antidepressants, and lithium. Drugs with marked anticholinergic effects can reduce sweating and thus raise body temperature. Cardiac arrhythmias, seizures, and death can be produced by extreme fevers so that immediate cooling must be applied. Treatment must be vigorous and includes full-body ice packs, cooling blankets, alcohol sponging, or cold water immersion. Chemotherapy, including aspirin to control fever and intravenous diazepam for seizures, has been used; and chlorpromazine, 25 mg IV, has been suggested in stimulant-induced fever for its hypothermic and hypotensive effects; for atropine poisoning or severe anticholinergic toxicity, physostigmine, 1 to 2 mg IV, should be used.[36]

Cyclic relapse. Cyclic relapse following overdose occurs most frequently with glutethimide, tricyclic antidepressants, and phencyclidine. Enterohepatic and enteroenteric circulation may be the most significant factors in this process since secretion into the gut and subsequent reabsorption can produce a fluctuating clinical course. Also, recovery from shock can increase visceral blood flow, thus resuming absorption and renewing coma. Close following of neurologic signs yields the most results in detecting other contributing causes.

Although coma may be protracted with some drugs, notably phencyclidine, even a week-long period of unconsciousness may still be compatible with complete recovery.[37]

Third-priority problems

The reactions to substance abuse that require emergency treatment but do not pose an immediate threat to vital functions may be considered third-priority problems. Indeed, these problems also represent a third class in that they often make their appearance after the first- and second-priority problems have been treated. A patient with cyanosis and apnea may be managed through stages of lighter coma and persisting hypertension but may regain consciousness only to display the third-priority problem of a combative delirium.

Various medical, surgical, and psychiatric emergencies may represent third-priority problems, but they will not be dealt with in this outline as they are covered in depth elsewhere in this text. Syndromes of disordered behavior frequently associated with substance abuse will be considered in detail, however, since different categories of drug-induced problems may require different approaches. With the exception of extremely suicidal or violent patients, behavioral disorders can be dealt with after physiologic functions have been stabilized and drug decontamination initiated. Once again, however, priorities must ultimately be assessed in each case on an individual basis.

Behavioral toxicity. Behavioral toxicity refers to aberrations in behavior caused by drug actions.[38] Drugs produce a wide spectrum of behavioral alterations, including changes in activity, mood, perception, thought processes, orientation, and memory. Significant medical problems may also occur in substance-abuse reactions that produce behavioral toxicity. The approach to the patient follows basic principles of psychiatric interventions: most important is an empathic relationship with the patient, augmented by manipulation of environmental effects, treatment of medical disorders, and judicious chemotherapy. As applied to substance abuse problems, these measures should include the following:

1. *Form a working diagnosis* based on available information and provide specific treatment if possible. Occasionally drug-induced behavioral toxicity can be treated with specific antidotes, such as physostigmine for atropine psychosis. Medical disorders known to produce behavioral aberrations, such as hypoglycemia, hepatic coma, uremia, or myxedema should be treated if present.

2. *Stabilize environment.* Measures to support vital functions and minimize drug absorption may create a confusing environment that is unsettling for any patient, let alone one whose mental functioning is impaired. Try to keep this stimulus load at a level comfortable for the patient. Lighting levels influence mood; a room that is excessively bright may seem more threatening. Likewise, the presence of unused medical hardware, such as respirator machines or IV stands, produces a potentially menacing scene. An ideal quiet room should be as much like a home or office as possible. It should have moderate lighting and noise levels and a minimum of breakable objects. The use of such a nonstimulating environment often makes the management of patients with even severe behavioral toxicity much easier.

3. *Establish a relationship* with the patient. Although this may seem impossible with very confused individuals, repeated orientation by the same staff persons maximizes chances for adequate control. *Explicit* expression of empathy is the key to rapport. Although difficult to describe, empathy can best be gauged by the patient's reaction. A frightened, confused patient may be calmed when the staff shows they understand how he feels. "You sound like you are really worried about being here," conveys more explicit empathy than, "Don't worry, everything will be all right." Voice, tone, and manner are even more important than what is said. Even frankly delirious patients may still have some ability to cooperate that can be mobilized by staff people who show that they empathize and understand.

4. *Set clear limits* on acceptable behavior. In many patients with behavioral toxicity, this is the biggest problem area. Limit setting is best achieved by having one staff person make frequent or continuous contact with the patient. Many emergency department disruptions, in part, represent attempts by patients to get attention and help. Giving attention before the disruption is the prudent course. Neglect fosters agitation. Be consistent with rules; do not tolerate destructive or assaultive behavior. Use restraints or assistance from security guards as necessary.

5. *Avoid drug solutions to drug problems.* Always use human contact first to treat problems of behavioral toxicity with talking down, reassurance, environmental stabilization, and clear limit setting. In extreme agitation or when experienced personnel are unavailable, tranquilizing drugs can be employed. Phenothiazines should be avoided since they may produce severe hypotension or exacerbate confusion caused by anticholinergic drugs. Diazepam, 30 mg IM or PO, is safe and effective. Chemotherapy should be adjunctive, but unfortunately, tranquilizers are often used to the point of inducing coma under the euphemism of sedation. Keep in mind that giving drugs can encourage the taking of drugs.

Behavioral toxicity may produce varying clinical pictures based on contributions of drug-specific, dose-related, individual, and environmental effects. Specific interventions can best be considered in terms of the most common reaction to the most widely abused drugs.

Intoxication with depressants. Drugs can interfere with brain metabolism in a variety of ways to produce confusion, disorientation, amnesia, or other signs of organic brain syndromes. Severe global impairments of cerebral function can be produced by minute amounts of some drugs, such as the synthetic anticholinergic Ditran. Others produce such symptoms only at toxic levels or in susceptible individuals. Among the first functions affected by drug-induced organicity are memory and judgment. Abusers often seek these actions to produce amnesia and disinhibition—a high of forgetting and not caring. Commonly abused drugs with such actions include the following.

Alcohol and the hypnotic sedatives. These drugs are the most popularly abused drugs in this group, and their disinhibiting effects can lead to argumentativeness and assaultive behaviors. Hypnotic sedatives, in particular, often produce agitation similar to the emergence delirium that may occur as a patient awakes from surgical anesthesia or other drug-induced coma. Concurrent metabolic disorders, previous cerebral injury, or predisposing psychiatric factors may increase the risk of development of delirium. For some drugs, such as alcohol, specific states have been described, including pathologic intoxication, alcoholic paranoia, and the *International Catalog of Diseases* diagnosis of "alcoholic jealousy." Such states are rarely observed in pure form. Rather than distinct entities, they probably represent the expression of underlying psychopathology through the disinhibiting effects of the drug delirium.

Hydrocarbon solvents and fluoroalkane gases. These agents have been widely abused by those whose age or purchasing ability has made acquisition of other drugs more difficult. The preferred route of administration is usually inhalation, but oral ingestion also occurs when a solvent-soaked rag is held in the mouth. Model airplane glue was previously a widely available source of solvents, but in many areas paint thinners and lacquer removers have become favorites. Toluene is often regarded as the connoisseur's choice, although halogenated hydrocarbons have enjoyed popularity. Gasoline, which contains some toluene along with other aromatics and aliphatic hydrocarbons, is popular among young abusers in disadvantaged areas, from American ghettos to Australian aboriginal tribal lands.

Volatile solvents. Volatile solvents dissolve well into body fat and may affect neuronal myelin or membrane lipids. Long-term hazards are unclear, but use of gasoline does carry increased risk of poisoning with organic lead compounds used as antiknock additives. Tetraethyl lead and related substances are quite lipid soluble, passing into the CNS more readily than nonorganic lead compounds, and may produce severe lead encephalopathy in adults. Fluoroalkane gases, which previously were considered inert, do exert pharmacologic effects such as sensitization of the heart to aphyxia-induced arrhythmias.[39] Substances in this group, especially Freon, are associated with a syndrome of sudden death in which the abuser, after inhaling the drug, abruptly begins running, then falls dead, presumably from cardiac arrhythmias.[40]

Dissociative anesthetics. Dissociative anesthetics such as phencyclidine and ketamine frequently produce delirium. Phencyclidine showed marked analgesic and anesthetic properties in early animal studies. On further investigation it proved unsuitable for human use, as it often produced agitation and panic. It is a useful anesthetic for other primates, however, and was released under the trade name Sernyl for veterinary use. Almost simultaneously it became widely available as a street drug, usually sold as PCP or angel dust. Substances sold as THC (tetrahydrocannabinol, the purified active ingredient of marijuana) are almost invariably phencyclidine or other drugs. The isolation or synthesis of true THC is elaborate to the point of heroism, whereas phencyclidine can be easily made in a cheap bulk process. Phencyclidine analogs may appear in street drugs. Ketamine has largely been abandoned for induction of anesthesia since emergence delirium was a frequent result. When it sporadically appears as a street drug it is usually well received. TCP, a thiophene analog, is more widely available, and users claim its effects are more marked. Another potent analog, PCC, may be produced by careless PCP synthesis and is reputed to regularly produce adverse reactions.

Phencyclidine has met with excellent consumer acceptance on illicit markets and regularly appears as an adulterant or major ingredient in a vast variety of street drugs. Its effects vary with dose or drug-drug interactions ranging from sedative to psychedelic actions. Phencyclidine can be consumed by a variety of routes: oral ingestion, application to the nasal mucus (snorting), or smoking with marijuana or tobacco. It is often used along with hypnotic sedatives or alcohol, which seem to potentiate its delirium-producing effects. Abusers describe a state of anesthesia combined with vivid hallucinations of movement, noises, and flashing light. Clinical signs include slurred speech, ataxia, and peculiar blank stare, sometimes with facial grimacing and drooling of saliva. Users often describe feeling brain damaged or like a sick animal; this effect of the drug may be reflected in its street names of horse tranquilizer or hog. At higher doses a more severe syndrome is produced with stupor, muscle rigidity, grunting, and moaning, along with the peculiar finding of spontaneous vertical nystagmus.[41]

Protracted coma is frequent, and pro-longed recovery the rule. Fluctuating levels of consciousness, disorientation, terrifying hallucinations, and depression with suicidal ideation may occur as the patient recovers from a phencyclidine overdose.

Anticholinergic agents. These drugs tend to produce confusion, hallucinations, and extreme agitation. Since antiquity, substances such as stramonium (jimsonweed) and the belladonna alkaloids (atropine, hycosine, scopolamine) have been used to induce states of intoxication. Today they most frequently appear as adulterants in psychedelic drugs and are occasionally used to increase the kick of marijuana. Many over-the-counter sleeping remedies contain significant amounts of scopolamine. Toxicity may occur with inadvertent or intentional overdose. Extremely potent synthetic anticholinergic drugs, such as the JB series or Ditran, enjoyed a brief street popularity but are now quite rare.[42] Many psychoactive compounds, particularly phenothiazines and tricyclic antidepressants, exert significant anticholinergic activity and may cause or exacerbate a delirium.

Management of depressant intoxication. General measures for the management of behavioral toxicity should be employed for drug-induced delirium, with particular emphasis on the following:

1. *Stabilize environment.* Reduction of stimuli by a quiet room and moderate lighting and noise levels helps reduce excitement and agitation in delirious individuals.

2. *Periodically orient the patient.* Delirium twists one's experiences of the world into kaleidoscopic distortions. Memory impairment breaks those experiences into a terrifying chaos. Warm, reassuring contacts by the same staff person at periodic intervals help to calm the patient. "Now, John, I can see you are frightened, but I want to tell you that you are in a hospital and we are doing our best to help you." If family members, friends, or even familiar objects from home are available, they can

help the patient focus his attention and remain more organized.

3. *Beware of rapid movement or thoughtless physical contact* with the patient; keep in mind the reality he is experiencing. Some delirious patients desperately want physical contact: a pat on the shoulder, a squeeze of the hand. Others are in such a state of terror that any touching is interpreted as an assault. Drug-induced delirium frequently brings feelings of depersonalization, hopelessness, and confusion. Disorders of perception may cause hallucinations ranging from hearing threatening voices to seeing crawling insects. Severely hallucinating patients are often in states of extreme terror and should receive a minimum of physical contact. Ultimately, the decision on when to touch a patient must be based on intuition. Give "space" if the patient seems threatened. If, on the other hand, he seems to want the reassurance of touch, begin gently with a light pat on the arm. Rapidly evaluate his response; if the patient needs distance, he will let you know by jumping or withdrawing. If procedures requiring more contact or physical restraint become necessary, move decisively. Hesitation will only make the patient more frightened. When physical immobilization is necessary, use an adequate number of personnel; one to each limb and one extra seems to work best.

Withdrawal from depressants. Depressant drugs are among the most frequently abused substances so that withdrawal syndromes are quite common. Since intoxication with these drugs generally produces euphoria, relaxation, and somnolence, withdrawal yields anxiety, insomnia, irritability, tremulousness, and in extreme cases, seizures and death. The commonly abused drugs producing serious abstinence syndromes include alcohol, narcotic analgesics, sedative hypnotics, and minor tranquilizers. Withdrawal symptoms from volatile solvents may occur in an unusual case, but these materials tend to be so poisonous

that signs of acute toxicity probably appear before tolerance occurs. General measures for emergency treatment of withdrawals include the following:

1. *Diagnose degree of withdrawal* as accurately as possible. Consider history and symptoms but rely mainly on physical signs.

2. *Avoid overtreatment* of withdrawal symptoms. Use drugs sparingly. Although hypnotic sedative withdrawal may require medication to prevent seizures, emergency treatment of withdrawal symptoms is frequently unnecessary. Severe alcohol withdrawal may require chemotherapy; narcotic analgesic withdrawal almost never does.

3. *Refer patients* to appropriate detoxification facilities if available. Admit patients in whom concurrent problems make more intensive care necessary. Prescribing drugs for detoxification on an outpatient basis rarely has any beneficial effect other than giving the patient a "legitimate" connection.

Narcotic analgesic withdrawal. Narcotic analgesic withdrawal is characterized by malaise, gastrointestinal distress, diarrhea, anxiety, insomnia, joint pains, lacrimation, rhinorrhea, mildly dilated pupils, and piloerection. This last sign is quite frequent in opiate withdrawal and through its common name of "goose bumps" has lead to the street expression "cold turkey." Withdrawing addicts may request almost any drug with the insistence that it has helped before, but after the crisis has passed, they often confide that heroin withdrawal is no worse than a bout of the flu. The withdrawal from longer acting narcotics, such as methadone, appears to be more severe, with some symptoms such as joint pain occurring intermittently for several months. When a mixed addiction or other medical problems make admission necessary, drug detoxification is indicated and methadone is clearly preferable over nonnarcotic drugs. In general, since specialized treatment facilities for narcotic addicts are present in most communities, withdrawing addicts should be referred to appropriate facilities whenever possible.

Hypnotic sedative withdrawal. Hypnotic sedative withdrawal can produce dysphoria, tremors, muscular weakness, postural hypotension, hyperreflexia, and seizures. Degree of tolerance can be assessed with a challenge dose of pentobarbital elixir, 200 mg (elixir or other liquid forms minimize placebo effects). Examination of the patient in one hour allows an estimate of daily hypnotic sedative requirement in equivalent doses of pentobarbital. Patients who claim to be withdrawing but are sleeping one hour after this dose do not require detoxification. Patients who are awake can be assessed by the following signs: drowsiness, slurred speech, nystagmus—400 to 600 mg pentobarbital equivalent daily; fine lateral nystagmus without other signs of intoxication—800 mg; signs of intoxication absent—greater than 1,000 mg. Individuals using the equivalent of 600 mg of pentobarbital daily have significant risk of withdrawal seizures and should either be admitted or transferred to appropriate facilities.[43] Occasionally longer observation is necessary since this test may be confounded by recently consumed drugs. Barbiturate withdrawal should be managed by titration with a longer acting barbiturate, such as phenobarbital. Subintoxicating doses sufficient only to reduce tremulousness and hyperreflexia are most useful since mild intoxication increases the likelihood of abusive or combative behavior.[44]

Minor tranquilizer withdrawal. Minor tranquilizer withdrawal represents a subclass of hypnotic sedative withdrawal and presents similar hazards of seizures. Abstinence symptoms are likely when daily use exceeds the equivalent of 0.5 g of chlordiazepoxide. Challenge testing does not seem to be particularly useful. Titration with periodic reevaluation is the safest

approach. Chlordiazepoxide, 50 mg, or diazepam, 15 mg PO or IM, should be given to control extreme agitation, tremulousness, and hyperreflexia. When severe prior use seems likely, patient should be admitted or transferred to appropriate facilities.

Alcohol withdrawal. Alcohol withdrawal is a complex clinical entity. The contributions of alcohol-related disorders, such as vitamin deficiencies or malnutrition, have not been adequately delineated, and considerable diagnostic confusion exists regarding the elements of the alcohol abstinence syndrome. Vague, but widely used terms, such as "impending DT's," perpetuate the imprecision. Signs and symptoms should be clearly recorded in each individual case and treatment based on the whole clinical picture. Of the various diagnostic schemes, division into two broad categories seems most useful.

Mild alcohol withdrawal is manifested by dysphoria, irritability, agitation, insomnia, tachycardia, diarrhea, and confusion. Symptoms typically begin 12 to 24 hours after the last drink and may develop to a peak of moderate severity. Although mild withdrawal can also represent early symptoms (impending DT's) that appear before the full-blown picture, the mild syndrome often subsides spontaneously and can be suppressed by further alcohol intake. Patients with mild signs should be transferred to specialized programs where they can be detoxified on an inpatient or outpatient basis. Although it is often common to discharge mildly withdrawing patients from the emergency department with a few days' prescription for a minor tranquilizer, this practice should be avoided. Detoxification programs can supply medication if appropriate. The routine dispensing of tranquilizers in the emergency department probably reduces the chances that the patient will bother with follow-up in counseling at all. When other medical problems make detoxification necessary, titration with diazepam or chlordiazepoxide produces the most satisfactory results. Since vitamin deficiencies often accompany alcoholism, thiamine, 100 mg IM, folic acid, 2 mg IM, and intramuscular multivitamin supplements should be given.

The *severe alcohol-related abstinence syndrome* (delirium tremens) was first described in the early 1800's. Since then the literature has been voluminous, contradictory, and quite confusing. Although the pathophysiology is still unclear, especially regarding the roles of vitamin deficiency and electrolyte disorders, it seems clear that the classic syndrome of delirium tremens is produced by abstinence in a tolerant individual.[45] Withdrawal may also occur in an individual who is still drinking, perhaps caused by stresses, such as intercurrent infections, or the physical difficulty of consuming a large enough volume of alcohol to overcome tolerance.

The definitions and etiologies of other alcohol-related disorders are in many cases even more obscure. Diagnostic entities have often been generated without adequate research and with little consideration for the pathophysiology of other drug-related disorders. "Rum fits" or "alcoholic epilepsy" are grand mal seizures that may occur following the abrupt withdrawal of alcohol in tolerant individuals. Although the diagnostic picture is often complicated by other seizure-producing factors, such as head trauma or preexisting epilepsy, rum fits are probably only another form of drug withdrawal seizures. Another confusing diagnostic category is alcoholic hallucinosis, which is characterized by hallucinations, usually auditory, in a calm, well-oriented patient. This disorder is probably extremely rare in its pure form and may represent combined effects of alcohol withdrawal, a chronic brain syndrome from long-standing alcohol abuse, and underlying personality disorders.

Severe alcohol withdrawal represents a genuine medical emergency. Even with aggressive care, however, the severe syndrome is quite lethal, with an overall mortality rate of approximately 15%. Concurrent medical problems fostered by personal neglect are also common, and prompt care is necessary.

1. *Admit or transfer* to inpatient care patients with severe withdrawal or serious medical complications. These include a history of seizures in a patient without prior epilepsy, recent history of head trauma with unconsciousness, or a history of previous episodes of severe withdrawal with medical complications. Ominous signs include stupor or coma, Wernicke's syndrome (ataxia, nystagmus, ophthalmoplegia), fever, severe malnutrition, or evidence of serious respiratory, gastrointestinal, or other medical problems.

2. *Sedate the patient*, titrating dosage to achieve mild drowsiness. It is unclear whether sedation significantly alters the final, often lethal course of severe alcohol withdrawal. Nevertheless, sedation makes the patient more comfortable and cooperative with the various examinations that must be performed. The degree of controversy regarding the drug of choice for alcohol detoxification emphasizes the fact that no one medication is clearly superior. Chlordiazepoxide, 50 mg PO, or diazepam, 30 mg PO, titrated every two hours seems to be the current first choice. Chlordiazepoxide is superior since it offers more sedative effect and a longer duration of action. Hydroxyzine, 100 mg IM or PO, has been advocated by some authors, but its anticholinergic properties could contribute to fever or delirium. Paraldehyde, 10 ml PO, was previously the drug of choice, and many alcoholics prefer it to all other sedatives. Its drawbacks are numerous, including its chemical instability, tendency to produce toxic by-products, and its irritating properties that make parenteral administration hazardous. Occasionally major tranquilizers may be necessary to control psychotic symptoms and haloperidol,

5 mg tid, is probably the drug of choice. Chlorpromazine should be avoided as it may induce serious hypotension or precipitate seizures.

3. *Vitamin supplements* should be given to all individuals with severe withdrawal syndromes. Vitamin deficiencies are typical in all chronic alcoholics, either from poor nutritional habits, malabsorption, or impairments of hepatic metabolism. All patients should receive thiamine, 100 mg IM, folic acid, 2 mg IM, and multivitamin supplements, IM, IV, or PO, daily during the course of detoxification. Vitamin K, 10 mg IM, should be given when prothrombin times are three seconds greater than control.

4. *Correct electrolyte disturbances.* Although dehydration is common in alcoholics, it is not an invariable finding. Tailor fluid replacement to the individual patient and use diuretics such as furosemide, 40 to 80 mg, as needed. Cautiously correct electrolytes, especially during the first 24 hours; replacing half of each initial deficit the first day is a safe rule. Diarrhea and other effects of withdrawal frequently produce potassium deficits, but since potassium is largely intracellular, the true severity may not be reflected by the serum levels. In hypokalemia, observe serum potassium levels closely and replace 100 mEq daily. Potassium choride is the best form and should be given orally, if possible. Intravenous replacement rate should not exceed 20 mEq per hour since lethal arrhythmias may be produced. The role of magnesium in alcohol withdrawal is still unclear, but replacement of body magnesium stores may have salutory effects. Magnesium sulfate, 2 ml (50% solution) IM q 6 h for six doses, may return magnesium stores to normal and reduce the likelihood of seizures.[46] Hypoglycemia frequently occurs in the course of alcohol withdrawal, so adequate oral or intravenous supply should be assured.

5. *Avoid prophylactic anticonvulsants or antibiotics.* Phenytoin probably does not prevent withdrawal seizures and should be reserved for individuals with posttraumatic or idiopathic epilepsy. Prophylactic antibiotics do little other than guarantee that when infections do occur they will be drug resistant. Frequent medical complications of alcohol use, such as pneumonia, hematopoietic disorders, pancreatitis, and gastrointestinal hemorrhage should be treated promptly when present.

Intoxication with stimulants. Compounds that tend to increase task vigilance and general motor activity or to oppose sleep have been called stimulant or analeptic drugs. In moderate doses these drugs produce a state of wakefulness, often with increased enthusiasm, feelings of energy, and mild pressure of speech. Amphetamines and closely related compounds are the most widely abused drugs of this group. Their stimulant actions are accompanied by appetite-supressing effects leading to their wide use for temporary weight loss. The monoamine oxidase (MAO) inhibitors, whose effects are similar to those of amphetamines but much milder, are rarely abused. Cocaine is often classified as a simulant, for in addition to its local anesthetic properties it produces feelings of excitement and energy. Caffeine may be consumed in its purified form but is more often used for its stimulant effects in coffee and soft drinks. Theophylline is the major stimulant ingredient of tea and related beverages. Strychnine, a general CNS stimulant that can produce seizure discharges directly within the spinal cord, is infrequently abused. Periodically this extremely poisonous substance is used by individuals with broad tastes in drugs ("garbage heads"), resulting in dramatic emergency department presentations that can include opisthotonus and status epilepticus. Adverse reactions to stimulant drugs can be grouped into the following categories.

Dysphoric reactions ("amped out," "caf-

feine jitters"). Almost any stimulant drug can produce dysphoric reactions, which are characterized by fatigue, depression, anxiety, or panic. These reactions occur when an individual who has been taking stimulants continuously finds that euphoria can no longer be produced by an increase in dosage. Although sleep usually intervenes at that point, some individuals may become so apprehensive that they seek medical attention. Reassurance and empathy provide the most appropriate treatment, although users may present credible arguments or even threaten suicide in an effort to obtain more drugs. Administration of stimulants is never indicated. When agitation is severe, diazepam, 30 mg PO, can be used, but administration of hypnotic sedatives only tends to perpetuate drug use of the upper-downer variety. Acidification of the urine enhances excretion of amphetamines, and many users claim that it allows "crash" to proceed more smoothly. Stimulant withdrawal rarely requires emergency department chemotherapy, but profound depression may occur following extended use of stimulant drugs. Psychiatric evaluation or admission may be appropriate.

Psychotic episodes. Psychotic episodes occur with a variety of stimulant drugs. Although these reactions can be produced by a single dose, they typically follow repeated administration of the drug, suggesting a cumulative psychototoxic effect. Paranoid ideation is quite common and may be as mild as ideas of reference or as severe as organized persecutory delusions. Since stimulant drugs in moderate dosages produce improvements in the performance of tasks requiring vigilance, paranoid ideation may, in part, represent the extreme range of alertness, a "toxic vigilance." In dealing with these patients, keep in mind their experience of a world where paranoid thinking makes the most benign gesture an ominous threat.

Amphetamine psychosis. Amphetamine psychosis is the classic, full-blown, stimulant psychosis and typically is seen as a paranoid state with motor stereotypy and hyperactivity. Although first described in amphetamine abusers, it may also be produced by other drugs such as methylphenidate (Ritalin) or phenmetrazine (Preludin).[47,48] A similar syndrome occurs with heavy cocaine use, but signs of an organic brain syndrome may also be present. Cocaine may produce terrifying hallucinations of vermin infestation ("cocaine bugs") or other signs consistent with delirium. Most other stimulant psychoses, particularly the amphetamine psychosis, show a sparing of orientation and memory, a finding quite unusual in toxic psychoses. The absence of organicity can aid in making the diagnosis but has also led to overlooking the role of drugs entirely so that patients with amphetamine psychosis have been misdiagnosed as suffering from paranoid schizophrenia.

Classic signs of amphetamine psychosis include loosely organized paranoid delusions, with stereotyped motor movements that include such activities as repeated opening and closing of containers, manipulation of equipment within the emergency department, and face scratching or lip licking. Other clinical signs include auditory hallucinations such as threatening whispers, and visual illusions such as movements in the peripheral visual fields. True visual hallucinations are unusual and suggest concurrent use of other drugs or, in rare instances, a toxic brain syndrome produced by a large overdose of amphetamine. Evidence of chronic amphetamine use may provide helpful signs since, although paranoid reactions from amphetamines can occur in anyone, risk probably increases with exposure to the drug.[49] Chronic use usually leads to weight loss, dry scaling skin, thinning hair, poor dental hygiene, and often a distinct acrid body odor ("speed sweat"). Venous scarring and other signs of intravenous drug use may also be present.

Treatment should always include frequent verbal reassurance since a warm empathic voice is still the best way to make contact. Give the patient space by maintaining a large physical distance and avoiding needless touching. Patients with stimulant-induced psychoses are occasionally armed with hidden weapons and, after an imagined assault, may suddenly begin fighting for their lives. Avoid physical restraints if possible, but use them decisively if other measures fail. Haloperidol, 5 mg PO or IM, is probably the drug of choice for controlling amphetamine psychosis since it does not interfere with the detoxification of amphetamines as does chlorpromazine.[50] If diagnosis is uncertain, diazepam, 30 mg PO, should be used. Management should also include urine amphetamine screens to confirm the diagnosis, and acidification of the urine with ammonium chloride to enhance excretion.

Patients with marked impairment of reality or persistent persecutory delusions should have psychiatric evaluation or admission. Most stimulant psychoses subside spontaneously within a week, but postpsychotic depression is common, and suicide risk may be significant. Patients with milder paranoid states who do not require admission should nevertheless have careful follow-up since continued drug use inevitably brings progression to frank psychosis.

Intoxication with psychedelics. A typical psychedelic drug intoxication is almost impossible to define. For most substances, drug-specific effects can account for most of what is observed; barbiturates, for example, are capable of producing somnolence in almost everybody. But for psychedelic drugs, individual-specific and environmental effects depend on the user's expectations. Indeed, a terrifying bad trip can often be completely reversed by simple reassurance and manipulation of the environment.

The controversy over these drugs in the last two decades has reflected both the social polarization regarding their use and the basic confusion regarding their effects. This confusion has been reflected in the proposed names for the class. Hallucinogenic was one of the early terms but is essentially inaccurate since true hallucinations from these drugs are uncommon, though perceptual distortions occur regularly. "Psychodysleptic" and "psychotomimetic" have been used by investigators who felt these drugs produced a state that modeled schizophrenia or other psychoses. Subsequent research has not found much support for such simplistic biochemical models of schizophrenia so these terms have fallen into disuse. Psychedelic (mind-manifesting) was proposed by Sir Humphrey Osmond in 1957 to reflect the enhanced state of awareness these drugs often produce. This term has been felt by some to condone or glamorize use of these drugs, but it has survived as the most adequate description of their effects.

The essential psychedelic drug–specific effect seems to be a change in the process of perception. Even at small doses, feelings of an immediacy of perception, as though one were directly experiencing something or seeing it for the first time; are often reported. Objects may appear to grow, melt, or disappear into a network of geometric patterns. Visual illusions are the most common, although occasionally true hallucinations of plaidlike patterns may appear. Different senses may be combined in a phenomenon of *synesthesia*, so that one can "see" sound or "feel" color. Perception of one's self is often altered, yielding a profound sense of union with the entire universe, an experience not unlike that described by religious mystics. This ineffable state described by R. Gordon Wasson and Aldous Huxley formed the basis for the drug cult later popularized by Timothy Leary.

Since prehistoric times man has used leaves, roots, bark, and seeds containing psychotropic chemicals. Some of these plant materials contain poisonous drugs such as physostigmine or atropine and produce states of delirium with confusion, disorientation, and hallucinations. By contrast, psychedelic drugs, such as the naturally occurring peyote cactus and psilocybin mushroom yield marked perceptual alterations without delirium. These drugs are still used in native religious rituals in parts of the world.

LSD-25, a synthetic derivative of the barley mold ergot, was accidently discovered in the course of investigating migraine remedies. It is one of the most potent drugs known, with observable effects beginning at doses as low as 1 $\mu g/kg$. The massive social upheavals of the 1960's brought a fondness for perception-altering chemicals, and LSD rapidly became a household word. It was easily manufactured from the cheap and then widely available ergot fungus. Illicit laboratories were spawned in basements and kitchens. Moreover, since 1 g (roughly a teaspoonful) of LSD could be divided into 10,000 doses, its production was an enormously profitable enterprise. Income from LSD production may have helped finance the burgeoning marijuana distribution industry but also allowed illicit chemists to turn their attentions to other psychedelic drugs. In the space of a few years, research efforts, both legitimate and underground, developed manufacturing techniques for a bewildering variety of psychedelic drugs, some naturally occurring and some wholly synthetic. Drugs were designed to mimic brain amines or combine the structure of other psychedelics and stimulants. A zoo of alphabetic names appeared, DMT, DET, PPT, MDA, MMDA, and DOM (STP).

Marijuana continues to enjoy ever increasing use and seems to have easily survived while the dinosaurs of the psychedelic era have perished. In the United States the drug is usually available as the dried leaves and flowers of the marijuana plant *Cannabis sativa*. Other preparations such as hashish or Thai sticks, which contain more concentrated amounts of drug resins, also appear. The active ingredients in marijuana are the family of tetrahydrocannibinols with the delta-9-THC isomer accounting for most of the activity. It may be possible that individual subtleties between different samples of marijuana depend largely on the concentration of delta-9-THC, analogous to the percentage of ethanol as the primary indicator of the intoxicating properties of an alcoholic beverage. Most of the marijuana available in the United States has a relatively low concentration of delta-9-THC (1% to 3%), but hashish and marijuana from foreign sources notably Jamaica, Columbia, and Southeast Asia, have significantly higher concentrations (3% to 15%). Hash oil, a centrifuged steam distillate of hashish, is probably the most concentrated form available (25% to 40%). Adverse reactions seem to be more common with the more potent derivatives so that the social perception of marijuana as a benign drug is, in part, a reflection of the relatively mild forms available. Medical complications with marijuana use have not been demonstrated, although the foreign literature frequently reports many varieties of respiratory, gastrointestinal, and other disorders attributed to its use.[51,52] An unusual syndrome has recently been reported, however, in which the use of marijuana has been associated with the development of ketoacidosis in an individual not previously diagnosed as diabetic.[53] Adverse reactions to psychedelic drug intoxication fall into several broad categories.

Acute dysphoric reactions. Intoxication with psychedelic drugs may produce dysphoric reactions ranging from mild anxiety to floridly psychotic states. During the years of peak use, acute dysphoric reactions or bad trips were commonly seen in the emergency department. Lately they have become rather rare, probably since users have become more sophisticated and use of powerful psychedelic drugs is low. Marijuana, on the other hand, seems to enjoy steadily increasing popularity and since more potent forms are increasingly available, dysphoric reactions from its use may become common.

In addition to altered perceptions, psychedelic drugs tend to produce loosening of associations, altered concepts of time and space, marked emotional lability, increased suggestibility, and a loss of ego boundaries. This last effect seems to be the key to bad trips since a loss of ego boundaries can be perceived as a joyous union with the universe or as a terrifying psychological death. Thus, individuals with rigid personality styles, obsessive-compulsive, or schizoid traits are more at risk of developing adverse reactions to psychedelic drugs. Floridly psychotic behavior is typical of these acute dysphoric reactions, with patients appearing "too crazy to be schizophrenic." A history of drug ingestion is almost always admitted.

Placing the patient in a nonstimulating, nonthreatening environment is an effective first step. Quite often an individual who is agitated and psychotic in the mayhem of a rock concert will improve considerably when taken to a quiet room. Personal contact by a warm empathic individual, preferably of the patient's age group, encourages rapport. Since loss of ego boundaries can induce feelings of being out of control, the relationship with the patient is the best avenue for reassurance. Statements like "you look frightened, I'd like to help you flow with the experience you're having" seem to get better results than brusque put-offs like "don't worry about anything, you're going to get a tranquilizer." Medication should be used sparingly, diazepam, 30 mg PO, or intravenously in cases of severe agitation. Patients with psychedelic drug intoxications are extremely suggestible so that panic or fear on the part of the health care personnel can be contagious. A calm, confident manner goes a long way in reassuring the patient. Phenothiazines should be avoided since massive hypotension may be produced and anticholinergic effects may be exaggerated. Physical restraints should be avoided unless absolutely necessary.

Prolonged adverse reactions. These are somewhat unusual problems that may be present hours to days after ingestion of the drug. These reactions probably represent precipitation of latent psychiatric disorders so that reassurance or minor tranquilizers are less effective. Confusion, memory loss, and disorientation are more common in this group than in the acute reactions. With some psychedelic drugs, such as marijuana, syndrome of frank organicity and paranoia have been described.[54] A history of psychotic behavior lasting more than 24 hours following drug ingestions suggests poorer prognosis. Psychiatric evaluation is in order, and inpatient care may be necessary.

Chronic syndromes. Chronic psychiatric conditions have often been attributed to drug use. Street lore describes the stereotype of the burned-out acidhead who has had one too many trips. Such individuals tend to be withdrawn, poorly motivated, and so apathetic that they rarely perceive anything as an emergency, let alone come to an emergency department. Investigators in India, Africa, and the Caribbean have described similar chronic conditions associated with use of cannabis derivatives. Unfortunately, adequate studies of the long-term hazards of these drugs are lacking since the effects of chaotic life styles, poverty, malnutrition, other drug use, and preexisting psychiatric disorders cannot be ruled out. Early reports that marijuana use produces an amotivational syndrome have not been supported by later studies.[55,56] Although it is possible that long-term hazards of psychedelic drug use would be demonstrated, research in this area has been inconclusive.

Flashbacks. Flashbacks are episodes in which the individual reexperiences the psychedelic state. This can be interpreted as a delightful remembrance of a past trip or as a terrifying loss of control. Shick and Smith have described three categories of flashbacks—perceptual, somatic, and emotional.[57] The perceptual variety are the most common and can produce pleasant hallucinations of geometric patterns, halos around objects, or intensification of color perception. Somatic flashbacks are more disturbing and may produce paresthesias, numbness, or feelings of depersonalization. Emotional flashbacks are often quite disturbing, bringing experiences of loneliness, panic, or hopelessness, and possibly leading to suicidal ideation.

Although it is possible that permanent biochemical alterations may produce flashbacks, they seem more likely to represent learned behaviors similar to hyperventilation attacks. Like conversion reactions, flashbacks often have important psychological payoffs—the patient may gain attention, avoid responsibility, or escape from a difficult interpersonal situation by having flashbacks. Counseling, using a crisis intervention model, is the best approach and may help the patient solve the underlying problem for which the flashbacks are a partial solution. Obviously the routine dispensing of tranquilizers should be avoided.

Special problems

The following special problems are not necessarily a consequence of substance abuse. Nevertheless, they frequently appear, usually as third-priority problems, in the course of caring for substance abuse patients. Suicide and psychiatric syndromes are covered in the chapter on psychiatric emergencies.

The uncooperative patient. The uncooperative patient can be maddening to deal with. While comatose patients are simply unable to cooperate, other individuals actively resist treatment. Uncooperative patients come in many varieties: withdrawn, sullen, whining, argumentative, boisterous, violent. Providing care for such individuals first requires inducing the patient to assist in his own treatment (or at least not to obstruct care), and second preventing the patient from harming himself or others. Listing these goals is easy; attaining them is another matter.

Although principles of interaction in such cases are dealt with in the chapter on psychiatric emergencies, some points can be made here. In almost every case of patient uncooperativeness, some substance intoxication is present. Occasionally, psychedelic or anticholinergic drugs may be involved, but the general rule seems to be hypnotic sedatives or alcohol intoxication.[20] While it may be impossible to gain the cooperation of every patient, some will respond to empathic intervention. Uncooperativeness represents a continuum from mild to severe, and patients may improve or worsen, depending on staff behavior.

For example, an unkempt muttering paranoid schizophrenia patient may come in with a chronic cough and be quite cooperative until a physician, attempting to examine his chest, approaches him from behind. His predisposing psychiatric disorder may lead him to perceive this movement as a serious threat, and sudden physical violence may result. An intoxicated barbiturate addict, on the other hand, may be noisy and combative until the nurse firmly but empathically sets limits on his behavior (leaving the rest of the staff wondering "how she does it").

More often than not, uncooperative patients are surly and argumentative rather than openly assaultive. When the staff ignores verbal aggression, however, it may escalate into physical violence. Uncooperativeness is usually played to an audience: patients, even delirious ones, are usually looking for some kind of response. Ignoring the problem often only makes it worse.

Management of the uncooperative patient should include the following points:

1. *Diagnose* the contribution of various factors to aid in planning intervention. These factors are drug-specific effects: intoxication, withdrawal, emergence delirium; individual effects: organic brain syndromes, preexisting psychiatric disorders; environmental effects: sociocultural valuation of violence as a display of manhood, and the like. Since drugs usually impair judgment, emotional factors may become prominent. Experiential questions should be considered: What does the patient feel? Is he afraid? Angry? Sad? Does he want reassurance? Limit setting? How do I feel while dealing with him? The answers help one to understand the patient as a human being and thereby can enhance rapport.

2. *Explicit empathy* shows the patient you understand how he feels. Uncooperative or violent patients may be apprehensive or panicked. Show you are human too with statements such as, "You sound pretty angry, but I want you to know we are trying to help you." Don't just *be* empathic, *show* it with words and actions.

3. *Set clear limits.* Make sure the patient understands what you want. Condescending baby talk like, "Now we know we shouldn't do that," is asking for trouble. If you want something, empathically say so. "You've pulled your IV out twice and I'm getting mad. I think you need that IV and I'm going to restrain you if you pull it again." All but the most psychotic patients can handle the truth of your feelings. If you are angry or scared, say so. They probably know it all ready. Acting like a robot in the name of professionalism just does not work with uncooperative patients. Individuals with impaired mental functioning need clear communication. Don't fake it. Show what you feel.

Escalation of uncooperative behaviors may be an indirect way of asking for further limits. A show of force, isolation in a private room or bed restraints, may be needed but can never substitute for frequent staff contact. Ignoring the patient asks for trouble. Use physical restraints only when necessary, but then use them quickly and decisively.

4. *Use chemotherapy* judiciously. Diazepam, 30 mg PO or 15 mg IV, is usually effective. Sodium thiopental (Pentothal), 100 to 500 mg IV, may produce respiratory depression but is needed in rare cases. Minor tranquilizers and crises counseling have been advocated for individuals with "episodic dyscontrol syndrome."[58] This disorder is characterized by periodic violence and impulsivity often provoked by minimal amounts of alcohol. Such patients can often develop enough control to come to the emergency department before episodes develop fully, thus using it as a sort of specialized outpatient clinic.

5. *Follow-up treatment* is usually indicated. Mildly uncooperative patients may be looking for help but are unable to ask. Violent individuals may need treatment to reduce the risk of harm to themselves or others.

Children. Substance abuse emergencies involving children were once limited to household caustics and other poisons. Times have changed: the 8 year old with an intravenous heroin reaction has become a reality. In home, at school, and on the street, drugs have become more available. As a result, both intentional abuse and accidental poisonings are more frequent. For the most part, substance abuse problems in children are managed like those of adults. Some common patterns are worth noting.

Accidental ingestion. Accidental ingestion of substances occurs most often with children age 10 or younger. Children may ingest tablets or capsules found at home, taken from older siblings, or obtained from schoolmates. Such cases are not always true accidents but often represent the child's attempt to imitate adults by eating pills. Curiosity or oral exploratory behavior is probably involved in many instances. Children put almost anything in their mouths. The accident is caused by adults' making poisons so accessible. Hypnotic sedatives, tranquilizers, antidepressants, and street drugs in pill form are the most frequently consumed. Illicit drugs in powder form do not find much favor with children, who are usually limited to the oral route. Some drugs, such as opiate narcotics, are poorly absorbed through the gut and infrequently produce poisonings in children. Methadone is an important exception, as it is well absorbed orally and children seem to find the 40 mg "diskit" tablets attractive. Psychedelic drugs have largely faded in popularity, but phencyclidine is increasingly used and may produce bizarre, violent behavior in children.

When young children take pills, they usually lack a well-formed concept of "drug." Candy is about as close as they can get, but they know that drugs, like sex, have some deeper meaning to adults. Children may imitate their parents, "I took some pills because I wanted to be like Mommy," or "Everybody in my family takes medicine." A more ominous case is that of the young child who wishes to escape from a painful life, "I just wanted everything to stop." Although a particular child may need individual care, follow-up family counseling is almost always indicated. At the least, the parents need help in setting clearer guidelines for the child. Frequently a child's drug taking is an attempt to communicate to the parents feelings that are difficult to articulate:

An 8-year-old female had consumed a capsule of unidentified substance she obtained at school. Her mother brought her to the emergency department that evening when she became panicky and agitated. On examination she appeared floridly psychotic, screaming that "everybody will be killed," and that snakes and spiders were in the air. She was found to have a pulse rate of 90 with dilated but reactive pupils and mild hyperreflexia.

Since she seemed more cooperative with her mother out of the room, she was examined alone by a physician and nurse. She was given frequent reassurance that her hallucinations were only a dream and could not hurt her. Conversation about school was well tolerated, and as she spoke, she became more coherent and oriented. She expressed anger toward a teacher but then quickly added that she was never angry at her mother. As soon as she had considered the subject of anger toward her mother, she became agitated again.

The patient's father had died the previous year, and recently her mother had planned to remarry. The day of the drug ingestion the patient's mother had finalized plans to take a brief trip with her husband-to-be. The patient, if angry, had not expressed it openly, but probably in a gesture to get attention and indirectly express her own anger, she took the available drug. Her anger toward her mother then became too frightening to feel, as she was afraid it might cause her only remaining parent to die also.

Since the patient seemed to be clearing from the intoxication, family counseling was employed. Through crisis intervention the patient was reassured that it is all right to be mad at somebody you love. As she spoke further about her anger toward her teacher and then later her anger toward her mother, her bizarre behavior receded. During the session with her and her mother she was able, after some encouragement, to express her fears regarding her mother's health and her anger over the planned trip. At discharge she was well oriented but sleepy. Outpatient follow-up care was arranged to help prevent further episodes.

Unfortunately the significance of a child's drug taking is often overlooked by adults. Since drug use in children is often used as communication with parents or other adults, attempts should be made in the emergency setting to intervene in this process before the crisis seals over and a pattern of chronic drug abuse begins.

Suicide attempts. Suicide attempts by children are not rare and usually suggest severe underlying disorders. Adolescents frequently make suicide attempts with antecedent events that may be as obvious as a broken romance or as ominous as feelings of emptiness. Even when augmented by wrist slashing, drugs (aspirin, tranquilizers, sedatives) are the usual means employed.

When younger children make suicide attempts, serious psychopathology and inner torment are suggested. In any child or adolescent in whom a suicide attempt is suspected, psychiatric consultation is mandatory

The young user. Children and adolescents tend to have patterns of use that reflect availability of drugs. Glue sniffing and other inhalant abuse seem almost uniquely the province of the young, but when available, the full array of drugs from narcotics to psychedelics finds eager acceptance. Some larger population centers regularly experience heroin abuse emergencies in children, but the suburban choice has tended to be pills. Geographic patterns are useful, but one can be deceived by the first 10-year-old patient whose coma is from snorted cocaine and heroin. With older children a reverse-bias stereotype may occur.

A 19-year-old male was brought to the emergency department by college friends. They claimed he was having a bad trip—crawling on the floor, screaming, and perspiring heavily—following use of "some heavy microdot" (alleged to be LSD). Samples for testing were not available. His friends insisted that all he needed was "a little Valium."

On examination the patient was incoherent, irritable, crying and mumbling to himself while picking at his clothing. Temperature was 39° C (102° F) with chest clear. Examination was consistent with simple drug intoxication except for nuchal rigidity. Brudzinski's and Kernig's signs were positve, and spinal tap later confirmed the diagnosis of bacterial meningitis.

Children generally require the same approaches as adults, but one should beware of stereotypes. In dealing with children strive to treat each patient as an individual. Keep in mind the child's experience of the world. The emergency department can be a terrifying place. In addition to prompt specific intervention, reassurance and empathy are vital.

Staff health. In our furious devotion to helping others, we in the healing arts often overlook ourselves. Nowhere is this more evident than in the health care systems we have created. Hospitals and emergency departments can be some of the sickest settings in which to work. Pettiness, thinly veiled hatreds, hopelessness, and futility seem almost basic features of many medical teams.

Some readers will doubt this proposition; others, perhaps with a particular head nurse or physician in mind, will exclaim to themselves, "Yes! That's just how they are." But the "they" are "us." We are part of the team, we help shape it. After a trying shift, it is all too easy to kick the cat or take it out on one's spouse, but we are part of what goes on. Putting up with a bad work situation only perpetuates the conflicts. All too often frustration is what we get for our hard work; frustration and that nagging question, "How much longer can I take this job before it kills me?"

Patients are not exposed to our systems as long as we are, but nonetheless, they feel effects. One young drug user put it well during an emergency department visit, "I want to get some help, but I was afraid to come here. These medical people are so uptight—who wants to be like them?" Ultimately, our health care systems and we ourselves are advertisements for a way of life. Not one particular philosophy but rather health and freedom as opposed to addiction and habits. Abusers, both street and "respectable," often live in an underground of drug use so that the emergency department is the first contact with the outside. We do not offer people much hope when our staff interactions are a poor parody of daytime television doctors' shows. Even white uniforms can not hide what we feel.

Using the hypothesis that a job situation that makes us miserable may be less than optimal for the patient, let us consider some interventions for ourselves:

The staff as a group. A collection of people in contact for a period of time begins to exhibit the features of a group. Their behavior is affected not only by the others as individuals but also by the group as a whole. The values, aspirations, and rules of the group, although invisible, are still quite powerful. Health care personnel in general and emergency department teams in particular tend to develop group values that compensate for the inherent stresses of working with life and death problems. Mistakes can easily have devastating consequences so the value system says, "Make no mistakes." Not making mistakes is impossible, so the values say, "At least be dedicated." That way, if we make mistakes, nobody can say we did not try hard enough.

All too often these values become woven into a mythology about how medicine must be practiced. The one on top (staff physician, charge nurse, etc.) adopts a general attitude of impatience and exasperation as though the subordinate (intern, RN, vocational nurse, etc.) just cannot get things right. An atmosphere of tension and hostility is created, not unlike a home where a parent acts like a child is not quite good enough. The communications are often nonverbal, loud sighs and head-shaking, so that reading between the lines becomes standard operating procedure. Direct, honest confrontation of feelings is rare, and gradually the staff breaks into competing factions with shifting alliances.

Overall, the benefits of this "sick" system are impressive. Nobody ever really says what is on his or her mind so that when things do go wrong, as they inevitably must, there is always someone else to blame. The subordinate blames the boss for not saying what he wanted in the first place, and the superior blames the subordinate for not being up to par. Even better, the superior gets to play the part of an impatient prima donna, and the subordinate can wallow in the role of the long-suffering Cinderella.

Such twisted interactions would hardly matter if they occurred in private between consenting adults. Unfortunately, they go on between people who are supposed to be helping others. A person with a myocardial infarction may not notice that a nurse is quietly enraged at a doctor. But a person hiding in the world of drugs, on the other hand, would feel the effect of such hidden tensions and find little reason to come back to a drug-free life: "Who wants to be like them?" The group processes in emergency teams often go unnoticed because they seem irrelevant or impossible to change. Irrelevant and impossible no, but dangerous, maybe. If you ever did try to talk truthfully to that doctor who drives you up the wall, you might get fired. Some of the nastiest people have the most power. It is much easier, but not necessarily better, to ignore it and just put up with each shift.

There may be a way, however—organize. Not just us against them, but organize the whole team. Sit down together once a week, once a month, whatever works best. Talk about how you feel toward each other. Avoid unsolicited diagnoses, "You're screwed up because you . . . ." Show what *you feel*. "I get *angry* when you . . . ." "I'm *scared* to say this but . . . ." Experiment, find what works. It is not necessary to make the team into ongoing group therapy, but at least talk.

Important themes often include the expression of feelings, particularly anger and the sharing of power over decisions that affect the whole staff. Social contact between staff members outside work is not a requirement for improved relationships. If anything, the ability to say "no" to each other is vital to good communication. Spend only as much social time with other team members as *you* want to.

The emergency department does not have to be oppressive. Contrary to most myths, people are *not* more efficient in uptight settings; fear of rejection and reprimand does not decrease the frequency of mistakes. Rather it only reduces care to the mechanical and perfunctory. A staff accepting of each other as people can catch mistakes early and help each other learn. What is most important is the creation of a work environment that is both good for the team and optimal for patient care.

The staff as individuals. Although research data in this area is lacking, it is probably fair to say that many health care professionals tend to be drudges who panic when they are not being "productive." People with this syndrome of overwork, often called "workaholics," have a wide range of symptoms ranging from feelings of hopelessness and futility to nagging boredom and fatigue. The number of hours worked is not critical; rather it is the quality of the rest of one's life that counts.

A balance between work and play is vital, but health care professionals often seem to feel that they must work constantly to justify their existence. It is easy to become a workaholic and make one's self-esteem dependent on constant productivity. But overwork gradually deteriorates the quality of one's productivity and the quality of everything else in one's life. Many marriages have been weakened or destroyed by a workaholic spouse. Risks of heart attacks, hypertension, and ulcers are probably increased for workaholics.

A simple challenge test is to take three hours over the next week and goof off; do something entirely unproductive (sleep does not count), lie on the beach, take a walk, anything; just take it easy. If you become frantic or guilty when you consider your unfulfilled obligations, you may be addicted to work. Slack off, goof off regularly, even brag about it. Overwork is a serious disorder. Do not take it lightly. When you work, work; when you play, play. Even the Creator took a day off.

Overwork may also be a sign of underlying troubles in one's life so that escapes to work can cover up marital, family, or individual problems. It is hard to change habits, staying in a rut is often easier. Health care professionals (who *should* know better) are often loath to change life-

long habits and instead try to "hang in there." Sometimes they break.

The need to earn feelings of self-worth is dangerous when one is dealing with problems of substance abuse. Almost everyone in the health professions wants to help people and feel like they are doing something worthwhile and important. It is also quite human to desire to be appreciated and accepted for one's efforts. Yet drug abusers are often uncooperative, unruly, and rude. Even worse, they may interfere with our ideas about how the healing game is supposed to be played: often they do not get better. If we base our self-respect on whether people are healed by our touch, we resent them when they do not.

Staff factors in health care cannot be reduced to a simplistic list. Nevertheless, we must consider what is going on with us since how we feel and think dramatically affects treatment. Overwork and hidden feelings are common, but other problems are also possible. Some health professionals rarely review their actions, as though every thing they do is automatically therapeutic. Good intentions should never replace critical self-evaluation. Rather, it is a balance of head and heart that is needed.

Disposition. There is great art to managing a smooth flow of patients through an emergency department. Some individuals require admission; some must be held for consultants; some need transfer to other facilities. Each route of patient intake or disposition makes the job more complex; each link with an outside agency is another source of mishap. Little wonder that emergency departments have an almost limitless potential for chaos.

Emergency department care proceeds in stages, with intake and treatment as the first order of business. These two stages may contain urgencies of the highest order. Significantly, legal guidelines for responsibility in these stages are well established. Disposition, on the other hand, is often only an afterthought. Clinically and legally the attitude often seems to be that it is someone else's problem now—as though through deft buck passing a "reasonable referral" is the end of the job.

Substance abuse patients are not dealt with so neatly. A brief note accompanying a comatose patient might suffice for admission or transfer. Awake individuals need more. The ambulatory outpatient referred to a counseling center with a slip of paper and a few hurried words may not bother to make his first appointment. If we do not think follow-up care is important, why should the patient take it any more seriously?

Substance abusers tend to have long-term, chronic problems that periodically spawn acute emergencies. Adequate treatment of the underlying disorders is vital. Resuscitation of a patient from grade IV coma becomes a heroic Band-aid when disposition is marginal. Yet, with substance abusers, disposition may often be overlooked because it seems so futile. "What can an emergency department do for such problems if other agencies have failed?" Possibly nothing, but here and there a substance abusing patient filled with the pain of a life that is going nowhere may be reached. The crisis that precipitated the emergency department visit may just destabilize his old habits enough for him to ask, "Is this really the life I want?"

To be certain, some substance abuse problems are depressingly chronic; some patients come back so frequently that they become known as regulars. As they cycle between the emergency department, detoxification centers, counseling programs, and back, they truly seem to be going nowhere. For some, their orbits through these various community agencies become almost as predictable as Haley's comet (but of course cycle far more frequently). Each month "old George," an alcoholic epileptic, may be brought in after his latest drinking bout provokes yet another group of seizures. Routinely sending him off to detoxification

after his fiftieth neurologic consultation may not be optimum care. He may be drunk and dazed after a seizure, but empathic, intrusive efforts by the staff might get through to him. Of course, this is a worst-case example, and such efforts may not produce much impact. But consider this: when was the last time a member of the emergency department staff spoke to him with dignity, respect, and empathic involvement rather than a condescending, condemning, verbal pat on the head for "old George"—"hopeless old George." If *we* think he is hopeless, what is *he* going to think?

Blind hope is not the answer, but showing the patient respect and faith that he *can* do something for himself goes a long way. The common staff pattern toward such patients is to harbor unspoken resentment that covers ambivalence. "Are these patients making their own problems by overindulging or is addiction really an illness?" "Are they really trying to get better or are they just making themselves worse?" These questions have no simple answers, and the result is frequently an aloof condescending attitude toward substance abusing patients and a tendency for the staff to joke covertly with nonverbal winks and nods, "Oh, no . . . it's old George again!"

For substance abusing patients, disposition is often the most critical stage. But it is easier for the staff to avoid the complexities of ensuring adequate follow-up care. The complexities of dealing with the next emergency are quite sufficient to keep everyone busy. In an ideal world a special staff clerk or social worker could handle such tasks. In this flawed real world, limitations of money and manpower form a familiar refrain. Emergency departments seem to have a primary charter to save victims of automobile accidents and resuscitate the near dead. Complex social problems, such as substance abuse that involves crisis or family counseling, are often too much to deal with. Listed below are some approaches that might be considered radical in communities where emergency department functions are restricted. On the other hand, the staff that is tired of seeing the same old patients might push for more vigorous involvement with follow-up care. Since emergency department work is typified by lulls and crises, the slack times may provide opportunities for following up patient dispositions.

1. *Disposition begins with admission.* Treating the acute emergency is the beginning, not the end. Planning for disposition should start with the initial patient assessment and be modified as care progresses. At the time of presentation a barbiturate overdose should be evaluated with such questions as, "Will this patient be likely to require admission? Will consultations be needed? Will emergency department discharge be feasible?" Definitive answers may not be possible at first, but waiting too long makes disposition even more awkward.

2. *Keep a register of available resources.* Options for disposition include hospital care, detoxification centers, outpatient clinics, short- and long-term residential centers. Obvious factors include the patient's condition and availability of beds, but often many other items need to be considered in selecting the best disposition. A list of resources may be quite large but must be kept up to date. Over the last decade, enormous amounts of public money have been channeled into the drug abuse treatment industry, and competition is fierce. Agencies appear and vanish at a startling rate so that the register must be frequently revised. For this reason a loose-leaf binder works best. Resources can be referenced both by name and by problems treated. Each page can display the agency's name, telephone number, address, hours of service, admission criteria, fee structure, and most importantly, the name of an agency staff person who can be contacted by the emergency department.

3. *Develop an effective relationship with the patient.* Aloofness is fine if patient is comatose, but if he is awake, empathy works better. Your relationship with the patient is the most powerful tool for gaining his cooperation. Even grossly delirious patients have some ability to cooperate. Whether he is to sit in a wheelchair until admission or call a counseling center on his own, his perception of you as caring and involved will motivate him.

4. *Do for the patient only what he cannot do for himself.* Show him respect; gain his cooperation by rewarding his efforts. Substance abusers are often manipulative and devious, but as much as possible involve the patient in planning his follow-up care.

5. *Do not make the mistake of thinking empathy means pity or hiding anger.* All but the most paranoid patients can accept your feelings if you express them free of judgment; "I'm angry at you for throwing your bedpan on the floor" gets through far better than, "How long have you had these problems of self-control, Mr. Smith?" Substance abusers are often crippled by poor self-esteem. See through their habits and manipulations to the person trapped inside. Your respect and honesty can gain their help—and give them hope.

6. *Follow up discharged patients.* This step is usually seen as someone else's job. Treating the emergency may be what the emergency department is for, but follow-up is often necessary to ensure later care is adequate. For patients discharged home with an outpatient referral a phone call to the patient a few days later is a good nudge into treatment. Substance abusers often feel that nobody cares, and a phone call to see how they are doing encourages them to help themselves. Rather than resent the intrusion, patients often seem touched that an emergency department staff member remembered them and cared enough to call.

Make follow-up contact with agencies. With the patient's written release of information, a copy of the emergency department record can be sent to the agency along with a phone call to a staff person. Agencies should be checked periodically to assess such questions as, Are they still in business? What kinds of problems are they treating? What kind of job did they do with the last few patients we sent them?

Make follow-up contact with physicians whose patients are seen in the emergency department. This is a ticklish area, however, and may be part of why emergency department follow-up in general is avoided. Community physicians and the emergency department often have less than optimal relationships. Difficult or annoying patients, especially those whose care is provided by public money, are infrequently seen by private physicians when they develop emergencies. Instead, they go to hospital emergency departments, and the staff, usually deprived of adequate patient history, struggles to cope. Emergency departments in private hospitals often provide brief care and then pass on such patients to county or teaching hospitals. "Ipecac and transfer" is one expression; "dump referrals" is another.

"Dumping," like much of the rarely printed slang of everyday medicine, is a term that displays staff resentment. All too often, rather than express anger at the primary physician or the first emergency department that dumped the patient, the staff will subtly punish the patient who started it all by taking drugs. Research data are lacking, but it is possible that such behavior is ineffective in gaining patient cooperation or even maintaining one's own sanity. It *might* be appropriate to call the "dumper" and express anger at them for transferring the patient after such cursory care. It *might* also be appropriate to call physicians who prescribe such excessive amounts of sleeping medications that they become suppliers for addicts and suicides alike. But then again it might be safer to stick to giving ipecac and monitoring CVP. Follow-up can be messy.

CONCLUSION

Substance abuse emergencies demand our best. The acute crises are severe, but often they are only symptoms underlying chronic disorders. A comprehensive approach to the patient—medical, psychiatric, and social—is needed to effect real change. Medical care of these emergencies requires a working comprehension of pharmacology and physiology, along with a command of current treatment. Psychiatric care calls for recognition of the patient as a person, involving him in his care and assisting him in finding ways to reduce involvement with drugs. Social care demands an approach to the patient as part of a larger interpersonal matrix, guiding him to follow-up care and helping him to restructure his life. Emergency care of substance abusers cannot be sharply demarcated from follow-up treatment. Rather, substance abuse emergencies are but the first contact in the beginning of a long process. Other areas of health care have better defined problems and require less from us as professionals. But then again, no one chooses to deliver emergency care because it is easy.

REFERENCES

1. Jaffe, J. H.: Drug addiction and drug abuse. In Goodman, L. S., and Gilman, A., editors: Pharmacological basis of therapeutics, New York, 1969, Macmillan Publishing Co., pp. 285-294.
2. Weil, A. T., Zinberg, N. E., and Nelsen, J. A.: Clinical and psychological effects of marihuana in man, Science **162**:1234-1242, 1968.
3. Chambers, C. D., Imciardi, J. A., and Siegal, H. A.: Chemical coping: a report on legal drug use in the United States, New York, 1975, Spectrum Publications.
4. Oswald, I., and Thacore, V. R.: Amphetamine and phenmetrazine addiction. Physiological abnormalities in the abstinence syndrome, Br. Med. J. **5354**:427-431, 1963.
5. Johnson, D. W., and Gunn, J. W.: Dangerous drugs: adulterants, diluents and deception in street samples, J. Forensic Sci. **17**(4):629-639, 1972.
6. Garriott, J. C., and Sturner, W. Q.: Morphine concentrations and survival periods in

acute heroin fatalities, N. Engl. J. Med. **289:** 1276-1278, 1973.

7. Levine, L. H., Hirsch, C. S., and White, L. W.: Quinine cardiotoxicity: a mechanism for sudden death in narcotic addicts, J. Forensic Sci. **18:**167-172, 1973.

8. Baselt, R. C., Allison, D. J., Wright, J. A., et al.: Acute heroin fatalities in San Francisco. Demographic and toxicologic characteristics, West. J. Med. **122**(6):455-458, 1975.

9. Cherubin, C., McCusker, J., Baden, M., et al.: Epidemiology of death in narcotic addicts, Am. J. Epidemiol. **96:**11-22, 1972.

10. Hahn, H., Schweid, A., and Beatty, H.: Complications of injecting dissolved methylphenidate tablets, Arch. Intern. Med. **123:** 656-659, 1969.

11. Hopkins, G. B.: Pulmonary angiothrombotic granulomatosis in drug offenders, J.A.M.A. **221:**909-911, 1972.

12. AtLee, W. E., Jr.: Talc and cornstarch emboli in eyes of drug abusers, J.A.M.A. **219:** 49-51, 1972.

13. Louria, D. B., Hensle, T., and Rose, J.: The major medical complications of heroin addiction, Ann. Intern. Med. **67:**1-22, 1967.

14. Cherubin, C.: Management of acute medical complications resulting from heroin addiction. In Bourne, P. G., editor: Acute drug abuse emergencies: a treatment manual, New York, 1976, Academic Press, pp. 69-86.

15. Thompson, W. R.: *H. vaginicola* endocarditis in a heroin addict, J.A.M.A. **215:**982, 1971.

16. Mills, J., and Drew, D.: *Serratia marcescens* endocarditis: a regional illness associated with intravenous drug abuse, Ann. Intern. Med. **84**(1):29-35, 1976.

17. Dreisbach, R. H.: Handbook of poisoning: diagnosis and treatment, Los Altos, Calif., 1974, Lange Medical Publications.

18. Stephenson, H. E., Jr.: Cardiac arrest and resuscitation, ed. 4, St. Louis, 1974, The C. V. Mosby Co.

19. Dole, V. P., Foldes, F. F., Trigg, H., Robinson, J. W., and Blatman, S.: Methadone poisoning. Diagnosis and treatment, N.Y. State J. Med. **71:**541-543, 1971.

20. Read, R. A., and Rusk, T. N.: The uncooperative psychiatric patient, J. Emerg. Nurs. **2:**47-49, 1976.

21. Tinklenburg, J. R.: The treatment of acute amphetamine psychosis. In Bourne, P., editor: A treatment manual for drug abuse emergencies, Washington, D.C., 1974, National Clearing House for Drug Abuse Information.

22. Reed, C. E., Driggs, M. F., and Foote, C. C.: Acute barbiturate intoxication, Ann. Intern. Med. **37:**290-303, 1952.

22a. Mandy, S., and Ackerman, A. B.: Characteristic traumatic skin lesions in drug-induced coma, J.A.M.A. **213**(2):253-256, 1970.

22b. Plum, F., and Posner, J.: The diagnosis of stupor and coma, Philadelphia, 1972, F. A. Davis Co., p. 25.

23. Burns, R. S., Lerner, S. E., Corrado, R., et al.: Phencyclidine—states of acute intoxication and fatalities, West. J. Med. **123**(5): 345-349, 1975.

24. Mark, L. C.: Analeptics: changing concepts, declining status, Am. J. Med. Sci. **254:**296-302, 1967.

25. Dimijian, G. G., and Radelat, F. A.: Evaluation and treatment of the suspected drug user in the emergency room, Arch. Intern. Med. **125:**162-170, 1970.

26. Schofferman, J. A.: A clinical comparison of syrup of ipecac and apomorphine use in adults, J. Am. Coll. Emerg. Phys. **5:**(1):22-25, 1976.

27. Gard, H., Knapp, D., Walle, T., et al.: Qualitative and quantitative studies on the disposition of amitriptyline and other tricyclic antidepressant drugs in man as it relates to the management of the overdosed patient, Clin. Toxicol. **6:**571-584, 1973.

28. Hayden, J. W., and Comstock, E. G.: Use of activated charcoal in acute poisoning, Clin. Toxicol. **8**(5):515-533, 1975.

29. Adamson, J. S., Jr., Flanigan, W. J., and Ackerman, G. L.: Treatment of bromide intoxication with ethacrynic acid and mannitol diuresis, Ann. Intern. Med. **65:**749-752, 1966.

30. Schreiner, G. E., Maher, J. F., Argy, W. P., et al.: Hemodialysis. In Brody, B., editor: Handbook of experimental pharmacology, New York, 1971, Springer-Verlag.

31. Waldron, V. D., Klint, C. R., and Seibel, J. E.: Methadone overdose treated with naloxone infusion, J.A.M.A. **225:**53, 1973.

31a. Spiker, D. G., and Biggs, J. T.: Tricyclic antidepressants. Prolonged plasma levels after overdose, J.A.M.A. **236**(15):1711, 1976.

31b. Sedal, L., Korman, M. G., Williams, P. O., et al.: Overdosage of tricyclic antidepressants: a report of two deaths and a prospective study of 24 patients, Med. J. Aust. **2:**74-79, 1972.

31c. Tobis, J., and Das, B. N.: Cardiac complications in amitriptyline poisoning: successful treatment with physostigmine, J.A.M.A. **235** (14):1474-1476, 1976.

32. Clemmesen, C., and Nilsson, E.: Therapeutic trends in the treatment of barbiturate poisoning. The Scandinavian method, Clin. Pharmacol. Ther. 2:220-229, 1961.

33. Duberstein, J. L., and Kaufman, D. M.: A clinical study of an epidemic of heroin intoxication and heroin-induced pulmonary edema, Am. J. Med. 51:704-714, 1971.

34. Tinklenburg, J. R.: The treatment of acute amphetamine psychosis. In Bourne, P., editor: A treatment manual for drug abuse emergencies, Washington, D.C., 1974, National Clearing House for Drug Abuse Information.

35. Kane, F. J., Jr., Keeler, M. H., and Reifler, C. B.: Neurological crises following methamphetamine, J.A.M.A. 210:556-557, 1969.

36. Ellinwood, E. H., Jr.: Amphetamine psychosis. Description of the individuals and process, J. Nerv. Ment. Dis. 144:273-283, 1967.

37. Schibanoff, J.: Personal communication, 1977.

38. Fingle, E., and Woodbury, D. M.: General principles. In Goodman, L. S., and Gilman, A., editors: Pharmacological basis of therapeutics, New York, 1975, Macmillan Publishing Co., p. 28.

39. Taylor, G. J., and Harris, W. S.: Cardiac toxicity of aerosol propellants, J.A.M.A. 214:81-85, 1970.

40. Bass, M.: Sudden sniffing death, J.A.M.A. 212:2075-2079, 1970.

41. Burns, R. S., Lerner, S. E., Corrado, R., et al.: Phencyclidine—states of acute intoxication and fatalities, West. J. Med. 123:(5): 345-349, 1975.

42. Ketchum, J. S., Sidell, F. R., Crowell, E. B., Jr., et al.: Atropine, scopolamine, and ditran: comparative pharmacology and antagonists in man, Psychopharmacologia 28:121-145, 1973.

43. Wikler, A.: Diagnosis and treatment of drug dependence of the barbiturate type, Am. J. Psychiatry 125:758-765, 1968.

44. Smith, D. E., and Wesson, D. R.: Phenobarbital technique for treatment of barbiturate dependence, Arch. Gen. Psychiatry 24:56-60, 1971.

45. Victor, M., and Adams, R. D.: The effect of alcohol on the nervous system, Assoc. Res. Nerv. Ment. Dis., Proc. 32:526, 1953.

46. Knott, D. H., Beard, J. D., and Wallace, J. A.: Acute withdrawal from alcohol: a diagnostic and therapeutic problem, Postgrad. Med. 42:A109-114, 1967.

47. Connell, P. H.: Amphetamines psychosis. Maudsley monograph no 5, London, 1958, Oxford University Press.

48. Kalant, O. J.: The amphetamines—toxicity and addiction, Springfield, Ill., 1966, Charles C Thomas, Publisher.

49. Griffith, J. D., Cavanaugh, J., Held, J., et al.: Dextroamphetamine. Evaluation of psychomimetic properties in man, Arch. Gen. Psychiatry 26:97-100, 1972.

50. Davis, W. M., Logston, D. G., and Hickenbritton, J. P.: Antagonism of acute amphetamine intoxication by haloperidol and propranolol, Toxicol. Appl. Pharmacol. 29:397-403, 1974.

51. Dupont, R. L.: Marihuana: a conversation with NIDA's, Science 192:647-649, 1976.

52. Tennant, F. S., Jr., Preble, M., Prendergast, T. J., et al.: Medical manifestations associated with hashish, J.A.M.A. 216:1965-1969, 1971.

53. Bier, M. M., and Steahly, L. P.: Emergency treatment of marihuana complicating diabetes. In Bourne, P. editor: Acute drug abuse emergencies New York, 1976, Academic Press, pp. 163-173.

54. Talbott, J. A., and Teague, J. W.: Marijuana psychosis: acute toxic psychosis associated with the use of cannabis derivatives, J.A.M.A. 210:299-302, 1969.

55. McGlothlin, W. H., and West, L. J.: The marijuana problem: an overview, Am. J. Psychol. 125:370-378, 1968.

56. Mendleson, J. H., and Meyer, R. E.: Behavioral and biological concomitants of chronic marijuana smoking by heavy and casual users. In Marijuana: a signal of misunderstanding (Report of the National Commission on Marijuana and Drug Use) Washington, 1972, U.S. Gov. Printing Office, pp. 68-246.

57. Shick, J. F., and Smith, D. E.: Analysis of the LSD flashback, Psychedelic Drugs 3:13-19, 1970.

58. Mark, V. H., and Ervin, F. R.: Violence and the brain, New York, 1970, Harper & Row, Publishers.

CHAPTER 14

Emergency orthopedics

Michael F. Rodi, M.D.

A simple fracture or dislocation may become a devastating injury resulting in severe, permanent disability. A moderate sprain, if inadequately treated, may likewise result in an unnecessarily prolonged disability, leading to recurrent injuries. The first person rendering care to a patient with a fracture, dislocation, or severe sprain will often determine the ultimate results occurring as a consequence of the injury.

As in all emergency situations, proper initial care is based on a thorough understanding of the principles of care and diligent practice.

MUSCULOSKELETAL SYSTEM

A basic understanding of the musculoskeletal system and its relationship to other organ systems is essential to proper management of orthopedic emergencies and, therefore, to the welfare of the patient as a whole.

Bone

Bone is a living structure with its own blood supply, innervation, and capacity for repair. The skeleton protects the body and vital organs. Even an injury as seemingly innocuous as fractured ribs should bring to mind what lies beneath; there is always the possibility of a ruptured spleen or traumatic pericardial effusion, as well as hemothorax or pneumothorax. Care for such life-threatening emergencies is discussed in Chapters 24 and 29, but if the diagnosis is not made, the patient may die. The skeleton functions also as the supporting structure of the body along with joints, ligaments, muscles, nerves, and arteries and veins. As a whole, these various parts of the musculoskeletal system enable the individual to move in daily activities. However, a slightly stiff finger resulting from an injury could permanently ruin the career of a flamenco guitarist. An injured elbow could bench a pitcher permanently. Likewise, a brick mason could be disabled from an inadequately treated minor shoulder injury, which would be inconsequential to a clerk. Without proper movement, therefore, there is no artisan, and without the artisan there is no art.

Arteries, veins, nerves

In varying but generally close proximity to the bones are the arteries, veins, and nerves. An unstable fracture or dislocation places these structures in jeopardy.

Joints

Joints are specialized junctions (articulations) between bone ends that allow for varied and specific motions. They are stabilized by ligaments and moved by the muscles. The blood vessels and nerves are always closely approximated to the joints. If these structures were to be placed at a distance from the joint, they would be required to stretch greatly with normal motions of the joint.

TRAUMA
Direct or indirect violence

Fractures and dislocations may be caused by direct or indirect violence. Direct violence implies that the force or blow is received directly on the bone that is fractured or joint that is dislocated. When a fracture or dislocation is caused by a direct blow, there may be severe damage to the overlying skin, muscles, and vessels that will not become apparent for several hours.[1]

When the fracture or dislocation occurs at a distance from the force or blow (i.e., a dislocation of the elbow as a result of landing on the hand), indirect violence is said to have occurred, and the majority of the associated soft tissue damage will come from within, from stretching and tearing by the dislocated or fractured bone end. Other examples of indirect violence are fractured ribs from a violent muscular contraction, a dislocated shoulder from a convulsive seizure, and an avulsion fracture where a tendon or ligament pulls away from a fragment of bone.

The clinical signs of fractures and dislocations are predictable:
1. Clinical signs of fracture
   a. Deformity
   b. Local swelling
   c. Point tenderness
   d. Crepitus (not to be tested for)
   e. Protrusion of bone end through the skin (open fracture)
2. Clinical signs of dislocation
   a. Gross deformity at joint
   b. Nearly complete inability to move affected joint
   c. Point tenderness about disrupted ligaments

It should be emphasized that palpation for tenderness should be *gentle*. Not only is deep palpation unnecessary and painful, but gentle palpation will yield much more information as to the location and severity of the fracture, dislocation, or sprain. Also, early swelling comes from lacerated vessels, later swelling comes from bone hemorrhage, and further swelling comes from accumulation of tissue fluid in the damaged soft tissues, particularly in the surrounding musculature.

Fractures

Fractures are any break, complete or incomplete, of a bone. They are described as being open if there is a wound extending from the fracture through the skin and closed if the skin has not been broken. Fractures are also defined by their radiographic appearance as being greenstick, transverse, oblique, spiral, comminuted, impacted, or displaced (Fig. 14-1).

A pathologic fracture is a break through an abnormal portion of bone, which may be associated with a tumor, infection, or underlying bone disease such as rickets.

A stress fracture is a fracture caused by repeated trauma, such as extended marches in young recruits, and generally occurs about the proximal femur, proximal tibia, or distal metatarsals.

Dislocations

A dislocation is a complete displacement of the normal articulating ends of two or more bones, implying severe disruption of the stabilizing ligaments of that joint. When the displacement is incomplete and a portion of the articulating surface remains in contact, the joint is subluxed.

Sprains

Sprains may be defined as mild when the supporting ligaments of the joint are stretched but remain intact; or severe when the ligaments are partially or completely ruptured.[2] Stretched or torn ligaments may render a joint all but useless. Any degree of swelling and the early appearance of ecchymosis around or distal to a joint implies hemorrhage from the vessels in and near the injured ligament. The findings of swelling and ecchymosis, therefore, are a measure of the severity of the sprain. The area of maximum tenderness to light palpation will identify the site of rupture and the specific ligament(s) torn. The mere application of an Ace bandage to a severe sprain does more harm than good, leading to the permanent disability of an unstable joint if its application delays proper orthopedic evaluation and care. Severe pain with a minimal sprain should lead one to suspect the potentially devastating problem of Sudeck's atrophy,[3] Volkmann's ischemic contracture,[4] or a coincidental septic arthritis (particularly gonococcal).

Tendon injuries

In evaluating trauma to the musculoskeletal system one must also be cognizant of tendon injuries.

Open lacerations of tendons about the

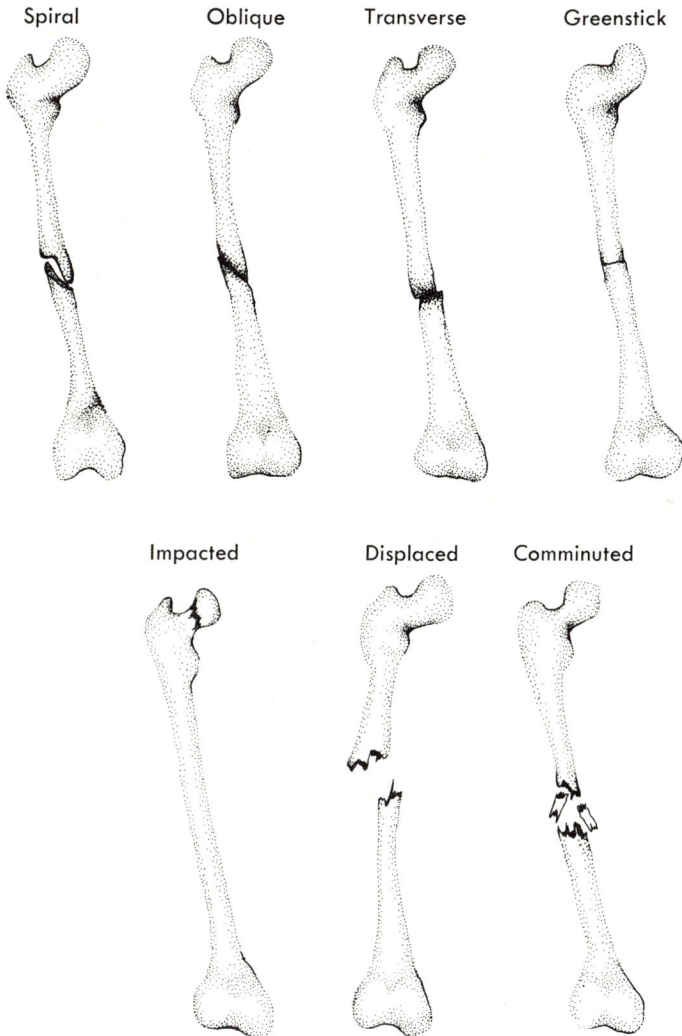

Fig. 14-1. Fractures by radiographic appearance.

wrist and hand with the attendant loss of function may be obvious. However, one must be cognizant also of the possibilities of less obvious tendon ruptures.[2] There may be partial or complete rupture of the rotator cuff (the tendons of the supraspinatus, infraspinatus, and teres minor) girdle about the shoulder as well as the long head of the biceps. Possible ruptures of the biceps tendon and brachialis should be considered in elbow injuries. To miss the diagnosis of an acutely ruptured tendo Achillis may lead to an extended and perhaps permanent disability. Because the tendon sheath is rapidly filled with blood from local hemorrhage, the tendon may appear to be clinically intact. However, if the patient is placed on his or her abdomen with the foot off the end of the stretcher, the diagnosis of an acute rupture of the tendo Achillis may be made. The patient's gastrosoleus is squeezed firmly, and if the tendo Achillis is ruptured, there will be no plantar flexion of the ankle. If there is dorsiflexion of the ankle, the tendo Achillis is at least partially intact.[4]

EMERGENCY CARE OF FRACTURES AND DISLOCATIONS

Emergency care of fractures and dislocations requires careful inspection of the injured part, local wound care, and splinting.[5]

Inspection

Careful inspection is directed at the circulatory and neurologic status of the area distal to the deformity, swelling, and point tenderness.

In an evaluation of the circulatory status the absence or presence of the pulses distal to the injury should be noted and recorded. Paleness, mottled cyanosis, and coolness distal to the injury are indications of severe circulatory impairment. These findings may be secondary to pressure, attenuation, or laceration of major vessels, and the fact that a physician is urgently needed is ob-

vious. The neurologic status is evaluated by testing for numbness to pinprick distal to the injury. The presence of paralysis at the time of the injury or ensuing paralysis on repeated examination is of great importance in determining the optimal course of definitive care. Circulatory and neurologic status observations of the extremity should be repeated at frequent intervals while the patient is in the emergency department (Fig. 14-2).

Wound management

Local wound care is initiated by assessment of the wound for evidence of severe hemorrhage, debris, and the presence of bone ends protruding through the skin. These findings should be noted on the chart, and a dry, sterile dressing should be applied so as not to further embarrass the circulation; there should be no attempt at wound cleansing or pulling the bones back beneath the skin. Any cleansing should await definitive debridement in the operating room because of the danger of increasing the contamination deep within the wound. Severe hemorrhage is generally controllable by direct pressure over the wound or over the arteries just proximal to the wound. The control of severe hemorrhage is more completely outlined in Chapter 6.

Amputations or partial amputations require special handling. When a patient with a partial amputation arrives in the emergency department, the amputated part should be immediately aligned in an anatomic position, covered with a sterile saline-soaked dressing, and splinted. Proper personnel should be notified immediately.

In the event that a patient is admitted with a complete amputation of a fingertip, the amputated part should be placed immediately in saline solution. Some clinicians consider the addition of antibiotics or heparin or both to be of help. In facilities where there is a team that performs major reimplantation surgery, the team should be consulted immediately as to preference in handling the amputated part.

A brief note should be made regarding puncture wounds that might conceivably have penetrated a joint. These wounds should be evaluated before being dismissed as being of no consequence. A decision must be made as to whether this joint should be explored (opened operatively); irreparable damage rapidly follows bacterial or foreign body invasion of a joint.

Management for children

Before discussing the final steps in emergency orthopedic care, special mention should be made of fractures and disloca-

tions in children. Because of open epiphyses (growth plates) and the inherent difficulty in evaluating the injury, there is potential for secondary growth deformities resulting from misdiagnoses or improper care.

Fractures through epiphyses may be difficult or impossible to determine radiographically[1] because of minimal displacement of the epiphyseal fracture. Comparison x-ray views of the opposite extremity should be routinely obtained. Even these may be of no help. Again, point tenderness, in this instance over an epiphysis, is sufficient reason for the emergency application of a rigid splint.

Fractures of the unossified capitellum,

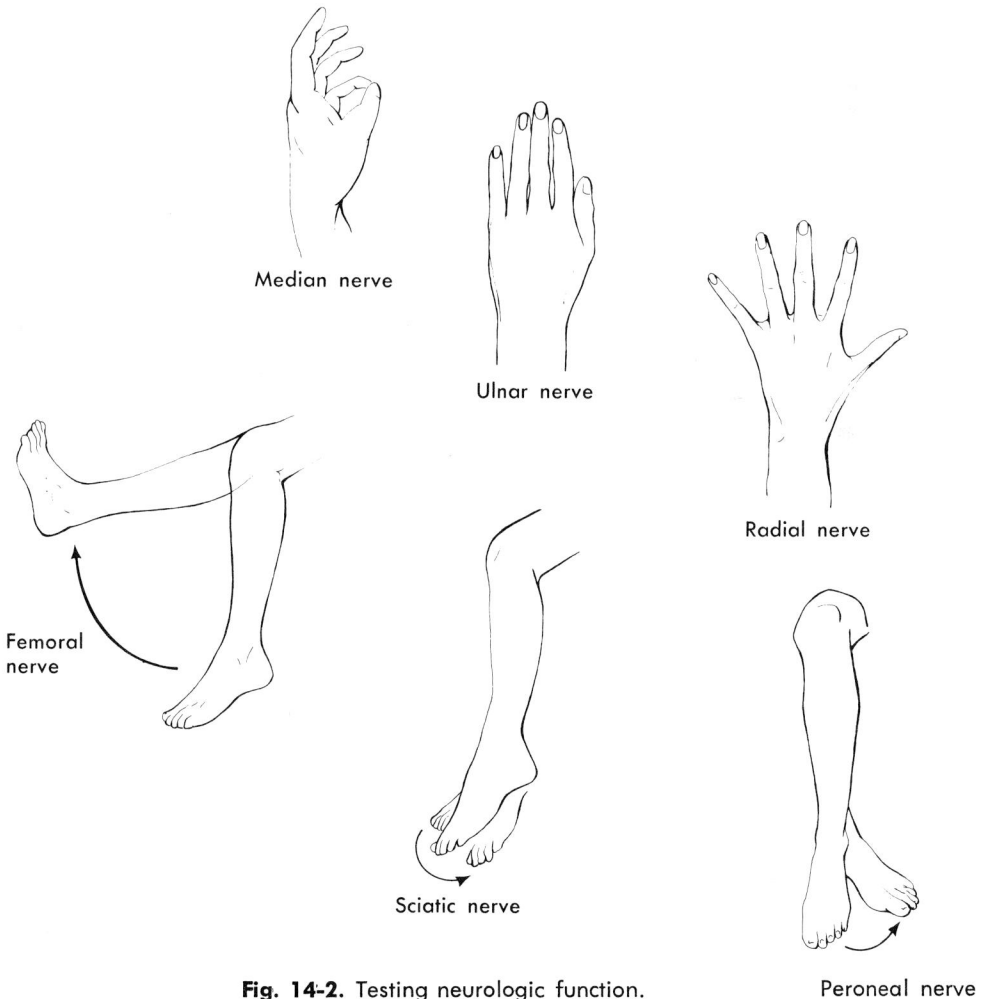

Median nerve

Ulnar nerve

Radial nerve

Femoral nerve

Sciatic nerve

Peroneal nerve

Fig. 14-2. Testing neurologic function.

lateral humeral epicondyle, or medial humeral epicondyle, or a dislocation of the unossified radial head in a child may likewise be a purely clinical diagnosis as there may be no positive radiographic abnormalities. Again, point tenderness, swelling, or clinical deformity indicates the necessity for application of a rigid splint to prevent further damage to the injured parts prior to definitive orthopedic evaluation and treatment. The diagnosis of a sprained elbow or ankle in the absence of radiographic abnormalities is a dangerous diagnosis if the patient is not properly splinted and referred for definitive care. If a fractured lateral humeral condyle has been mistakenly diagnosed as a sprained elbow, the injury may result in severe permanent disability. Unless recognized early, before healing has begun, there will be disability despite the best orthopedic management.

Again, the evaluation of fractures about epiphyses or unossified portions of the skeleton must rest largely on a high index of suspicion and careful examination since the x-ray studies may not be helpful. A rigid splint and orthopedic consultation are required if there is any doubt as to the presence or absence of a significant injury.

Splinting

The purpose of splinting is to prevent motion of fractured bone fragments or dislocated joints, thereby preventing the following:

1. Further damage to local blood vessels with attendant hemorrhage, ischemia, and tissue death
2. Further damage to nerves by inadvertent excessive traction, contusion, or laceration resulting in possible permanent loss of sensation and paralysis
3. Further damage to muscles with subsequent necrosis, scarring, and permanent disability
4. Further damage to skin with the danger of increasing contamination of the wound, infection of bone, and extreme extended disability
5. Further excessive pain
6. Shock
7. Delayed union or nonunion, which may result from excessive local tissue damage to all the above-noted structures

A fracture, dislocation, or severe sprain should be splinted before the patient is moved further. The splint should be applied after careful inspection of the circulatory and neurologic status distal to the injury, after local wound care, and after straightening a severely angulated fracture (except fractures at the shoulder, elbow, wrist, or knee). Do *not* straighten a dislocated joint.[6] A dislocated joint should not be straightened because of the danger of further damage to the nerves and blood vessels that travel in close proximity to the joint. The joint should be splinted in the position in which it is found. A severely angled fracture, except at the shoulder, elbow, wrist, or knee, should be straightened (not reduced) in order to relieve pain and allow for improved circulation. Severely angulated fractures at the shoulder, elbow, wrist, and knee should not be straightened, again because of the danger of further attenuation or laceration of the nerves or blood vessels in close proximity to the fracture (Fig. 14-3).

Types of splints. In general, there are three types of splints: soft, rigid, and traction.

Soft splint. A soft splint is one that has no inherent rigidity, such as a pillow or blanket.

Rigid splint. Rigid splints, by definition, have inherent rigidity. Rigid splints utilized at the scene of an accident by bystanders might include wood, rolled newspapers, or other convenient materials. Rigid splints available to ambulance attendants and emergency department personnel might include cardboard splints, padded board splints, various aluminum splints, ladder splints, hinged splints, and air splints. Each of these types has advantages and disadvantages beyond its availability. Board splints must be carefully padded with soft materials such as Kerlix, blankets, or towels in order to afford even pressure throughout the injured part and to avoid excess pressure over bony prominences. Likewise, the cardboard and ladder splints should be carefully padded. Ladder splints have the additional advantage of being malleable, so they may be made to conform to some degree to the contour of the extremity. Occasionally, the use of hinged splints is advantageous since they are hinged at the level of a joint, hence more easily conforming to the position of that joint. These

splints must also be padded. Air splints, when applicable, have the great advantage of affording even pressure over the entire injured extremity without increasing pressure over bony prominences. They also provide excellent immobilization of the injured part.

Assuming all the above rigid splints to be well padded and properly contoured, application of these splints to the injured extremity runs a great risk of further compromising the circulation to the injured extremity. This danger is avoided to a large extent by the use of an air splint. It should be inflated by *mouth* to the point where the thumb will cause a slight dent if pressed against the splint with modest pres-

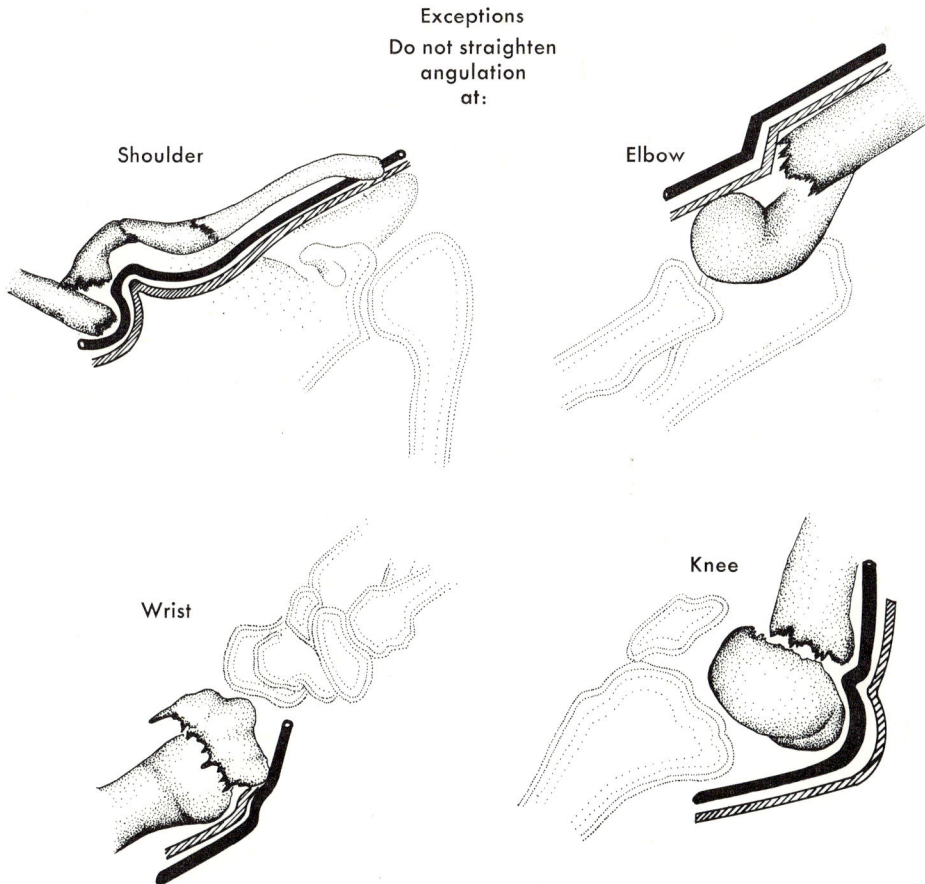

Fig. 14-3. Close approximation of neurovascular structures to fractures around joints.

sure. When using other types of rigid splints further embarrassment to the circulation is avoided if the extremity beneath the wrappings is well padded, if the wrappings are applied just firmly enough to afford immobilization, and if elastic bandages are avoided.

The availability of plaster splints in an emergency department and the ability of plaster to conform to an injured extremity justify its inclusion in this discussion as a rigid splint. Frequently, fractures about the arm, forearm, wrist, or ankle are difficult to splint with the aforementioned splints, or they may be more satisfactorily splinted with the use of plaster. Six to ten thicknesses of plaster splints of appropriate width and length may be applied with careful attention to adequate padding and careful wrapping. The injured extremity must be supported until the plaster sets.

Traction splint. The traction splint not only affords rigid support of the injured extremity but also gains further immobilization and control of angulation of a fracture by the use of traction. Traction splints should *not* be used on the upper extremity because of the danger of further injuring nerves or impeding circulation. Examples of traction splints are the hinged half-ring splint and its newer competitor, the Hare splint.

Application of splints. After careful inspection of the injured part and local wound care, one is ready to apply a splint. The splint should be well chosen, well padded, well adjusted, and applied without endangering the circulation and tissues above, at, or below the injury. The first step in the application of a splint is to correct the severe angulation of the fracture if it is not at the shoulder, elbow, wrist, or knee. The angulation is corrected by one individual's stabilizing the extremity proximal to the angulation, and by a second individual's applying gentle, steadily increasing traction to the extremity below the level of angulation. If traction is applied slowly

and steadily and the patient is constantly reassured verbally, the angulation can be reduced with little discomfort and no tissue damage. The angulation should not be changed forcibly. No attempt to fully correct the angulation should be made. The traction should be maintained by both individuals until the splint has been applied under, alongside, or on top of the limb and the limb has been secured to the splint. The splint should be of sufficient length to include and immobilize the joint above and the fracture, or the bone above and the bone below the dislocation. Again, do not change the angulation of a dislocated joint.

Steps in application of the rigid splint (board, cardboard, aluminum, ladder, and plaster) are as follows[6]:

1. Reduce severely angulated fractures except at the shoulder, elbow, wrist, or knee as described above.
2. Gently support the limb and apply slight traction (or continue traction as required for the severely angulated fracture).
3. Have an assistant place the splinting device under, alongside, or on top of the limb.
4. Apply padding to assure even pressure and to protect any bony prominences.
5. Apply the binding so as not to further impair circulation or cause local pressure damage to soft tissues.

Steps in the application of the air splint are as follows[6]:

1. Straighten severely angulated fractures as described previously and maintain traction.
2. Place the splint on your own arm and hold it open.
3. Help support the patient's limb.
4. Slide the splint onto the patient's limb.
5. Inflate by *mouth* to the point where the thumb will cause a slight dent if pressed modestly against the splint.
6. If the air splint is a zippered type, lay the gently supported limb in the

unzippered splint, zip it, and inflate as above.

Steps in application of the traction (Hare) splint are as follows[6]:

1. Gently apply the ankle hitch, being careful to see that no soft tissue damage will occur; leave the shoe on if one is being worn.
2. Apply sufficient traction to the limb to correct any major angulation at the fracture site and afford (with the local muscle spasm) substantial stability at the fracture site.
3. While traction is maintained a second individual carries out the following:
   a. Slides the traction splint into position, fastening the strap over the padding at the groin, avoiding pressure in the genital area and over the femoral vessels; the padded ring at the proximal end of the splint should be pressed against the ischial tuberosity
   b. Arranges the pulling device (windlass rope, etc.) and applies traction equal to or more than being exerted by hand
   c. Places four or more cradle slings under and around the thigh and legs, starting at the ankle
   d. Carefully pads and binds the entire leg and splint with a circular bandage, and places a support under the traction splint

Specific methods of splinting

With this background, one is now able to consider methods of splinting (immobilizing) specific fractures and dislocations of the upper and lower extremities.

Fractures of the upper extremities. Fractures of the clavicle generally occur at the junction of the middle and distal thirds from a blow over the lateral or posterolateral aspect of the shoulder. Swelling, tenderness, and deformity are generally evident. Supporting the extremity in a sling and binding the extremity against the thorax with a swathe will sufficiently immobilize the fracture pending definitive orthopedic management. However, severe, direct violence over the clavicle, such as often occurs in motorcycle or automobile accidents, may fracture the clavicle more medially and force one or more of the fractured ends into the thoracic outlet, injuring the lung, subclavian artery or vein, and brachioplexus as they traverse the thoracic outlet passing downward into the upper extremity. The pulmonary and neurovascular injuries then become of paramount importance.

Fractures of the upper end of the humerus may occur with or without a concomitant dislocation of the glenohumeral joint. Since severe pain will prevent any active abduction, the axillary nerve continuity should be tested. The absence of sensation to pinprick in an area the size of a half dollar over the lateral deltoid indicates that the axillary nerve has been injured, and this finding should be noted and recorded in the chart. If there is gross angulation at the fracture site, the extremity should be splinted in the position found, utilizing padded boards and pillow splints until x-ray films are taken and definitive orthopedic care can be initiated. In most instances fractures of the upper end of the humerus demonstrate little gross angulation and may be splinted with the use of a sling to support the extremity and a swathe to bind it to the chest.

Fractures of the midshaft of the humerus endanger the radial nerve, the status of which may be checked by the patient's ability to extend the fingers and by the presence or absence of sensation to pinprick over the dorsum of the forearm. If angulation is present, it may be reduced by gentle constant traction along the side of the body. A sling then may be applied, and while traction is maintained, a padded board or plaster slab may be placed along the outer border of the humerus. A swathe is applied to hold the humeral shaft against the thorax. A fracture of the midshaft of the humerus without angulation is likewise best treated with a sling and a padded rigid splint along the lateral border of the humerus, followed by application of a swathe bandage.

Fractures about the elbow place the radial, ulnar, and median nerves, as well as the brachial artery, in great jeopardy. The fractures should be splinted using a rigid splint in the position of deformity without attempting to decrease the deformity. If possible, the extremity should be bound to the side to add additional support.

After reduction of any severe angulation, fractures of the radius or ulna should be splinted with a padded board or an air splint immobilizing both the wrist and the elbow.

Fractures occurring about the wrist should be splinted in the position of deformity without any attempt being made to change the angulation. A well-padded board splint or plaster splint will suffice to stabilize the fracture. Extending the splint above the elbow will alleviate pain and further displacement of the fractured fragments by preventing supination and pronation.

It should be emphasized that a "sprained wrist" is frequently a fractured navicular in which there is no x-ray evidence of a fracture for 10 to 14 days. The "sprained wrist" should be splinted and the patient referred for further observation and definitive care.

A very common fracture about the wrist is the Colles' fracture. This fracture involves the distal radius wih volar angulation and dorsal tilt of the distal fragment and fracture of the ulnar styloid. Definitive care for such a fracture may vary from the application of a well-molded, short-arm plaster in a minimally displaced fracture, to closed reduction under anesthesia (axillary block, local infiltration, or general anesthesia). A short-arm cast, long-arm cast, or sugar tongue plaster splint for more com-

plicated fractures may be used depending on the severity of the fracture, the amount of swelling, and the preference of the orthopedic surgeon. These fractures are frequently seen in older individuals with relative osteopenia, severe comminution, and deformity. They tend to recur even after adequate closed reduction and immobilization. Therefore, following reduction, the fracture may be treated with pins introduced percutaneously into one or more of the metacarpals distally and into the radius or ulna proximally. These pins are incorporated into plaster to avoid late recurrence of deformity.

Fractures of the hand are best treated with a bulky fluff dressing and a padded board or plaster splint immobilizing the hand and wrist.

Dislocations of the upper extremities. Eighty-five percent of the dislocations about the shoulder girdle are anterior dislocations, wherein the humeral head comes to lie anterior to the glenoid, compressing the axillary nerves and vessels against the thorax. These dislocations should be splinted in whatever fashion necessary to obtain maximal stability without changing the deformity. Pillow splints, and frequently the help of a second individual in supporting the extremity in the displaced position, will be sufficient to stabilize the extremity until x-ray films can be taken and orthopedic care is available.

Approximately 15% of dislocations about the shoulder are posterior dislocations wherein the humeral head comes to lie posterior to the glenoid. In posterior dislocations of the shoulder, the extremity is adducted and the forearm is held across the chest or abdomen, and there is little gross deformity at the shoulder. All that is required is a sling and swathe to maintain the position until definitive orthopedic management is carried out. Of particular note with posterior dislocations is the importance of obtaining an axillary, transthoracic, or transscapular view to demonstrate the dislocation. Posterior dislocations are frequently missed on routine anteroposterior x-ray studies, which can lead to prolonged and sometimes permanent disability.

Dislocations about the elbow must be splinted with a rigid, well-padded splint in the position of deformity. The splint should extend to the axilla and include the wrist. In the event that the rigid splint will not conform to the deformity, the splint may have to "bridge" the elbow joint using soft dressings and padding in order to accomplish sufficient stabilization before the patient is taken to the x-ray department. Here, special mention should be made of the young child who, following a pulling injury to the upper extremity, refuses to move the arm because any motion causes pain. X-ray films may show no abnormality and the diagnosis of a dislocated radial head from beneath the annular ligament remains a clinical one. These injuries should be appropriately cared for after x-ray evaluation before the child leaves the emergency department.

Dislocations about the wrist are attended in the same fashion as fractures about the wrist, and dislocations of the fingers are generally sufficiently stable so as not to require any splinting prior to treatment.

Fractures of the lower extremities. Fractures of the pelvis generally result from a severe external force directly on the pelvis or from an indirect force transmitted from the femur into or through the acetabulum. Because the pelvis is a bony ring, it is generally fractured in at least two separate places, and there may be a separation of one or both sacroiliac joints. One can expect approximately 500 ml of blood loss from each fracture, and an immediate type and crossmatch of an appropriate amount of blood is required upon admission to the emergency department. An IV should be started immediately for volume replacement to prevent shock. Again, one must be aware of the contents of the pelvis when evaluating fractures of and about the pelvis. Fractures of the pubic ramus may lacerate the urethra; fractures of the brim of the pelvis may obstruct or disrupt the ureters; and the bladder itself may be ruptured. An indwelling Foley catheter should be placed in the bladder, and a cystogram and intravenous pyelogram should be considered as emergency measures.

Generally, no splinting is required for the fractured pelvis unless the symphysis is severely disrupted and the pelvis has "opened like an oyster shell." Pillows and sandbags generally suffice to support the fractured pelvis until treatment is undertaken.

Fractures of the hip or proximal femur are generally divided anatomically into two types: fractures of the neck of the femur (transcervical) and fractures through the trochanters (intertrochanteric). Clinically, there is pain and swelling about the hip, pain on hip motion, and a variable degree of shortening and external rotation. In the emergency department the fractured hip is generally best splinted with sandbags or pillows until x-ray films can be taken and further care is instituted. However, if the patient is to wait several hours or requires further transportation, a traction splint, such as the Hare splint or Thomas ring splint, should be applied.

Special mention should be made of the "occult" fracture of the hip. The patient with an occult fracture of the hip may be ambulatory and complain only of the hip or knee pain. The x-ray films of the hip may show no abnormality, only to have the fracture "fall apart" several hours or days later.

If there is pain on internal rotation of the hip and any suspicion of a fracture, x-rays must be taken after several days of bed rest. Tomograms of the hip, or x-ray films obtained of the hip with traction applied to the extremity, may be required to make the diagnosis.

Stress fractures of the proximal femur

are not an infrequent occurrence, particularly among military recruits. These patients generally complain of groin, hip, or knee pain following prolonged marches.[1] The initial x-ray studies may be entirely negative, or careful inspection may reveal a tiny infraction through the medial cortex.

In considering injuries about the hip in children, it is important to realize that the complaint of a limp, a limp and pain in the hip, or a limp and pain in the knee are of paramount significance. These symptoms are not to be ignored, even though the clinical findings may be minor or absent. The diagnoses of slipped capital femoral epiphysis, Legg-Perthes' disease, traumatic synovitis, or nonspecific synovitis of the hip must be considered, and comparison x-rays obtained of both hips. These children should not be dismissed from the emergency department without orthopedic consultation.

Fractures of the femoral shaft should be splinted with a Hare or Thomas ring traction splint and kept in the splint until definitive orthopedic care is carried out. Gross angulation should be corrected by traction prior to the application of the splint.

Fractures about the knee should be splinted as found, using a padded board, air splint, or plaster splint depending upon which best conforms to the injured extremity. Severe gross angulation may be decreased to some degree by gentle traction if no resistance is met.

Fractures of the patella are easily managed with a padded board, air, or aluminum splint with the knee in extension.

Fractures of the tibia, likewise, are generally easily splinted with an air splint, padded board, or aluminum splint after correction of severe angulation by traction. Great care must be taken not to cause the bone ends to penetrate through the skin. The ankle and knee joints must be included in the splint, which is best carried as high as the groin.

Fractures about the ankle, if severely angulated, should be straightened by traction applied to the heel and forefoot immediately upon entering the emergency department to restore the impaired circulation to the foot. The foot and ankle may then be easily splinted in an air or padded plaster splint. Reduction of the angulation by traction is most easily accomplished if the knee is allowed to bend 90 degrees over the end or side of the examining table.

Fractures of the foot are splinted with an air or padded plaster splint to include the ankle and leg.

Dislocations of the lower extremities. Hip dislocations are described as anterior, central, or posterior, depending upon the relationship of the femoral head to the acetabulum. A central dislocation implies a fracture of the acetabulum with displacement of the femoral head through the acetabulum into the pelvis. Dislocations of the hip are splinted in the position of existing deformity with sandbags and pillows. Because of the proximity of the sciatic and femoral nerves to the acetabulum, immediate and repeated evaluation of the neurologic status of the limb is exceedingly important.

Dislocations about the knee are splinted in the position of deformity with a padded board or pillows as required. Again, plaster splints may be very helpful.

Ankle dislocations rarely occur without associated fractures and should be aligned and splinted as described for fractures of the ankle.

Dislocations of the foot are rare and may be splinted with air, plaster, or aluminum splints. Toe dislocations are inherently stable and require no splinting.

After splinting, where possible, the extremity should be elevated and ice placed on the injured part. If the ice is crushed and in a large plastic bag, it will not only help to prevent further swelling but also will make the patient more comfortable and enhance the splinting device.

Following splinting the patient is sent to the x-ray department for appropriate films. The patient then returns to the emergency department. These films should be evaluated by someone who has had adequate training in reading and interpreting injuries of bones and joints unless the films have already been interpreted by a competent radiologist. It is the responsibility of emergency personnel to report these findings to the physician responsible for care of the patient. If there is any question as to necessary treatment, the advice of a competent orthopedic surgeon should be sought.

Septic joints are an orthopedic emergency.[3] The painful joint is generally swollen, red, and hot, and all motion is exceedingly painful. X-ray films should be obtained and the joint splinted in the position of maximum comfort. Management will include a complete blood count, sedimentation rate, joint aspiration, and probably surgical drainage.

Treatment of fractures

Once a fracture has been adequately splinted and sufficient x-ray films have been obtained to define the type and severity of the fracture, definitive orthopedic care of the fracture is instituted. Accurate reduction and stabilization of the fractured bone or bones is provided until the fracture has united by callus formation sufficient to provide enough inherent stability to allow removal of the stabilizing devices. These devices may be external supports such as casts or cast braces, internal support such as intramedullary rodding and plate fixation, or a combination of internal and external supports, such as internal fixation rods, plates, or pins in combination with plaster casting. The length of time required for satisfactory union depends upon variables such as the inherent stability or instability of the fracture site, the severity of associated local tissue damage, the amount of inherent circulation at the level of the fracture, and the presence

or absence of contamination or infection.

If an external support such as a cast is applied, the patient should be taught important aspects of home care. The patient must be advised to elevate the injured part for 24 to 72 hours, depending on the severity of the fracture. This prevents swelling distal to the plaster. If there is any severe swelling, intense pain, loss of sensation, or persistent cyanosis distal to the plaster, the patient should immediately consult the physician or return to the emergency department. Further advice should be given regarding keeping the cast dry at all times. Motion of all joints of the injured extremity which are not immobilized in plaster should be encouraged.

Care of hand injuries

Because of the vital importance of the hand and fingers, the complex anatomy, and frequent permanent disability following inappropriate or incomplete treatment, even of minor injuries, special consideration must be given to the injured hand.

The skin of the palm is closely adherent to the palmar aponeurosis, a dense fibrous layer that protects the nerves, tendons, intrinsic muscles, and vessels. The dorsal skin of the hand is loose and overlies the veins and lymphatics draining the hand; hence, any infection in the palm and fingers generally results in swelling of the dorsum of the hand. The dorsal swelling is generally lymphedema and very rarely is purulent; therefore, nothing is gained by draining the dorsum of the hand alone. Location of the infection in the fingers or palm must be identified and drained appropriately. These infections, generally arising from puncture wounds, may be confined to (1) the tendon sheaths enclosing the flexor tendons from the base of the distal phalanx to the distal flexion crease of the palm; (2) the radial or ulnar bursa encompassing the flexor tendons in the proximal palm and at the volar aspect of the wrist beneath the transverse carpal ligament; and (3) the underlying midpalmar or thenar spaces lying deep to the flexor tendons and adjacent lumbricales, and superficial to the metacarpals and interossei. One or more of these individual spaces or bursae may be connected.

If the infection involves the peritenon of one or more of the tendons in the hand, pain, redness, and exquisite tenderness may be found to extend proximally into the forearm overlying the tendon, and extreme pain is experienced on active or passive motion of the involved finger or fingers. Appropriate drainage, antibiotics, moist compresses, and immobilization followed by appropriate physical therapy are required if one is going to avoid severe permanent damage and disability from any of these infections. As a rule, these infections require hospitalization, appropriate anesthesia, and surgical drainage under tourniquet control. As inappropriate incisions for drainage may themselves cause further damage, a well-trained surgical specialist is required.

A *paronychia* is an abscess beneath the cuticle at the base of the nail. If minor, it may be treated with moist soaks. However, if there is significant purulence and swelling, the cuticle must be elevated and the root of the nail incised traversely across its base and removed without damaging the nail bed.

A *felon* is an abscess confined to the volar aspect of the distal phalanx trapped between the multiple septa extending from the skin to the periosteum. It requires drainage utilizing a midradial or midulnar longitudinal incision, avoiding the digital nerves and transection of these fibrous septa to allow free drainage. Drainage is followed by appropriate moist compresses and immobilization.

Paint-gun injuries are a new category of hand injuries. With the advent in recent years of exceedingly high-pressure paintguns, small, seemingly innocuous particles of paint or cleaning fluid enter the fingers and hand. In these injuries the paint or cleaning fluids entering through the fingertip may dissect as far proximal as the midforearm. Immediate radical surgical intervention is required, frequently opening the entire palm and forearm to prevent loss of digits and even late amputation of the hand.

Puncture wounds involving the joints may result in complete loss of function of that joint and must always be presumed to leave contaminated material within the joint. Probably one of the frequently encountered and worst open injuries is that from the human tooth, in hand-to-mouth combat. These joints must be surgically opened, debrided, and irrigated, followed by appropriate antibiotics and splinting.

SUMMARY

In a mass disaster and triage, most fractures, if well splinted in the absence of circulatory embarrassment, may "wait their turn" with little detriment, behind pulmonary and abdominal emergency cases. The important life-threatening exception is the severe pelvic fracture with unseen hemorrhage and urinary tract injury.

REFERENCES

1. Watson-Jones, R.: Fractures and joint injuries, vols. 1 and 2, ed. 4, Baltimore, 1962, The Williams & Wilkins Co.
2. O'Donoughue, D. H.: Treatment of injuries to athletes, Philadelphia, 1970, W. B. Saunders Co.
3. Mercer, W., and Duthie, R. B.: Orthopedic surgery, ed. 6, Baltimore, 1966, The Williams & Wilkins Co.
4. Thompson, T. C., and Doherty, J. H.: Spontaneous rupture of the tendon of achilles: a new clinical test, J. Trauma 2(2):126-129, 1962.
5. American Academy of Orthopaedic Surgeons: Initial emergency care and transportation of the sick and injured. Sponsored by the Committee on Injuries of the Academy for the September 13-16, 1967, program in Portland, Oregon.
6. "Emergency medical care," American Academy of Orthopaedic Surgeons.

CHAPTER **15**

Vascular emergencies

Gordon Sproul, M.D.

Major blood vessel rupture, thrombosis, and injury are common causes of emergency admission. Overlooked, such disease states may lead to therapeutic disaster or death. All the skills needed for vascular reconstruction are available in most hospitals, but lack of recognition or timidity in evaluation and care remains prevalent.

Successful repair of vital arteries can be accomplished to the level of the wrist and ankle with expectation of continued patency. Graft replacement is an everyday art and can be utilized when direct repair is not possible. Ligation of major vessels has no place in modern surgery except in traumatic amputation or hopelessly infected vessel disruptions. Vascular abnormalities can be discovered by careful observation, palpation, and auscultation. When these basic tools are supplemented by angiography, significant blood vessel disease or damage can always be detected. With the advent of safe angiography and availability of skilled angiographers, one should utilize this method of diagnosis on the slightest suspicion.

The absence of a pulse calls for angiograms: waiting for the "spasm" to remit or using vasodilating drugs as primary treatment may lead to costly delays in diagnosis and possibly jeopardize a salvageable limb.

A major amount of persistent bleeding either apparent externally or manifest by shock, hematoma, or falling hematocrit demands serious consideration for exploration and hemostasis.

It seems useful when considering vascular emergencies to review them as outlined below. It may help bring them to the mind of the examiner who sees the emergency patient.

I. Vascular injury
   A. Arterial
   B. Venous
      1. Penetrating
      2. Blunt
      3. Fracture-associated
II. Thrombosis
   A. Arterial
   B. Venous
III. Rupture—arterial
   A. Aneurysm with rupture
   B. Aneurysm with dissection

VASCULAR EXAMINATION

Careful observation, palpation, and auscultation can lead to the correct diagnosis in most vascular disorders. This important examination can be rapidly done and serves as the basis for continued observation or immediate therapy.

The patient's general appearance is helpful, since most significant arterial obstructions or ruptures are accompanied by severe pain. The further from the site of the obstruction, the more severe the pain appears to be. Immediate bilateral arm blood pressures are taken; disparate blood pressures may signify either preexisting arteriosclerotic obstructive disease or dissections of the aorta which might mimic myocardial infarction. Shock is likewise not a "one-armed" diagnosis. The erroneous diagnosis of shock, which occurred because the pressure reading was taken on a chronically obstructed arm, may result in serious diagnostic and therapeutic errors. One next palpates the pulses bilaterally from the superficial temporal arteries, which are found just anterior to the ear top, down to include the carotids, the subclavian arteries, the axillary and brachial arteries, and the radial and ulnar arteries (Fig. 15-1).

Attention is then directed to the abdominal aorta. Steady, deep pressure with slightly separated thumb and fingers in the midepigastrium with the patient relaxed will give a measure of the aortic width and thrust.

Femoral, popliteal, and pedal pulses are then evaluated. Popliteal pulses seem best felt with the leg extended and relaxed; the examiner should use both hands to feel for the pulse. The thumbs are placed on the patella and the fingers are placed posteriorly over the tibial condyles, slightly lifting the knee and flexing it with exertion of fairly heavy pressure with the examining fingers. The pulse will be felt slightly lateral low in the popliteal area (Fig. 15-2). Width and strength of the popliteal pulse are estimated. This is important in detecting popliteal aneurysms, which can be associated with catastrophic thrombosis of the distal vessels.

Pedal pulse locations are relatively constant. The dorsalis pedis is in the midportion of the dorsum of the foot just lateral to the extensor tendon of the great toe; the posterior tibial pulse is best felt just behind the medial malleolus.

It is of great benefit in evaluation of pulses to compare by simultaneous or rapid sequential palpation both paired vessels. Temporal, carotid, radial, femoral, and pedal pulses lend themselves to this com-

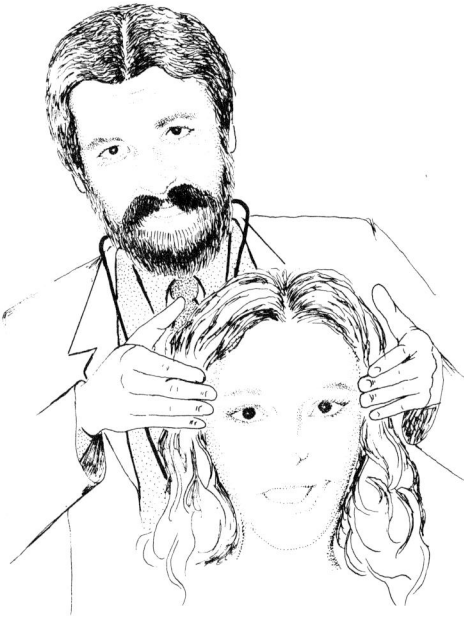

Fig. 15-1. Palpating the temporal artery.

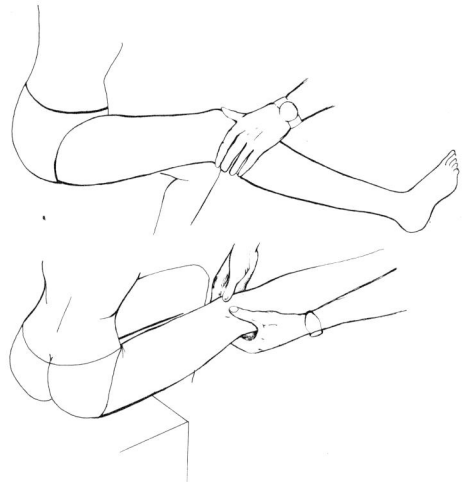

Fig. 15-2. Palpating the popliteal pulse.

parison and give the clinician an estimate of relative strength.

Auscultation of the carotid bifurcation just below the angle of the jaw, and auscultation of the supraclavicular region, the area over the abdominal aorta in the midline of the abdomen between the xiphoid and the umbilicus, and over the femoral arteries in the groin may lead to discovery of bruits. These sounds signify flow interference secondary either to stenosis of the vessel, excessive tortuosity, or increased flow. In addition, communications between artery and vein may be detected by similar sounds, which tend to be to and fro in character, heard at the same sites, and are indicative of turbulence and rapid flow. It is important also to remember that auscultation of hematomas with associated arterial or venous injuries may make early diagnosis of a traumatic arteriovenous fistula possible by hearing these sounds.

Observation of the skin for pallor, cyanosis, sweating, venous collateral, and edema is important, since these features may help one differentiate arterial or venous disorders.

Temperature changes on the same extremity or differences in temperature in paired extremities are easily detected within 2 or 3 degrees by the back of the examiner's hand. These differences may also be indicative of impaired circulation.

Simple pinprick sensitivity should be tested on the distal portions of the extremities, comparing both sides, as well as proximal and distal on the same limb. Neurologic deficits frequently occur in conjunction with trauma to vessels or acute obstruction with severe ischemia. Traumatic injuries are frequently accompanied by nerve injuries, since major arteries and nerves are closely associated anatomically. Occult diabetes is sometimes discovered by the alert examiner who finds diminished distal sensation in the lower extremities. Diminished sensation may also accompany trauma to vessels or acute thrombophlebitis

with peripheral vascular spasm. The common denominator in all these states, with the exception of direct injury to accompanying nerves, is that of arterial insufficiency to the distal extremity with secondary ischemia of the nerve.

Capillary filling can easily be assessed by light pressure quickly withdrawn from the palmar aspect of the finger or plantar aspect of the toe. The pale area produced should rapidly turn pink with normal circulation. Delay may signify vasoconstriction caused by reflex as in thrombophlebitis, or poor volume or poor cardiac output with general vasoconstriction; or more commonly it is the result of actual obstruction from embolus or thrombosis or pressure on vessels secondary to fracture displacement.

Elevation of the paired extremities (overhead elevation of the arms or 30-degree elevation from the horizontal of the legs) can give one a comparison of filling pressures in the involved extremities; differences are usually apparent by paleness of the involved extremity.

Palpation is also a primary tool in detecting aneurysms, be they in the extremities, neck, or abdomen. Grossly widened arteries and tender, pulsating masses make the diagnosis secure. It is well to remember that popliteal aneurysms frequently present with sudden onset of distal ischemia suggesting embolic phenomenon, and if the popliteal space is not felt and the aneurysm discovered, the wrong diagnosis and treatment may be instituted. Embolectomy is not successful under these circumstances.

More involved patency testing, such as the Allen test for continuity of the palmar arterial arch or the Adson maneuver for compression between the first rib and the clavicle, is more appropriate to leisurely elective investigations and will not be discussed here. One must remember during the examination that acute venous thrombosis may show signs easily confused with arterial insufficiency, with reflex vasospasm and minimal edema making pulses impalpable. Usually, however, the accompanying edema is either grossly obvious or measurable by comparing circumference increases between the involved and uninvolved limbs. Acute ischemia is not accompanied by edema but rather it is an accompaniment of venous blockage. In addition, the presence of engorged venous collateral at the proximal end of the involved arm or leg should give one a clue to the diagnosis of deep venous obstruction.

ARTERIAL INJURIES

Major arterial injury is strongly suspected in the face of (1) continuing copious hemorrhage from an open wound, (2) rapidly accumulating hematoma in penetrating trauma, (3) shock persisting or occurring after initial resuscitative volume replacement, or (4) when major peripheral nerve injury occurs. This latter association results from the close anatomic proximity of major blood vessels and nerves. Worth emphasis is the fact that acute vascular occlusion secondary to trauma may masquerade as purely neurologic deficit if pulses are not noted. The numb paralyzed leg can well be from acute ischemia, and spinal cord injury can be simulated or produced by acute aortic thrombosis either in the chest or in the abdomen.

Penetrating injuries

In the presence of a penetrating injury, one considers the path of the wound and probable tract of injury to determine the likelihood of vessel damage. Such injuries as the boning knife injury of the butcher and the horn wound of the matador both tend to injure the femoral vessels in the groin.

Wounds of the neck are particularly prone to produce major vascular damage because of the close proximity of many major vascular structures.[1-3]

In the face of continuing bleeding or hematoma, exploration appears to be the safest course in care. In both neck and groin injuries one must be prepared to attain proximal control in chest or abdomen. However, use of Fogarty or Foley catheter tamponade within the vessel lumen can be achieved by introduction of these catheters into the proximal artery via the wound. Balloon inflation will permit repair without other proximal control.

Major vessel injury within the chest and abdomen causes massive, continuing bleeding and requires vigorous resuscitative measures. However, the best resuscitative measure is proximal and distal control, so all haste is made in the preparation for immediate surgical exploration. Urinary output and blood pressure cannot always be restored to normal levels; these will return with repair and further volume replacement.

An interesting complication of missile penetration of major vessels or of the heart is remote embolization of the missile. Small-caliber, low-velocity missiles such as .22-caliber bullets are particularly prone to this sort of accident. They may enter a large artery or vein and come to lodge either in the lung or in a peripheral artery, depending on the site of entry. Usually the location within the lung is asymptomatic, but location in an artery may be accompanied by signs and symptoms of arterial obstruction as from any other cause. Left atrial wounds may result in perplexing bullet locations if this possible complication has not been considered. The heart wound gives access to the left-sided circulation, and embolization occurs anywhere within the peripheral tree. A frequent site of this embolization is the common femoral artery where diameter reduction to form the superficial and profunda arteries occurs. This is likewise a site common in embolization of clot from the heart.

Penetrating injury by knife, ice pick, or sharp glass fragments occasionally results in acute arteriovenous fistula with communication between artery and vein and very little external evidence of injury. The close approximation of major veins, particularly in areas where major veins pass posterior to major arteries, such as in the groin, makes such an injury possible. The fistula can usually be detected early, however, by auscultation over the area of injury. A harsh systolic bruit or a continuous systolic-diastolic murmur is usually heard over the area. Such a finding indicates the need for exploration and repair. There may be signs of arterial insufficiency or venous engorgement of the involved limb as well.

Diagnostic aids. The routine use of a central venous pressure in major injuries, monitoring of urinary output at timed intervals, and monitoring of pulse rates, hematocrits, and blood pressure will help determine the extent of volume loss and whether bleeding is continuing. Plain x-ray films may show evidence of occult free hemorrhage in the chest or abdomen. Soft tissue masses or displacement of normal organs suggests hematoma. Missile location and wound of entry or exit may help determine possible location of major vessel injury. Associated organ injuries such as of the esophagus or trachea can be suspected by adventitious air.

Angiography. Angiography may be helpful if the site of injury or presence of injury is in doubt. Frequently, the time spent is not worth the additional hazard of delay unless a complicated approach can be avoided or preparation for unusual support, such as the use of the pump oxygenator, can be determined.

Blunt trauma

With 50,000 fatal accidents occurring on the highways yearly, one can well imagine the traumatic effects of rapid deceleration on the survivors. Arteries that are tightly bound over bony prominences, such as the common femoral artery and the aorta or the carotid artery over the transverse process of the cervical spine, are particularly subject to crushing. This injury may result in thrombosis of the vessel, usually from intimal fracture with folding in a downstream direction and occlusion (Fig. 15-3). Blunt objects such as fists or surfboards are capable of producing these injuries, as are the more common industrial accidents. The findings are those of acute arterial occlusion without blood loss. Acute aortic thrombosis produced in this way may present as paraplegia due to spinal cord ischemia. Angiography usually is not necessary unless confusion exists as to the presence of preexisting arteriosclerotic vascular disease. Acute thoracic aortic injury can also occur with severe deceleration. Injuries include total transection of the aorta as well as lesser injuries with false aneurysm or aortic thrombosis. The mechanism depends on the fixation of the transverse aortic arch by major vessels and the relatively unsupported descending aorta. When a sudden stop occurs, the descending aorta continues on and shears at the level of the left subclavian artery because of the differences in fixation (Fig. 15-4).

Progressive widening of the mediastinum, continuing left hemothorax, and shock indicate traumatic aortic rupture. Obscure cases may require angiography, since major chest injury is frequently present, clouding the clinical picture. In addition, angiography will hopefully document the exact site of rupture to allow for planning the surgical approach. Early repair is mandatory. Paraplegia may also accompany this injury if there is sufficient disruption of the spinal cord blood supply from intercostal arteries or if total thrombosis of the aorta occurs.

Fracture-associated arterial injuries

The mechanism for penetrating or blunt trauma is readily apparent in fracture-associated vascular injuries. Frequently, the

A

B

C

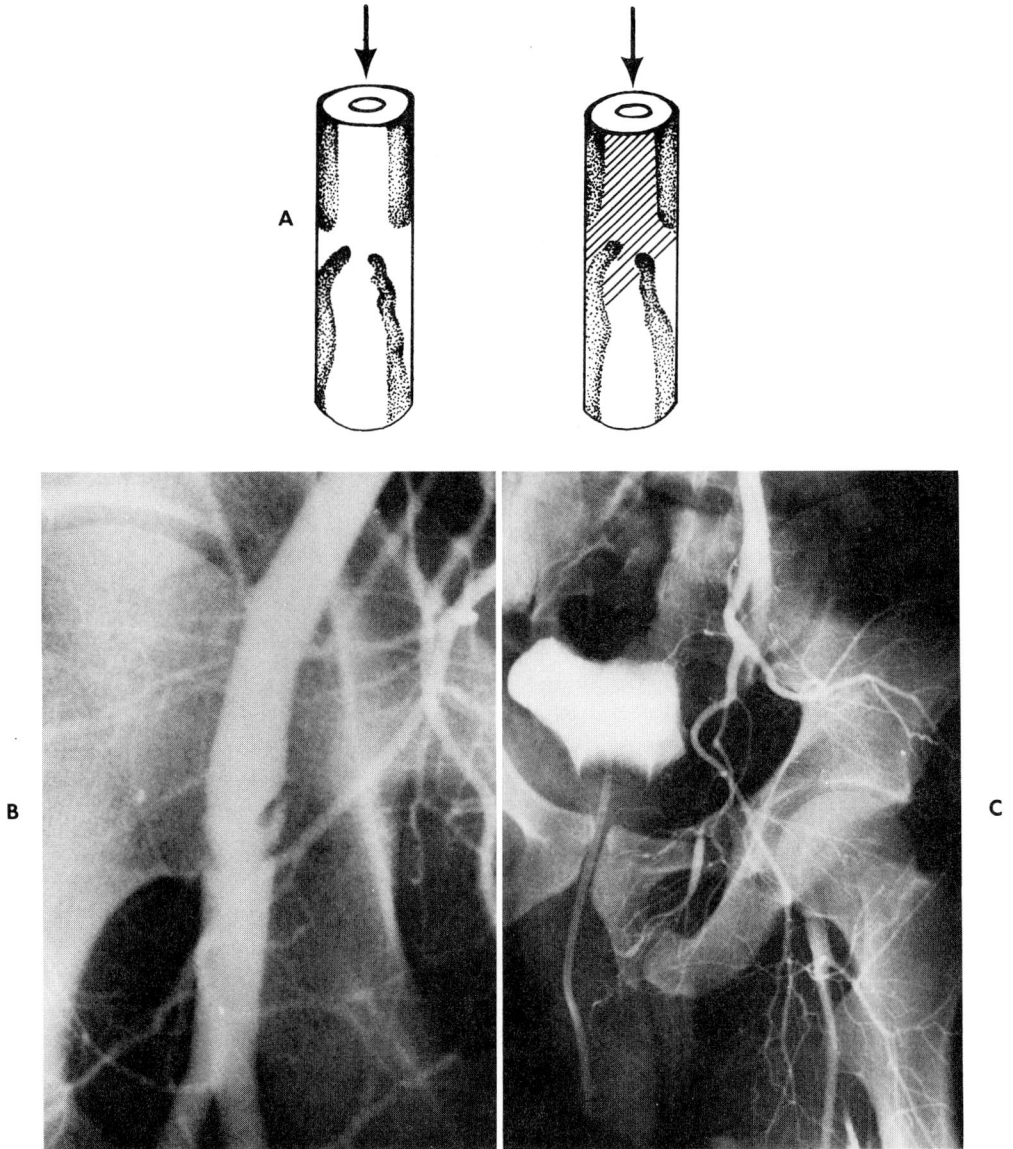

Fig. 15-3. A, Fracture of intima with secondary thrombosis. **B,** Left angiogram shows intimal fracture. **C,** Right angiogram shows thrombosis secondary to such injury.

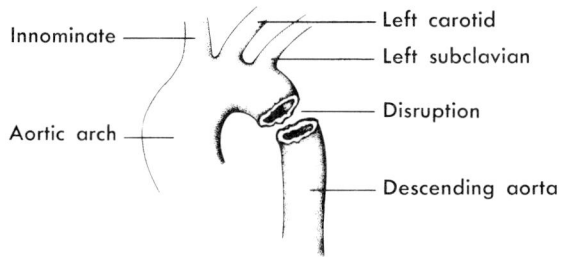

Innominate —

Left carotid

Left subclavian

Disruption

Aortic arch —

Descending aorta

Fig. 15-4. Common site of traumatic aortic aneurysm.

major neurovascular structures are closely applied to bone, and though this is a protection in some injuries, it may be a hazard in others. Displacing forces that cause fractures may also stretch vessels or compress them against angulated bony segments. Penetration by bone fragments can occur, producing injuries identical to other penetrating wounds, except frequently without evidence of external bleeding. The massive blood loss into the tissue in femoral shaft fractures, for instance, is likely the result of injury to one or several of the major branches of the profunda femoris within the muscular mass surrounding the femur.

Fracture dislocations about the knee and elbow are likely to be associated with some vascular compromise.[2,4] Volkmann's contractures, thought to be due to compression of the artery, may well be better defined by angiography as actual traumatic thrombosis of the brachial artery. Major vessel damage about the knee is not rare and, if overlooked, can result in limb loss, since acute popliteal artery occlusion is very poorly tolerated and gangrene frequently results.[4] Clavicular fracture may be associated with traumatic aneurysm of the subclavian artery secondary to crushing of this vessel against the first rib.[5]

Pelvic fractures with extreme displacement may result in iliac or femoral vessel damage, but more commonly venous tearing occurs with secondary retroperitoneal hematoma.

Fractures associated with signs and symptoms of vascular embarrassment require arteriography to assess the need for vascular repair. The hazard of these injuries lies in overlooking the arterial damage. Rather than splitting the cast or decreasing the flexion for "arterial spasm," it would seem wise to resort to angiography early. Spasm does occur, but the patient would be best served by demonstrating arterial continuity under these circumstances.

Arterial embolus and acute thrombosis

Acute obstruction to flow, whether caused by embolus or acute thrombosis, gives rise to all the symptoms and signs enumerated in the preceding sections.[6] Obviously, these conditions are not associated with trauma but with preexisting cardiac arrhythmias, myocardial infarction, or progression of arteriosclerotic vascular disease. The use of the electrocardiogram is mandatory to discover the presence of atrial fibrillation or previous myocardial infarction or evidence of rheumatic heart disease as a source of intracardiac thrombus. Mitral stenosis and underlying rheumatic heart disease should be considered in the younger patient presenting with embolic obstruction. Atheromata within great vessels or laminated thrombus within aneurysms, either aorta or peripheral vessels, can be associated with sudden embolic obstruction caused by the breaking off of fragments of the intraluminal clot.

The history of onset is acute with pain and paresthesias, which are often described by the patient as the involved part's being "asleep." Coldness with paleness and mottling and motor paresis are often noted. Pulses are usually absent beyond the area of obstruction, though occasionally an embolus is not totally occluding, allowing a diminished blood flow and a weak pulse. Common sites of lodgment are areas of bifurcation because of the decrease in vessel diameter. The brachial artery at the elbow and the common femoral artery are the most common sites, with the aortic bifurcation and the popliteal artery trifurcation the next most common areas. Plain x-rays may show calcium in the vessel walls of arteriosclerotic origin, and lateral x-ray of the abdomen may actually show the outline of an abdominal aneurysm. Chest x-ray may show mitral heart configuration with left atrial enlargement or even valvular calcification.

Angiography can be helpful but frequently is not necessary to the diagnosis.

If there is a question of acute thrombosis versus embolus, angiography should be done, since evaluation of the distal tree or other areas of disease may cause the surgeon to prepare for a full-scale reconstruction rather than a simple embolectomy. Clues to the possibility of acute thrombosis lie in a history of previous arterial insufficiency in the extremity and the absence of pulses in other locations where ischemia is not present. Bruits likewise signify flow disturbance and likely arteriosclerosis. Such findings should make one consider angiography first, since attempts to extract emboli by Fogarty embolectomy catheters when a lesion is really an acute thrombosis may lead to vessel damage and possible limb loss.

Acute thrombosis is usually tolerated by the limb while the diagnosis and care are planned, since collateral has been forming while stenosis of the vessel has been progressing prior to the occlusion. This fact may also help in the diagnosis; the limb which appears only mildly ischemic but is without distal pulses usually does not represent an embolus. Acute embolic obstruction of a previously wide open vascular tree is manifested by severe signs and symptoms of ischemia.

Visceral emboli

Renal embolus. The sudden onset of severe flank and costovertebral angle pain with colic in the presence of atrial fibrillation, recent myocardial infarction, or mitral valvular disease with or without accompanying hematuria may signify renal embolus. Frequently, the urine will have microscopic or gross signs of blood and oliguria may occur. This sequence of events followed by a developing mass and fever is indicative of renal embolus with infarction. Bilateral renal emboli with anuria occasionally occur. The kidneys are capable of being revascularized if this condition is detected even after a considerable period of time. Emboli to the renal artery may

occur as discrete emboli to both kidneys, or in the presence of old aortic thrombotic disease a large embolus may lodge, occluding both renal arteries by its aortic position. Frequently, emboli to the kidneys are associated with emboli to the extremities, and this should be considered when there is an embolus to the extremity with some vague abdominal or back pain. The emergency pyelogram will show nonfunction or poor function of the involved kidney. In the presence of oliguria or anuria, retrograde pyelography is in order to rule out the possibility of obstructive uropathy as a cause for the anuria. Angiography here is of paramount importance and should precede other studies, particularly if the urine flow is down. Although ischemia of the kidneys is occasionally tolerated for long periods of time, early intervention will save renal tissue.

Mesenteric embolus. This catastrophe usually occurs in the elderly arteriosclerotic patient with atrial fibrillation and has its onset with severe, crampy, diffuse, abdominal pain. Early in the clinical course diarrhea may occur for one or two movements because the ischemic distal gut has hyperactive peristalsis, but later ileus supervenes. A rising white blood cell count and temperature and general signs of peritonitis and shock make the diagnosis obvious. Unfortunately, at this late stage the salvage rate is very low and one should strive for early recognition. At first x-ray studies may show little, perhaps a loop or two of small bowel gas without particular distension. At this time angiography can be life saving because it can quickly demonstrate patency of the visceral vessels. If an embolus is present, early embolectomy can then be carried out and will avoid extensive bowel resections or death. Perhaps nowhere else is the demonstration of an embolus and its extraction at the earliest possible time so important. Once irreparable damage occurs, mortality rapidly approaches 100%. One should never hesitate to use angiography on suspicion of this condition, since after acute onset the course may be insidious until too late for treatment.

Arterial rupture

The primary cause of arterial rupture is the arteriosclerotic aneurysm. Weakening of the supporting elements of the vessel wall allows dilatation, and dilatation causes turbulence and increasing lateral pressure. This is produced by forward flow striking the relatively stagnant area of slower flow and producing abnormal stresses on the arterial wall (Fig. 15-5). This tends to be a vicious circle with further dilatation occurring in the weakened wall and eventual rupture. The rupture may be free with total disruption of the wall into the abdomen, but more often it is confined within the retroperitoneum for a period of time, or in the groin or popliteal area within the soft tissues.

Occasionally, mycotic aneurysms occur when bacteria from the bloodstream aggregate in plaques or aneurysms and cause infection and bursting of the vessels. These, however, are rare and may be indistinguishable clinically from the usual type of aneurysm. Aneurysms of the abdominal visceral branches such as the splenic and hepatic arteries do occur with rupture.

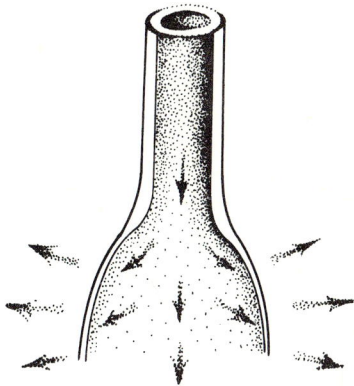

Fig. 15-5. Mechanism of aneurysm enlargement.

Rupture of femoral and popliteal aneurysm is unusual.

Abdominal aneurysms

Abdominal aneurysm rupture causes severe abdominal pain combined with shock and signs of blood loss. This may be preceded by lesser pain for a week or so, or may occur as an acute catastrophe. Patients with aortic aneurysm often have a history of lumbosacral back pain from retroperitoneal extension or actual bony erosion of the lumbar spine. There may be radiation of the pain into the groin or down the legs, and occasional misdiagnosis of renal colic or strangulated hernia may occur if careful evaluation is not carried out. More rarely, the signs and symptoms of progressive arterial insufficiency of the legs may occur as the aneurysm bursts and deforms the outflowing vessels. Occasionally, complete aortic obstruction can result from aneurysm, usually when accompanied by preexisting, severe, obstructive disease. Physical examination will often reveal a pulsatile mass, and the patient may have noticed rather prominent pulsations in the abdomen, particularly when lying on his or her back in bed.

X-ray studies of the abdomen may be helpful in an obscure case, especially in the obese patient; approximately 50% of aneurysms will be visualized anterior to the lumbar spine as calcified outlines. Occasionally, circular epigastric calcium or left upper quadrant calcium is seen in visceral vessel aneurysms. The incidence of visceral aneurysms, especially those of the splenic artery, appears to be greater in females. Rupture is often the first presentation of these aneurysms. Strangely enough, splenic artery aneurysm rupture appears in young age groups and may accompany pregnancy. Angiography can locate the site of visceral vessel aneurysm, but frequently the precipitous course of a rupturing aneurysm does not allow leisurely diagnosis; most often the diagnosis remains obscure as to location until surgical exploration is carried out.

Aortic dissection

Dissections of arteries other than the thoracic aorta have been reported. However, this disease is primarily one of the thoracic aorta. It results from tearing of the inner linings of the aorta, usually just above the aortic valves or just beyond the left subclavian artery. Following the tear, blood dissects between the outer and inner layers, causing a double lumen, which may occlude important branches of the aorta as it progresses (Fig. 15-6). Rupture frequently occurs into the pericardium and results in death from acute cardiac tamponade. The most common cause of this disorder is arteriosclerosis with hypertension. It is also seen in Marfan's syndrome in younger people in which there is a genetically transmittable connective tissue defect with weakness of the elastic lining of the major vessels. The vessels with their weakened elastic layers are prone to dissection, which is a frequent cause of death in these patients.

Aortic dissection is frequently misdiagnosed as a myocardial infarction because the onset is heralded by severe chest pain and interscapular pain. Shock may occur, but this is not usual. Frequently, there is electrocardiographic evidence of injury to the myocardium. When such a misdiag-

nosis is made and anticoagulation therapy is used, it may result in a speedy death. The pain associated with this condition may pass down into the epigastrium, and often there is a blood pressure difference or pulses are weak to absent in an extremity. Acute stroke may result from occlusion by the dissection of the major branches to the brain. Oliguria or anuria can occur, as can intestinal infarction; the cause is interference with the blood supply either to the gut or to the kidneys. Pain is severe and there is stepwise progression of the symptoms. One should think of this entity when such a progression occurs.

X-ray examination of the chest may show mediastinal widening or, in the patient with Marfan's disease, enlargement of the ascending arch of the aorta. There may be a small amount of pleural fluid. Serial films may be helpful, showing changes in the aortic configuration. The x-ray films, however, may give no clue, and a secure diagnosis rests on angiography. Determination of the point of tear is important as well in planning surgical approach. Good angiograms will prevent unnecessary surgery if a dissection is not present, and may be life saving, since the surgical approach is formidable. Some authorities feel that if no major visceral vessels are involved and hypertension is present, treatment with vasodepressing drugs such as trimethaphan camsylate (Arfonad) may allow stabilization or permanent healing, and they recommend this as primary treatment. Generally, however, the approach is surgical.

VENOUS INJURIES

Trauma to veins by missiles, stabbing, blunt trauma, or fracture has all the potential for major hemorrhage that arterial injury presents, but bleeding tends to be less because of the low pressures involved and the elasticity of the venous walls. Usually major venous injury has a less dramatic course, and evidence of continued hemorrhage or obstruction may be subtle.

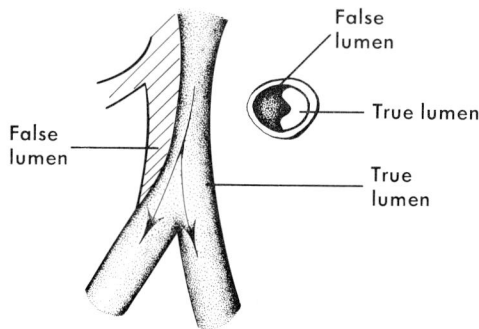

Fig. 15-6. Dissection of aorta.

Bleeding usually is self-limited though it may be extensive, except in major venous injury within the chest or abdominal cavity where free bleeding can continue due to the large potential space. Rather heavy blood loss with tissue infiltration in various planes does occur with venous injury, and alertness to the degree of this loss is necessary for replacement, although actual surgical intervention may not be warranted.

Vena caval injury or tears of large visceral veins, such as the hepatic, portal, or mesenteric vein, usually present as continuing hidden blood loss and progressive distention. These injuries are frequently not diagnosed primarily, but discovered on exploration for clinical evidence of blood loss. They are frequently associated with major organ trauma as well. Because of the low pressure, high capacity system, veins are not usually subject to rupture by compressive forces in direct trauma as are arteries.

Penetrating injuries

These injuries are evidenced by continuing blood loss. They are often associated with nerve or artery damage as well because of anatomic proximity, as mentioned previously. Reconstruction of all major veins of the extremities and trunk excluding the smaller mesenteric branches should be attempted, although single major veins can usually be ligated with impunity if there has been no previous venous disease. Venography as an aid to repair of trauma is seldom, if ever, needed.

Blunt trauma

Crushing injury to a vein over a bony prominence may cause the same sort of intimal damage as seen in arteries. The resulting thrombosis may then propagate secondary to bed rest necessitated by other accompanying injuries, and the presentation may be either acute thrombophlebitis in the involved extremity or evidence of pulmonary embolus secondary to occult venous clotting.

Such patients may not be aware of venous obstruction; however, they may complain of numbness and coolness of the extremity secondary to vasospasm, and with acute edema there may be associated aching discomfort. The leg may appear cyanotic or pale and mottled and have diminished or absent pulses. Motor power, however, will not be compromised; and edema, either grossly evident or indicated by measurement, will give a clue to the underlying problem. One should always look for venous collateral about the shoulder or hip, depending on the extremity involved, as an additional clue to thrombosis of deep venous channels. This particular collateral frequently appears early in the course of venous thrombosis. Although venous thrombosis usually does not require surgical care except for limb-threatening massive obstruction, differentiation from arterial injury and recognition of its presence will lead to early elastic compression and elevation of the involved extremity. Although heparinization would seldom be advisable because of associated injuries, Dextran may be used for its prophylactic effect without the danger of major bleeding.[2]

Fracture-associated injuries

These injuries appear to be of minor importance except when associated with crushing or tearing of veins; then the major concern is that of continuing blood loss. Pelvic fractures frequently are accompanied by major venous hemorrhage retroperitoneally, but rarely require more than active blood replacement in large volumes.

Other conditions

Two venous disorders that frequently present as emergencies are "effort thrombosis" of the upper extremity and massive acute venous obstruction of the lower extremity, or "phlegmasia cerulea dolens."

These are both the result of sudden thrombosis of major veins with the onset of severe swelling, pain, and evidence of vasospasm. These conditions may require urgent thrombectomy.

Effort thrombosis. This disorder usually occurs in an active adult, often following muscular effort associated with work or athletic endeavor, particularly overhead work or strenuous arm activity. Patients frequently state that they felt something pop or pull in the shoulder followed by almost immediate coolness, tingling in the hand, and, very shortly, progressive swelling of the hand and arm. Pain may be severe or mild. It often seems more related to the evidence of vasospasm, with coolness and sweating of the hand, than actual swelling. The hand and arm may appear quite cyanotic but may also be relatively normal in color. Engorgement of the collateral veins about the shoulder usually is seen, and pulses may be difficult to palpate because of edema, but capillary filling appears adequate. X-ray studies may be helpful if there is a cervical rib suggesting an element of thoracic outlet compression. Chest x-ray should be done to rule out lung or mediastinal masses with compression of the vein at the thoracic outlet or in the mediastinum. Thrombectomy has been advocated early in this disorder to restore venous drainage. Established treatment appears to be compression, elevation, and anticoagulation, with the use of vasodilating drugs when spasm is a significant component.

Phlegmasia cerulea dolens. Spontaneous thrombophlebitis may be so mild as to be clinically undetectable, or it may occur as a fulminating thrombosis of most of the major veins of the leg. The latter form presents a bona fide emergency to avoid actual tissue necrosis. Although most frequent in women in the postpartum period, the condition does occur at all ages. The pathology entails venous thrombosis, usually secondary to stasis, but occasionally seen with trauma. The thrombosis very rapidly progresses to involve all the major venous channels of the leg. This massive venous obstruction with normal arterial inflow results in a very rapid extravasation of fluid to the extravascular compartment. Massive swelling of the leg then occurs, and blistering and skin necrosis can also result from severe venous outflow obstruction. Considerable pain accompanies this rapid swelling. The leg may be warm, but generally is cool and pale with blotchy areas of cyanosis. Tenderness may be felt along the course of major veins such as in the groin along the medial thigh and in the midline posterior of the calf. Early in the course numbness and tingling of the extremity may occur, particularly of the foot, secondary to vascular spasm and sympathetic overactivity. Later these findings may be due to actual ischemia of the part. Although motor loss is not common, some impairment of this function may occur secondary to muscle swelling. Usually rather prominent venous collateral is seen about the hip. Fever and elevated white blood counts are also seen. X-ray studies are not particularly helpful; venography does not materially aid the diagnosis and is not clinically feasible.

Early vascular decompression by thrombectomy of the iliac and femoral veins is necessary to avoid tissue necrosis.[8] Considerable blood loss is inherent in thrombectomy of the distal and proximal venous tree, so adequate quantities of blood should be available. Frequently, caval clipping and postoperative anticoagulation are added to prevent pulmonary emboli from clots loosened but not removed by the procedure. If the decision is made for nonsurgical treatment, massive doses of heparin and vasodilators, and compression and elevation with careful skin protection are in order. If adequate care is not begun early, at the very least, prolonged, significant disability of the extremity will ensue.

COMPARISON OF ARTERIAL AND VENOUS CONDITIONS

By comparing the two lists below, one may note a general similarity between venous injury or thrombosis and arterial injury. Although the two entities are pathologically distinct, the examiner must be alert to a disorder in one system simulating the other. Careful vascular examination will help to differentiate the two, since the treatment is frequently direct in arterial problems and indirect in venous problems.

Signs and symptoms of arterial injury

Hemorrhage—wound and concealed
Shock
Neurologic manifestations—motor and sensory or spinal cord
Pain—distal and severe
Temperature—cool
Color—pale, blotchy, cyanotic
Blood pressure differences in the extremities
Capillary filling—poor
Pulses—absent or diminished

Signs and symptoms of venous injury or thrombosis

Hemorrhage—concealed or wound
Edema
Pain—general and local along course of veins
Temperature—cool or warm
Color—may be mottled and have patchy areas of cyanosis
Neurologic manifestations—paresthesias distally with sweating
Capillary filling—generally good though may be impaired
Pulses—may be diminished secondary to spasm, or impalpable due to edema

All the findings indicative of vascular injury, particularly arterial injury, may be elicited without the aid of any sophisticated equipment or highly specialized knowledge. The placement of "pulses" as the last item on each list is not by accident, but rather serves to emphasize that the careful examiner should be almost certain of the presence or absence of a pulse by the time the first portion of the list is completed. Occasionally, major obstructions or injuries to vessels will occur with distal pulses present, but this is not usual, and other findings should lead to the correct diagnosis. A frequently neglected but simple step is the taking of the blood pressure in both arms. Differences of 20 mm Hg consistently indicate pathologic obstruction, and this may be the only clue to major vascular trauma or preexisting arteriosclerosis.

Summary—vascular injuries

A high degree of suspicion in fractures, particularly fracture dislocations, should be maintained to detect potentially disastrous arterial injuries. The early use of angiography when appropriate is both safe and helpful in many vascular disorders. Neurologic manifestations frequently are associated with ischemia, from whatever cause, and should not lead one astray from the basic diagnosis. Although vascular spasm does occur, I am loath to attribute all signs and symptoms of vascular insufficiency to spasm until other causes are thoroughly ruled out, and ruling them out usually includes the use of angiography. Remember that *edema* distinguishes acute venous insufficiency from acute arterial insufficiency despite an otherwise similar clinical picture. The final point to bear in mind is that expeditious diagnosis and treatment is of paramount importance in all acute vascular injuries or obstructions. The viability of the extremity or organ involved may depend on the speed with which the diagnosis is made and care is undertaken. Attempts to totally resuscitate patients with ruptured major arteries are ill advised. It is much better to make rapid preparation for massive support and get them to the operating room where control of the hemorrhage can be carried out and replacement becomes effective.

STROKE

Although the origins of stroke are various, they usually fall into the categories of thrombosis, hemorrhage, and embolus that are common to other vascular emergencies. The subtleties of neurologic diagnosis need not concern the emergency personnel. Any patient who gives a history of transient paralysis or aphasia or arrives in the emergency department with a residual paralysis of sudden onset can be categorized as having had a stroke. Although the pathology may vary from intracerebral hemorrhage or thrombosis to the extracranial obstruction or embolus, the clinical picture is frequently similar.

Two main thrusts of assessment and intervention should be used. First, determine by history, examination, and all helpful radiologic or laboratory tests whether this "stroke" requires primary supportive care or vigorous diagnostic approach and perhaps some surgical intervention.[9] Second, having reached a tentative diagnosis, meticulous support of vital functions must be maintained during preparation for intervention or continued observation.

It should be emphasized that stroke is not a diagnosis of discards and hopelessness. Many patients recover and lead useful and worthwhile lives without residua even after what appears at first to be catastrophic brain damage. Only time can tell eventual recovery limits.

It must also be recognized that certain types of stroke, particularly those of transient nature or a mild deficit, may benefit by surgical intervention with prevention of more disabling strokes. Many of these patients have extracranial obstructive arterial disease, and the lesions are amenable to repair. Control of hypertension in others may prevent further problems. Specific causes, such as intracranial aneurysm, may be corrected surgically.

Diagnosis

History. A history of high blood pressure is frequently associated with those strokes caused by either intracranial hemorrhage or progressive arteriosclerosis with obstruction of vital vessels.

Most often the event is of sudden onset. The patient may remain completely paralyzed or show progressive recovery; or there may be progressive paralysis and loss of consciousness. This latter sequence is usually ominous. Headache frequently accompanies or precedes stroke. The patient may have had premonitory symptoms, such as brief episodes of aphasia and transient clumsiness of an arm or leg. Drooping of the corner of the mouth may have been noted by relatives or friends. Sometimes episodic blindness called "amaurosis fugax" heralds thrombosis of the ipsilateral carotid artery weeks prior to frank stroke. Sudden diplopia accompanied by vertigo and nausea may precede other signs of basilar artery thrombosis. The age of the patient may be helpful in diagnosis; cerebral aneurysms and strokes secondary to embolus from rheumatic heart disease occur more frequently in younger age groups. A history of atrial fibrillation or myocardial infarction in the older patient would make one consider an embolus as the underlying cause.

Physical examination. Hypertension is found in about one half of all stroke patients. Bilateral arm pressure should always be taken to alert the examiner to the possibility of dissection of the aorta as the cause for the stroke. Underlying arteriosclerotic vascular disease with obstruction of the arm vessels may cause differences in arm pressures and suggests carotid obstruction as the cause of the stroke. Subclavian obstruction may produce a "subclavian steal," with symptoms of basilar artery insufficiency.

If the subclavian artery or innominate artery obstruction occurs proximal to the origin of the vertebral artery, blood may be shunted from the base of the brain to the arm. The "steal" is produced by the reduced pressure in the arm beyond the obstruction and the unique direct connection of the vertebral arteries to the basilar artery. Blood then flows up one vertebral artery and down the other toward the low pressure side, reducing the effective flow to the brain stem (Fig. 15-7). This condition is corrected by restoring pressure to the distal subclavian artery by bypass from the carotid artery, or less often by direct removal of the obstruction by endarterectomy. The latter is a much more formidable procedure requiring thoracotomy and is seldom used.

Noting the patient's state of consciousness is important, since only the more profound strokes or those involving the brain stem render the patient unconscious. Intracerebral hemorrhage can also produce coma and neck rigidity. The patient with cerebral thrombosis usually does not have a stiff neck.

The common neurologic manifestations of the internal carotid distribution are motor loss on the opposite side of the body (including the face) and aphasia if the stroke involves the left hemisphere in the right-handed person. Other more subtle types of stroke and their manifestations need not be discussed here. It is impossible to tell from the patient's appearance whether the obstruction is intracranial or extracranial and, at a given moment, whether it represents profound brain damage. If the patient is completely flaccid on the involved side and has diminished consciousness, it is extremely likely that there has been a major brain infarction. If this state persists, it becomes certain.

Angiography. If the patient has had a transient attack of paralysis, many authorities feel that four-vessel angiograms should be obtained. If these demonstrate significant obstruction in one or both internal carotids, I would suggest surgical repair immediately. Visualization of the head vessels is also desirable and may show unexpected sources of neurologic symptoms, such as aneurysm or tumor, or document severe, intracranial disease. The latter situation makes surgical repair of the extracranial obstruction unwise. In the case of cerebral hemorrhage, most authorities feel a period of stabilization prior to angiography and treatment is in order.

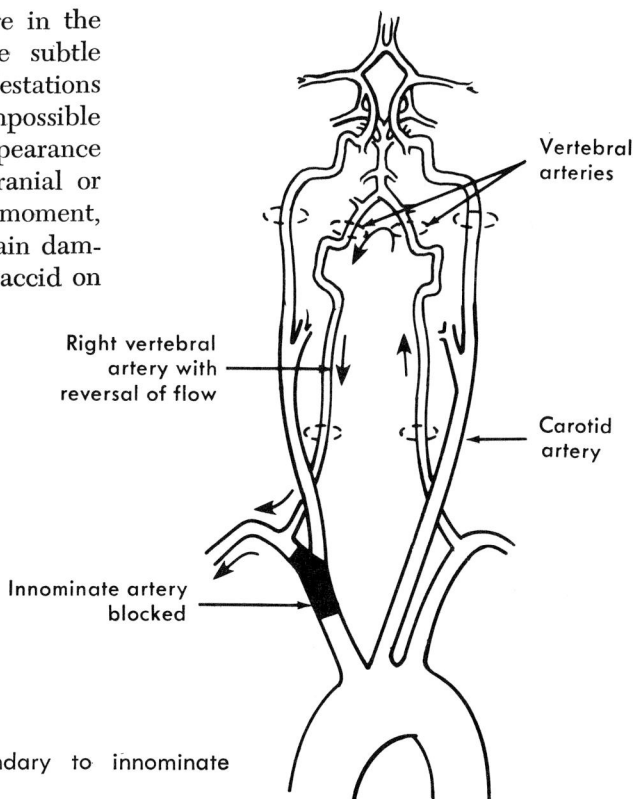

Fig. 15-7. Subclavian "steal" secondary to innominate artery thrombosis.

Embolus, if discovered by angiography, lodged in the extracranial carotid is surgically approachable.

Laboratory tests. Cerebral spinal fluid examination is usually in order in the emergency department unless there is evidence of increased intracranial pressure by ophthalmoscopic examination. Bloody fluid will bring further manipulative maneuvers to a halt and call for neurosurgical evaluation. Increased protein may be an indication for careful intracranial arteriograms to rule out mass lesions. A coagulation panel consisting of prothrombin time, clot retraction, and partial thromboplastin time will occasionally uncover a bleeding problem of which the stroke is a manifestation; these tests may also serve as a guide if anticoagulation therapy is contemplated. An electrocardiogram is important because it may show rhythm disturbances or recent myocardial infarction, which could serve as a source of embolus. The presence of degrees of heart block might unmask such syndromes as the Stokes-Adams syndrome wherein transient heart block causes symptoms of cerebral vascular insufficiency caused by poor cardiac output.

X-ray studies. Skull films may be helpful but usually are not. Occasionally, they may show a midline shift or undiscovered fracture or metastatic deposits. Calcified aneurysms or vessels may be seen, or primary tumors may contain calcium. The usual stroke has none of these. Chest x-ray should never be omitted, however, since lung cancer or metastatic tumor with cerebral metastasis is not rare and may give an entirely different direction to the diagnosis and treatment.

Supportive management

After the various steps mentioned above have been carried out little more is required of the emergency department personnel by the patient who has had a mild stroke. Vascular or neurosurgical help may be sought. However, the severely ill patient, whatever the etiology, requires more support.

Airway. Usually a soft nasopharyngeal airway will be sufficient to avoid respiratory obstruction in the paralyzed or semi-stuporous patient. Occasionally, the placing of a nasotracheal tube will be more satisfactory, particularly if a degree of respiratory depression is present. There is considerable question, however, whether continued respiratory support is warranted if spontaneous respirations cease, since this is almost always a fatal problem. Placing an airway (either oral or naso-oral) allows easy suctioning of secretions.

A urinary catheter is often useful because overdistention of the bladder is common.

Pressure protection. Padding the elbows and heels can avoid troublesome pressure points.

Nasogastric tubes. Some authorities feel that passage of a nasogastric tube is helpful to avoid aspiration in a patient unable to adequately protect the airway.

Positioning. Although traditionally the patient is placed on his or her back for observation and care, the lateral position has several advantages. Aspiration can be avoided if vomiting occurs and the tongue does not tend to drop back into the pharynx with consequent respiratory obstruction. Frequent turning is helpful to avoid pooling of secretions in the lungs as well as to avoid pressure on the bony prominences on the back.

Perhaps the greatest early hazard to the stroke patient is hypoxia and hypercapnia secondary to respiratory obstruction. Therefore, careful positioning, suctioning, airway care, and supplemental oxygen are extremely important.

Summary—stroke

Stroke is frequently seen in the emergency department. Personnel should view it as a diagnostic and therapeutic challenge and institute early preventive and diagnostic measures as appropriate. Perhaps one half of all stroke patients are capable of excellent recovery either by natural course of events or by surgical intervention preceded by accurate angiography.

REFERENCES

1. Weil, P. H., and Steichen, F. M.: The treatment of penetrating injuries of the neck, J. Trauma **11**:590-594, 1971.
2. Brink, B. E.: Vascular trauma, Surg. Clin. North Am. **57**:189-196, 1977.
3. Smith, R. F., Elliot, J. P., Hageman, J. H., Szilagyi, D. E., and Xavier, A. O.: Acute penetrating arterial injuries of the neck and limbs, Arch. Surg. **109**:198-205, 1974.
4. Singh, I., and Gorman, J. F.: Vascular injuries in closed fractures, J. Trauma **12**:592-598, 1972.
5. Bricker, D. C., Noon, G. P., Beall, A. C., and DeBakey, M. F.: Vascular injuries of the thoracic outlet, J. Trauma **10**:1-15, 1970.
6. Edwards, E. A.: Acute peripheral arterial occlusion, J.A.M.A. **223**:909-912, 1973.
7. Rowen, M., Dorsey, T. J., and Hepps, S. A.: Primary venous obstruction of the upper extremity, Calif. Med. **118**:18-23, 1973.
8. Rich, N. M., Hobson, R. W., II, Wright, C. B., and Fedde, C. W.: Repair of lower extremity venous trauma—a more aggressive approach required, J. Trauma **14**:639-652, 1974.
9. Dye, W. S., and Brown, C. M.: Surgical correction of carotid and vertebral artery stenosis, Surg. Clin. North Am. **53**:241-251, 1973.

Additional readings

Fields, W. S., and others: Joint study of extracranial arterial occlusion, J.A.M.A. **203**:955-959, Mar. 11, 1968; **21**:1993-2003, Mar. 23, 1970; **222**:1139-1143, Nov. 27, 1972.

Gomensoro, J. B., and others: Joint study of extracranial arterial occlusion, J.A.M.A. **224**:985-991, May 14, 1973.

Hunt, J. L., McManus, W. F., Haney, W. P., and Pruitt, B. A., Jr.: Vascular lesions in acute electric burns, J. Trauma **14**:461-473, 1974.

Rich, N. M.: Vascular trauma, Surg. Clin. North Am. **53**:1367-1392, 1973.

CHAPTER 16

Emergency management of burns

Hugh A. Frank, M.D.

The first task of emergency department personnel is to separate those burn patients who can be successfully treated on an outpatient basis from those requiring hospitalization. This distinction is usually clear cut; but where doubt exists, it is often safer to admit the patient for 48 to 72 hours.

TRIAGE—ASSESSING THE PATIENT AND THE INJURY

Care required for thermal burns is based on determining the following factors[1,2]:
1. Estimated depth of the surface wound
2. Area of body surface affected
3. Particular areas of the body that are injured
4. Age of the patient
5. Presence of preexisting disease
6. Additional trauma
7. Patient's life-style, personality, and home environment

Depth of surface wound

A scheme for classifying the depth of the burn wound[3] is summarized in Fig. 16-1. The depth of a burn wound is often difficult to determine immediately, but an initial estimate should be made as a guide to prognosis and therapy. The distinction between partial thickness (second degree) and whole thickness (third degree) skin loss may require many days' observation *or tangential excision as described* by Janzékovic.[4] Subsequent injury from pressure or surface wound infection may quickly convert a relatively superficial burn wound to one of full thickness skin loss or deep tissue destruction. Improper treatment can cause such injury. For simplicity, the classification of burn depth is a rough appraisal of those areas that appear to be first, second, or third degree in character (Fig. 16-2).

Area of body surface affected

The area of body surface involved in each degree of injury should be sketched on a diagram,[1,5] such as that shown in Fig. 16-2. This diagram, together with the data relating patient age to the relative surface area of the various body parts, allows determination of total body surface percentage involved in the various depths of the burn. This figure is critical in making the initial decision to treat and send home, admit to the hospital, or transfer to a specialized burn treatment facility. It is also part of the data needed to plan fluid replacement during the shock phase of serious burns.

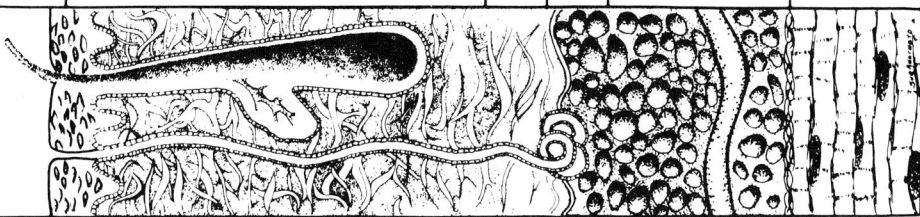

Depth of burn		Pain and pinprick sensitivity	Appearance	Healing time	End result of healing	Treatment
1°	Erythema only, no loss of epidermis	Hyperalgesia	Erythema		Normal skin	Allow to heal by natural processes Protect from further injury and infection
2° (Partial skin loss)	Superficial, no loss of dermis	Hyperalgesia or normal		6-10 days	Normal skin	
2°	Intermediate, healing from hair follicles	Normal to hypo-algesia	Erythema to opaque, white blisters are characteristic	7-14 days	Normal to slightly pitted and/or poorly pigmented	
2°	Deep, healing from sweat glands	Hypoalgesia to analgesia		14-21 days	Hairless and depigmented. Texture normal to pitted or flat and shiny	
3° (Whole skin loss)	Deep dermal, occasionally heal from scattered epithelium	Analgesia	White opaque to charred, coagulated; subcutaneous veins may be visible	More than 21 days	Poor texture Hypertrophic Scar frequent	Elective skin grafting may save time and give better end result
3°	Whole skin loss, healing from edges only			Never if area is large	Hypertrophic scar and chronic granulations unless grafted	
4° (Deep tissue loss)	Deep structure loss	May be some algesia				Skin grafting mandatory

Fig. 16-1. Classification of burns according to depth of burn.

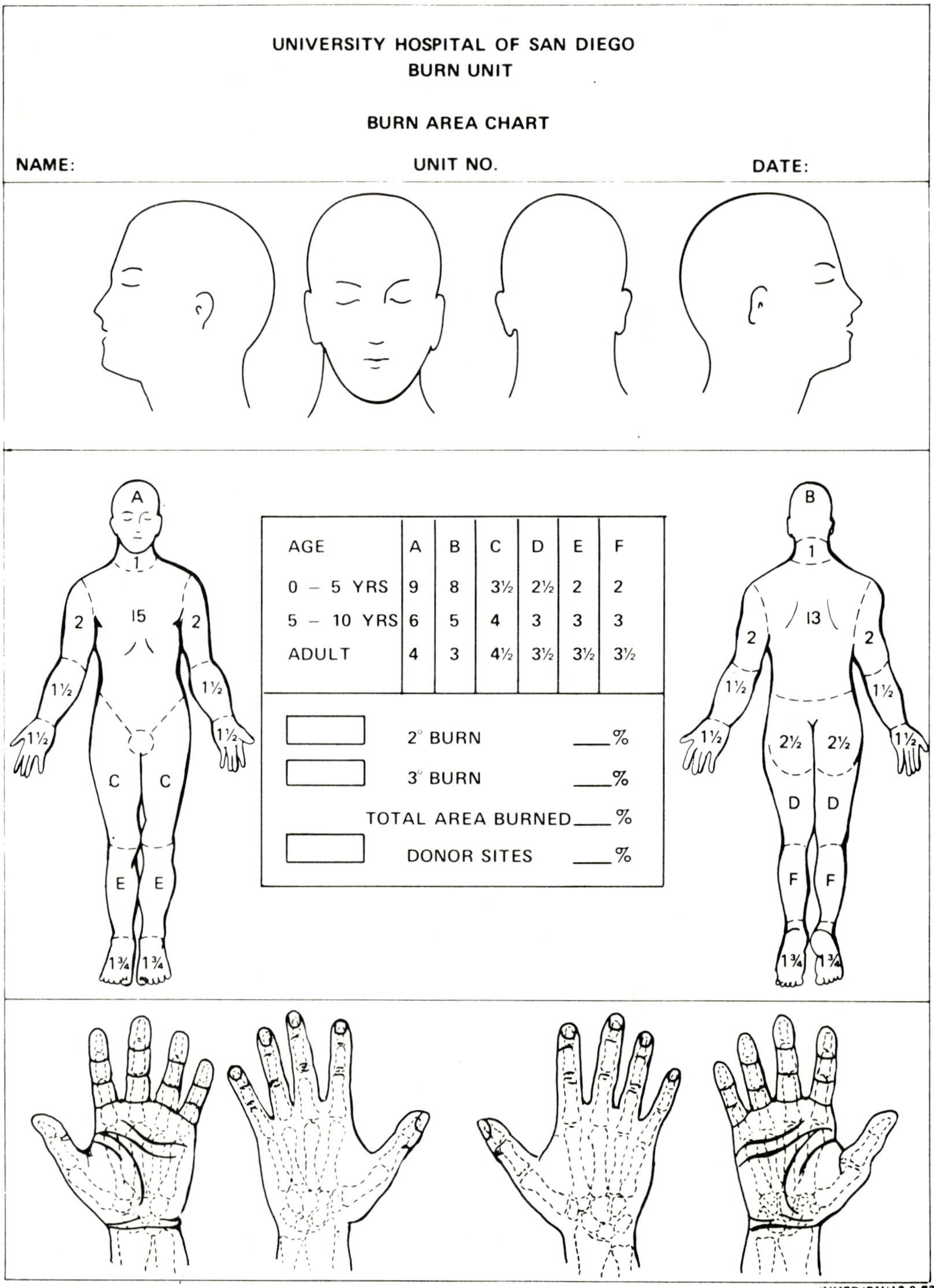

UNIVERSITY HOSPITAL OF SAN DIEGO
BURN UNIT

BURN AREA CHART

NAME: UNIT NO. DATE:

AGE	A	B	C	D	E	F
0 – 5 YRS	9	8	3½	2½	2	2
5 – 10 YRS	6	5	4	3	3	3
ADULT	4	3	4½	3½	3½	3½

2° BURN ____%

3° BURN ____%

TOTAL AREA BURNED____%

DONOR SITES ____%

(UHSD/BU/12-8-72)

Fig. 16-2

Parts of body injured

The involvement of certain critical areas affects the severity of the injury. Burns of the face, hands, feet, or genitalia and perineum, even though relatively small in area, constitute serious injury and may, by themselves, be an indication for hospital admission.

Age

Patient age not only affects the relative surface area of the body parts, but, more importantly, it also affects the ability to survive. Burns in infants and children under 18 months or in adults over 45 years produce a sharp increase in mortality and morbidity.[6,7] Such patients are more critically ill than young adults with burns of similar size and depth.

Preexisting disease and additional trauma

Other factors that may lead to a critical classification include preexisting conditions such as heart disease, emphysema, diabetes, and the presence of associated injuries, such as fractures, internal injuries, and severe lacerations. The most significant and a frequent concomitant injury is pulmonary damage caused by the inhalation of smoke and noxious gases. The probability that a pulmonary injury has occurred should always be considered if two or more of the following criteria are present[8,9]:

1. The burn occurred in a closed space

2. Flame burns occur on the face, nose, and mouth
3. Nasal hair is singed
4. Carboxyhemoglobin is present in the admission blood sample

If three or more of these criteria are present, pulmonary injury is virtually certain, and the prognosis is serious.

Life-style

The patient's life-style and social environment may affect hospital admission. A patient with both hands burned and in bandages may be sent home if the family will provide needed care, while a person living alone may require hospital admission for the same injury.

Burn categories

General criteria for where to treat are summarized in Table 16-1. This triage plan is generally applicable to heat energy burns (scalds and flame burns). Special categories of burns may require special consideration.

Electrical burns. Electrical burns[10,11,12] are more severe and extensive than the surface appearance would indicate. Often there is occlusion of major vessels or damage to nerves, muscles, and bones away from the wound of entry. These burns should be considered as serious until observation over several days proves otherwise. Usually hospital admission is required.

Table 16-1. Classification of burns according to severity

Burn category	Description
Minor burns—treat in emergency department; send patient home	Second and third degree burns total less than 15% body area; third degree burns less than 2% body area; none on critical areas of hands, face, or genitalia
Major burns—admit to hospital	Second and third degree burns total between 15% and 30% body area; third degree burns total from 2% to 10% body area; minor electrical and chemical burns
Critical burns—transfer to major burn center if possible	Total area of second and third degree burns more than 30% body area; major electrical and chemical burns; patient under 18 months or over 45 years of age; complicating illness or concomitant injuries present

Chemical burns. Chemical burns[1,13] are frequently combined with heat burns when hot acid or alkali solutions are splashed on the skin. The continuing action of the injurious chemical or the toxicity of the chemical absorbed into the body makes some of these injuries serious, even though a small area is involved. Notable among such chemicals is hydrofluoric acid,[14] which is used in a number of common industrial processes. Burns with this agent may seem trivial at first, but continuing action of the chemical even after thorough washing may result in progressive damage. A day or two later this becomes apparent unless suitable early treatment has been carried out.

Radiation. Patients with various forms of acute radiation injury may be admitted to the emergency department. Most common, of course, is sunburn.[15] While sunburn is usually not serious, occasionally a patient may be ill enough to require hospital admission. It is wise not to dismiss such a patient with superficial evaluation, especially if the body temperature is over 38° C (101° F) or if much blistering is apparent over large areas. Acute injuries caused by ionizing radiations (x-rays and radioactive isotopes) are rare, but they do occur.[16-18] Patients with such injuries should be hospitalized for observation and treatment. The degree and extent of radiation injury are often not fully apparent for two to three weeks. With the proliferation of the use of radioisotopes and of nuclear power the hazard of accidents in which patients are not only burned but also contaminated with radioactive materials exists. Fortunately, such accidents are rare. Nevertheless, each emergency department should have a plan of management for decontamination to protect the hospital and its personnel while treating the patient. Good programs for this are available and will not be detailed here.[19] Laser injuries[20] usually result in small areas of deep burn and may be evaluated like similar injuries from splashes of molten metal or other heat sources. Microwaves emitted by radar installations, television sets, and electronic ovens produce heat energy on passage through tissues. They are potentially dangerous, but to date no injuries have been reported.[21,22]

Other burnlike injuries. The friction and abrasion injuries of "street burns" caused from sliding on pavement, or grinder injuries in industry, share some of the characteristics of mechanical injuries and heat injuries. They are often complicated by contamination with dirt, tiny particles, and bacteria. Their management is, in many ways, similar to burn treatment, and they may be classified similarly to heat burns for emergency department triage purposes.

Cold injuries[23] (frostbite) share many burn characteristics. Such injuries often involve both hands and both feet as well as the face—all critical areas—and require hospital admission.

Finally, in our current drug culture, pressure injuries, which occur when a person lies immobile for many hours "tripped out" on a drug, may result in areas of whole-thickness skin loss and even underlying tissue necrosis similar to deep burns. These patients usually require hospital admission for both the pressure injuries and primary drug intoxication.

In less severe injuries a detailed and more leisurely evaluation of patient and injury can be carried out. In the more seriously ill, however, both evaluation and treatment are urgent and must be started immediately and carried forward concurrently.

INTERVENTION IN THE EMERGENCY DEPARTMENT
Critical burns—preparation for safe transfer to a special burn treatment facility

The chances for survival of a critically burned patient are significantly improved if he or she can be cared for in a specialized burn treatment facility where a team of experienced medical and paramedical personnel is prepared to deal with the many difficult aspects of burn care.[5,24] Patients can be moved to such a facility easily and safely in the first few hours after the injury if the proper procedures for stabilization are carried out at or near the scene of the accident. Suitable life support vehicles and teams available to attend to the transfer are mandatory. The following must be done prior to transfer:

1. Assure an adequate airway and oxygenation. If necessary, a nasotracheal tube can be passed or a tracheostomy done. Oxygen therapy should be begun. Adequate equipment for suctioning the airway, ensuring ventilation, and administering oxygen must be in the transfer vehicle (refer to Chapter 26).

2. Hemorrhage, if any, must be controlled. A central venous line of large caliber must be placed and vigorous fluid replacement started. Adequate equipment for intravenous therapy and supplies of replacement fluid must be available in the transfer vehicle. Blood is not usually needed in the early stages of burn shock.

3. A urinary catheter is placed and connected to a container for measuring urine output. Urine flow should be established prior to transfer if possible.

4. A gastric tube is passed and the stomach emptied. Equipment for maintaining gastric suction should be available in the ambulance.

5. Sedation, preferably a *small* intravenous dose of morphine, is given prior to transfer.

6. Tetanus toxoid or human antitoxin is administered in appropriate amount. Penicillin or broad-spectrum antibiotic therapy is initiated.

7. No attempt should be made at local care nor medication applied to the burns. The patient's clothing can be cut away and the patient laid on a clean sheet and covered with a clean sheet on the stretcher. Definitive care of the burn wound found is delayed until after transfer.

8. Any fractures are splinted to prevent further injury in transit.

9. It is often useless to waste time on laboratory work and x-rays prior to transfer unless such problems as possible ruptured spleen or collapsed lung need evaluation and management.

Most burn patients can be prepared for transfer within the first half hour at an emergency facility and be safely on their way at the end of that time. If properly prepared and managed in transit, journeys requiring many hours can be safely accomplished.

Major burns—preparation for hospital admission

The following protocol[1,5,8] was developed for the guidance of the staff at the University of California, San Diego, Medical Center for the admissions to its burn unit. Physicians who plan to care for burned patients might do well to evaluate their own skills against those needed to care for such patients, as suggested in *Emergency Department Organization and Management.*[25]

I. Call the burn service house staff immediately on patient's arrival.

II. Management (in order of priority)

  A. Respiratory support—call the respiratory care service for help if needed.

    1. Inspect for burn injury of the face and upper airway.

    2. Establish an airway; clear the passages.

    3. Assist respiration as needed. Use supplemental O_2 through mask, prongs, or catheter. Place endotracheal tube, and use mechanical ventilation support if necessary. Defer tracheostomy for definite indications later on. If carbon monoxide poisoning is present, administer 5%[26] carbogen to assist its wash-out.

  B. Circulation support—administer shock therapy.

    1. Insert a central venous catheter

of large bore and attach a venous pressure manometer.

2. Start Ringer's lactate solution pending calculation of the patient's fluid requirements. Run this fast enough to establish a urine flow of 30 to 75 ml per hour (in adults).

C. Attend to urgent concomitant injuries.
   1. Control hemorrhage.
   2. Attend to chest wounds.
   3. Temporarily splint fractures.
D. Place a catheter in the bladder.
   1. Send the initial urine to the laboratory; measure its volume.
   2. Attach a urinometer and measure the urine hourly.
E. Place a sump tube in the stomach; empty the stomach and keep it empty with suction.
F. Draw blood for initial laboratory data.
   1. Type blood and screen serum for abnormal antibodies
   2. Complete blood count
   3. Blood sugar
   4. Blood urea nitrogen and creatinine
   5. Albumin and globulin levels
   6. Bilirubin and alkaline phosphatase levels
   7. Calcium and phosphorus levels
   8. Electrolytes and venous pH
   9. Arterial blood gases including carbon monoxide level if indicated
G. Take an initial chest x-ray.
H. Take as complete a medical history as possible including the following:
   1. Details of the accident resulting in the burn
   2. Any known drug idiosyncrasies
   3. Any preexisting health problems or regular medications
I. At this point, *small* doses of intravenous morphine may be used.
J. Complete the physical examination.

K. Record areas of burn on a burn chart and calculate area of burn.
L. Calculate fluid requirements and adjust intravenous fluid rates according to the "new" Brooke formula.[27]
   1. First 24 hours estimate 3 ml of Ringer's lactate times kilograms of body weight times percent of surface burned. Plan to give half that amount in the first eight hours and the other half over the next 16 hours. Adjust amount and rate of flow to maintain an hourly urine output of 0.5 to 1.0 ml per kilogram of body weight.
   2. During the second 24 hours, administer glucose in water and Plasmanate as required to maintain the same urine output.
   3. The above formulas are good first approximations of the actual requirements in burns between 20% and 50% of body surface area, but are not very reliable in larger burns.
   4. The results of fluid calculations are approximations only and must be modified by the patient's response to therapy as indicated by the continued monitoring.
M. Start data flow sheets, monitoring at frequent intervals the following:
   1. Pulse
   2. Blood pressure
   3. Central venous pressure
   4. Respiratory rate and, if necessary, tidal volume, minute volume, and O_2 of inspired air
   5. Temperature
   6. Urine output
N. Then, and only then, attend to the surface wounds.
   1. Cut away any clothes.
   2. Clean patient, preferably in a tub or tank. Wash thoroughly with copious amounts of water

or saline and small amounts of iodophor soap.

3. Shave all hair in and around burn areas.
4. Remove all blister debris. Do not break intact blisters.
5. Weigh patient.
6. Photograph all wounds after cleansing and prior to dressing.
7. Perform escharotomies to relieve compression from circumferential, constricting, full-thickness burn if needed.
8. Decide on and begin topical antibacterial therapy. (Our mainstay at present is Betadine ointment [povidone iodine ointment] or silver sulfadiazine cream applied on a single layer of fine mesh gauze and held in place with elastic netting or a minimum of adaptive gauze. This is essentially exposure treatment. It is supplemented by frequent hydrotherapy.)
9. Splint and elevate hands and feet as required; occlusive dressings may be required.

O. Administer tetanus toxoid or human immune globulin or both.
P. Start penicillin therapy using large doses for 72 hours. If the patient is allergic to penicillin, use vancomycin.
Q. In infants and small children give a dose of prophylactic gamma globulin.
R. Send patient to the burn intensive care unit.

For some burns this general protocol may be modified, but in any burn large enough to warrant admission to the hospital, it is better to be complete and stay ahead of the problem than to try to come from behind when a crisis has developed.

It is obvious that such an involved treatment program requires the facilities and personnel team of a major hospital if it is to be accomplished at all. In order to accomplish it with efficiency and economy, burn units have been organized at a number of centers in this country and abroad.

Minor burns—outpatient management

The relief of pain from small areas of surface burn may result from application of cold water or ice as a first aid measure. It does not reverse the damage done by the burning agent, and if continued too long, may increase the damage. Once the burn has been evaluated, the wound should be gently but thoroughly cleaned with warm water and soap. Currently, iodophor soaps are used for their antibacterial effect. All hair in and adjacent to the burned area should be shaved so that subsequent cleansing of the wound will be easier and less painful. Blister debris should be removed. Unbroken blisters may be left alone or punctured and drained and allowed to fall back against the wound.

Exposure treatment is widely used for the management of major burns in the hospital environment, but it is seldom suitable for outpatient management of burns. Occlusive dressings are more reliable to protect burns and prevent introduction of infection in the highly variable and unpredictable environment of home and shop. Most of the burns treated on an outpatient basis will be second degree burns and, if protected, will heal. Small areas of whole skin loss can be skin grafted on an outpatient basis or during a short admission when the wound is ready for grafting. It is not necessary to change dressings frequently on these injuries. Usually a first redressing can be done at four or five days. Thereafter, redressing at weekly intervals may suffice. Further debridement and wound cleansing can be done at redressings as needed. The details of the dressing itself are important.

Dressings. A layer of fine mesh gauze should always be placed closest to the wound. This has about 40 threads per inch.

Ordinary roller gauze with about 20 threads per inch is too coarse, and batiste or linen is too fine to be suitable. Coarse gauze allows the threads to be incorporated into granulations and causes excessive pain and bleeding on removal. Tightly woven materials quickly become impervious with coagulum and exudate and allow secretions to accumulate between the wound and the dressing, leading to bacterial growth and wound damage.

The first layer of fine mesh gauze can be applied sterile and unmedicated if desired, but many prefer to apply it impregnated with an antibacterial ointment or cream. This material should have a water-soluble base so that the ointment base will not act as an impervious layer. The medications commonly used are nitrofurazone (Furacin Soluble),[28] xeroform, neomycin, or bacitracin. All are suitable. Sulfamylon cream,[29] Betadine ointment, and silver sulfadiazine cream are not suitable as topical antibacterial agents when used under occlusive dressings that are changed infrequently because they soon lose their topical effectiveness. They are useful for the exposure treatment combined with frequent hydrotherapy and reapplication of the material.

The first layer of medicated or non-medicated fine mesh gauze should be held in place with a gauze dressing smoothly and firmly applied. Over this, bulky dressings of sterile cotton are placed. These are prepared by dividing the standard 1-pound roll of surgical cotton in half to provide two long rolls about 6 feet long and 6 inches wide. The cotton is then rerolled without its paper, wrapped, and sterilized. Over the cotton, bias cut stockinette is wrapped tightly to produce a firm, slightly compressive, immobilizing dressing. The area of dressing should be considerably larger than the area of injury. Often plaster slabs are incorporated between the cotton and the bias cut stockinette to assist immobilization in a func-

tional position. The whole dressing is then secured with tape. A properly applied dressing should be protective and comfortable. Pain usually subsides shortly after the dressing is applied.

Positioning is particularly important in the hand, which is a frequent site of burn injuries. The usual functional position of the hand is with the wrist dorsiflexed about 20 degrees. The fingers are close together and are partly flexed at all three joints into a gentle curve that brings the tips of the fore and middle fingers to a point about 2.5 cm from the tip of the thumb, which is widely abducted, slightly flexed, and opposed. For burns this position is altered so that the finger metacarpophalangeal joints are more fully flexed while the interphalangeal joints are fully extended, including the interphalangeal joint of the thumb. This is the duck-bill position and is designed to prevent development of the clawed position so often seen after disastrous hand burns (Fig. 16-3).

Some authorities recommend the use of allografts (cadaver skin) or xenografts (pigskin) as dressing materials[30] directly on the areas of second degree burn rather than fine mesh gauze. While these materials are very useful, they are not readily available in every emergency depart-

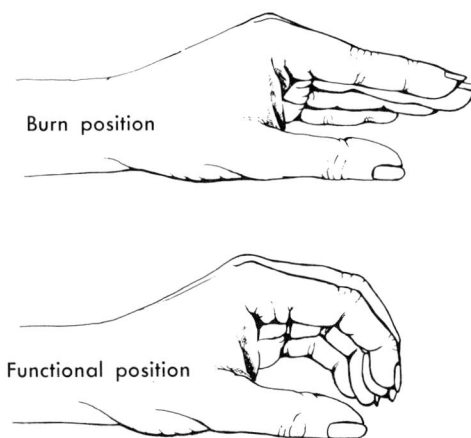

Fig. 16-3. Positioning the hand in dressings.

ment. Another recent suggestion has been the use of micropore tape directly applied to the burned surface[31] as a primary dressing for second degree burns.

As with more serious burns, one should avoid the excessive use of pain medications. The administration of tetanus prophylaxis is a must. The prophylactic use of penicillin or a substitute is sometimes indicated.

Chemical burns. Certain specific types of burns and related injuries require special consideration as was indicated under triage. Chemical burns resulting from acids or alkalies getting on the skin should be thoroughly washed with copious quantities of flowing water at or near body temperature.[32,33] A shower is an excellent method. Flowing water removes the chemical by dilution and mechanical action. It decreases the rate of chemical reaction, decreases the inflammatory reaction, minimizes the hygroscopic effects of the agent, and restores the pH of the skin toward normal. Finally, it removes any heat generated by the chemical reactions that occur. Neutralization of the injurious agents by chemical means has never been shown to be more effective and may produce further injury through heat generated by the neutralization reaction. The one exception to this is hydrofluoric acid burns where chemical neutralization is essential.

Hydrofluoric acid[14] requires the use of calcium solutions to stop its action. The fluoride ion rapidly penetrates skin and becomes incorporated into tissues, producing continuing damage. It combines with calcium and magnesium ions to form relatively insoluble and inactive compounds. Any fluoride ion remaining on the surface should be washed off with lime water (calcium hydroxide solution). Any fluoride ion that has penetrated the tissues should be neutralized by infiltrating the injured skin and the subcutaneous tissue with calcium gluconate solution, which is available in 10 ml ampules for injection.

When acids or alkalies enter the eye,

copious irrigation is difficult or impossible. The use of a hypertonic (0.5 molar) phosphate buffer solution to supplement the irrigations is useful.[34]

Tar burns. Tar burns are another common type of combined heat and chemical injury. Removal of the tar in the emergency department presents a problem. Not only is it painful, but it may result in further injury. Sometimes tar can be removed by first applying ice to make it hard and then peeling it off. It has been shown, however, that immediate removal of the tar is not essential. Tar is soluble in petroleum greases, and ordinary petrolatum jelly can be used to dissolve and remove it. The burns can be dressed with polymyrine B sulfate (Neosporin) ointment (in petrolatum base) and gauze dressings. Any residual tar will be dissolved and absorbed by the gauze. Several redressings at 12-hour intervals will remove the residual tar painlessly, while the antibiotic will suppress bacterial growth.[35]

Sunburn. Sunburn deserves consideration because it is so common. Fortunately, it is usually first degree (erythema) or superficial second degree (blisters). A multitude of over-the-counter remedies for sunburn are available. Some contain various local anesthetic agents. Neither their safety nor effectiveness has been well studied. Placebo effect is significant as indicated by the fact that shaving cream delivered to the burn surface from a spray can labeled "burn cream" was highly effective in relieving pain, but not when delivered from a can labeled shaving cream.[36] Sunburn produces dermal hyperemia, and the burned surface is hot to the touch. The patient's body temperature may be elevated. This heat can be dissipated and local pain relief achieved simply by evaporative cooling. A single layer of wet cloth is applied to the burn area, and a fan is blown over it. As soon as it dries, the wet cloth is replaced with another. For a torso burn, a wet cotton T-shirt works well. After a period of evaporative cooling, a bland oily lotion may be helpful. Topical and systemic corticoids have been recommended for reducing the inflammatory process in severe sunburn[15] and may be helpful. Treating areas injured by sunburn (ultraviolet radiation) with infrared radiations has been described through the years. Such treatment is said to reduce the erythema of sunburn,[37] and it may be beneficial.

Abrasion injuries. Street burns, grinder injuries, and other abrasion injuries are similar to burns, and may be first, second, or third degree in depth. They are usually small in area and suitable for outpatient care. As with other "burns," thorough cleansing is important. Anesthesia, local or general, may be required to make this possible. All particulate matter must be removed at the primary treatment or it may be incorporated during healing and become a permanent deep tattoo. Hydrogen peroxide is useful to loosen particles and aid in their removal. Brushes may be required to remove some of the debris. A binocular loupe for magnification and time-consuming removal of particles with a needle or a knife point may be required. After cleansing, dressings can be applied as with a second degree thermal burn. Antibiotic ointments are especially helpful in abrasive injuries. Third degree abrasion injuries may require skin grafting.

SUMMARY

Severe burns constitute a critical illness involving the skin, respiratory, cardiovascular, and renal systems. Support of vital systems takes precedence over wound management. Prevention and treatment of infection is of paramount importance. Management of the burned patient demands a team, a plan, and the material and equipment needed for treatment of critically ill patients with multisystem disease. A few simple measures, available in every emergency department, make it possible to resuscitate these patients until they are transferred to a facility that offers extensive and intensive burn care. Minor burns can be managed on an outpatient basis using a few simple principles.

REFERENCES

1. Artz, C. P., and Moncrief, J. A.: The treatment of burns, ed. 2, Philadelphia, 1969, W. B. Saunders Co.
2. American Burn Association: Patient severity classification, 1976.
3. Jackson, D. MacG.: In search of an acceptable burn classification, Br. J. Plast. Surg. 23:219-226, 1970.
4. Janz'ekovic, Z.: The burn wound from the surgical point of view, J. Trauma 15:42-62, 1975.
5. Stone, N. H., editor: Profiles in burn management, Miami, 1968, Industrial Medicine Publishing Co.
6. Feller, I., and Crane, K.: National burn information exchange, Surg. Clin. North Am. 50:1425-1436, 1970.
7. Barnes, B. A., Constable, J. D., and Burke, J. F.: Mortality of burns at the Massachusetts General Hospital, 1955-1969. In Matter, P., Barclay, T. L., and Koničková, Z.: Research in burns, Berne, 1970, Hans Huber Medical Publisher, pp. 430-433.
8. Polk, H. C., and Stone, H. H.: Contemporary burn management, Boston, 1971, Little, Brown & Co., pp. 109-138.
9. Zikria, B. A., Weston, G. C., Chodoff, M., and Ferrer, J. M.: Smoke and carbon monoxide poisoning in fire victims, J. Trauma 12:641-645, 1972.
10. Sturim, H. S.: The treatment of electrical burns: Collective review, Surg. Gynecol. Obstet. 128:129-133, 1969.
11. Sturim, H. S.: The treatment of electrical injuries, J. Trauma 11:959-965, 1971.
12. Hunt, J. L., McManus, W. F., Haney, W. P., and Pruitt, B. A.: Vascular lesions in acute electric injuries, J. Trauma 14:461-473, 1974.
13. Curreri, J. W., Asch, M. J., and Pruitt, B. A.: The treatment of chemical burns: specialized diagnostic, therapeutic, and prognostic considerations, J. Trauma 10:634-642, 1970.
14. Iverson, R. E., Laub, D. R., and Madison, M. S.: Hydrofluoric acid burns, Plastic Reconstr. Surg. 48:107-112, 1971.
15. Goldman, M. S., Leon, A. J., and Rand, G. L.: Topical and systemic corticosteroids in severe sunburn, Dermatol. Intern 5:75-78, 1966.

16. Sweet, R. D.: Acute accidental superficial x-ray burns, Br. J. Dermatol. **74:**393-402, 1962.

17. Sweet, R. D.: Treatment of acute local radiation injuries, Clin. Rad. **15:**55-58, 1964.

18. Lewis, G. K., and Landa, S.: Radiation burns, Int. Coll. Surg. **37:**237-259, 1962.

19. United States Energy and Development Administration: Emergency handling of radiation accident cases, ERDA-17, April 1975.

20. Fine, B. S.: Burn injury after carbon dioxide laser irradiation, Arch. Surg. **98:**219-222, 1969.

21. Michaelson, S. M.: Biomedical aspects of microwave exposure, Am. Ind. Hyg. Assoc. J. **32:**338-345, 1971.

22. Odland, L. T.: Observations on microwave hazards to USAF personnel, J. Occup. Med. **14:**544-547, 1972.

23. Owens, J. C.: Treatment of cold injuries, Postgrad. Med. **48:**160-165, 1970.

24. Kirksey, T. D., Dowling, J. A., Pruitt, B. A., and Moncrief, J. A.: Safe, expeditious transport of the seriously burned patient, Arch. Surg. **96:**790-794, 1968.

25. American College of Emergency Physicians, Jenkins, A. L., editor: Emergency department organization and management, St. Louis, 1975, The C. V. Mosby Co.

26. Dinman, B. D.: Management of acute carbon monoxide intoxication, J. Occup. Med. **16:**662-664, 1974.

27. Artz, C. P.: Burns updated, J. Trauma **16:**3-15, 1976.

28. Hunter, G. R., and Chang, F. C.: Outpatient burns: a prospective study, J. Trauma **16:**191-195, 1976.

29. Harrison, H. N., Boles, H., and Jacoby, F.: The behavior of mafenide acetate as a basis for its clinical use, Arch. Surg. **103:**449-453, 1971.

30. Miller, T. A.: The second-degree burn: a reevaluation, Burns **1:**207-211, 1975.

31. Miller, T., and White, W.: Healing of second degree burns: Comparison of effects of early application of homografts and coverage with tape, Plast. Reconstr. Surg. **49:**552-557, 1972.

32. Bromberg, B. E., Song, I. C., and Walden, R. H.: Hydrotherapy of chemical burns, Plast. Reconstr. Surg. **35:**85-95, 1965.

33. Wolfort, F. G., DeMeester, T., Knorr, N., and Edgerton, M. T.: Surgical management of cutaneous lye burns, Surg. Gynecol. Obstet. **131:**873-876, 1970.

34. Poser, E.: Emergency treatment of chemical injuries, Ill. Med. J. **127:**161-162, 1965.

35. Asbell, T. S., Crawford, H. H., Adamson, J. E., and Horton, C. E.: Tar and grease removal from injured parts, Plast. Reconstr. Surg. **40:**330-331, 1967.

36. Lewis, S. S.: In Goldman, L., and Gardiner, R. E., editors: Burns: a symposium, Springfield, Ill., 1965, Charles C Thomas, Publisher, p. 74.

37. Everett, M. A., Doran, C. K., Everett, H. D., and Anglin, J. H.: Modification of sunburn by infrared rays, J.A.M.A. **186:**778-779, 1963.

CHAPTER **17**

Poisons

Melvin A. Ochs, M.D.

It is estimated that there are approximately 10 million cases of poisoning in the United States each year; in 1971 just over 5,000 deaths occurred in the United States. Of these fatalities, more than 4,000 occurred in and around the home. The National Safety Council[1] has provided the figures shown in Fig. 17-1.

From ages 1 to 4 years, poisoning is the fourth leading cause of death, a reflection of the child's newly discovered mobility and curiosity. The incidence drops significantly until ages 15 to 24 when it again rises to fourth place, perhaps a reflection of depression or experimentation. The San Diego Poison Information Center, which supplies information to the general public as well as to medical personnel, reports an incidence of 58% of poisonings from household product ingestion, 23% from drug ingestion, 9% due to plants, and 10% miscellaneous.

It is important to realize that there are few specific antidotes for poisons, and therefore a thorough history of the exposure coupled with a rapid assessment of the patient's physical status should, in most instances, direct the examiner along the course of proper care. There are five basic principles to follow in any case of suspected poisoning: (1) identify the poi-

son, (2) stop absorption, (3) hasten elimination, (4) give symptomatic care, and (5) give appropriate antidote.

IDENTIFYING THE POISON

In identifying the poison, an attempt should be made to discover both the name of the poison and some estimate of the quantity ingested or time of exposure. Record the time elapsed since ingestion along with the patient's age, weight, a brief description of the progress of symptoms in the preceding interval, and any previous treatment. Friends or relatives may be asked to bring in empty containers or may be sent to search for these important clues when the diagnosis is obscure. A previous drug abuse history or knowledge of current drug fads may also be helpful in diagnosis. With or without the aid of a history, the physical examination should narrow the field of suspect toxins. Table 17-1 lists some physical signs that may be caused by various toxins.

STOPPING ABSORPTION

Generally, material may be recovered from the stomach for up to two and perhaps four hours. Notable exceptions are (1) salicylate, which causes pylorospasm resulting in recoverable amounts as long

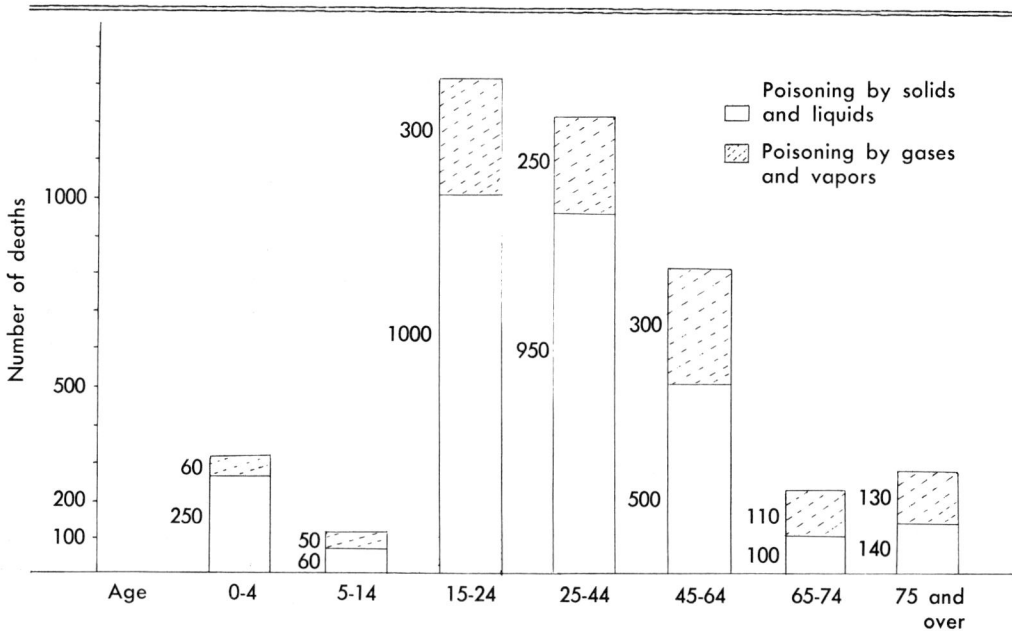

Fig. 17-1. Deaths from poisons, 1971. (From National Safety Council: Accident Facts, 1972.)

Table 17-1. Physical signs that may be caused by various toxins

Presenting symptom	Some poisons to be considered
Vomiting	Heavy metals (lead, arsenic), alcohol, corrosives (iron, acid, alkali), aspirin, phenol, fluoride, parathion, plants, iron, digitalis
Changes of consciousness	Barbiturates, alcohol, tranquilizers, narcotics, benzene, carbon monoxide, carbon dioxide, antihistamines, sedatives, bromides, chloroform, ether, diphenoxylate, tricyclic antidepressants
Convulsions	Strychnine, parathion, dextropropoxyphene, camphor, amphetamines, hydrocarbons, lead, tricyclic antidepressants
Dilated pupils	Belladonna, plants, alcohol, cocaine, amphetamines, nicotine, ephedrine
Myosis	Morphine, dextropropoxyphene, diphenoxylate, parathion
Cyanosis	Acetanilid, nitrites, aniline dyes, phenacetin
Pink skin	Carbon monoxide, atropine (flushed)
Acidosis (Kussmaul respiration)	Aspirin, salicylate, methanol, ethanol, mercuric chloride
Dry mouth	Belladonna, morphine, antihistamines
Hematemesis	Iron, phosphorus, fluoride
Diaphoresis	Parathion, alcohol, insulin, fluoride, aspirin, mercuric chloride, arsenic
Parkinsonism	Phenothiazines

as six hours after ingestion, and (2) narcotics, which, because of depressed gastric motility, are recoverable for longer periods of time. Gastric lavage with a large-bore, multiple-hole tube is useful for gastric emptying. In children, lavage should be performed with half-normal saline to prevent water intoxication from excess absorption. Emetics have been shown clearly superior for complete gastric emptying. They also empty the proximal small bowel, which is an advantage. Syrup of ipecac, 15 to 30 ml orally with ½ to 2 glasses of warm water and repeated at 15-minute intervals to three doses if needed, will generally cause an emesis in 18 to 20 minutes. Do not give more than two glasses of water before emesis occurs to avoid flushing the poison through the pylorus. After emesis has occurred, it can be restimulated by giving additional water.

For a more rapid, controlled emesis, apomorphine, 0.03 mg per pound subcutaneously, will cause emesis almost uniformly in three to ten minutes and may be promptly terminated with administration of naloxone.[2] Apomorphine will cause sedation; therefore, it is not indicated in patients already stuporous or with respiratory depression. Emesis is contraindicated in corrosive ingestion, ingestion of petroleum distillates, and in the sedated patient. In all instances the airway must be protected with ready suction and endotracheal intubation if protective reflexes are depressed (Table 17-2). Because of sedation, this is not commonly used.

A charcoal slurry, using activated charcoal (not burnt toast) will neutralize many poisons and may be given as an adjunct. Since it also absorbs ipecac, activated charcoal should be given only *after* emesis from

Table 17-2. Apomorphine as an emetic

Apomorphine dosage* 0.03 mg/lb or 0.066 mg/kg	Weight		Naloxone dosage 0.4 mg/ml or 0.01 mg/kg
	Pounds	Kilograms	
0.39 mg (0.39 ml)	13	6	0.06 mg (0.15 ml)
0.81 mg (0.81 ml)	27	12	0.12 mg (0.3 ml)
1.20 mg (1.2 ml)	40	19	0.19 mg (0.5 ml)
1.65 mg (1.65 ml)	55	25	0.25 mg (0.6 ml)
2.1 mg (2.1 ml)	68	31	0.31 mg (0.7 ml)
2.5 mg (2.5 ml)	82	37	0.37 mg (0.9 ml)
2.85 mg (2.85 ml)	95	43	0.40 mg (1.0 ml)
3.3 mg (3.3 ml)	110	50	0.5 mg (1.1 ml)
3.7 mg (3.7 ml)	123	56	0.56 mg (1.4 ml)
4.1 mg (4.1 ml)	137	62	0.62 mg (1.5 ml)
4.5 mg (4.5 ml)	150	68	0.68 mg (1.6 ml)
4.65 mg (4.65 ml)	155	70	0.70 mg (1.75 ml)
5.0 mg (5.0 ml)	165	75	0.75 mg (1.8 ml)

NOTE: DO NOT REPEAT APOMORPHINE DOSE

NOTE: IT IS SAFE TO DOUBLE THIS NALOXONE DOSAGE OR IT MAY BE REPEATED

*Apomorphine is used to induce emesis. When adequate emesis is developed, the emesis can be terminated and any side reactions of the apomorphine can be neutralized by the narcotic antagonist, naloxone.

To prepare apomorphine, crush a 6 mg tablet with the plunger of the syringe. Draw up 6 ml (cc) of sterile saline or water. Shake for ½ to 1 minute until dissolved.

The correct dose can then be found in the "established dose schedule." For a child's dosage, a tuberculin syringe or a 2 ml syringe with a needle can withdraw the apomorphine solution through the needle hub of the larger syringe. 1 ml (cc) = 1 mg.

From Rauston, D. S., and Ochs, M. A.: Apomorphine-naloxone controlled rapid emesis, J. Am. Coll. Emerg. Phys. **2**(1):44-45, Jan.-Feb., 1973.

ipecac has occurred. Do not forget that plain water can act as a diluent or flooding agent. Following is a list of drugs well absorbed by charcoal. Fifteen to thirty grams may be mixed in water as a slurry. If desired, cherry syrup may be added to increase palatability.

Alcohol	Nicotine
Amphetamine	Opium
Antimony	Oxalates
Antipyrene	Parathion
Atropine	Penicillin
Arsenic	Phenol
Barbiturates	Phenolphthalein
Camphor	Phenothiazine
Cantharides	Phosphorus
Cocaine	Potassium
Digitalis	permanganate
Glutethimide	Quinidine
Iodine	Salicylate
Ipecac	Selenium
Malathion	Silver
Mercuric chloride	Stramonium
Methylene blue	Strychnine
Morphine	Sulfonamides
Muscarine	

HASTENING ELIMINATION

Cathartics such as magnesium sulfate, sodium sulfate, and Phospho-Soda will accelerate material through the intestinal tract that has already progressed beyond the reach of lavage or emesis.

Volume loading and diuretics increase urine output for those toxins excreted by the renal route. Alkalinization of the urine will markedly enhance the excretion of some toxins, such as salicylate and phenobarbital. Peritoneal dialysis or extracorporeal dialysis may be required in some cases, and exchange transfusion may be necessary. Charcoal perfusion filters may also be useful in removing agents directly from the blood.

SYMPTOMATIC MANAGEMENT

Central nervous system depression requires only supportive care. Previously rec-ommended stimulants, such as methylphenidylacetate (Ritalin), pentylenetetrazol (Metrazol), and picrotoxin are dangerous and may cause seizures.

Hypotension is best treated with fluid loading, followed by central venous pressure monitoring. Pressor agents play a secondary role but may be of vital importance if the central venous pressure is elevated. Seizures are best controlled with intravenous administration of diazepam (Valium) or amobarbital (Amytal) as a second choice. Phenobarbital is used for immediate prophylaxis since phenytoin (Dilantin) is absorbed too slowly to be of value in the emergency situation.

Intracranial hypertension

Intracranial hypertension or cerebral edema, which may result from hypoxia, methanol poisoning, or carbon monoxide poisoning, may be treated with methylprednisolone (Solu-Medrol) or dexamethasone (Decadron). Urea and mannitol will produce an immediate improvement but are followed by a rebound increase in pressure as their osmotic pressure draws interstitial fluid into the intravascular space.

Renal failure

Renal failure, associated with nephrotoxins or prolonged shock, may require peritoneal or renal dialysis.

MEDICATIONS AND APPROPRIATE ANTIDOTES

It must be remembered that there are few specific antidotes available for most medications. However, Table 17-3 lists several specific ones.

Overdose of medications accounts for a large percentage of poisonings. The causes range from the childhood tendency to taste or ingest all things that are handled, to adolescent experimentation with drugs, to mistaken use of the wrong drug, or unknowing overdose based on the philosophy that "if one is good, two are better."

Table 17-3. Specific antidotes available for medications

Poison	Antidote
Morphine, narcotics, propoxyphene (Darvon)	Naloxone (Narcan); also nalorphine (Nalline) and levallorphan (Lorfan)
Iron (ferrous salts)	Desferoxamine
Organic phosphate insecticide	Atropine, 2-PAM
Cyanide	Nitrite
Mercury, arsenic, lead	British anti-Lewisite (B.A.L.)
Lead	Versene, penicillamine
Anticoagulants (warfarin, Dicumarol)	Vitamin K
Tricyclic antidepressants, scopolamine, belladonna alkaloids, diphenhydramine (Benadryl), jimsonweed	Physostigmine

Analgesics

Eighty-five percent of all children poisoned are below the age of 5, and salicylates are the most common agent. Although aspirin is the usual offender, oil of wintergreen is a highly concentrated source; as little as 5 ml is a potentially fatal dose.[3-5] Salicylates have a direct stimulatory effect on the respiratory center with a loss of CO_2 and consequent respiratory alkalosis. Salicylates also induce metabolic derangements leading to accumulation of organic acids and metabolic acidosis.

Excretion occurs almost entirely by the renal route and can be trebled if the urine pH is maintained above 7.0. With good diuresis and maintenance of alkaline urine pH, the salicylate level may be reduced by one half in a 6-hour period. A serum level greater than 30 mg/100 ml at four to six hours postingestion is considered toxic. The syndrome of salicylate intoxication is marked by progressively developing hyperpnea, vomiting, tinnitus, acetone odor on the breath, abdominal pain, delirium, incoordination, restlessness, seizure, coma, uremia, and respiratory failure.

Initial treatment involves delaying absorption by simple water dilution or a charcoal slurry or both. However, large amounts of water should be avoided to prevent (if possible) washing of the salicylate through the pylorus. Gastric emptying should be accomplished at the earliest possible time, while salicylate levels and arterial blood gases are being obtained. In mild cases, treatment may consist only of oral bicarbonate, increased intake of carbohydrate beverages such as sweetened soft drinks, and salty broth. If the P_{CO_2} is less than 20 and the pH below 7.25, the condition is considered serious and intravenous fluids with an alkaline diuresis may be necessary or dialysis may be needed.

Acetophenetidin

Acetophenetidin (phenacetin) is another commonly used analgesic. This drug converts hemoglobin to methemoglobin and sulfhemoglobin resulting in cyanosis. There is also central nervous system stimulation and damage to the kidneys and liver.

The overdosed patient may be cyanotic with sweating, chills, tinnitus, circulatory collapse, polyuria, coma, seizures, and respiratory failure, leading to death. Treatment involves gastric lavage and support of circulation. Methylene blue may be administered intravenously to reduce methemoglobin to hemoglobin. In children use 1.5 to 2 mg/kg. This should be in a 1% solution administered intravenously at a slow rate.

Anesthetics

Cocaine has become a popular drug for abuse but has been around for a long time as a local anesthetic. The fatal dose may be 30 mg, and therefore solutions stronger than 5% generally should not be used. It is much less toxic orally than intravenously, but is rarely fatal. Cocaine causes an initial stimulation of the central nervous system followed by depression spreading from higher to lower nervous centers.

An overdose is characterized by restlessness, excitability, hallucinations, tachycardia, dilated pupils, chills, fever, sensory aberration, abdominal pain, vomiting, numbness, and muscle spasm. This may be followed by irregular respirations, seizure, and circulatory failure. The potent topical vasoconstricting properties may tend to cause septal perforation in the nose when the drug is chronically abused by sniffing.

Initial care involves decontamination, lavage, or the placement of a venous tourniquet above the injection site. Seizures may be controlled with intravenous administration of diazepam (Valium) or barbiturate. If the victim survives beyond three hours, the prognosis is good.

Lidocaine is a most useful local anesthetic and valuable for the treatment of cardiac arrhythmias. The toxic dose is 75 ml of 1% solution for an adult. The basic toxicity and treatment are the same as for cocaine.

Depressants

Among the most commonly abused drugs are the barbiturates, which cause generalized, progressive, central nervous system depression starting with the cortex and progressing to the medullary areas. This may be followed by pulmonary edema, pneumonia, cerebral edema, and subsequent death from respiratory failure. Overdose victims show signs and symptoms beginning with lethargy, progressing to coma, followed by respiratory depression and loss of reflexes. Terminally, respiratory and cardiac depression occur. Chronic use followed by complete abrupt withdrawal will result in a reaction characterized by seizures, which occur 36 to 72 hours later.

Initial care of the overdose victim consists of gastric emptying. If the protective reflexes are absent or depressed, endo-

tracheal intubation with a cuffed tube is necessary to prevent aspiration. Long-acting barbiturates are excreted mainly through the kidneys, and excretion is enhanced by alkaline diuresis. Short-acting barbiturates are cleared mainly by liver metabolism; however, a lesser amount may be cleared in the urine in direct proportion to the amount of diuresis. Subsequent treatment is entirely symptomatic. Central nervous system stimulants should be avoided because of the danger of precipitating seizures. Two exceptions to this are doxapram (Dopram) and ethamivan (Emivan); these respiratory stimulants, under intermittent or constant intravenous infusion, may be used to increase rate and depth of respirations. Hypotension should be treated with fluid loading. Pressor agents should be avoided in the absence of elevated central venous pressure.

Narcotics and narcotic derivatives such as morphine, meperidine (Demerol), opium, codeine, propoxyphene (Darvon), oxycodone (Percodan), diphenoxylate (Lomotil), nalorphine (Nalline), levallorphan (Lorfan), or methadone cause central nervous system depression. The patient may be initially lethargic, progressing to coma with complete respiratory depression. Pupils are pinpoint until terminal stages when they dilate due to hypoxia. The duration of heroin effect is eight hours; however, methadone may last from 24 to 48 hours, and the overdose patient must be observed for a sufficient time to ensure that depression does not recur. Tolerance develops with continued use, leading to maintenance doses in multiples of ordinary use.

Ventilation and respiratory support are the vital points of initial care and must be given prior to drug therapy.

Naloxone (Narcan) is a narcotic antagonist that reverses all effects of the narcotic. Unlike nalorphine (Nalline) and levallorphan (Lorfan), which themselves cause respiratory depression, it has no side effects of its own and can be used when the diagnosis is in doubt. Abrupt narcotic withdrawal produces a "super-flu" syndrome characterized by rhinorrhea, abdominal cramping, sweating, vomiting, diarrhea, and myalgia. In the event of methadone overdose the patient must be observed for 24 to 48 hours, since the duration of the antagonist effect is much less than the duration of the methadone effects.

Antihistamines, such as diphenhydramine (Benadryl) and various antimotion sickness medications, cause a complex central nervous system stimulation and depression characterized by drowsiness, tachycardia, flushing, dry mouth, urinary retention, and in higher doses lead to hallucinations, stupor, coma, and subsequent seizures. Gastric emptying should be accomplished as quickly as possible and blood pressure supported. Stimulants are to be avoided.

Phenothiazines such as prochlorperazine (Compazine), chlorpromazine (Thorazine), trifluoperazine (Stelazine), promazine (Sparine), thiethylperazine maleate (Torecan), and thioridazine (Mellaril) will cause lethargy, postural hypotension due to alpha-blocking effects, tachycardia, and ataxia. High doses or idiosyncratic reactions may produce extrapyramidal effects characterized by nuchal rigidity, muscle spasm, trismus, dysphagia, spinal rigidity, oculogyric crisis, salivation, seizures, and parkinsonism.

Intravenous administration of diphenhydramine (Benadryl), 50 mg, should result in prompt remission of extrapyramidal symptoms. Epinephrine should be avoided in the treatment of hypotension because of the resultant paradoxical hypotension produced by the alpha-blocking effect of the phenothiazine. Levarterenol (Levophed) is recommended for the treatment of hypotension.

Autonomic nervous system drugs—atropine and related compounds, such as belladonna, scopolamine, propantheline (Pro-Banthine), isopropamide (Darbid), and glycopyrrolate (Robinul)—block the action of the effector cells of acetylcholine at nerve endings resulting in delirium, tachycardia, fever, dilated pupils, flushing, tachypnea, urinary retention, and seizures. Physostigmine (Antilirium) can be used to reverse the symptoms of anticholinergic crisis resulting from these drugs. The dosage must be titrated by effect. Further treatment is symptomatic and is aimed chiefly at body cooling and control of seizures. Attention should be directed to possible urinary retention and precipitation of acute glaucoma attacks. Excretion is by the renal route.

Epinephrine, ephedrine, and amphetamines stimulate cells located in muscles and glands that are innervated by the sympathetic nervous system and cause central nervous system stimulation. Large doses lead to nausea, vomiting, chills, irritability, tachycardia, dilated pupils, seizure, coma, respiratory failure, hypertension, hallucinations, paranoid psychosis, and arrhythmias. Initial care is directed at gastric emptying and control of seizures. Sedatives may be helpful.

Drugs of the physostigmine group—neostigmine, pilocarpine, bethanechol (Urecholine), edrophonium (Tensilon), and pyridostigmine (Mestinon)—block the effect of acetylcholinesterase or stimulate the receptor site to produce a parasympathetic overactivity. This is manifest in salivation, lacrimation, urination, defecation, pinpoint pupils, vomiting, wheezing, and bronchial constriction, muscle twitching, thready pulse, seizures, and death from asphyxia and bradycardia. Airway care is of primary concern and ventilation and suctioning of secretions must be accomplished prior to drug therapy. Atropine in large doses may be used to titrate the effects, using cardiac rate to judge adequacy of atropinization. Pupillary size is an unreliable index for treatment. If atropine is administered prior to adequate oxygenation, cardiac arrhythmias may be precipitated.

Antidepressants

Tricyclic antidepressants such as amitriptyline (Elavil) and imipramine (Tofranil) can cause sedation, tachyarrhythmias, seizures, coma, cardiovascular collapse, and death. These drugs prevent the reuptake of norepinephrine at the nerve ending and thereby cause a catecholamine-excess phase marked by tachyarrhythmias, excitation, and seizures, followed by a catecholamine-depletion phase marked by cardiovascular collapse and death.

Treatment consists of immediate gastric emptying. Physostigmine (Antilirium) should be administered if the pulse is greater than 140/min, or symptoms are progressive. Peripheral and central blood pressure should be closely monitored and supported with volume expansion followed by a dopamine (Intropin) infusion with the addition of levophed (Levarterenol) if necessary to maintain pressure. Cardiac monitoring is necessary for up to 72 hours due to delayed arrhythmias.

Antiseptics

Iodine and iodide cause precipitation of protein, which results in irritation and erosion of the mucosa of the gastrointestinal tract, along with renal damage in the form of glomerular and tubular necrosis. Victims exhibit vomiting, diarrhea, thirst, fever, anuria, vascular collapse, delirium, coma, uremia, and subsequent death. The fatal dose is approximately 2 g. Treatment involves lavage with starch water until no blue color returns. (Starch plus iodide produces a blue color.) Prognosis is good if survival exceeds 48 hours; however, esophageal strictures may occur at a later time.

Phenol and disinfectants such as creosotes, caustics, germicides, and surface antiseptics denature and precipitate protein, and small doses may simulate salicylate toxicity. Necrosis of mucosal surfaces and central nervous system edema occur, resulting in vomiting, collapse, coma, seizures, and pulmonary edema. Absorption should be delayed and gastric emptying accomplished followed by administration of 60 ml of castor oil, which dissolves phenol and retards its absorption. This is followed by a saline cathartic. For topical exposure the area should be washed for 15 minutes with repeated applications of castor oil or 10% ethyl alcohol.

Cardiovascular drugs

Digitalis in normal doses increases myocardial contractility; however, higher doses produce increased myocardial irritability characterized by multiple arrhythmia patterns. There are also central nervous system effects typified by nausea, vomiting, "yellow vision," and delirium. The pulse may be slow or irregular, and heart block, ventricular tachycardia, or ventricular fibrillation may be precipitated. For an acute overdose, gastric emptying should be accomplished. Increasing serum potassium levels counteracts the effect on the myocardium. Intravenous infusions of lidocaine, potassium, or phenytoin (Dilantin) are effective in controlling arrhythmias, and propranolol (Inderal), by its beta-adrenergic blocking effect, is also effective in arrhythmia control.

Quinidine causes a slowing of myocardial conduction and prolongation of the refractory period leading to heart block. The overdose patient may exhibit tinnitus, nausea, diarrhea, hypotension, nystagmus, or bradycardia. If hypotension occurs, it should be treated with pressor agents. Intravenous lactate will antagonize the effects of quinidine.

Propranolol produces a beta-adrenergic blockade. In larger doses it produces cardiac failure, nausea, vomiting, diarrhea, dizziness, and constipation; it may precipitate asthma attacks in susceptible individuals. Intravenous administration of isoproterenol (Isuprel) will competitively inhibit the effects of propranolol.

Stimulants

Theophylline and aminophylline, if administered intravenously at too rapid a rate, produce cardiac inhibition, vascular collapse, and death. Large doses may result in generalized seizures and some subsequent central nervous system depression. Initial care involves oxygenation, support of blood pressure, and treatment of seizures.

Strychnine, which is found in tonics and some rodenticides, is fatal in doses of 15 to 30 mg. This drug causes increased reflex excitability in the spinal cord. This results in simultaneous contraction of all muscles due to the loss of normal inhibition of the spread of motor cell stimulation. Doses less than necessary to cause acute poisoning are without toxic effect. The toxic individual exhibits increased deep tendon reflexes followed by stiffness progressing to muscle spasm, which is elicited by any sensory stimulation. Death follows from respiratory failure. Initial care involves lavage unless the patient is seizing, in which case treatment consists only of control of seizures with intravenous administration of diazepam (Valium) and supportive care. The prognosis is good if survival exceeds 24 hours.

MISCELLANEOUS AGENTS
Carbon monoxide poisoning

Carbon monoxide, a colorless, odorless, tasteless gas, is the product of incomplete combustion. Its bond to hemoglobin is approximately 250 times as strong as that of oxygen, and consequently it displaces oxygen from the hemoglobin molecule. Carbon monoxide also shifts the oxyhemoglobin dissociation curve to the left, resulting in less availability of oxygen at the cellular level.

Carboxyhemoglobin has a bright red color and imparts this color to the skin of the victim—a true red herring in a patient who may actually be severely hypoxic. A normal arterial oxygen tension may also mislead since it will be unaffected by the carbon monoxide and may be in the normal range despite high carboxyhemoglobin levels. A metabolic acidosis, however, will reflect the severity of the cellular hypoxia.

Significant symptoms begin at carboxyhemoglobin levels of 20% to 30% and start with severe headache. At levels of 30% to 40% the patient will show weakness, dizziness, diplopia, and nausea and may collapse and act intoxicated. With levels of 40% to 70%, coma, seizures, Cheyne-Stokes respirations, and death may occur.

A positive history and the presence of symptoms justify treatment immediately since central nervous system damage from the cellular hypoxia is devastating and irreversible, and one cannot wait for the results of laboratory confirmation. Treatment involves simply displacing the carbon monoxide by high concentrations of oxygen.

Administering 100% oxygen for four hours will assure return to safe levels, or if it is available, the victim may be placed in hyperbaric oxygen at 2.5 atmospheres pressure for one hour with similar results. Residual symptoms are due to cerebral edema and hypoxic damage.

Carbogen should not be used since the resultant hyperventilation does not assist in carbon monoxide removal. It also superimposes a respiratory acidosis from exogenous carbon dioxide on a preexisting metabolic acidosis, which is equally undesirable.

Correction of the metabolic acidosis with sodium bicarbonate is a complex problem since it also would further shift the oxyhemoglobin dissociation curve to the left and decrease availability of oxygen at the tissue level.

Disulfiram

Disulfiram (Antabuse) blocks the enzymatic breakdown of ethanol at the acetaldehyde level, allowing it to accumulate in the system. In mild reactions, flushing, sweating, tachycardia, breathlessness, hyperventilation, hypotension, nausea, vomiting, and lethargy may occur. More severe reactions are accompanied by severe hypotension, arrhythmia, air-hunger, cardiac pain, and possible myocardial infarction. Primary care involves respiratory support, maintenance of blood pressure with pressor agents, and the use of ascorbic acid to ameliorate the alcohol-disulfiram reaction. This reaction may be fatal especially in the presence of preexisting heart disease, diabetes, pregnancy, atherosclerosis, or hypothyroidism.

Iron salts

Iron salts are absorbed only in the ferrous form. The fatal dose for a 2-year-old child ranges from 5 to 10 g. There is also a corrosive effect on the mucosa. Initial signs may be lethargy, vomiting, tarry stools, diarrhea, fast, weak pulse, fall in blood pressure, and circulatory collapse. If not immediately fatal, the symptoms clear in four to six hours, leading to a 6- to 24-hour asymptomatic period during which there is a temporary binding of the iron salts in the reticular cells. This is followed by disruption of the cells with the release of the iron into the system once again, causing a relapse with cyanosis, vasomotor collapse, pulmonary edema, coma, and death within 12 to 48 hours.

Initial care involves delay of absorption and gastric emptying by emesis. A 1% sodium bicarbonate solution may be given orally or by nasogastric tube to precipitate remaining iron. Transfusions may be needed if hemorrhage occurs. Confirmation of ingestion or the adequacy of gastric emptying may be obtained with an x-ray of the abdomen since the pills are radiopaque. If serum levels are greater than 500 mg/100 ml, deferoxamine (Desferal) is administered to chelate the iron. The recommended dose of 1 g should be given intramuscularly; however, if the patient is in shock, the

intravenous route should be used to ensure absorption. The rate of infusion should not exceed 15 mg/kg/hr. Serum iron levels should be checked periodically. If serum levels are greater than 500 mg/100 ml, the urine will turn a rosé color after administration of deferoxamine. Prognosis is good if survival exceeds 48 hours; however, death may occur up to one week after ingestion. Strictures in the small bowel may occur as a late complication leading to intestinal obstruction.

Household chemicals

Bleaching solutions are 3% to 6% sodium hypochloride. These solutions cause severe irritation by inhalation or ingestion of the chemical resulting in coughing and choking and progressing to pharyngeal edema. Initial treatment consists of dilution, either topically by flooding or orally by administration of water, followed by the administration of sodium thiosulfate, 5 to 10 g in 200 ml of water, which causes a decomposition of the bleaching solution. An alternative is to give sodium bicarbonate and a cathartic.

Insecticides

Insecticides of the chlorinated hydrocarbon group, such as DDT, methoxychlor, aldrin, Dieldrin, Endrin, and chlordane, block nerve function. They act directly on the cerebellum and motor cortex leading to vomiting, tremor, and seizures. They are also associated with hepatic and renal damage and cause edema and hemorrhages in the brain, liver, and kidneys. If ingestion has occurred, the stomach should be emptied as soon as possible and cathartics given. Skin contamination should be treated at once with a shower and shampoo with careful attention given to areas beneath nails and in the ear canals. Respiration must be supported and anticonvulsants administered as needed. No stimulants should be given. If tremor is the only manifestation, the patient will probably be asymptomatic in two to three months. If seizures occur, the prognosis is questionable.

Cholinesterase inhibitors

Another group of insecticides or nerve gases are the cholinesterase inhibitors such as parathion, malathion, metacide, TEPP, and EPN. These insecticides are phosphate esters and combine with and inactivate acetylcholinesterase. This results in (1) increased parasympathetic activity characterized by salivation, lacrimation, urination, defecation, and cardiac slowing; (2) depolarization of skeletal muscles resulting in tremor and paralysis; and (3) stimulation progressing to depression of the central nervous system. The effects are cumulative over a period of four to six weeks.

Mild toxicity is manifest as headache and dizziness, some weakness and tremor, and impairment of visual acuity with miosis. Moderate toxicity is characterized by gastrointestinal hyperactivity with nausea, vomiting, cramping, and salivation. There is also cardiac slowing, sweating, tearing, and muscular fasciculation. Severe toxicity is marked by respiratory difficulty, pulmonary edema, loss of sphincter control, pinpoint and nonreactive pupils, diarrhea, seizures, coma, and heart block. Because of the cumulative effects, a single, relatively small exposure may result in sudden severe symptoms out of proportion to that specific contact.

Initial care is directed at the respiratory system with suctioning and oxygenation. This is followed by large intravenous doses of atropine given in 1 mg increments every three to five minutes until the pulse rate is above 80 per minute. Other signs of atropinization, such as pupil size, are less reliable. NOTE: Do not give atropine prior to oxygenation since fatal arrhythmias may occur. Simultaneously with the above treatment, begin thorough decontamination by shower and shampoo and gastric emptying if indicated. To reactivate cholinesterase,

2-PAM (Protopam) may be given in a 1 g dose intravenously, repeated twice within each 24-hour period, but only for organic phosphate cholinesterase inhibitor intoxication. It may be harmful in carbamate cholinesterase inhibitor intoxication. This drug should be administered only with maximum atropine administration.

Lead

Lead is often found in the paint of older buildings and may be chewed from the walls and furniture by small children. Other sources include glazes and fumes from such materials as storage batteries, industrial compounds, and painted objects. Acute poisoning causes inflammation of the gastrointestinal tract and renal tubular degeneration. Chronic poisoning is associated with cerebral edema and degeneration of nerve and muscle cells. In acute poisoning the patient exhibits abdominal pain, vomiting, diarrhea, black stools, oliguria, collapse, and coma. Chronic poisoning results in a progression of symptoms from anorexia and weight loss, gastrointestinal upset, fatigue, headache, weakness, and anemia to more persistent vomiting, nervousness, incoordination, stupor, and lethargy. Peripheral sensory disturbances progress to encephalopathy, cranial nerve paralysis, delirium, seizures, and coma. Symptoms suggestive of incipient encephalopathy should be considered an emergency. Laboratory studies showing a blood lead level above 0.1 mg/100 ml and the appearance of radiopaque material on a plain film of the abdomen or lead lines in the wrists and knees on x-ray films are sufficient indication to start therapy. Gastric emptying and catharsis should be followed by diuresis. If symptoms of lead poisoning are present, dimercaprol, 4 mg/kg intramuscularly every four hours for 30 doses, should be initiated. Beginning four hours later, calcium disodium edetate, 12.5 mg/kg, is administered intramuscularly every 4 hours in a 20% solution for a total of 30 doses.

INDUSTRIAL COMPOUNDS

Methanol is found in solvents, denaturants, antifreeze, and paint remover. It is metabolized to formic acid and formaldehyde in the cells and distributed within the water throughout the body, thus accounting for its particularly destructive concentrations within the eye. The patient exhibits visual disturbances, acidosis, vomiting, diarrhea, and central nervous system depression. The stomach should be emptied, and ethyl alcohol may be given as an antidote since it competitively inhibits the metabolism of methanol. Acidosis should be corrected and fluids administered. There is a 50% mortality if the Pco_2 is below 20. Vision that has not improved after one week has a poor prognosis.

Ethanol is metabolized at 15 to 30 ml per hour and results in central nervous system depression. Chronic use is associated with liver, renal, and cerebral damage. With blood alcohol levels from 0.05 to 0.10 mg/100 ml there is mild visual impairment, slightly impaired coordination, and some decrease in reaction time. Blood alcohol levels of 0.15 to 0.3 mg/100 ml are associated with slurred speech, incoordination, sensory loss, and definite visual impairment. Severe intoxication with blood levels of 0.3 to 0.5 mg/100 ml is associated with marked incoordination, diplopia, stupor, and possible severe hypoglycemia with seizures, especially in children. Fatalities begin in this range, and with blood alcohol levels greater than 0.5 mg/100 ml, coma or respiratory depression and death occur. Intervention consists of gastric emptying and supportive care. Differential diagnosis in a patient with the odor of liquor present must include postictal states, hypoglycemia, head injury, psychosis, and ingestion of other drugs.

Hydrocarbons, such as kerosene, gasoline, petroleum distillates, naphtha, paint thinner, and benzene, are irritants that dissolve fat and lead to central nervous system depression. Aspiration causes dispersion over a large surface area of the lung resulting in lipid pneumonia. The patient exhibits coughing, choking, nausea, vomiting, and progressive pulmonary edema. Gastrointestinal upset and bronchial pneumonia may occur. Liver, kidney, and bone marrow damage are seen with benzene ingestion particularly. Doses in excess of 1 ml/kg are associated with central nervous system depression, seizures, and coma. The prevention of aspiration should be of primary concern in the initial treatment. Liquid petrolatum, once felt useful in delaying absorption, is now felt to add undue risk of aspiration and to be of little benefit. If the amount ingested exceeds 1 ml/kg, careful gastric emptying should be accomplished. If protective reflexes are depressed, the trachea should be intubated to prevent aspiration. Following lavage, a cathartic such as magnesium sulfate or sodium sulfate should be left in the stomach.

If the patient is alert and cough and gag reflexes intact, less risk of aspiration occurs simply by giving ipecac to induce emesis. Signs of aspiration should be treated with cortisone and antibiotics. After 24 hours, the severity is directly proportional to the pulmonary involvement.

CORROSIVES

Acids and acidlike chemicals, such as sodium acid sulfate (a toilet bowl cleaner that produces sulfuric acid and nitrogen oxide), are chemicals that precipitate protein. The resultant corrosion is associated with perforation of the esophagus and stomach; intense vascular stimulation also occurs, resulting in a vascular collapse. Hematemesis, shock, peritonitis, and mediastinitis are associated with perforations. Inhalation causes choking, dizziness, and weakness progressing in six to eight hours to pulmonary edema. Skin burns and corneal destruction are associated with topical contamination. Initial care involves diluting the acid with milk, water, or egg followed by lavage if ingestion occurred less than one hour previously. Shock and pain are treated symptomatically. Topical contamination, particularly ophthalmic, is treated by flooding with water for 15 minutes.

Alkalies denature protein and convert fat to soap. The particular hazard here is the persistent penetration of the chemical because of its solubility; damage is directly proportional to length of exposure. Topical irrigation and washing should continue until the "soapy, slippery" feeling is gone from the skin. Milk, citrus juices, and diluted vinegar may be used for ingested alkali and must be administered at once. All patients who have ingested lye should be admitted to the hospital. Steroids and antibiotics should be given until esophagoscopy has ruled out any esophageal lesions. If these are present, then the patient must remain on steroids and antibiotics and be fed via a small, thin tube.

ANIMAL TOXINS

Refer to Chapter 18. For stingray toxin refer to Chapter 19.

PLANTS

Personnel involved in providing emergency care should be familiar with the more common varieties of poisonous plant life in their area. Whenever the toxicity of a particular plant is not known, it should be treated as potentially hazardous, and gastric emptying should be accomplished.

Castor beans

These seeds contain ricin, a toxic albumin, which causes agglutination and hemolysis of red blood cells and is associated with hemorrhage and edema of the gastrointestinal tract and the kidneys. Vomiting and diarrhea, associated with circulatory collapse, will occur. Symptoms may be delayed one to three days and are accompanied by abdominal pain, disorientation, cyanosis, and oliguria progressing to uremia. Gastric emptying and cathartics are indicated along with support of circula-

tion. The urine should be alkalinized to prevent precipitation of hemoglobin, and a diuresis should be maintained. There is a 5% mortality rate, and death may occur up to 14 days following ingestion.

Mushrooms (Amanita)

The two most dangerous species of mushrooms are the *Amanita muscaria* and *Amanita phalloides*. The first contains two alkaloids, one of which has atropinelike effects, and the second has effects similar to those of parasympathetic stimulation. The latter alkaloid is called muscarine. Signs and symptoms of *Amanita muscaria* ingestion begin within one to two hours and are characterized by excitement, delirium, salivation, lacrimation, vomiting, diarrhea, bradycardia, varying pupillary reaction, and muscle tremor. In *Amanita phalloides* toxicity there is a latent interval of 12 to 24 hours followed by severe gastrointestinal reaction including nausea, vomiting, diarrhea, hematemesis, and melena. Hepatomegaly, jaundice, pulmonary edema, confusion, hypoglycemia, coma, and seizures may occur. Initial care involves gastric emptying and catharsis. Atropine in large doses, such as 2 mg followed by 1 mg increments at 3- to 5-minute intervals, may be given with caution and repeated as needed. Symptomatic treatment of electrolyte imbalance and hypoglycemia should be given. Liver function may return in six to eight days. There is a 50% mortality associated with liver damage.

Oleander

This popular flowering shrub is found in many yards as well as in great abundance as a road divider along many of the nation's highways. All parts of this plant are toxic. Ingestion is treated with gastric emptying and then as for digitalis overdose.

Arum family

Plants of the Arum family (calla lily, dieffenbachia, philodendron) all contain oxalic acid crystals, which produce severe irritation of the mucous membranes and may be associated with nausea, vomiting, and diarrhea. Treatment involves flooding the area with water and gastric emptying if ingestion has occurred.

Marijuana

Marijuana contains the chemical cannabinol, a mild hallucinogen that is found in the leaves and flowering tips. The chemical produces altered awareness of time, variable drowsiness, lack of coordination, and inflammation of the mucous membranes. Its effect on the nervous system produces a state of intoxication with a feeling of well-being, some confusion, loss of judgment, and some feeling of levity. There may be a depression, moodiness, or anxiety. Treatment involves observation, reassurance, and mild sedation if anxiety is significant.

Jimsonweed

Jimsonweed contains belladonna derivatives and produces hallucinations, arrhythmias, flushing, tachycardia, mydriasis, hyperpyrexia, and possibly seizures and coma. Treatment is gastric emptying, with physostigmine given as for tricyclic antidepressants. Arrhythmias may occur for up to 24 to 48 hours.

SUMMARY

It should be remembered that there are a significant number of poisonings yearly and that adequate preparation must be made in advance to expedite their treatment in the emergency department. Education of the personnel involved in providing emergency care of poison victims, provision of needed medication and equipment, and acquisition of a basic toxicology library provide the groundwork for efficient handling of cases.

REFERENCES

1. National Safety Council: Accident facts, 1972.
2. Rauston, D. S., and Ochs, M. A.: Apomorphine-naloxone controlled rapid emesis, J. Am. Coll. Emerg. Phys. **2**(1):44-45, 1973.
3. Dreisbach, R. H.: Handbook of poisoning, Los Altos, Calif., 1969, Lange Medical Publications.
4. Goodman, L. S., and Gilman, A.: The pharmacologic basis of therapeutics, London, 1970, Collier-Macmillan Publishers.
5. Gleason, M. N., et al.: Clinical toxicology of commercial products, Baltimore, 1969, The Williams & Wilkins Co.

ADDITIONAL READINGS

Rumack, B. H., and Temple, A. R., editors: Management of the poisoned patient, Princeton, N.J., 1970, The Science Press.
Weil, M. H., and Shubin, H., editors: Critical care medicine handbook, Baltimore, 1974, The Williams & Wilkins Co.

CHAPTER 18

Poisonous reptiles and insects

W. T. Soldmann, Jr., M.D.

There are about 2,500 species of snakes in the world. Of these, about 200 are dangerous. They are dangerous either because of tremendous strength and weight or because of the presence of toxins and an effective means of administrating these toxins.

There are 30 species and 66 subspecies of rattlesnakes, two species and four subspecies of coral snakes, and one species of Gila monster. Some species of rattlesnakes are found in countries other than the United States.

Good statistical records of the incidence of venomous snake bites in the United States or the world have never been tabulated. It has been estimated that approximately 30,000 persons are killed by venomous snakes each year in the world; 5% of these persons are in Bombay, India. However, these figures are estimates and are not verified by registered deaths. It has also been estimated that there are approximately 1,000 persons bitten by poisonous snakes in the continental United States each year.[1] Approximately 30 of these bites, or 3%, will be fatal. Another statistic, gathered in 1968, revealed that fewer than 7,000 persons in the United States suffered venomous snake bites with some degree of poisoning and of these only 15 died.[2] Of those bitten, the ratio of men to women

is about 2:1. About 50% of the victims are children (60% are less than 20 years old). Bites usually occur from April to October with the peak in July and August. The greatest concentration of snake bites occurs in the southern United States. Maine, Delaware, Alaska, and Hawaii claim that there are no snakes in these states.

By far the most numerous bites occur on the limbs, with more bites occurring on the lower than on the upper limbs.[3] Bites on the limbs are less serious than those on the body because of isolation of venom, ease of treatment, and relatively slow absorption of the toxins. However, when the venom enters a vascular area or directly into a vein, the bite is much more serious regardless of what part of the body is envenomated.

PIT VIPERS
Anatomy

The only poisonous reptiles indigenous to the United States are pit vipers, coral snakes, and Gila monsters. The pit vipers include all poisonous snakes that have a "pit" in their head. This is a depression that lies distal to and below the eye and between the eye and the nostril. There is one depression on each side of the head (Fig. 18-1). In a broad sense this group includes rattlesnakes and snakes without

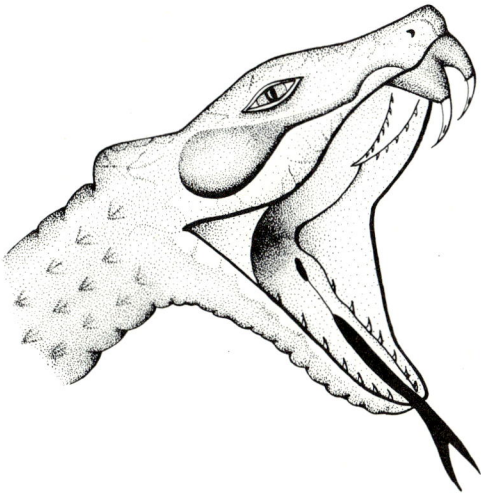

Fig. 18-1. Pit viper.

rattles, such as moccasins and copperheads.

The pit vipers may have front fangs or back fangs. The front-fanged snakes are more common and more dangerous to man. The back-fanged snakes rarely bite people, and when they do, they must literally chew before they can inject their venom.

Striking mechanism

The fangs of pit vipers are efficient hypodermic needles. They are curved, and the discharging opening is just above the tip of the tooth on the front surface. In the process of biting, the fangs are driven into the victim by one set of muscles. The venom sacs are then evacuated by another set of muscles; the venom is forced into the fang and finally into the victim. Therefore, it is possible to be bitten and still not receive any venom into the tissues. The fangs may vary from 0.5 to 2.5 cm (¼ to 1 inch) in length. They are retractable, similar to a cat's claw, and are kept at rest in a depression in the upper jaw of the reptile. There are six fangs on each side of the maxilla in various stages of development. The most mature of these projects out of a sheath in the front of the upper jaw. In the forepart of the snake's

head are four sockets. Two of these are used by the most mature of the fangs. The other two will receive the next two fangs to mature. Fangs are shed, and when this happens, the next most mature fangs replace them and seat themselves in the empty sockets. Fangs are shed approximately every six to eight weeks. Because of shedding and because fangs are delicate, it is conceivable that at times a snake will have one or no fangs present.

Anatomic findings that do not always indicate a poisonous snake are a triangle-shaped head, vertical elliptical pupils, the presence of rattles, and a heavy, thick body.

It is not necessary for a snake to be coiled before it can strike. The forepart of the body needs only to be in the attitude of flexion for striking. The snake can then strike to a distance of one third to one half of its body length. It does not jump into the air. The speed of the strike has been estimated at approximately 8 miles per hours. The snake will usually strike and then recoil, but it may strike again. Because the snake can open its jaws to about 180 degrees, it can strike a flat surface. There has been some discussion as to whether a snake strikes or bites. However, it is evident that the snake thrusts its body forward as a strike, and as soon as it touches an object, its jaws close in the attitude of biting.

Venom

The venom of a poisonous snake is a highly sophisticated mixture of poisons and enzymes for the twofold purpose of killing and digesting its victims.

Pit vipers are viviparous; newborn snakes have venom in their glands, but this venom is not as poisonous as the venom of adult snakes. The potency of the venom also varies with the species of snake and supposedly with the seasons, although this is disputed by authorities.

The largest pit viper ever measured was

an eastern rattlesnake *(Crotalus adamanteus).* It was 255 cm in length and weighed about 10 kg.

Signs and symptoms of snake bite

Immediate and usually intense pain followed in a very few minutes by swelling and subsequent bleeding is almost always diagnostic of snake venom poisoning. Classically, the signs and symptoms of snake envenomation are as follows:

1. There will usually be two puncture wounds above and two below. The upper two are almost always the largest and represent the wounds from the fangs.
2. An intense, burning pain is almost always present.
3. Swelling and edema occur very rapidly and progress rapidly.
4. A bloody discharge appears around the wound.
5. Ecchymosis of the tissues begins early and spreads extensively over the limb and trunk of the victim.
6. If untreated, pain will last for hours, but it may be followed by numbness. The edema and swelling may engulf a great deal of the body. Ecchymosis continues, and as the venom is absorbed into the body, hemorrhages can occur in internal organs with resulting hematuria and intestinal bleeding.
7. Muscle fasciculation and twitching usually occur and may begin immediately after the bite. It is frequently seen circumorally.
8. The victim may have difficulty articulating, and the speech will be slurred.
9. Nausea and vomiting frequently occur.
10. Blisters and bleb formation usually begin in about one hour. The blebs become very large and later will be hemorrhagic.
11. Syncope and coma are common.
12. Sweating occurs.
13. The pulse becomes very rapid and the blood pressure drops.
14. Respirations become shallow, and respiratory failure can occur.

When signs and symptoms occur rapidly, one can assume that (1) there has been a great deal of venom injected, (2) it is of a toxic nature, (3) absorption has been rapid, and (4) the condition of the victim warrants rapid and heroic treatment.

Variables

Because of the many variables when a person is bitten, prognosis and treatment are difficult to estimate. A snake bite is not a simple affliction producing uniform results. There are variations in the size, age, sex, and health of both the victim and the snake. There will be variations in the rate of absorption of the venom and the sensitivity of the victim to the venom. The patient may be allergic to the proteins in the venom. An emotional and excitable individual may increase absorption of the venom by activity. The general body reaction to a bite will be less severe if the bite is at the distal end of an extremity or if it is in a fatty area. The bite may be a deeply penetrating wound or merely a scratch. If the victim is dressed in heavy clothing or leather boots, the fangs may not penetrate the skin. Variables concerning the snake also are present. The snake may strike and puncture the skin with only one fang. When the weather is cold (snakes are poikilothermic), snakes are sluggish, and even though they may strike, the fangs may not penetrate the skin. When snakes are irritated or agitated, they are more dangerous. If the snake has just killed an animal, it may have emptied part or all of the venom sac and not have much venom left if it strikes again. The size and health of the snake also affect the severity of the bite. The venom of certain pit vipers is more toxic than others.

Therefore, the gravity of a snake bite

cannot be easily prognosticated unless one knows all the circumstances pertaining to the bite. Even if all these variables are known, we still have to deal with the psychologic impact that the bite has on the victim. Even the type of first aid will affect the outcome. In some cases folklore treatment may have a deleterious effect on the ultimate outcome of the condition. The condition of the victim is greatly modified also by the period lapsed between the time the bite occurred and the time the patient reaches the emergency department.

Management

In caring for the victim, one strives to (1) remove as much venom as possible, (2) prevent further absorption, (3) neutralize any venom that has been absorbed, (4) treat any condition that has resulted from the envenomation, and (5) prevent complications so that rehabilitation will not be protracted.

Field and first aid care. Slow down the absorption of the venom. The victim should be out of the sun in a cool spot and should lie down if possible. The affected limb should be dependent. A tourniquet should be applied just tight enough to constrict the venous and lymphatic flow but should not constrict the arterial flow. The tourniquet should be placed at a soft muscular area of the body and never on a digit or over a bony prominence. It should be moved approximately every 15 to 20 minutes. When it is reapplied, it should be moved proximally on the limb in advance of the swelling. When the tourniquet is moved, some of the venom will leak into the general circulation. This will not severely harm the victim, since the body is capable of handling small amounts of venom. The affected part should be washed, since some of the venom may be deposited on the skin.

Incision and suction. This must be done as soon as possible and definitely within the first hour. The incision should be made along the long axis of the limb and should be approximately 0.5 cm deep (or through the layers of the skin) and approximately 1.5 cm long. It should traverse each of the holes made by the fangs. Cruciate incisions are not advisable. Suction should then be applied and continued for at least one hour. It is not advisable to use mouth suction unless no other method is available.

Ice or ice water may be applied to the wound. Do not add salt or other chemicals to the ice water. Do not apply the ice with pressure. Ethyl chloride or other freezing agents should not be applied to the wound. However, these agents may be used to freeze a wet piece of cloth and this may be applied.

Apply dressings to cover the wound. Field dressings are applied to prevent further contamination of the wound.

If possible, portage the victim out of the area and to a medical facility. The victim should never run and should move as little as possible. *Never cauterize the wound with either heat or medicaments.*

Hospital management. Any person who has been bitten by a poisonous snake should be hospitalized for at least 24 hours. Although most of the cardinal symptoms occur rapidly and are recognizable, delayed symptoms can and do occur. In fact, when one is bitten by the Mohave (*Crotalus s. scutulatus*) rattlesnake the initial symptoms are usually mild, and the severe symptoms, such as respiratory failure, do not appear until 24 hours later.

Antivenin. The only specific therapy for poisonous snake envenomation is the administration of antivenin. In the United States two kinds of antivenin are available: antivenin (Crotalidae) polyvalent (Wyeth), and antivenin (*Micrurus fulvius*) (equine origin) North American coral snake (Wyeth Pkg. No. 62A139). The Crotalidae polyvalent antivenin is taken from horses injected with prepared venom from *Crotalus d. terrificus, C atrox, C adamanteus,* and *Bothrops atrox* (fer-de-lance). The antivenin is lyophilized and will keep unrefrigerated as long as five years.

Because the antivenin is made from horse serum, the victim must be tested for sensitivity to the serum. Directions for the testing will usually be found in the package insert. In the event that the instructions are lost, follow these steps:

1. Before beginning the testing have epinephrine on hand.

2. Get a good history of any sensitivity to horses or horse serum. Ascertain if there is any history of allergy to food, pollens, and the like, and if the patient has had attacks of hay fever or asthma.

3. Using a short 27-gauge needle and a small syringe, inject approximately 0.10 ml of a 1:10 dilution of the horse serum intradermally. This will be sufficient to form a small wheal in the skin. The wheal will be white at first. If the patient is sensitive to horse serum, the area will become red within 10 to 15 minutes. If the patient develops any local or systemic reactions (usually within 20 minutes), do not give the antivenin.

In the event that a history of allergy or sensitivity to horse serum is discovered, the test material should be diluted to a 1:100 dilution before testing.

4. If the individual shows signs of severe reaction to the test (irritability, urticaria, sneezing, edema of the eyelids, face, or lips, respiratory distress, or cyanosis), inject 0.3 to 0.5 ml of a 1:1,000 dilution of epinephrine subcutaneously and observe the patient closely. Because of the possibility of respiratory failure, be prepared to give resuscitation and oxygen. Also, be aware that shock may ensue.

5. An alternate method of testing is to drop one or two drops of a 1:0 solution of horse serum on the conjunctiva of the eye. If the test is positive, the conjunctiva will become red. If the reaction is severe, one or two drops of a 1:1,000 solution of epinephrine may be placed on the conjunctiva to neutralize the effect of the horse serum.

The amount of antivenin needed to treat any given case is empirical. The determining factors are the severity of the signs and symptoms and the rapidity with which they develop (Table 18-1). The amount to be used is also inversely proportionate to the size of the victim. Other determining factors are (1) the amount of venom injected that must be neutralized; (2) the quantity of venom that the patient's body can take care of by its own inherent defense (relative to the patient's weight and the minimal lethal dose); and (3) the quantity of venom eliminated by such accessory methods as incision and suction. It is better to give too much antivenin than too little, and it is better to give a large dose at one time than to give a series of injections.

The antivenin may be given subcutaneously, intramuscularly, intravenously, or intraarterially. When administering antivenin, particularly via the intravenous or intraarterial route, it is advisable to have on hand and ready for use a corticosteroid that can be given intravenously.[4,5] It is well, when giving antivenin via the intraarterial[6] route, to mix the corticosteroid with the antivenin before administering it.

Antivenin is never given in or around a digit; nor does there seem to be any benefit in injecting the antivenin around a wound.

Antibiotics. Antibiotics and antitetanus will be necessary. The snake's mouth harbors many different types of bacteria, and the victim will be inoculated with these.

Shock. Be aware that shock may ensue, fluid balance must be watched, and pain should be treated. If morphine is used, respiratory failure is not uncommon. Oxygen and respiratory support must be on hand.

The patient should be typed and crossmatched for whole blood. Frequently there is a considerable loss of blood into tissue. The enzymes of the venom will decrease the coagulability of blood, destroy blood vessels, any lyse red cells. Hemorrhage and ecchymosis are common to all snake bites.

Steroids should always be used when giving antivenin intraarterially.[4] They should also be used to prevent and alleviate the toxic symptoms of envenomation.

Surgery. The steps in surgery directly to the wound and fasciotomy are as follows:

1. Apply sterile technique when cleansing the wound and surrounding area. Venom is frequently spattered around the wound.

2. If there are signs and symptoms of severe reaction to the venom, even though as much as two hours have elapsed since the patient was bitten, it is well to make a 2.5 to 3 cm elliptical incision around the puncture wounds and remove this skin. This will allow for better suction and will also provide for better drainage. It will help to prevent further edema and swelling.

3. After antivenin has been started, discontinue the tourniquet.

4. Dress the wound. Use copious dressings as there will be a great deal of drainage. If the hand is involved, use a full hand dressing covering the hand and the wrist. The fingers should be in anatomic flexion, and the tips of the fingers should be exposed so that circulation can be observed.

5. The large blebs and blisters that form will be filled with serum at first, but later these will become hemorrhagic. They should be opened, debrided, and drained,

Table 18-1. Grading of envenomation

Grade	Clinical findings	Amount of antivenin needed
0	History of suspected snake bite; presence of fang wound(s); no evidence of envenomation; minimal pain may be present; also minimal edema and erythema; no systemic manifestations during first 12 hours	None
I	Estimated minimal envenomation; history and signs of snake bite; moderate pain or throbbing localized at fang wound(s) surrounded by 2.5-12.5 cm of edema and erythema; no evidence of systemic involvement after 12 hours of observation	IM anterolateral should be given in thigh or buttocks; 1 vial
II	Moderate envenomation; symptoms and signs of grade I rapidly progress during first 12 hours; pain becomes more severe and widely distributed; edema spreads toward trunk; petechiae and ecchymoses limited to area of edema; systemically, nausea, vomiting, giddiness, and mild elevated temperature usually present	Part IV (50%), remainder IM; 2-4 vials
III	Severe envenomation; signs and symptoms begin like I and II but rapidly progress in severity; shock may ensue soon after the bite; within 12 hours edema spreads up extremity and may involve part of trunk; petechiae and ecchymoses may be generalized; systemic manifestations include rapid pulse, shocklike state, subnormal temperatures	All IV; 5 or more vials
IV	Very severe envenomation; seen especially after envenomation by a large rattlesnake; symptoms and signs of sudden pain, rapidly progressive swelling that may reach and involve trunk within a few hours with ecchymoses, bleb formation, and necrosis; systemic reactions often start early and usually include weakness, nausea and vomiting, tingling of lips and face; muscular fasciculation, painful muscular cramping, pallor, sweating, cold and clammy skin, rapid and weak pulse, incontinence, convulsions, and coma also may be observed; death may occur	All IV; 10 or more vials

since this fluid will probably contain some venom. The tissue under the blisters will appear very hemorrhagic and resemble a severe burn. The dressings should be changed daily because there will be much discharge.

6. Fasciotomy[4] was previously discouraged because it was delayed until three to four days after the bite occurred; by this time the limb was severely damaged and a great deal of tissue was already destroyed. However, whenever intense swelling and edema are present and these conditions are progressing rapidly, fasciotomy should be done immediately. The time for this procedure is within the first two or three hours after the bite. The incision should be carried proximally beyond the edema and deep enough to open the muscle compartments to relieve pressure.

The wound may be closed in five to ten days.

Follow-up management—amputation, reconstruction, and rehabilitation. Orthopedic consultation is advisable. Amputations and contractures should be treated immediately when they arise. Contractures may continue to appear months after the bite. Physiotherapy will probably be necessary. During the acute phase of the condition always be alert for delayed respiratory failure and injury to internal organs. Urine examinations should be done at least daily. The plasma fibrinogen level should be measured daily, and fibrinogen may be needed.

Harmful procedures. Anything that will excite the victim, raise the blood pressure, or increase circulation, particularly in the injured limb, is contraindicated. Therefore, do not administer caffeinated drinks, stimulants, alcoholic drinks, or hot drinks. Do not allow the patient to run. He should walk when necessary and walk slowly. Have the injured area in a dependent attitude.

Do not apply a tight tourniquet. A soft rubber tubing is the best tourniquet, but a piece of cloth or a shoelace may be used

if it is applied so that it constricts only the venous and lymphatic flow. Never apply a tourniquet to a digit or over bony prominences. If an incision is to be made, make it along the long axis of the body or the afflicted member. Do not make cruciate incisions.

Ice, ice water, or cooling solutions may be applied to the wound area, but do not use cryotherapy (emersion of the limb in ice water for days). Do not apply ethyl chloride or freezing agents to the wound.

If medication is necessary to relieve pain, use meperidine, if possible. If morphine is used, be alert for respiratory failure.

CORAL SNAKES
Species and distribution

There are two genera of the family Elapidae found in the United States: *Micrurus micruroides* and *Micrurus fulvius*. The latter has four subspecies. *Micrurus fulvius euryxanthus* (Kennicutt), the Arizona or Sonora coral snake, is found in Arizona. *Micrurus fulvius tenere*, the harlequin or Texas coral snake, is found in southwest Arkansas, western Louisiana, and from Texas to Mexico. *Micrurus fulvius fulvius* is found from southern Florida to Alabama, South Carolina, and the southern parts of North Carolina. *Micrurus fulvius barbouri* is found in southern Florida.

Color

The snakes usually have black, red, and yellow bands about the body. In general, the black and yellow bands are wider than the red bands. The forepart of the head is black ("black head means dead"), which distinguishes the coral snake from the nonvenomous king snake.

Melanistic (all black) and albino (all white) and partially pigmented forms are occasionally seen.

Anatomy

The coral snakes are usually under 50 cm long; however, one specimen of the *M f fulvius* was recorded at 157.5 cm. The contour of the body is usually slender. The head is bullet shaped and is approximately the same circumference as the neck and body. The fangs are fixed, small, and erect and are located in the anterior maxilla. They are partially covered by a sheath. The eyes are round and black and do not have an elliptical pupil like the Crotalidae.

Coral snakes are oviparous and lay their eggs in the early summer.

Habitat

Coral snakes are burrowing snakes and live in gardens and loose soil. They are shy and elusive, but are found in settled areas.

Envenomation

Good statistics are not available as to the number of persons bitten or the number of deaths that occur. In general, it is believed that there are relatively few people bitten and few of those who are bitten die. Thirty-three bites were recorded in a six-year period, and there were no deaths. The low incidence of deaths is probably due to the fact that the coral snake has tiny, short fangs, and when it bites it must chew to force the venom over the surface of the fang and into the victim's flesh. However, the venom of the coral snake is the most toxic of any snake in the United States.

The effect of the venom is almost purely paralytic. Characteristically, there are few or no symptoms until 12 or more hours have elapsed after the bite. When the symptoms and signs do occur, the damage is irreversible. If there is a good possibility that a person has been bitten by a coral snake, it is well to start care immediately, although no symptoms or signs are apparent.

Clinical findings

Locally, there may be scratch marks or tiny punctures with or without minimal to moderate edema, erythema, and pain. There may be paresthesias. As previously mentioned, there may be no local reaction. Systemic symptoms of euphoria, lethargy, abnormal reflexes, nausea, vomiting, excessive salivation, ptosis of the eyelids, dyspnea, convulsions, and weakness or paralysis, motor or sensory or both, usually will develop in one to seven hours, but these symptoms can be delayed for as long as 18 hours. When symptoms do occur, they can progress very rapidly.[8]

Management

If there is any conclusive evidence that the victim was bitten by a coral snake, he or she should be hospitalized for 48 hours. Adequate care should begin even though at first there are few if any local or systemic signs or symptoms. In any event, the area around the wound should be washed thoroughly to remove any venom splattered on the skin. If any fang marks are present, incision and suction should be done. A tourniquet is advisable if there is a waiting period until antivenin is started. Observe the patient carefully and follow the general procedures used for the care of snake bites from venomous snakes. Because respiratory paralysis is common, it is well to have an anesthesiologist, mechanical respirator, and oxygen equipment ready and to be prepared to do a tracheostomy.

Antivenin

Coral snake antivenin (antivenin *Micrurus fulvius;* Wyeth) must be started. The patient must be tested for sensitivity to horse serum before the antivenin is given. When it is given, it should be administered intravenously. Start with a sodium chloride intravenous solution and add the antivenin directly into the tubing of the intravenous solution. Give the first 2 to 3 ml slowly and observe for allergic reactions. If they do not occur, give three to five vials of antivenin.

As symptoms and signs develop, follow the routine prescribed above for pit viper envenomation. However, because respiratory failure is common in coral snake envenomation, respiratory depressants such as morphine derivatives are contraindicated.

In summary, if there is any possibility of a coral snake bite, begin antivenin care immediately. Pathologic conditions, when they arise, are most often irreversible.

MYTHS, SUPERSTITIONS, AND FOLKLORE

There are many myths and superstitions relative to snakes.[1] Since time immemorial, snakes have been both condemned and heralded by people all over the world. Statues have been designed around the images of snakes.

Parents condition their children against snakes by warning them against picking up a "slithering, slimy" snake; it may bite. Further, children learn about the asp in the Garden of Eden.

One of our American flags had a picture of a rattlesnake with the caption "Don't Tread on Me" on it. The medical caduceus has two snakes on its staff.

Various parts of rattlesnakes have been used as "cures" for many ailments. Rattlesnake oil or fat has been used in the form of an ointment or liniment for muscle and joint aches and pains.

In the United States many myths and legends were invented by hunters, guides, and cowboys to spoof the tenderfoot. These became magnified and after being told and retold, some became "factual." This perpetuation of myths can be very dangerous. An example is the old myth that rattlesnakes will not bite children until they reach the age of 7! Also dangerous is the myth that snakes will not strike a person from the rear or that they will not bite when in water.

Finally, rattlesnakes do not sting as some people believe. They bite and the poison comes from a fang similar to a hypodermic needle. The virulence of the snake venom is not proportionate to the anger of the snake.

GILA MONSTERS

The Gila monster[9] *(Heloderma suspectum)* is the only lizard found in the United States that has poison-producing glands and a means of administering the poison. Its center of distribution is central Arizona. It has a related species, the Mexican bearded lizard *(H horridum),* which is found only in Mexico.

Anatomy

The Gila monster has a beady skin that is black and coral in color. It has a heavy body, short legs, a waddling gait, and reaches a length of approximately 60 cm. The female is oviparous and deposits from 5 to 13 eggs 6.25 cm long in a sand hole, which she covers with moist sand.

The venom glands are in the lower jaw and have three to five ducts leading to approximately 20 grooved teeth in the lower jaw. Ordinarily, the Gila monster is not pugnacious and does not spit venom. However, when it is agitated, it will produce copious amounts of saliva and bathe both the upper and lower teeth in venom; venom may be forced out of its mouth when it snaps its jaws or thrusts out its tongue.

Biting mechanism

When the Gila monster bites, it hangs on and chews, milking the venom along the grooved teeth into the victim's tissues.[10] The most efficacious means of releasing the grip is to take a strong hold of the animal's body and forcibly jerk it loose from the victim. The teeth of the animal are loosely attached to the jaw and in pulling you will extract the teeth from the animal. The animal will at times flip over onto its back, probably to facilitate envenomation, but this is not necessary.

Signs and symptoms

A person who has been bitten by a Gila monster may not show any signs of poisoning. This occurs because the animal has not had time to grind the venom into the tissues. However, the venom is primarily neurotoxic in nature and reactions may be slow in arising. Anticoagulants are present in the venom, and therefore the wounds bleed readily. There will be swelling and ecchymoses at the site of the bite. Eventually, cardiac and respiratory failure will occur.

Management

Care and treatment of the victim are essentially the same as that administered to victims of rattlesnake bites. However, morphine is contraindicated because of its suppressive effect on the cardiac and respiratory centers.

INSECTS

Insects[11,12] are found in vast numbers all over the world. They have adapted themselves to all climates and have a phenomenal rate of reproduction.

The order Hymenoptera includes bees, wasps, hornets, and ants. In addition to the fact that these insects are at times pests and can give a painful sting, they can also cause death. Death can occur either because of the number of stings sustained by an individual at one time or because the person is allergic to the protein in the venom. It is said that if a person is stung approximately 500 times, death may result. Of course, this depends on the size, age, and health of the victim. On the other hand, there is on record a case of an individual who was stung 2,000 times at one time and survived.

Anaphylactic shock in persons allergic to insect venom appears to be the most severe manifestation of insect bites; on occasion, it is fatal. In the United States more people die each year from bee stings than from rattlesnake bites.[13] About 20% of the American population are believed to be hypersensitive to venoms of hymenopteran insects (including honeybees, bumblebees, wasps, hornets, and fire ants). These insects often sting with little provocation. From 1950 through 1959, half of the 460 deaths caused by venomous animals were the result of stings of Hymenoptera (especially the honeybee); 1.7% were caused by scorpion stings.[13]

The sting

Generally when one is stung by a honeybee, the stinging apparatus is torn from the bee and left attached to the victim. This apparatus will consist of the stinger and the venom glands. The stinger of the honeybee has barbs that catch in the skin, and when the bee flies away, the apparatus is torn free. The bee then dies. All the other stinging Hymenoptera have smooth stingers that can be removed from the victim, and therefore they can sting repeatedly.

Management

Before any therapy is begun, it is important to identify, if possible, the arthropod that administered the sting.[14] If the insect is a honeybee, examination of the sting area may reveal that the stinging apparatus is protruding from the skin. This should not be grasped because more venom will be squeezed into the tissues. The stinger should be scraped away with the blade of a pocket knife or some similar instrument. The stinging apparatus should be removed as soon as possible because contractions of the walls of the venom sac continue long after the stinger has separated from the body of the bee.

Once the stinger has been removed, the wound area should be cleansed thoroughly with soap and water and an antiseptic.

The application of ice may help prevent excessive swelling. Heat should not be applied. If a limb is involved, place it at rest and elevate.

Antihistamines are not effective unless urticaria develops around the sting site, and they should be given orally. Also, steroids are used only when the reaction to the sting is protracted or resistant to ordinary measures. However, steroids and antihistamines are a necessity when allergic symptoms occur or when the patient has a history of allergies.

Epinephrine should always be available whenever a patient is treated for insect stings. If mild symptoms occur or if the patient has a history of allergies, always be on the lookout for more profound symptoms and signs of severe allergic reactions and shock. In such cases, intravenous steroids, aminophylline, Aramine, (metaraminol bitartrate), or Levophed (levarterenol bitartrate) may be mandatory.[14]

As a follow-up in cases of allergy, consultation with an allergist is comforting. In long-term management hyposensitization may be necessary. A likely candidate for a severe generalized reaction should carry an insect sting kit.[*]

Ants

Harvester or agricultural ants will attack man if they happen to blunder upon him. They cause a stinging sensation locally but rarely have caused any severe reactions.

Fire ants, however, will produce a characteristic local lesion and severe systemic reactions. The ant grasps the skin with its strong mandibles, and by pivoting around this axis, it can sting in multiple areas. The insertion of the stinger causes immediate pain similar to that of a bee sting. The pain subsides in a few minutes and is then followed by the formation of a wheal. The wheal persists and grows, and within four hours it becomes a superficial vesicle containing a thin, clear fluid. Eight to ten hours later the fluid be-

comes cloudy and purulent. The process progresses, and in 24 hours the pustules become umbilicated and may be surrounded by a painful reddened area. The pustules are absorbed in three to eight days leaving a crust and scar.

Because most ants are found on the ground or low grasses, most stings will be on the legs.

Management. There is no efficacious local treatment known. However, one should watch for severe systemic or allergic reactions. They must be treated as described for bee stings.

Blood-sucking flies

Houseflies can neither bite nor sting. The other flies, such as the stable fly, horse fly, deer fly, black fly, sand fly, and biting midges, all cause some damage to man. These flies do not bite but cause damage by stabbing or piercing as a pin or needle. Besides the toxins that they carry in their saliva, they are vectors for serious diseases such as anthrax, tularemia, loiasis, and animal trypanosomiasis.

Management. The first order of treatment is thorough cleansing with soap and water to reduce the possibility of infection. If infection does occur, this should be treated with the ordinary measures of antibiotics, heat, and the like. Allergic reactions should be treated with antihistamines.

MITES

The two common mites causing toxic manifestations to man are the *Sarcoptes scabiei* causing scabies, and the chigger or "red bug." Their saliva causes local pruritus but on occasion may cause a sensitization reaction similar to serum sickness. The only threat to life occurs when these mites are vectors of pathogenic organisms.

The animal burrows into the skin and release a digestant that liquefies epidermal cells. This liquid is sucked up and

---

[*]Insect Sting Kit, Center Laboratories, Port Washington, New York.

the process repeated so that gradually a tube is formed. Finally, a small macule is formed with a red center. In 3 to 24 hours an urticarial papule forms surrounded by a small vesicle containing clear fluid. The process resembles chicken pox but is distinguished from this disease by the fact that it is more localized in distribution.

Management

Gamma benzene hexachloride (Kwell) is the drug of choice for scabetic infestation and can also be used effectively in all forms of pediculosis.[15] It kills the nits or eggs as well as the lice and chiggers. This drug is irritating to the eyes, skin, and mucous membrane and can be toxic if absorbed in excessive amounts. If irritation becomes evident after application of the drug, it should be washed off and not used again.

The usual dose for pediculosis corporis and scabies is 20 to 30 g of a 1% lotion or cream to all parts of the body except the face. Pat the skin dry and in 24 hours wash off thoroughly. Repeat the treatment eight days later.

For pediculosis capitis, first moisten the scalp with water, shampoo with a 1% solution of Kwell for five minutes and then rinse thoroughly. Repeat the procedure four and eight days later.

TICKS

Ticks are found everywhere in the world and in every type of environment. They possess the ability to regenerate lost parts and to repair mutilated organs. Ticks will attach themselves to a suitable host in all three stages of their life cycle—larva, nymph, and adult. They fasten themselves to the host with their teeth and then secrete a cementlike material reinforcing their attachment. The tick can quickly detach itself from the host; however, any attempt to remove the tick manually will result in removing the body and leaving the mouth parts imbedded. Also, squeezing the tick will result in injecting more toxins.

The toxins from ticks may cause tick paralysis. This is an acute, flaccid paralysis caused apparently by a neurotoxin. The paralysis starts as paresthesia and pain in the lower extremities followed in several hours by a symmetrical, ascending, flaccid paralysis. Rapid progression of this paralysis continues. Bulbar paralysis finally ensues and the patient may die of respiratory failure. However, once the tick is removed, the paralysis clears up spontaneously and dramatically.

Management

Make a careful search for the tick. It will be gray and oval. Examine the total body. When the tick is found, do not remove it manually. Apply gasoline or ether to the head or the hot tip of a match or cigarette to the body. Following this, wait a full ten minutes for the tick to disengage itself.

SPIDERS

Of the many spiders of the world, only two found in the United States are dangerous to man. They are the brown recluse spider, *Loxosceles reclusa*, and the female black widow spider, *Latrodectus mactans*.

Each of these spiders has a characteristic marking which makes it easily recognizable.

Black widow spider

The female black widow spider has an hour-glass-shaped marking on its abdomen, which is either orange or red in color. The remainder of the spider is coal black. The females are about 15 mm in length and about 10 mm across the abdomen. They are found everywhere in the United States except Alaska.

Clinically, a definite history of a spider bite usually cannot be obtained. However, after close questioning, the victim will recall a sharp pinprick sensation followed by a dull, somewhat numbing pain.

Further search will reveal a slight local swelling and tiny red fang marks. When the bite is on the lower extremity, the local pain will be followed by pain and rigidity of the abdominal muscles. If the bite is on the upper extremities, the pain and rigidity will be felt in the chest, back, and shoulder.

The pain and muscle rigidity increase in intensity for 12 to 48 hours and then gradually subside. When the abdominal muscles are involved, acute abdominal conditions must be ruled out. Other signs and symptoms such as a rise in temperature and blood pressure, increase in white cell count, albumin, and hematuria may develop. The spinal fluid is often under increased pressure. Mortality rate is 4% to 5%.

Management. Although the symptoms are usually self-limiting, their severity demands attention. Local treatment of the wound is useless except perhaps to apply ice to reduce and slow down the rate of absorption of the toxins.

Muscle relaxants will help to relieve the intensity of pain and spasms. Intravenous injections of 10% calcium gluconate are helpful. However, the effect lasts only one to four hours, and subsequent injections are less effective.

The best and only specific treatment is antivenin.* As with rattlesnake antivenin, this is made using horses as the experimental animal. Therefore, testing for hypersensitivity to horse serum must be done before treatment is instituted. When and if the test is negative, one dose of 2.5 ml restored serum is the usual dose and will cause subsidence of symptoms in one to three hours. Occasionally, a second dose is needed.

Brown recluse spider

The brown recluse spider is 10 to 15 mm long and 5 to 7 mm across and is

---

*Antivenin (Latrodectus mactans) Lyovac. Merck, Sharp & Dohme.

brown or tan. All spiders have a median band of darker color, which extends back from the eyes and is shaped like a violin. Peculiar to this spider is the presence of three pairs of eyes placed in a semicircle on the anterior part of the cephalothorax.

Local reactions to the toxins do not begin for two to eight hours. Then the area becomes painful and reddened and a bleb or blister forms surrounded by an area of ischemia. Later, in the third to fourth day, the center turns dark, violaceous, and firm to touch. By the seventh to fourteenth day the central area is depressed, sharply demarcated, and mummified. Separation occurs and an open ulcer forms. This ulcer can be several centimeters in size. It usually heals in about three weeks, but the skin may have to be grafted. Skin grafts are not always successful.

General reaction can be severe: fever, chills, malaise, weakness, nausea, vomiting, and joint pains; also, a petechial eruption can occur. Hemolytic anemia and thrombocytopenia have been reported. These symptoms are always worse in children.

Management. There is no known specific treatment. Excising the skin over the wound area immediately to remove tissues containing toxic material has been done with some success. The administration of steroids in all forms is helpful, especially when combined with antihistamines and antibiotics.

SCORPIONS

About 30 species of scorpions are found in the United States and are common in the southwestern areas. Only two of these are considered "deadly," *Centruroides gertschi* Stahnke and *C sculpturatus* Ewing. In Mexico several other deadly species are known. Most stings occur in the warmer months, and deaths are more common from scorpion stings than from rattlesnake bites.

The scorpion does not bite but stings by flicking its curved tail. The tail has a venom apparatus at the end, and the pointed tip is driven into the victim. The symptoms are either local or systemic. The sting of the nonlethal scorpion causes local symptoms only. These symptoms include a sharp burning sensation, swelling and discoloration at the sting site, and, rarely, anaphylaxis.

The venom of the lethal variety of scorpion will cause no visible local effect. There will be, however, sharp pain followed by hyperesthesia, and these symptoms progress very rapidly. The hyperethesia is followed by hypoesthesia, numbness, and drowsiness. Later, itching of the nose, mouth or throat will be noted. Speech becomes impaired because of sluggishness of the tongue. Trismus of the jaw may occur, and generalized muscle spasms follow along with pain, nausea, vomiting, incontinence, and convulsions. The convulsive episodes come in waves, and death may result from exhaustion. More commonly, death occurs from respiratory or circulatory failure. The symptoms may last from 24 to 48 hours or longer. When death does not occur, the last part of the body to return to normal during recovery is the original site of the sting.

Management

Prompt treatment is essential. A tourniquet should be applied near the site of the sting (i.e., if the sting is on the foot, place tourniquet on the ankle). The affected area should next be packed in ice water. The ice water should extend well above the tourniquet, and after the area has been immersed in ice water for five minutes, the tourniquet may be removed. If a tourniquet cannot be applied, use crushed ice around the wound. Keep the remainder of the body warm to maintain good circulation. Keep the ice on continuously for about two hours. "On and off" treatment is not advisable because sudden changes in temperature will cause pain. Morphine and codeine are contraindicated

because they increase the toxic effect.

Scorpion antivenin* is the only specific treatment and should always be used when the sting is from the deadly scorpions. This is available in lyophilized cat serum. Antivenin may be obtained in Mexico† for the Mexican varieties of scorpions. One 5 ml vial will neutralize 75 MLD *Centruroides* venom.

CENTIPEDES

Many centipedes are seen in the desert. The large poisonous desert centipede attains a length of 15 to 20 cm and has jaw muscles of sufficient strength to inflict a painful bite. Poison glands are located at the base of the jaw, and the toxins that they secrete will cause the inflicted area to swell and become hot and painful. It may remain this way for as long as several weeks and, at times, will become infected.

Management

Usually there will be no serious aftereffects from centipede bites. First aid, antiseptics, and antibiotics are usually all that is needed unless pain is great enough to require analgesics.

SUMMARY

The cardinal effects of envenomation from reptiles are usually pain, swelling, and bleeding. When these occur immediately following the bite, treatment must be seriously considered. If the victim may have been bitten by a Mohave rattlesnake or coral snake, consider adequate antivenin treatment even though the three cardinal symptoms or signs do not occur.

The first principle in treating wounds from venomous animals is first aid. This, of course, means soap and water to remove any venom deposited around the wound.

*Available from Poisonous Animals Research Laboratory, Arizona State University, Tempe, Arizona.

†Laboratories Myn. Av. Coyvocan 1707, Mexico 12, D. F.

Second, localize the venom at the site of the wound as well as possible and, third, whenever available, use specific antivenin. Finally, treat the complications as they arise. Be careful of folklore remedies, as these may complicate a simple wound.

REFERENCES

1. Klauber, L. M.: Rattlesnakes: Their habits, life histories and influence on mankind, 2 vols., ed. 2, Berkeley, Calif., 1972, University of California Press.
2. Leviton, A. E.: Reptiles and amphibians of North America, Garden City, N. Y., 1970, Doubleday & Co., Inc., p. 191.
3. Parrish, H. M.: Incidence of treated snakebites in the United States, Public Health Reports, vol. 81, no. 3, 1966.
4. Glass, T. G., Jr.: Intravenous hydrocortisone and immediate fasciotomy in the treatment of severe pit viper envenomization, University of Texas Medical School, San Antonio, Texas, July, 1971.
5. Glass, T. G., Jr.: Early debridement in pit viper bites, J.A.M.A. **235**(23):2513-2516, 1976
6. Longo, M. F.: Review of current management of snakebite, J. La. State Med. Soc. **123**(I):11, 1971.
7. Coral killer control. J. Florida Med. Assoc. **55**(4):348-350, 1968.
8. Dowling, H. G., and Menton, S.: Quick action to save the snake bite victim, Patient Care, June 1968, pp. 55-67.
9. Dodge, N. N.: Poisonous dwellers of the desert, 1961, p. 27.
10. Stahnke, H. L.: The treatment of venomous bites and stings, 1966, p. 23.
11. Frazier, C. A.: Diagnosis and treatment of insect bites, Ciba Clinical Symposia, Summit, N. J., 1968, Ciba Pharmaceutical Co.
12. Frazier, C. A.: Ten points to remember in managing insect bites and sting reaction. Consultant, April 1972.
13. Parrish, H. M.: Analysis of 460 fatalities from venomous animals in the United States, Am. J. Med. Sci. **245**:129-141, 1963.
14. Frazier, C. A.: Management of insect bites and stings, Mod. Med., July 14, 1969, pp. 62-68.
15. American Medical Association: Drug evaluation, 1971, Chicago, 1971, The Association, pp. 481-482.

CHAPTER **19**

Aquatic medical emergencies

William L. Orris, M.D.†

During a workshop on Biomedical Problems of Living Under the Sea (Department of Health, Education, and Welfare, 1967), Dr. Fred N. Spiess, head of the Marine Physical Laboratory of Scripps Institution of Oceanography, University of California, San Diego, stated, "Within fifty years, man will move onto and into the sea, occupying it and exploiting it as an integral part of his use of this planet for recreation, minerals, food, waste disposal, military and transport operations, and, as populations grow, for actual living space."[1] Dr. Spiess's prediction is probably well ahead of schedule.

With man's invasion of the waters of the world, there has been an attendant increase in aquatic medical emergencies. Aquatic medical emergencies by definition result from exposure to water and its organisms. Drownings now account for over 7,000 deaths in the United States yearly,[2] some of which occur in the estimated 10 million skin and scuba* divers; divers may also be victims of pressure-related diseases or dangerous and venomous aquatic animals. Water pollution contributes to an overgrowth of pathogenic viruses, bacteria, fungi, and parasites, some of which may cause aquatic emergencies. Table 19-1 gives a summary of 200 underwater accidents reported by Miles in 1967.[3]

To fulfill their responsibility to the public, medical personnel should acquaint themselves with the recognition, diagnosis, pathophysiology, and treatment of water-related emergencies. Assistance of a specialist in aquatic medicine may be necessary. A list of such specialties should be readily available; such a list appears each spring in *Emergency Medicine* magazine.

Detailed reports of water-related medical emergencies are urgently needed. Forms may be obtained from the University of Rhode Island Scuba Safety Project, 277 South Wales Hall, University of Rhode Island, Kingston, Rhode Island 02881. Sample forms are shown at the end of this chapter (see Fig. 19-9).

Three major categories of aquatic medical emergencies will be discussed:

I. Effects of the physical aquatic environment
   A. Drowning

---

†Dr. Orris, who suffered a fatal heart attack on February 1, 1977, contributed a great deal to the advancement of aquatic safety and understanding of aquatic medical emergencies. His contributions will long be remembered and respected. Dr. Orris was Director of Medical Services, Scripps Institution of Oceanography, University of California, San Diego, La Jolla, California. He was a member of the Aerospace Medical Association, the Undersea Medical Society, and the International Society on Toxicology.

*Self-contained underwater breathing apparatus.

Table 19-1. A summary of 200 underwater accidents*

Cause	Fatal	Nonfatal	Total
Asphyxia	22	11	33
Anoxia	8	16	24
Illness in water			
Coronary thrombosis	2	1	3
Acute pneumonia	2	1	3
Epilepsy	1	2	3
Oxygen poisoning	5	5	10
Syncope and collapse	—	46	46
Pulmonary barotrauma	5	14	19
Decompression sickness	—	35	35
Ears and vertigo	—	10	10
Shark bite	3	—	3
Other causes	3	8	11
Total	51	149	200

*From Miles, S.: Medical hazards of diving. In Davies, C. N., and others: The effects of abnormal physical conditions at work, London, 1967, E. & S. Livingstone Ltd.

B. Near drowning
  1. Without aspiration
  2. With aspiration
C. Hyperventilation leading to drowning or near drowning in underwater swimmers
D. Immersion hypothermia and paradoxical cooling
E. Cold allergy
F. Carbon monoxide poisoning
G. Pathologic effects of change in ambient pressure and the partial pressure of nitrogen in inhaled gases
  1. Squeeze
  2. Decompression sickness, pulmonary barotrauma, and air embolism
II. Aquatic organisms
  A. Dangerous and venomous organisms
    1. Bites
    2. Stings
    3. Spines
  B. Poisonous aquatic organisms
    1. Ciguatera poisoning
    2. Paralytic shellfish poisoning
    3. Scombroid poisoning
III. Miscellaneous
  A. Amebic encephalitis
  B. Algal allergic reaction
  C. Cercarial dermatitis

EFFECTS OF THE PHYSICAL AQUATIC ENVIRONMENT
Drowning

Approximately 140,000 people drown annually in the world (Table 19-2). Drowning is one of the three leading causes of accidental deaths in the United States.[2] Some drown without aspiration; that is, they die from respiratory obstruction and asphyxia while submerged in a fluid medium. Others drown with aspiration; that is, they die from the combined effects of asphyxia and changes secondary to aspiration of fluid while submerged.

Near drowning

The near-drowning victim survives, at least temporarily, the physiologic events (essentially hypoxemia and acidosis) which lead to cardiac arrest and death in drowning. It is impossible to estimate the number of near drownings annually. Near drowning with or without aspiration is characterized by acute asphyxia. The recently submerged victim will, therefore, have varying degrees of arterial hypoxemia, acidemia, and hyper-

Table 19-2. Drowning mortality

Country	Number of drownings per year	Rate per 100,000 population per year
United States	7,000	4.6
England	2,000	4.0
Australia	500	5.5
Japan	8,000	9.0
WORLDWIDE	140,000	5.6

capnia. Blood pH changes reflect a combination of respiratory and metabolic acidosis. Hypercapnia results in respiratory acidosis; anaerobic metabolism during hypoxemia results in metabolic acidosis. Aspiration of fluid is a complication of near drowning that may alter its pathophysiology, prolong hypoxemia and acidemia, and cause secondary infection.

Near drowning without aspiration. Laryngeal spasm or breath holding prevents water from entering the lungs, and death from asphyxia can result. About 10% of drowning victims die without having aspirated fluid.[2] If initial blood gases are within normal limits, there probably has been no aspiration of a fluid. Since there is no injury to lung tissues or vital organs, other than what may have developed from anoxia, prompt resuscitation usually results in full recovery without complications.

Near drowning with aspiration. Aspiration is the entry of fluid into the alveoli of the lungs. Because of inadequate reporting, there seems to be no way of determining the number of near-drowning victims who have aspirated fluid.

Following aspiration of a fluid, pathophysiologic changes result from the hypotonicity of fresh water or the hypertonicity of salt water, and the amount of fluid aspirated. Knowing the tonicity of the fluid aspirated makes it possible to predict, to some extent, tissue and organ response. The amount of fluid aspirated cannot be determined; therefore, it is impossible to predict the degree of tissue and organ response. The majority of victims, however, have probably aspirated less than 10 ml of fluid per pound of body weight[2] (about one third the total amount of fluid the lung could contain, exclusive of residual volume).

Because of the osmotic gradient, fresh water is rapidly absorbed into the circulation while salt water draws plasma from the circulation into the alveolar spaces (Fig. 19-1).

Greater hypoxia is seen with the aspiration of sea water than with an equal amount of fresh water because salt water and tissue fluids in the alveoli reduce ventilation mechanically. Persistent hypoxia accompanying aspiration may last for days and be present with or without positive x-ray findings. See Table 19-3 for a comparison of the effects of fresh and salt water aspiration.

If enough water has been aspirated to cause significant electrolyte changes, death occurs in approximately 85% of the victims.[2] Electrolyte changes in the near-drowing victim are generally insignificant, transitory, and return to normal spontaneously. Changes in the cardiovascular system are secondary to hypoxia. When large volumes of water have been aspirated, changes in blood volume as well as electrolyte concentrations contribute to cardiovascular effects. Neurologic changes result from acute asphyxia and persistent hypoxia; therefore, cerebral hypoxia is usually the cause of coma, and consciousness may return when arterial oxygen and pH are brought within normal limits. Although acute tubular necrosis secondary to severe lactic acidosis or hypoxia may occur,[4] intact renal function is seen in the majority of victims. Aspirated water may contain sand, mud, algae, chemicals, oil, or other pollutants capable of causing secondary problems. Aspiration pneumonitis with pulmonary edema, damage to the alveolar capillary membrane caused by fluid toni-

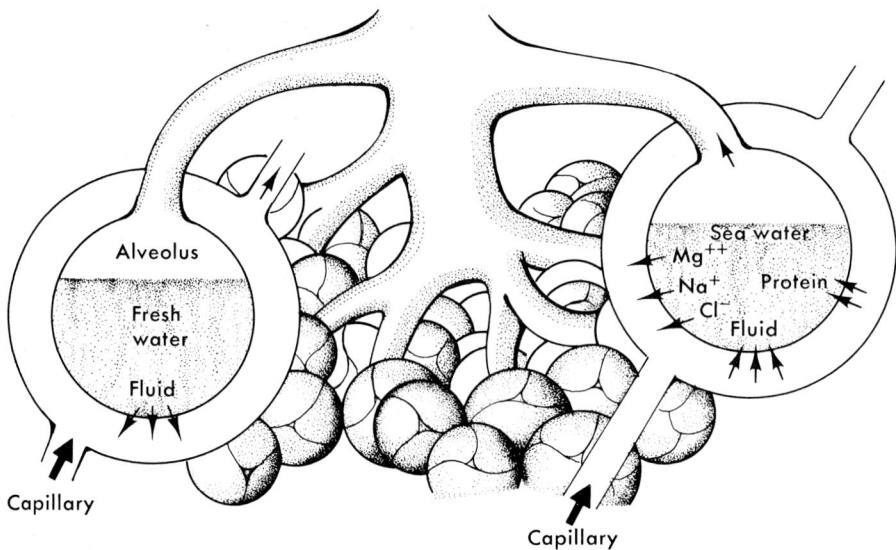

Fig. 19-1. Direction of fluid flow in fresh and sea water aspiration.

city or toxicity, and secondary infection can complicate fluid aspiration.

If initial blood gases are not within normal limits (arterial oxygen tension below 80 torr at $F_1O_2 = 0.21$), the patient has probably aspirated fluid (Tables 19-4 and 19-5). During the diagnostic phase it is well to keep in mind that near drowning may be a complication of other diseases seen in skin and scuba divers, such as air embolism, decompression sickness, or venomous animal injury.

For scientific and medical clarity, Modell[2] completes his list of definitions with "delayed death subsequent to near-drowning," which includes those victims who succumb subsequent to near drowning after apparent successful rescue or resuscitation.

Management of near-drowning victim. Effective ventilation, oxygenation, circulatory support, and use of buffers, singly or in combination, may restore normal arterial blood gas tensions and acid-base balance in the near-drowning patient. There is, however, no way to initially determine the presence or degree of aspiration; therefore, the apparent well-being or return to

consciousness of the victim does not necessarily mean normal recovery or survival. Delayed sequelae or even death from hypoxia may occur days to weeks later. Therefore, all near-drowning victims, with or without aspiration, should be hospitalized until normal arterial blood gas tensions and acid-base levels have been established and can be maintained while the patient is breathing room air. There can be no exceptions to this rule. In the hospital, pulse, blood pressure, temperature, ECG, urine output, serum electrolytes, pH, P_{CO_2}, P_{O_2}, bicarbonate, hematocrit, and hemoglobin should be monitored and recorded. Fifty milliliters of blood should be drawn from adults while the intravenous catheter is being put into place for laboratory studies, including a serum alcohol level and drug abuse panel. Serial chest x-rays should be started and continued even after the patient has been discharged. An analysis of blood gases synthesizes cardiac and pulmonary function; it is impossible to evaluate and properly care for the near-drowning patient without them.

Immediate artificial pulmonary resuscita-

Table 19-3. Significant differences between salt and fresh water aspiration

Salt water	Fresh water

Hypoxia

Greater degree of hypoxia; fluid in alveoli interferes with ventilation	Alteration of normal surface tension properties of surfactant with subsequent collapse of the alveoli; atelectasis; uneven ventilation and recurrent collapse continue until surface active material regenerates

Blood volume

Hypertonic fluid draws water into the alveolar spaces causing a persistent hypovolemia; increase in blood osmolarity and viscosity	Hypotonic water rapidly absorbed into the circulation; transient hypervolemia; decrease in blood osmolarity and viscosity; elevated CVP

Serum electrolytes

Changes usually insignificant; hyperkalemia may result from severe hypoxia and acidosis

Picture may be complicated by ingestion of large amounts of salt water

Hemoglobin

Hemolysis occurs after aspiration of at least 11 ml of fluid/kg body weight, with a possible decrease in hemoglobin

Hematocrit

Technical problems make correct measurements almost impossible and interpretation difficult

Cardiac changes

Sufficient water to cause ventricular fibrillation is seldom aspirated

Central venous pressure

An increase in CVP coincides with hyperventilation; falls rapidly to normal when only small amounts of liquid have been aspirated

Aspiration of large amounts of fluid results in initial rise in CVP, followed by a rapid drop to zero	Aspiration of large quantities of fluid results in a persistent rise in CVP

Neurologic effects

When sea water is ingested in large quantities, the magnesium ion may cause lethargy, drowsiness, and coma

Urinary system

Acute renal failure due to tubular necrosis resulting from hypoxia and hypotension	Acute renal failure due to hemolysis and hypotension

Table 19-4. Arterial blood gas and pH values found on admission to the hospital after near drowning in fresh water*

pH	Pa$_{CO_2}$ (torr)	Base excess (mEq/liter)	Pa$_{O_2}$ (torr)	F$_I$O$_2$
6.95	64	−19	245	1.0
7.01	38	−22	28	0.2
7.05	59	−16	40	1.0‡
7.13	30	−19	67	0.2
7.14	45	−14	68	0.2
7.18	33	−15	110	1.0
7.19	29	−16	108	±0.8‡
7.21	37	−13	175	1.0
7.22	54	− 7	123	1.0‡
7.28	54	− 3	35	0.4
7.33	41	− 4	127	1.0
7.40†	32	− 4	103	0.2
7.44	32	− 2	76	0.2
7.45†	35	1	84	0.2

*From Modell, J. H.: Drowning and near-drowning, Springfield, Ill., 1971, Charles C Thomas, Publisher.
†Patients likely did not aspirate fluid by clinical course.
‡Ventilation supported mechanically.

Table 19-5. Arterial blood gas and pH values found on admission to the hospital after near drowning in sea water*

pH	Pa$_{CO_2}$ (torr)	Base excess (mEq/liter)	Pa$_{O_2}$ (torr)	F$_I$O$_2$
7.03	36	−21	58	1.0
7.08	58	−14	21	1.0†
7.20	46	−10	27	0.2
7.29	49	− 4	364	1.0†
7.31	35	− 8	85	0.8†
7.35	47	− 1	45	0.2
7.46	25	− 5	71	0.2
7.47	26	− 3	82	0.4

*From Modell, J. H.: Drowning and near-drowning, Springfield, Ill., 1971, Charles C Thomas, Publisher.
†Ventilation supported mechanically.

tion is mandatory for the apneic patient. Mouth-to-mouth or mouth-to-nose resuscitation should be instituted immediately. No time should be wasted in attempting to remove water from the lungs or the stomach. Although adequate volumes of air are moved during resuscitation, the near-drowning victim who has aspirated water will remain hypoxic unless supplemental oxygen (100%) is ultimately used. The reason for this is the intrapulmonary shunt-

ing of blood, which results in hypoxemia. Hand-operated or controlled intermittent positive pressure ventilation should be started as soon as possible.

Po$_2$ levels should be maintained between 60 and 90 mm Hg. Prolonged exposure to high concentrations of oxygen should be avoided to prevent irreversible oxygen toxicity. If prolonged use of high concentrations of O$_2$ is indicated, positive end-expiratory pressure (PEEP) will allow adequate oxygenation at lower concentrations. PEEP will also help to keep the alveoli from collapsing in the absence of adequate surfactant. A Pco_2 greater than 50 mm Hg is an indication that the ventilator should deliver a greater volume or a greater rate.

Ventilatory support should be continued until the true or absolute intrapulmonary shunt has subsided. This is indicated by a satisfactory Po_2 when the patient is on less than 50% inspired O_2, the Pco_2 is within normal limits, and the physical signs of pulmonary edema are no longer present.[1] Continued used of mechanical ventilation exposes the patient to hospital infections, particularly *Pseudomonas;* pulmonary infection and sepsis are constant dangers.

Although ventilation of the patient is of primary importance, simultaneous restoration of circulation may be necessary. This will be indicated by the absence of a carotid, radial, or femoral pulse, and external cardiac massage should be started. If circulatory arrest is secondary to hypoxia, proper ventilation may reoxygenate the myocardium with spontaneous return of circulation. However, correction of severe acidosis or ventricular fibrillation (seen infrequently) may be necessary to bring about cardiac response. Neither the length of time the victim has been submerged nor the size of the pupils should be used as a criterion for determining physiologic status, that is, the probable success of resuscitative efforts. In near-drowning victims there may be small pupils with circulatory arrest, while in profound hypoxia the pupils may be dilated and fixed despite a functioning circulatory system.

The physiologic response to circulating blood volume is ideally monitored by observing pulmonary artery wedge pressure (which reflects left heart function) using a Swan-Ganz Pathfinder right heart catheter. Lacking this capability, monitoring of the central venous pressure (CVP) should

be used for this purpose, as well as to determine the adequacy of myocardial function.* Such measurements are important in differentiating pulmonary edema, that is, fluid in pulmonary cells and tissue, caused by circulatory overload from that caused by primary pulmonary injury. An increased wedge pressure (normal is 8 to 12 mm Hg), a CVP greater than 15 mm H_2O, and a decrease in platelet and white blood cell count are indications of pulmonary edema, namely, the "wet lung" syndrome. Methylprednisolone sodium succinate (Solu-Medrol), 30 mg/kg body weight given intravenously over a period of 5 to 10 minutes, is recommended both prophylactically and for the treatment of pulmonary edema. It reaches the cells in seconds, where it remains for a considerable period of time†; hence one dose is sufficient. Methylprednisolone may stimulate the production of surfactant, stabilizes lysosome, possibly increases the oxygen-carrying capacity of red blood cells, and maintains or improves the physiologic function of the alveolocapillary membrane. Sodium retention is minimal, and phagocytosis by white blood cells is not appreciably altered. A low CVP reflects the hypovolemia caused by a loss of blood plasma into the lungs, namely, pulmonary congestion. However, subsequent fluid replacement must be undertaken with care if pulmonary edema is to be controlled and not compounded.‡ Giordano[5] noted a decrease of serum albumin in patients with pulmonary inter-

---

*It is important to remember that the CVP reflects only *right heart function,* because pulmonary edema can occur from injury to lung parenchyma without cardiac involvement.

†See Wilson, J.: Cellular localization of ^{3}H-labeled corticosteroids by electron microscopic autoradiography after hemorrhagic shock. In Glenn, T. M.: Steroids and shock, Baltimore, 1973, University Park Press, pp. 275-300.

‡The reader is referred to Moss, Gerald: Shock lung: a disorder of the central nervous system, Hosp. Pract., Aug., 1974, p. 77, for a better understanding of the so-called wet lung syndrome.

stitial edema. No significant change in blood gases was obtained by his using IPPB, diuretics, or intubation. However, diuresis and significant improvement in Po_2 resulted from the use of massive amounts of intravenous albumin.

Vasopressors should be used in near-drowning patients only when specifically indicated, and their prolonged use should be avoided. Since alpha-receptors have the capability of compounding metabolic acidosis, the temporary use of a beta-receptor, such as isoproterenol in a slow intravenous drip, to increase cardiac output until blood volume can be established is recommended.

One of the most common findings in near drowning is acidosis. Intravenous sodium bicarbonate, 0.3 to 0.4 mEq/lb of body weight, should be given routinely and as soon as possible, preferably at the scene of the accident. Subsequent sodium bicarbonate should be given as indicated by laboratory results.

If the victim survives near drowning, the electrolyte changes are likely to be transient and spontaneously revert to normal[2] (Table 19-6). Hyperkalemia, probably secondary to hypoxia and acidosis, is the most frequent disturbance seen. An intravenous infusion should be started with Ringer's lactate and switched as soon as possible to the fluid indicated by laboratory results. Low molecular weight fluids go into the tissues easily and should be avoided when pulmonary edema is present.

Hyperventilation leading to drowning or near drowning in underwater swimmers

Even expert swimmers have drowned while swimming underwater after hyperventilating to lengthen the time they can hold their breath. The underlying cause is a delay in the reflexive need to breathe.

CO_2 buildup in the blood creates an irrepressible need to breathe, while low blood oxygen is a comparatively weak stimulus to breathe, which can consciously be repressed. During hyperventilation, virtually all CO_2 is removed from the blood. As the underwater swimmer continues to hold his or her breath, most of the blood oxygen may be used up before the CO_2 level rises to a point which forces the swimmer to seek air and breathe. The brain of the apneic underwater swimmer is deprived of O_2, and he or she loses consciousness, becoming, by definition, a drowning or near-drowning victim. Resuscitation and treatment are the same as for near drowning.

Immersion hypothermia and paradoxical cooling

Immersion hypothermia results from the loss of body heat into the surrounding liquid.[6] Water conducts heat about 25

Table 19-6. Means and standard deviations of serum electrolyte concentrations and specific gravities of samples obtained from the left ventricles of victims of freshwater drowning, saltwater drowning, or other causes (Control)*

	Freshwater victims (74)	FW vs. Control P value	Controls (24)	Control vs. SW P value	Saltwater victims (44)	FW vs. SW P value
Cl, mEq/l	89 ± 11.4	†	93 ± 8.7	< 0.001	120 ± 16.8	< 0.001
Na, mEq/l	128 ± 11.5	< 0.01	135 ± 9.9	< 0.001	150 ± 12.5	< 0.001
K, mEq/l	18.2 ± 7.4	†	18.6 ± 9.1	†	16.1 ± 6.6	†
Specific gravity	1.0280 ± 0.0040	< 0.01	1.0309 ± 0.0046	†	1.0307 ± 0.0037	< 0.01

*From Modell, J. H.: Drowning and near-drowning, Springfield, Ill., 1971, Charles C Thomas, Publisher. (Note: These are all postmortem findings.)
†No significant difference between groups, P > 0.10.

times faster than air, but wet suits (nylon or rubber) and clothing help to maintain a normal core temperature. However, respiratory heat loss may exceed the amount of heat being generated by the body. The working body loses more heat than the resting one, thus shivering and exercise accelerate death from hypothermia. Immersion hypothermia may be a severe complication of near drowning or other water-related illnesses[7] (Table 19-7).

Paradoxical cooling is caused by a drop in core temperature on exposure to warm air and may result in shock or even death. The hypothermic individual has a relatively bloodless "shell" (contraction of the blood vessels in the skin and subcutaneous tissues) on being removed from the water. Stimulated by warm air, these contracted vessels dilate, allowing flow of blood from the inner body to the outer "shell." Since this "shell" has about the same temperature as the water that surrounded it, the core blood moving to the periphery is further cooled before returning to the core, resulting in a lowering of the core temperature. As can be seen in Table 19-7, improper warming of a hypothermic individual could worsen his or her condition and even cause death.

Core temperatures are ideally determined by using an esophageal thermometer or telemetry (a transmitting capsule swallowed by the patient). Rectal temperatures can be used but tend to be inaccurate. Treatment consists of the immediate application of heat (hot water at 40°-41° C [104° to 106° F]), which must be contained close to the skin to be effective. Blankets, towels, or clothing can be kept hot by total immersion, shower water, or other means. For the scuba diver still in a wet suit, total immersion, allowing hot water to circulate between the suit and the skin, has been found to be the best method of warming. Hot drinks such as hot chocolate may be helpful, but whiskey precipitates the effects of paradoxical cooling by dilating peripheral blood vessels.

Cold allergy (primary acquired cold urticaria)

People allergic to cold are subject to urticaria or angioedema, lacrimation, sneezing, cough, or bronchial asthma. When a person who is hypersensitive to cold jumps into cold water, a reaction sufficiently severe to cause unconsciousness may occur. The care for cold allergy is the same as that for other allergies, but includes warming. Cyproheptadine (Periactin) may be effective prophylactically.[8]

Carbon monoxide poisoning

Breathing compressed air contaminated with carbon monoxide results in carbon monoxide poisoning if concentration and time of exposure are sufficient. A contaminated breathing medium should be suspected in every diving emergency.

Carbon monoxide combines with the hemoglobin in red blood cells, rendering them incapable of carrying oxygen to the tissues. Tissue hypoxia ensues even though the oxygen supply to the lungs is ample and arterial oxygen tension remains high. Hemoglobin combines with carbon monoxide 200 times as readily as with oxygen; hence, very small amounts can be dangerous.[9]

Symptoms are almost identical to those of other types of hypoxia. Weakness, dizziness, or confusion may precede unconsciousness. However, with high concentrations of carbon monoxide, unconsciousness can occur without warning. Symptoms may be alleviated by fresh air, but in more

Table 19-7. Pathology associated with abnormal core temperatures

Core temperature	Pathology
34° C (94° F)	Amnesia
32° C (90° F)	Cardiac arrhythmias
30° C (86° F)	Loss of muscle strength and unconsciousness
25° C (77° F)	Cardiac arrest and death

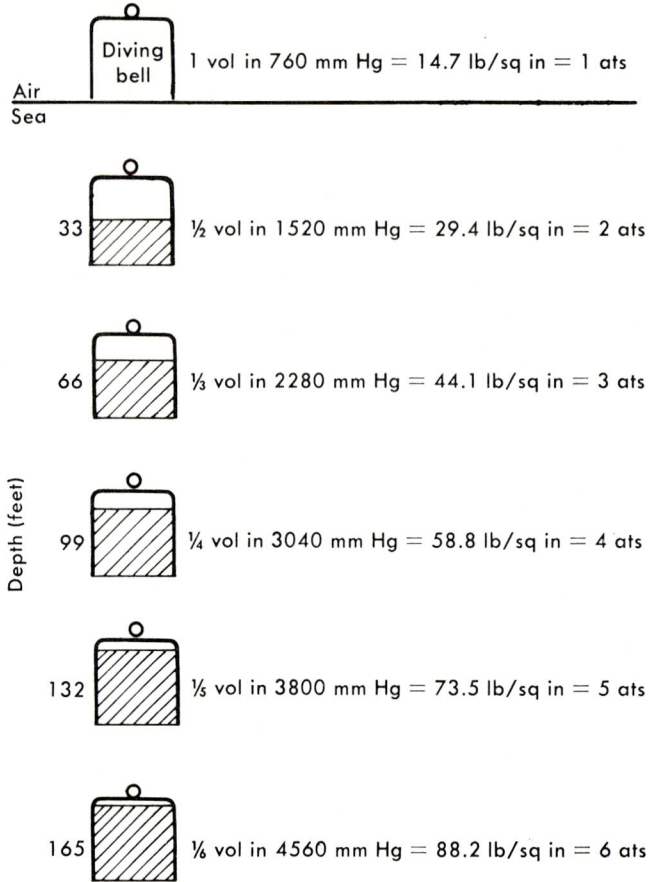

Fig. 19-2. Boyle's law: $P_1V_1 = P_2V_2$.

Fig. 19-3. The effect of ambient pressure (see Fig. 19-2) on enclosed body spaces, such as the middle ear when the eustachian tube is *not* patent, can be confusing, particularly in regard to whether enclosed air is trying to expand or contract, that is, exerting a positive or negative pressure on the container wall. With increased ambient pressure (descent) air inside a rigid sphere would like to occupy a smaller space. Essentially, it is compressing, but since the rigid container cannot get smaller, a relative vacuum is created and there is a negative force created on the inside of the container. With decrease in ambient pressure (ascent) air inside a solid container would like to occupy a large space. Essentially it is expanding, but since the rigid container cannot get larger, the air is compressed and there is a positive force exerted against the wall of the container. **A,** Descent. Water enters the open sphere as it descends (because of increased ambient pressure) to keep pressure on the inside and outside of the sphere equal. The air is neither expanding nor compressing, it is merely occupying the space it needs at any particular ambient pressure, and inner and outer pressures are always equal. As ambient pressure increases outside the closed sphere, the inner pressure becomes relatively less until the sphere finally implodes (bursts inward). The eardrum of the descending diver may *implode* if the eustachian tube is not patent and cannot allow air into the middle ear to equalize external and internal pressures. **B,** Ascent. As the open sphere ascends (decreased ambient pressure), air leaves the sphere to keep inner and outer pressures equal. As the closed sphere ascends, external pressure decreases and internal pressure becomes relatively greater. An explosion (burst outward) finally results. The eardrum of a diver whose eustachian tube suddenly closes as he is ascending may burst outward. Air in a balloon can expand or contract with changes in ambient pressure, thus the internal and external pressures remain equal with ascent or descent.

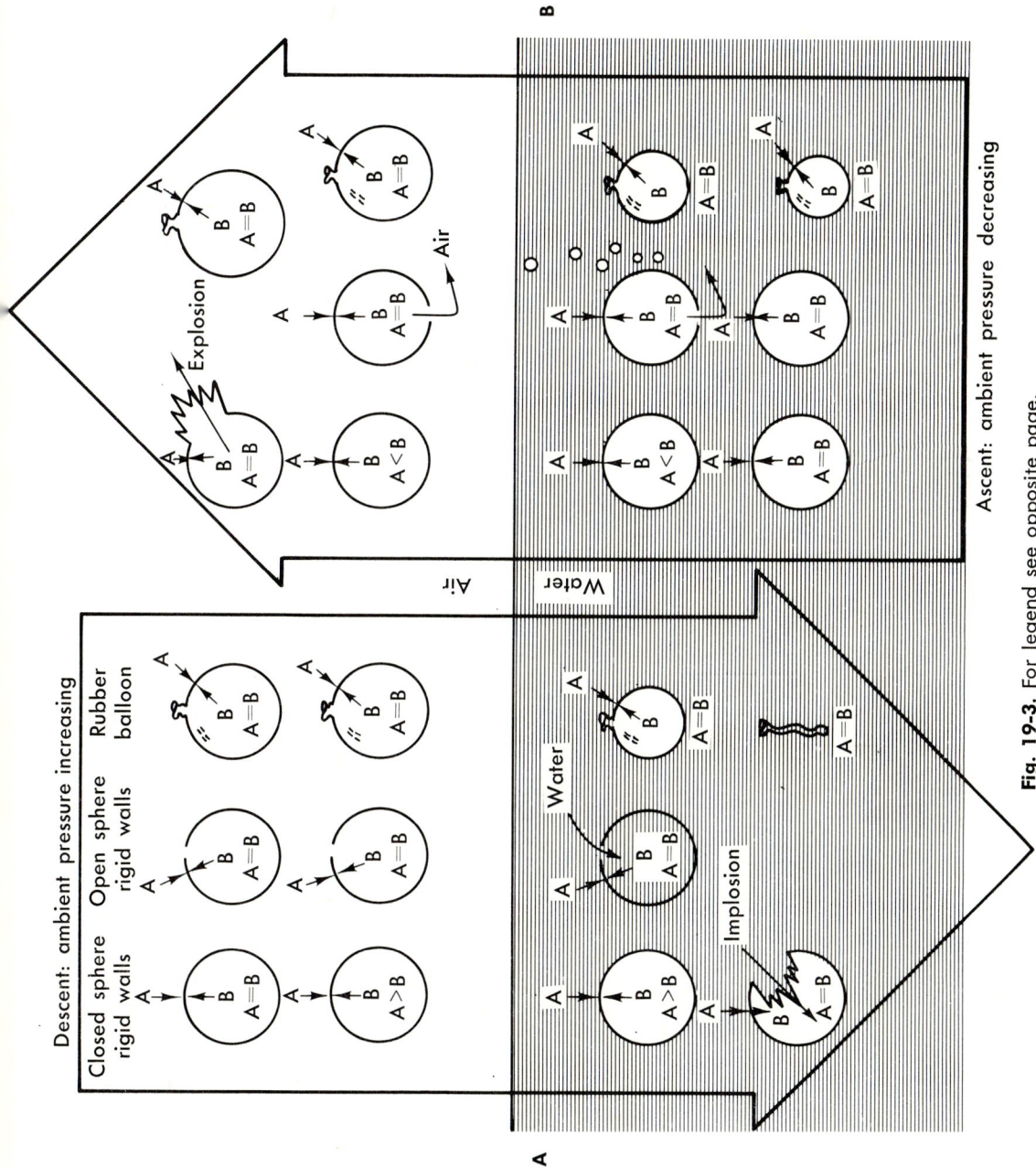

Fig. 19-3. For legend see opposite page.

severe cases artificial respiration and oxygen may be required. Hyperbaric oxygen, if available, provides the most effective treatment.

Pathologic effects of change in ambient pressure and the partial pressure of nitrogen in inhaled gases

On the surface of the earth the human body is in equilibrium with the ambient pressure (1 atmosphere) and the partial pressure of nitrogen in the air. Changes in these require compensatory changes in body spaces and tissues. Body spaces have vents to the outside, enabling them to maintain equilibrium with ambient pressure; for example, the middle ear and sinuses communicate with the external environment via tiny tubes and the lungs via the tracheal tube. When a vent from a noncollapsible body space is obstructed, injury may result from increased or decreased pressure (Fig. 19-2) within the space. The pressure within the space may be negative or positive depending on what direction air would flow were the vent to open (Fig. 19-3): negative (decreased pressure within the space) if the air would flow in; positive (increased pressure within the space) if the air would flow out. For clarity, one might picture what the air inside the noncollapsible space is trying to do. If it is trying to occupy a smaller space than that which it is in, which it does during descent as the ambient pressure increases, then the inside space pressure is negative and a relative vacuum exists; namely, water or air would flow into the space if the noncollapsible wall were punctured. If the noncollapsible wall were to break, an implosion would result. If the air is trying to occupy a space larger than it is in, which it does during ascent as outside pressure decreases, the inside pressure is positive and air would flow out if the noncollapsible wall were punctured. If the wall were to break, an explosion would result.

Air contains approximately 20% oxygen and 80% nitrogen. Nitrogen enters and leaves body tissues via the lungs and bloodstream (Fig. 19-4). The amount of nitrogen tissue can hold depends on the partial pressure of nitrogen in the breathing mixture and the type of cell involved. Fat cells can hold more nitrogen than water cells, but absorb and give it off more slowly. As the body descends and the partial pressure of nitrogen increases, tissues can absorb and hold more nitrogen. However, as the body ascends and the partial pressure of nitrogen decreases, body tissues cannot hold as much nitrogen and must give it off via the bloodstream and lungs (Table 19-8). At any particular ambient pressure, for example, at the earth's surface (1 atmosphere = 14.7 lbs/sq in), the amount of nitrogen in the tissues reaches a state of equilibrium with the partial pressure of nitrogen at that level, and the tissues are said to be saturated. Since it takes a certain amount of time for tissues to absorb and give off nitrogen, unless ascent or descent is very slow, there is always a lag between how much nitrogen the cells can hold and the rate at which they are absorbing or giving it off. This is of no consequence when the individual is descending. However, if the individual ascends faster than nitrogen can be given off by the cells, nitrogen bubbles form in the cells, tissues, and bloodstream triggering a sequence of pathologic events that constitute decompression sickness. This is true of ascent in both water and air (Table 19-9).

Diving emergencies related to changes in ambient pressure and the partial pressure of nitrogen may be divided into two major categories.

I. Blockage of vents normally open to outside (ambient) pressure
   A. Squeeze
   B. Pulmonary barotrauma
      1. Air embolism
      2. Pneumothorax
      3. Interstitial emphysema

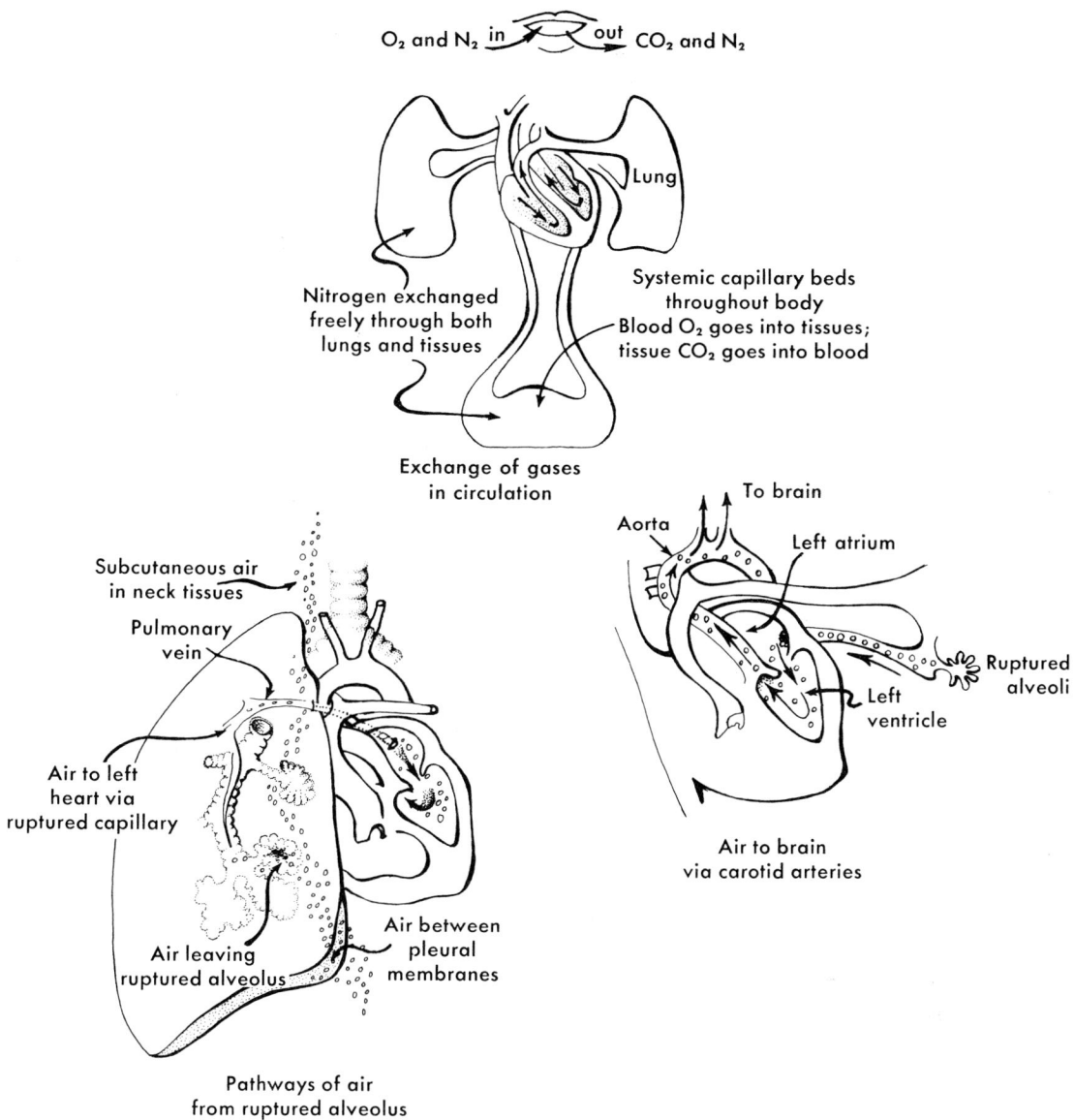

Fig. 19-4. Circulatory exchange of gases and bubble pathways.

Table 19-8. Amounts of gases dissolving in contact fluids at various partial pressures

Depth in feet	Total pressure		Partial pressure	
	Atmospheres	mm Hg	Nitrogen (mm Hg)	Oxygen (mm Hg)
0 (surface)	1	760	600	160
33	2	1,520	1,200	320
66	3	2,280	1,800	480
99	4	3,040	2,400	640
132	5	3,800	3,000	800

Table 19-9. Changes in pressure at various altitudes and depths

Altitude in feet	Pressure in atmospheres absolute
30,000	0.30
20,000	0.46
10,000	0.69
5,000	0.83
Sea level	1.00
Depth in feet	
100	4.00
250	8.55
500	16.15
1,000	31.30

II. Release of cellular or tissue nitrogen faster than it can be dissipated as the diver ascends—decompression sickness

Squeeze. According to Dr. Michael Strauss,[10] United States Navy Diving Officer, over 90% of the medical complaints seen in sports divers involve the ear. Some of these involve middle ear "squeeze" resulting from blockage of the eustachian tube because of infection, inflammation, or enlarged tonsils and adenoids. In these cases, negative pressure during descent may cause the eardrum to burst inward (implode, see Fig. 19-3, *A*), whereas positive pressure during ascent may cause it to burst outward (explode, see Fig. 19-3, *B*). Since a sudden hearing loss related to diving may result in permanent deafness if not immediately and properly cared for, an emergency exists.

Reactions include a feeling of fullness in the ear, tinnitus, pain, expectoration of blood, and dizziness. The eardrum becomes erythematous, injected, and may be ruptured. Profound or total hearing loss may result suddenly from mechanical damage to the ossicles or oval and round window membranes.

Closure of the eustachian tube usually responds to decongestants such as pseudoephedrine (Sudafed) or oxymetazoline (Afrin). If no response is obtained, the hearing loss may be the result of

inner ear damage, and proper care should be instituted immediately, aimed at decongesting the tissue and improving circulation. Histamine, nicotinic acid, anticholinergics, anticoagulants, and decongestants are recommended.[11] A mixture of 5% CO_2, 85% O_2, and 10% N_2, which is a potent dilator of cerebral vessels when inhaled, should be used for 15 minutes three times a day.

Decompression sickness, pulmonary barotrauma, and air embolism. Decompression sickness and pulmonary barotrauma with possible air embolism are two of the most potentially lethal diving medical emergencies. They both occur as the diver decompresses (ascends), and immediate recompression is mandatory to stop and reverse the pathophysiologic changes that would otherwise result in permanent injury or death. Since the emergency department probably will not have a recompression chamber, personnel must locate the nearest one and arrange transportation of the patient to it.

No time should be sacrificed to confirm a diagnosis. It is only necessary to recognize that decompression sickness or pulmonary barotrauma with the possibility of air embolism may be present to justify immediate action: *recompression in the nearest chamber capable of going to 165 feet (6 atmospheres)*, no matter where it is located. Competent duty officers, knowledgeable in the use of U. S. Navy Recompression Tables 3, 4, 5, 5a, 6, and 6a, as well as other current modes of therapy, will be present to take over the care of your patient. Permanent injury and death have resulted because of a reluctance to recompress promptly, whereas there is no record of a diver's having succumbed because of unnecessary recompression.

Decompression sickness or pulmonary barotrauma should be suspected when the following are present:

1. The diver has made a free ascent (NOTE: The greatest pressure changes

occur near the surface of the water; see Fig. 19-2.)

2. The diver has been making repeated dives
3. The diver has made a "fast" ascent after having been below 33 feet for some period of time
4. There is any indication of breath holding during ascent (NOTE: Divers are frequently unaware they have held their breath while ascending or are reluctant to admit it.)
5. There is a history of preexisting pulmonary pathology, for example, cysts, blebs, obstructive emphysema

One or any combination of the following reactions should alert personnel to the possibility of decompression sickness or pulmonary barotrauma and possibly air embolism in the patient: paralysis, pain and cyanosis, pain and convulsions, pain and dizziness, pain during ascent, hemiplegia aphasia, numbness, crepitance, swelling of the neck, change in voice quality, chest pain, uneven expansion of the chest, weakness of arms or legs, tingling, cough, hemoptysis, unconsciousness occurring during ascent or at the surface, unequal pupils, visual disturbances, hyperpnea, mottling of the tongue, decreased breath sounds during auscultation, disorientation, unexplained rash, or any unexplained pain, particularly around the joints.

Call the duty officer at the Navy Experimental Diving Unit, Washington, D.C.; phone 202-433-2790 to locate the nearest recompression chamber on land or sea and to obtain assistance with a diving medical emergency. This service is available 24 hours a day, seven days a week.

The United States Coast Guard will also assist in locating the nearest recompression chamber and transporting the patient to it. It should be kept in mind that transportation in aircraft incapable of being pressurized to ground (1 atmosphere) pressure is contraindicated.

While transporting the patient to a re-

compression chamber, supportive therapy may include cardiac massage, respiratory assistance (100% oxygen should always be given if available), and intravenous administration of sodium bicarbonate. The patient should lie down at all times, regardless of apparent condition, with the head lower than the feet and the body tilted 20 degrees longitudinally toward the left to reduce the possibility of bubbles entering the cerebral circulation.[12]

Pulmonary barotrauma. Pulmonary barotrauma is injury to lung tissues caused by overdistension of the alveoli that results from expansion of air forcibly held in the lungs as the diver ascends (see Fig. 19-3, *B*). Once lungs are damaged, air bubbles (emboli) entering the circulation via torn vessels are a continuing possibility until a certain amount of healing has taken place.

Air can be forcibly held in the lungs during ascent by breath holding, laryngospasm, or preexisting lung pathology. As lung tissue is stretched, the alveolar membranes may rupture with leakage of air causing the following:

1. Air embolism with cerebral or coronary infarction (Fig. 19-4, *B*)
2. Pneumothorax (NOTE: Spontaneous pneumothorax may occur in the diver from the rupture of preexisting lung cysts, etc., or it may be catamenial[13] in the female diver.)
3. Interstitial and subcutaneous emphysema (Fig. 19-4, *C*)

Cardiac or cerebral manifestations of air embolism usually occur within seconds or minutes of surfacing. Vertigo and limb tingling may be the only signs.[14] Other signs include sudden loss of consciousness, convulsions, spastic or flaccid paralysis (commonly vertical, i.e., involvement of one half the entire body longitudinally), bleeding from the mouth, or visual changes. Pneumothorax may be present with hyperpnea, blueness of the fingernails and lips, and cough or decreased breath sounds on the collapsed side of the chest. Interstitial and subcutaneous emphysema may be accompanied by chest pain.

Berhage[15] reported on over 1,000 barotrauma accidents that occurred in the U. S. Navy. Pathologic findings are shown in Table 19-10.

The presenting signs and symptoms in 30 cases of pulmonary barotrauma reported by Miles[14] are shown in Table 19-11.

It has already been stated that the care for pulmonary barotrauma is immediate recompression in a chamber. Pneumothorax and subcutaneous or interstitial emphysema are usually self-healing and require no attention other than rest. The difficulty is that in their presence the threat of air embolism exists; hence, extremely conservative measures are indicated.

Decompression sickness. As the diver ascends, ambient pressure decreases (Tables 19-8 and 19-9), and the nitrogen absorbed by body cells must be expelled. If the ambient pressure decreases too rapidly, nitrogen cannot be expelled fast enough and forms bubbles in cells (as yet hypothetical), tissue, and the bloodstream. The various pathophysiologic changes that occur when nitrogen forms bubbles before it can be expelled are collectively called decompression sickness.

The pathology of decompression sickness may involve any or all of the body systems. About 25% of decompression victims will have neurologic symptoms.[12] Edema in or around the spinal cord, if not resolved immediately, may result in permanent nerve injury. In about 2% of the cases respiratory symptoms called "chokes" develop.[12] This pulmonary condition is very similar to the "shock lung syndrome." Considerable changes in the hemostatic system and blood and urine chemistries have been noted by many workers. Philp[16] studied 16 human subjects and noted *increased* packed-cell volume, hemoglobin concentration, plasma-free fatty acids, and prothrombin time; *decreased* platelet counts, plasma cortisol, complement activity, serum lactate, euglobulin lysis time, and prothrombin consumption time. Other studies have shown a tendency toward red blood cell clumping.

There is strong evidence of decompression sickness if unexplainable itches, rashes, pains, respiratory distress, visual defects, paralysis, or signs and symptoms of cerebrospinal irritation appear in a decompressed individual. The evaluation is confirmed if signs and symptoms disappear on recompression of the patient.

As previously discussed, the care of decompression sickness is immediate recompression. Research evidence indicates that low molecular weight dextran 40 given

Table 19-10. Pathologic findings of 1,000 barotrauma accidents that occurred in the U.S. Navy*†

Findings	Percentage
Air embolism	45%
Mediastinal emphysema	20%
Subcutaneous emphysema	8%
Pneumothorax	5%

*Twenty-two percent of the cases were "suspected barotrauma" with no further diagnosis.
†Data from Berhage, T. E.: Summary statistics: U.S. Navy diving accidents, Res. Report 1-66, U.S. Navy Experimental Diving Unit, Washington, D.C., June 1, 1966.

Table 19-11. Presenting signs and symptoms in 30 cases of pulmonary barotrauma*

Signs and symptoms	Number of cases
Unconsciousness	16
Pain in the chest	13
Weakness and paralysis	13
Disorientation	9
Cough	6
Visual impairment	4
Convulsions	3
Breathlessness	2
Cyanosis	2

*Data from Miles, S.: Underwater medicine, Philadelphia, 1972, J. B. Lippincott Co.

intravenously has plasma-expanding, anti-sludging, and anti-platelet-adhesive properties. Whether this offsets the disadvantage of its contribution to pulmonary edema with decreased ventilation remains to be seen.* It might be best to start intravenous fluids only after the patient's blood volume can be monitored. Other supportive therapy should be used as indicated.

AQUATIC ORGANISMS

The survival of some aquatic animals is partly dependent upon protective or aggressive behavior and toxic mechanisms. Those that are potentially deadly and may cause an emergency will be discussed.

Dangerous and venomous organisms

Dangerous and venomous aquatic organisms may be divided into three categories: (1) animals that bite, (2) animals that sting, and (3) animals that have spines.

Each of the above three categories contains venomous aquatic animals. Generally, aquatic animal venoms fall into two classes: those used for defense and those used offensively to obtain food. Defensive venoms are usually not meant to kill but merely to warn the intruder to stay away; hence, they are quick acting and usually very painful, as in the stingray injury. Offensive or food-obtaining venoms are usually found at the oral pole, the mouth. They are generally neurotoxic, relatively painless, and contain poisons and enzymes meant to paralyze the prey and start enzymatic digestive processes. Examples include the venom of the sea snake and octopus.

Injuries from animals in all the above categories may be the source of secondary infection. Considerable bacterial and viral pollution is found in both fresh and salt water, particularly near large cities and river estuaries. Both gram-positive and gram-negative organisms may be present, so a broad-spectrum antibiotic is recommended prophylactically in the care of all water-related injuries. *C tetani* spores have not yet been found in any type of water, and tetanus is no more likely to occur in water-related injuries than in terrestrial ones. Routine caution should, of course, be used when caring for water-related injuries.

Generally, traumatic injuries are attended routinely. Injuries from venomous animals are cared for with heat, tourniquets, and antivenins. The total physiologic effect depends upon the toxicity of the venom, the amount injected, and the site of injection, as well as the age, state of health, and sensitivity of the victim. Death may result despite a wide variation in any one of these factors, including toxicity.

Venoms of most aquatic animals have at least one protein fraction that is heat labile. To obtain maximum benefits, heat must be used properly. Too little heat used for too short a time will have no effect on toxic substances in the tissues. The patient, particularly a child, will tolerate more heat if the temperature is raised slowly. Put the extremity into comfortably hot water, then add hotter water slowly to obtain the highest temperature the patient can tolerate, short of first degree burns. Temperatures between 43° and 46° C (110° and 114° F) should be maintained for a minimum of 30 minutes. Remember that the very young and very old cannot dissipate heat entering the body via the skin as well as the intermediate age group, and will, therefore, blister more easily. The process is repeated each time symptoms return, to effect complete and prolonged detoxification. Hot compresses or total body immersion may be necessary for parts of the body other than the extremities.

Some confinement of toxic substances to local areas may be obtained by slowing

*The reader is referred to Moss, G.: Shark lung: a disorder of the central nervous system, Hosp. Pract., Aug., 1974, p. 77, for a better understanding of the so-called wet lung syndrome.

down venous return using an elastic tourniquet; allow for the insertion of one finger between the tourniquet and the skin. The tourniquet should be loosened, not removed, for two to three minutes every 45 to 60 minutes. In cases of extreme envenomation or sensitivity, a properly applied tourniquet may be life saving.

Antivenins for sea snake, stonefish, and deadly sea wasp (jellyfish) toxins are available from the Commonwealth Serum Laboratories in Melbourne, Australia.

Bites. Aquatic animals that can inflict injury by biting include sharks, barracudas, moray eels, octopuses, sea snakes, sea lions, and killer whales. Care of these injuries is routine and may include deep exploration and x-ray studies for evaluation purposes and to determine the presence of foreign material, such as shark teeth.

All sea snake bites and octopus bites contain a neurotoxin of varying toxicity, depending on the species.[17] The sea snake uses its venom to obtain live food and is apparently reluctant to waste it. It probably can control the amount of venom injected at any one time; hence, defensive bites usually contain a minimal amount of toxin. Lethal bites in man are rare.

Local effects from sea snake and octopus bites are usually minimal and relatively painless. Systemic signs and symptoms may develop within two to six hours and include muscle stiffness, myoglobulinuria, paralysis, collapse, and death from respiratory arrest. Although *O rugosus,* an octopus found in Australian and nearby waters, is reported to have caused several deaths,[18] the bites of most octopuses are of minor consequence.

Initial emergency care consists of applying a tourniquet, controlling shock, and giving cardiac and respiratory support if required. Respiratory paralysis is managed as with bulbar poliomyelitis and may include intubation, tracheotomy, and the use of a respirator or iron lung.

Stings. All coelenterates, that is, jelly-fish, hydrozoans (Portuguese man-of-war), anemones, and corals, have characteristic nematocysts (stinging capsules). Each nematocyst contains an inverted threadlike stinger coiled within it that everts when the capsule "fires." Nematocysts may break loose from the main body of the organism and may be present in the water or on the beach; they can retain their ability to fire for months. Microscopic stinging capsules deposited on the skin may "fire" immediately or some time later. Under certain conditions, mechanical stimuli (rubbing the skin with sand), exposure to fresh water, or a change in pH may cause a nematocyst to "fire" and inject its venom (Fig. 19-5).[19]

Not all species have nematocysts capable of penetrating human skin, and the toxicity of injected venom varies with species; it may be innocuous or lethal to humans. Coelenterate toxins are allergenic, and sensitive individuals may exhibit allergic reactions, including anaphylaxis.

Nematocyst injuries are frequently misdiagnosed because the victim has not seen the offending organism. Microscopic evidence of nematocysts in skin scrapings will confirm the diagnosis and may identify the species. Lesions consist of burnlike welts, occurring singly, in clusters, or in whiplike streaks.

Initial pain is sudden, confusing, and may be of sufficient intensity to cause shock and collapse. It is probable that a number of drownings have indirectly resulted from contact with nematocysts. In addition to pain, the victim may experience a throbbing headache, cramps, paralysis, or sensations of suffocation.

Care for nematocyst wounds is almost specific, namely, alcohol to inactivate intact nematocysts (prevent them from firing), and a basic substance to neutralize the acid-reacting venom. Alcohol (isopropyl, perfume, liquor, etc.) is poured on the affected skin areas and left for six to eight minutes. A supersaturated solution of baking soda (sodium bicarbonate) is then ap-

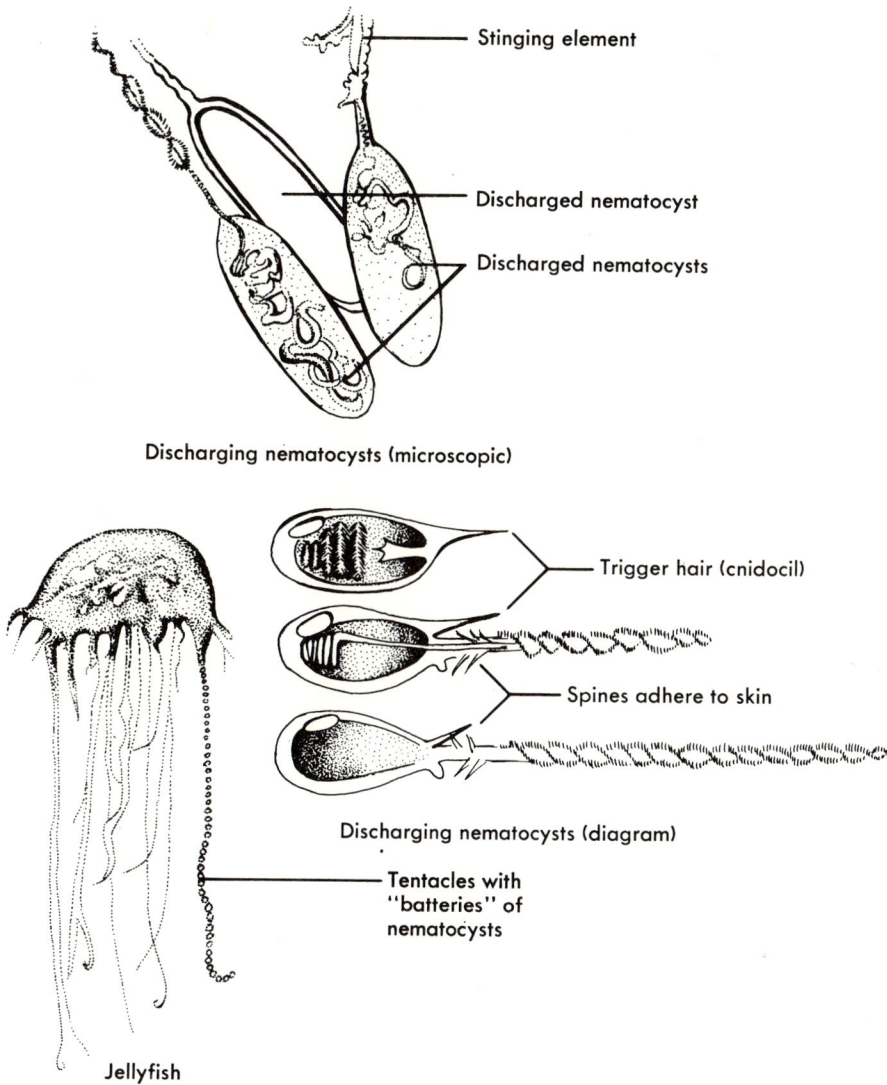

Fig. 19-5. All coelenterates, that is, jellyfish, corals, hydroids, and anemones, have stinging nematocysts.

plied and allowed to dry. In cases of severe envenomation or in hypersensitivity reactions tourniquets to restrict venous return may be life saving.

Spines. Many aquatic organisms such as the stingray, sea urchin, catfish, and scorpion fish have spines capable of inflicting traumatic and venomous wounds.

Stingray. Approximately 750 people are stung by stingrays each year along the North American coasts.[20] When stepped on, the stingray flips its tail into an arc, exposing a sharp spine covered by a thin and venomous integumentary sheath (Fig. 19-6). The barbed spine carries the venom into the skin creating a lacerationlike wound, which can be extensive and requires debridement and surgery.

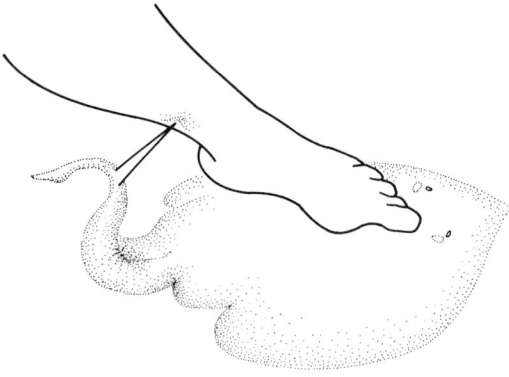

Fig. 19-6. Stingray injury.

The predominant symptom is a sharp, shooting, throbbing, or spasmodic pain, sometimes of extreme intensity. Although reactions are usually localized, the venom may produce changes in the cardiovascular, respiratory, nervous, or urinary systems. Low concentration of venom causes transient peripheral vasodilation or constriction; lethal amounts cause marked vasoconstriction and cardiac standstill, with secondary respiratory effects. Syncope, weakness, nausea, nervousness, arrhythmias, vomiting, tremors, generalized cramps, inguinal or axillary pain, and respiratory distress may be present.

Of 1,097 stingray injuries reported over a five-year period in the United States, 232 were seen by a physician at some time during the recovery phase.[21] Sixty-two victims were hospitalized; the majority of these required surgical closure of the wounds or treatment for secondary infection or both. At least ten patients were hospitalized for care because of over-exuberant first aid care (the use of potassium permanganate, ammonia, formaldehyde, or ice water). Only eight were hospitalized because of systemic effects suffered from the toxin. There were two fatalities.

Heat promptly and properly applied is the most effective treatment for stingray envenomation. Relief from pain is immediate and dramatic. Flushing the wound with normal saline removes some foreign material and toxin.

Scorpion fish. Scorpion fish, including the California sculpin, stonefish, and lionfish, have venomous fin spines capable of inflicting painful and potentially lethal injuries. They are found in the warmer North American waters and are popular in public and home aquariums. Approximately 300 Americans are stung each year by *Scorpaena guttata* (sculpin) or related species.[22] Scott Carpenter, astronaut turned aquanaut, was stung on the hand by a California scuplin during the U. S. Navy Sea Lab program off the coast of San Diego, California, in 1965. Extensive medication was required to control swelling of the entire arm.

Responses include immediate and intense pain and swelling, which may progress to the axilla or groin. In severe envenomation with systemic effects, excruciating pain, primary shock, pulmonary edema, and ECG changes will require hospitalization.

The proper use of heat and antivenin will neutralize the venom, and the wound should be managed as for stingray injuries.

Catfish. The catfish has venomous spines on its dorsal and pectoral fins capable of inflicting severe and potentially contaminated (because of life habits) injuries. Envenomation produces an instant stinging, throbbing pain which usually subsides in an hour. The wound should be cleansed and irrigated and a broad-spectrum antibiotic given to avoid secondary infection.

Sea urchins. Sea urchin spines and pedicellaries (tiny fanglike organs among the spines) may inflict venomous and traumatic injuries, depending on the species. When barbs are present on the spines of some species, they point toward the tip of the spine, making continued penetration almost impossible (Fig. 19-7, *B*). The ven-

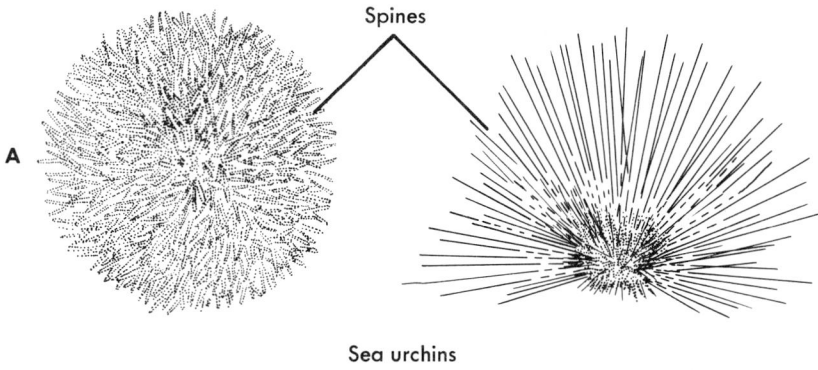

Spines

A

Sea urchins

B Tip of
spine

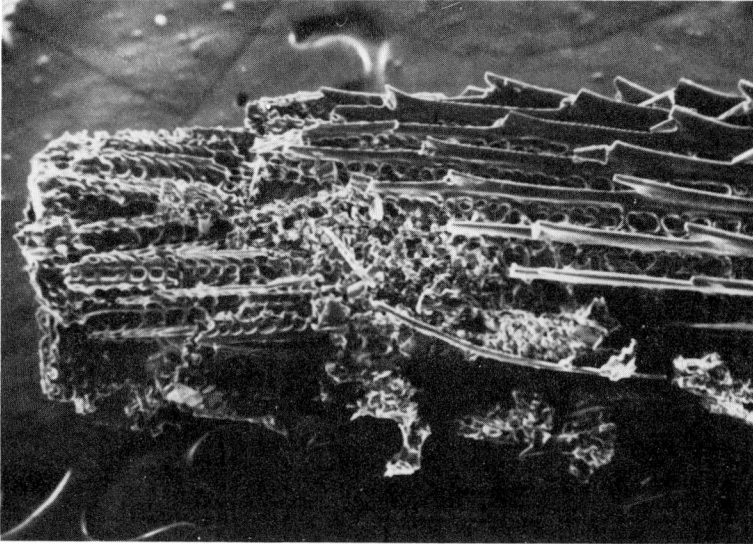

Forward-
pointing
barbs
←

Tip of spine taken from a purple sea urchin
(Stronglyocentrotus franciscanus)

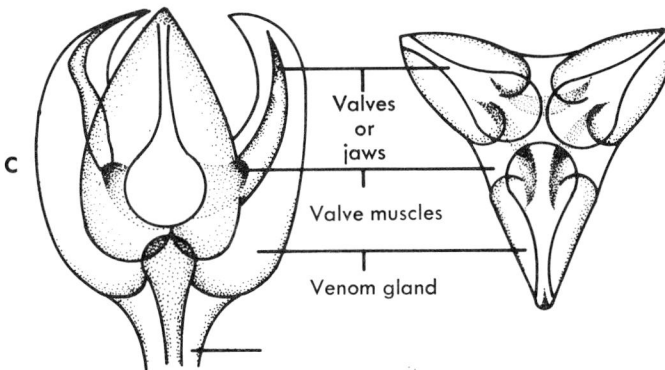

C

Valves
or
jaws

Valve muscles

Venom gland

Pedicellaria—found at base of spines

Fig. 19-7. Sea urchin spines and pedicellariae. (**B** from electronmicrophotograph by W. L. Orris, Scripps Institution of Oceanography.)

om of pedicellariae is apparently more toxic than that of venomous spines (Fig. 19-7).

Penetration of spines may produce immediate pain, followed by erythema, swelling, numbness, and possibly paralysis.[23] Pedicellariae (Fig. 19-7, *C*), encountered mostly in the short-spine urchins, may cause radiating pain, numbness, paralysis, respiratory distress, and death.

Envenomation responds to heat and supportive therapy. The spines are highly frangible and some contain a dye that makes it difficult to determine their presence in tissue. Most are readily absorbed; others require surgical removal, particularly if a granulomatous reaction has been stimulated. An attempt should be made to demonstrate the presence of spines by x-ray examination. Immediate attempts at surgical removal may be unrewarding and mutilating. A granulomatous lesion may result from an embedded urchin spine. This is probably the result of foreign protein reaction caused by the spiny integumentary sheath, which also may be instrumental in preventing absorption of the spiny skeleton.

Poisonous aquatic organisms

Aquatic gastrointestinal emergencies (ichthyotoxism). A wide variety of normally edible aquatic animals may suddenly become poisonous, probably because of environmental factors.

Ciguatera and paralytic shellfish poisoning. The toxic syndromes seen in ciguatera and paralytic shellfish poisoning are very similar, indicating the two toxins may be closely related, if not identical.

Ciguatoxin may be found in marine reef or shore fish between latitudes 35° N and 34° S.[22] Paralytic shellfish poison (saxitoxin) occurs spasmodically in the Alaskan butter clam, the California mussel, and other species along the Pacific coast and Gulf of Mexico, and in shellfish along the Atlantic coast. A true nerve poison with a curarelike action is involved. Pathognomonic reactions appear within one-half hour of ingestion and include tingling or burning of the face, lips, and tongue, which gradually spreads to the neck, arms, fingertips, legs, and toes. Paresthesia may progress to numbness, motor incoordination, paralysis, and death by respiratory failure—usually within 12 hours. Gastrointestinal symptoms, namely, vomiting, diarrhea, and abdominal pains, are not common.[19]

Care consists of immediate evacuation of the stomach or the use of absorbents and alkaline fluids or both. In severe cases maintaining respiration may be paramount. Forced diuresis helps to remove the toxin from the system. Nikethamide, neostigmine, and pyridoxine may be useful in combating respiratory depression by means of CNS stimulation, reversal of the curarelike effects and neurologic stabilization, respectively.

Scombroid poisoning. Scombroid fishes, that is, mackerellike fishes (tuna, bonita, mackerel, skipjack, etc.) have a considerable amount of histidine in their dark flesh. When improperly stored, bacterial action changes this to saurine, a histaminelike substance. When ingested, saurine causes symptoms similar to those of severe allergy, namely, nausea and vomiting, flushing of the face, intense headache, epigastric pain, burning of the throat with difficulty swallowing, thirst, and swelling of the lips. Symptoms usually subside within 12 hours.

Administration of an antihistamine and evacuation of stomach contents with catharsis is recommended if the patient is fully conscious and there is no respiratory distress. Intravenous administration of steroids may be necessary in severe cases.

MISCELLANEOUS REACTIONS
Amoebic encephalitis

Naegleria aerobii (formerly *N gruberii*), a free-living amoeba found in fresh water, reaches human nerve tissue via nasal membranes causing encephalitis. Bacterial pollution of fresh water is increasing, resulting in a proliferation of *N aerobii* and exposure of many swimmers, particularly younger ones, to this deadly disease.[24]

Symptoms usually start with a headache, which progresses rapidly in intensity to blindness, coma, and death within seven days. The patient becomes delirious as the fever mounts. Diagnosis is difficult and usually made at autopsy. A high index of suspicion and knowledge of the patient's swimming in fresh water prior to the onset of symptoms are helpful.

No specific therapy for this disease is presently available. The use of amphoteri-cin B (Fungizone) in the largest intravenous dosage possible is recommended.

Algal allergic reactions

When microscopic algal plants come into contact with skin or mucous membranes, an allergic rash or symptoms similar to a cold or hay fever may result. This is particularly true in areas of so-called "algal blooms," such as the Red Tides seen on the west coast of Florida. The algae may be either waterborne or airborne. Even persons with no previous history of allergic sensitivity may react to algae. Care is the same as for other allergic reactions, namely, antihistamines and steroids.[25-27]

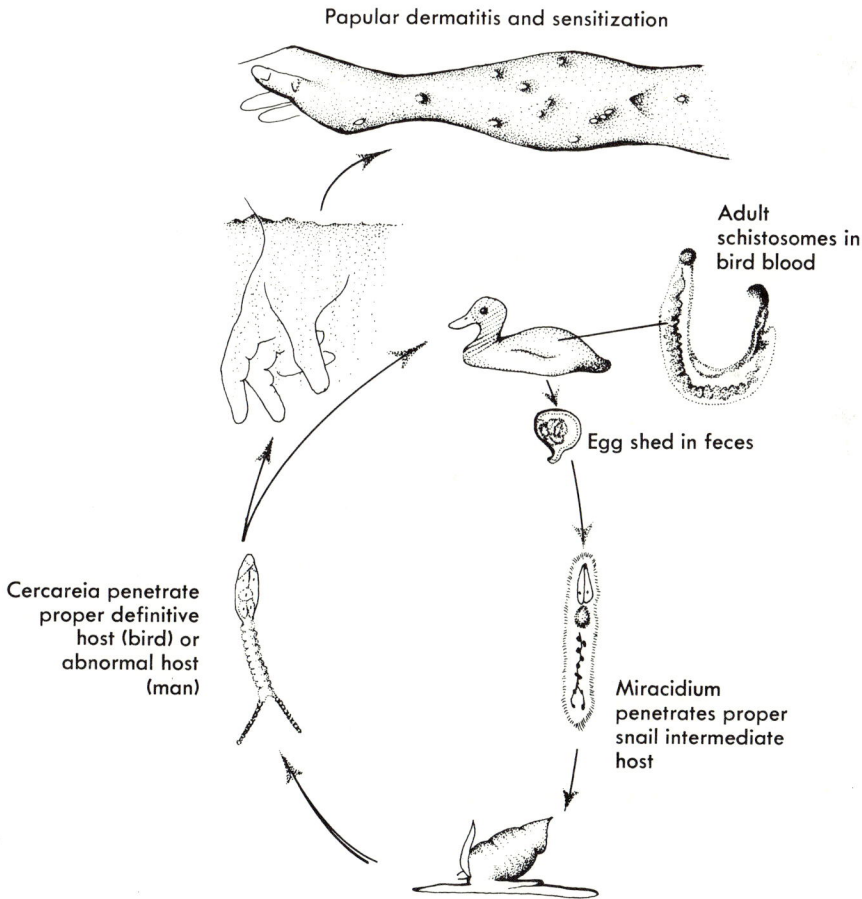

Fig. 19-8. Life cycle of schistosome, which causes cercarial dermatitis.

Cercarial dermatitis

Genera of the family Schistosomatidae are found in fresh and salt water in most places of the world.[28] Free-swimming cercariae, seeking a bird or mammal, are part of the life cycle of this parasite, which includes a species-specific water snail. When man intrudes into the water habitat, cercariae may penetrate the skin, causing a papular rash and subsequent sensitization. The rash may be accompanied by intense itching and swelling (Fig. 19-8).

This disconcerting disease is self-limiting, and palliative measures, such as isopropyl alcohol, Caladryl, antihistamines, or steroids, are usually effective.

SUMMARY

The number of aquatic medical emergencies is increasing because of an increase in water activities and water pollution. The speed of air travel makes it possible for medical personnel anywhere in the United States to be confronted with one of these emergencies. Recognition of these emergencies may require a high index of sus-

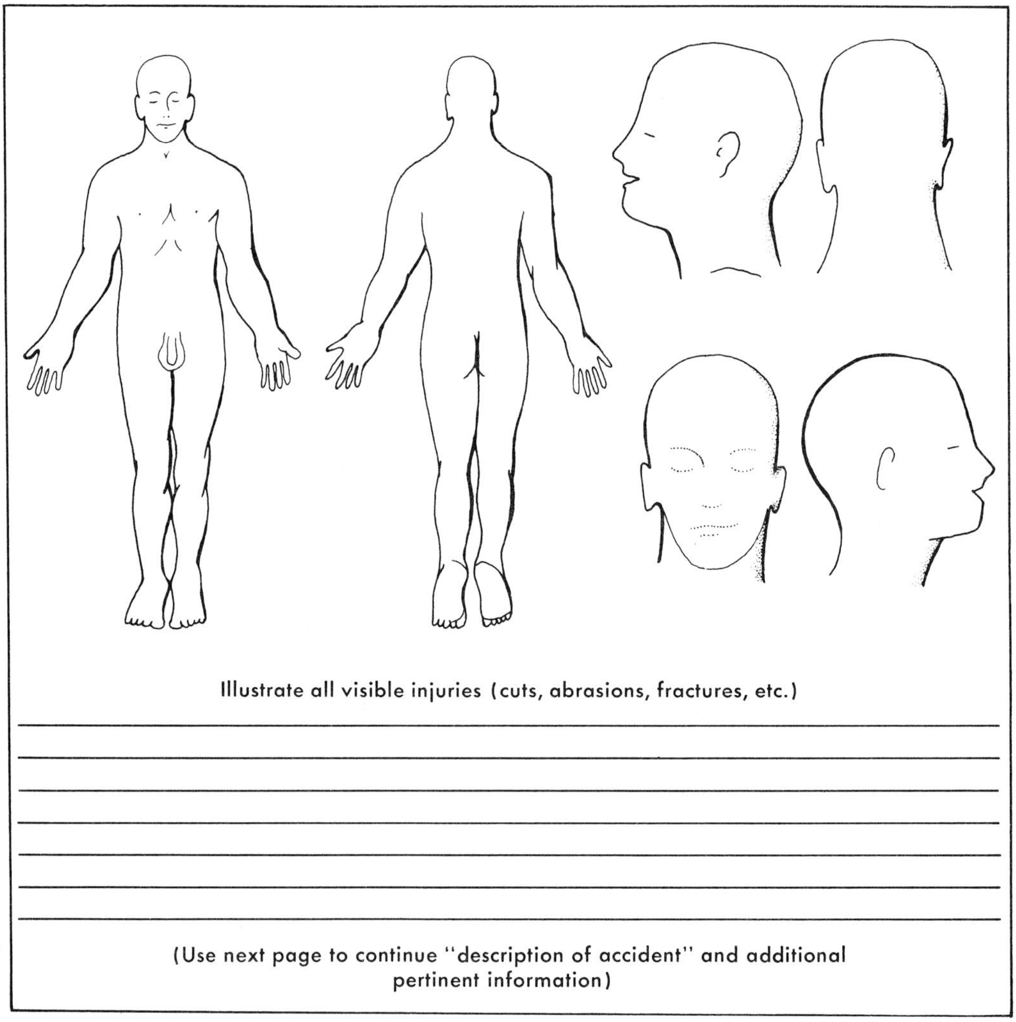

Illustrate all visible injuries (cuts, abrasions, fractures, etc.)

(Use next page to continue "description of accident" and additional pertinent information)

Fig. 19-9. Report forms available from URI Scuba Safety Project.

UNDERWATER ACCIDENT REPORT

Name of victim _____

                              Last   First   Middle

Address _____

_____ State_____

Location of accident _____
(use landmarks, distance
from prominent terrain _____
features. Attach chart
or map if available) _____

_____ State _____

Jurisdiction or organiza- _____
tion reporting

Address _____

_____ State_____

(Designate location
by code number)

1. Ocean, bay, sea
2. Minor lake, pond, slough
3. Quarry, pit, open mine   3A. Cave
4. River
5. Major lake, pond
6. Swimming pool
7. Great Lakes

Date and time of accident _____ _____
                              Day   Mo.   Yr.   (Use 24 Hour Clock)

Date and time of death _____

Date and time of recovery _____

Death occurred in water? _____
                                (Yes or No)

Victim's Sex___ Age___ Hgt. ___Wgt. ____

Marital Status M__ S__ D__ W__ UNK ___

Occupation_____

Employer_____

Cause of death_____

Autopsy performed:_____
                    (Yes or No)

Medical examiner_____
           Name   Address   Phone

Code for Nonfatal incident. Circle one only (A, B, C, or D) which best describes seriousness of incident. Important: Report all "incidents", however minor. Describe in detail below. Include equipment factors.

A. Incapacitating injury rendering person unable to perform normal activities as walking or diving or to leave scene without assistance.

C. Possible injury indicated by complaint of pain, blackout, limping, nausea, etc.

B. Nonincapacitating evident injury as loss of blood, abrasions, lump on head, etc.

D. Incident with no apparent injury (near miss, etc.)

Description of all dives within previous 12 hours including accident dive.

Depth	Time down	Surface interval
_____	_____	_____
_____	_____	_____
_____	_____	_____
_____	_____	_____

Type of diving: (explain if necessary)

Scuba___ Skin___ Other___ Unknown_____

At time of incident:
activities engaged in:

Recreational _____
Commercial _____
Under instruction _____
Instructing _____
Cave diving _____
Spear fishing _____
Photography _____
Night diving _____

At time of incident:
Buddy record

Diving alone_____
Diving with buddy_____
Buddy distance_____
Diving with more than one_____
Distance to next nearest diver_____

Others in accident _____
          (Yes or No)

Separate report filed _____
          (Yes or No)

Vessels involved _____
          (Yes or No)

U.S. Coast Guard aid sought _____
          (Yes or No)

WITNESSES AND OTHER SOURCES OF INFORMATION (Names, addresses, and phone)

(Give details in "description of accident" name, captain, address, phone, etc.)

_____
_____
_____
_____

Name and address of reporter _____ Phone_____

Describe in detail how the accident happened, including what the person was doing, any specific marine life or objects, and the action or movement which led to the event. Include details of first aid or resuscitation efforts. Describe any "decompression" and/or "recompression-treatment" in description of accident.

_____
_____
_____
_____
_____

(Use page four for additional reporting space)

Continued.

Fig. 19-9, cont'd. Report forms available from URI Scuba Safety Project.

ENVIRONMENTAL CONDITIONS

Sea: Calm_____Moderate_____Rough_____   Weather: Clear____ Cloudy____ Fog____ Snow____ Rain _____

Current: Slight____ Moderate_____Strong_____ Direction_____   Thunderstorms____Tornado, hurricane ____ Other_____

Wave height:_____Water depth:_____ Type bottom:_____   Wind force_____ Direction _____

Water temperature: (°F)_____   Air temperature: (°F)_____

HUMAN FACTORS

Swimming experience: Years _____ Scuba experience: Years _____

Skindiving experience: Years_____Courses and agency (1) _____Certification date_____

(2) _____ -DO- _____

Hours of sleep in past 24 hours____   (3) _____ -DO- _____

Time of last meal _____   What and how much?_____

Time of last alcoholic drink _____What and how much?_____

Any known physical ailments, disability or impairment _____

_____

Equipment data Date and time of Inspection	Brand, type	Present before diving (Yes or No)	Present at time of recovery (Yes or No)	Condition	Equipment	Brand, type, serial no.	Present before diving (Yes or No)	Present at time of recovery (Yes or No)	Condition
Diving suit					Knife (posit.)				
Hood					Ab iron				
Boots or socks					Flashlight				
Gloves or mits					Depth gauge				
Mask					Spear gun				
Snorkel					Compass				
Fins					Regulator				
Weight belt (lbs)					Tank				
Buckle					Reserve				
Flotation device					Watch				
Other equipment									

Flotation device: Used _____ Tested after event?_____   Results _____
                               (Yes or No)   (Yes or No)

Tank: Air left_____ MFG._____Date_____ Last hydro-test date_____ Last visual inspection date_____
      (PSIG)

Internal condition: Clean_____Slight corrosion_____Extensive corrosion_____Other_____

Regulator tested? _____   Results _____
                        (Yes or No)

By: _____
    Name   Address   Phone

Special comments: on equipment_____

Equipment inspected by: _____
                              Name   Address   Phone

Equipment: Released to/or/held by:_____
                                       Name   Address   Phone

Fig. 19-9, cont'd. Report forms available from URI Scuba Safety Project.

picion. Special training in modes of care and an understanding of the pathophysiology involved are prerequisites for effective attention and life-saving decisions. Victims of aquatic medical emergencies are usually young and in good physical condition. They are often more seriously ill than is apparent, and great care must be exercised to avoid underestimating their medical problems. Making a diagnosis implies putting a specific name to the patient's illness. This may, in fact, be impossible since the illness may have various etiologies with such combinations as near drowning with decompression sickness, decompression sickness with air embolism, or near drowning with a venomous aquatic animal injury. Since time is of the essence, it is obviously more important to synthesize the patient's signs, symptoms, and laboratory results than it is to waste time groping for a specific name for the illness. As is always true in the evaluation phase of an illness, an accurate and exact history from the patient or a witness will be extremely helpful. Heat is the one most useful tool in the care of envenomation by an aquatic animal. Inhaled oxygen and intravenous sodium bicarbonate are the two most useful drugs in the care of near drowning. Recompression in a chamber capable of going to 165 feet is mandatory for victims of pulmonary barotrauma or decompression sickness.

REFERENCES

1. Spiess, R.: The ocean environment, Astronautics Aeronautics 4(4):40-45, 1966.
2. Modell, J. H.: Drowning and near-drowning, Springfield, Ill., 1971, Charles C Thomas, Publisher.
3. Miles, S.: Medical hazards of diving. In Davies, C. N., and others: The effects of abnormal physical conditions at work, London, 1967, E. & S. Livingstone Ltd., p. 111.
4. Grausz, H., Amend, W. J., Jr., and Earley, L. E.: Acute renal failure complicating submersion in sea water, J.A.M.A. 217(2):207-209, 1971.
5. Giordano, J. M., Joseph, W. L., Klingenmaier, C. H., and others: The management of interstitial pulmonary edema, J. Thorac. Cardiovasc. Surg. 64:739-746, 1972.
6. Bullard, R. W., and Rapp, G. M.: Problems of body heat loss in body immersion, Aerospace Med. 41:1269, 1970.
7. Keating, W. R.: The physiology and treatment of immersion hypothermia and drowning, Oxford, 1971, Oxford University Press.
8. Wanderer, A. A., and Ellis, E. F.: Treatment of cold urticaria with cyproheptadine, J. Allergy Clin. Immunol. 48:366-371, 1971.
9. U. S. Navy Diving Manual, March 1970, NAVSHIPS 0994-001-9000.
10. Strauss, M.: Skin Diver Magazine, p. 16, Sept. 1971.
11. Deafness can result from damage to inner ear membranes, Medical News, July 5, 1971.
12. Department of Ocean Engineering: Scuba safety report series, Report 3, Kingston, R. I., 1971, University of Rhode Island.
13. Lillington, G. A., Mitchell, S. P., and Wood, G. A.: Catamenial pneumothorax, J.A.M.A. 219(10):1328-1332, 1972.
14. Miles, S.: Underwater medicine, Philadelphia, 1972, J. B. Lippincott Co.
15. Berhage, T. E.: Summary statistics: U. S. navy diving accidents, Research Report 1-66, Washington, D.C., U. S. Navy Experimental Diving Unit, June 1, 1966.
16. Philp, R. B., Ackles, K. N., Inwood, M. J., et al.: Changes in hemostatic system and in blood and urine chemistry of human subjects following decompression from hyperbaric environment, Aerospace Med. 43:498-505, 1972.
17. Pickwell, G., and Evans, W. E., editors: Handbook of dangerous animals for field personnel, Andersen Naval Center.
18. Cleland, J. B., and Southcott, R. V.: Injuries to man from marine invertebrates in the Australian region, Canberra, 1965.
19. Hyman, L. H.: The invertebrates, New York, 1940, McGraw-Hill Book Co., pp. 382-392.
20. Russell, F. E.: Stingray injuries, Public Health Rep. 74:855-859, 1959.
21. Russell, F. E.: Stingray injuries: a review and discussion of their treatment, Am. J. Med. Sci. 226:611-622, 1953.
22. Russell, F. E.: Poisonous marine animals, Neptune City, N. J., 1971, T. F. H. Publications, p. 144.
23. Halstead, B.: Dangerous marine animals, Cambridge, Md., 1959, Cornell Maritime Press.
24. Center for Disease Control, Morbidity and Mortality, vol. 20, no. 24, June 19, 1971.
25. Heise, H. A.: Symptoms of hayfever caused by algae, Ann. Allergy 9:100, 1951.

26. Natural gas, Environment, vol. 12, no. 2, 1970.
27. McElhenney, T. R.: Algae: a cause of inhalant allergy in children, Ann. Allergy **20:** 739-743, 1962.
28. Chu, W. T. C.: Pacific area distribution of fresh-water and marine cercarial dermatitis, Pacific Sci. **12:**299-312, 1958.

ADDITIONAL READINGS

Modell, J. H., Calderwood, H. W., Ruiz, B. C., and others: Effects of ventilatory patterns on arterial oxygenation after near-drowning in sea water, Anesthesiology **40**(4): 376-384, 1974.
Ruiz, B. C., Calderwood, H. W., Modell, J. H., and others: Effect of ventilatory patterns on arterial oxygenation after near-drowning with fresh water: a comparative study in dogs, Anesth. Analg. **52**(4):570-576, 1973.

CHAPTER 20

Head injuries

Randall W. Smith, M.D.

The initial diagnosis and early management of head injuries constitutes one of the most crucial emergency department functions. Lack of understanding in this area results in wrong diagnoses, inappropriate therapy, and inaction when minutes can mean the difference between recovery and brain death. When a head injury patient is dying in the emergency department, inaction is indefensible. Neither lack of training nor "waiting for the neurosurgeon" is sufficient reason for therapeutic immobility regarding patients with head injuries.

Initial diagnosis and therapy are based on a limited amount of historical material and a brief neurologic examination. The history can and should be taken by the nurse. In the temporary absence of a neurosurgeon the neurologic examination can also be performed by nurses. Armed with this information, a nurse is perfectly capable of reaching correct clinical impressions and instituting necessary, brain-preserving therapy.

WHAT IS A HEAD INJURY?

In order to understand the important diagnoses to be made in head injuries, it is necessary to appreciate how the head and brain become damaged.

All injuries result from the sudden application of force to the head and thus to the scalp, skull, and brain. These three structures are often but not always injured together. A patient may have severe scalp damage with little or no brain injury, while a badly damaged brain can result from trauma that does not leave a mark on the scalp or fracture the skull.

Scalp

Force applied to the scalp may bruise it (contusion), scrape off the outer skin layer (abrasion), result in a "goose egg" (hematoma), or tear the scalp open (laceration). These lesions, though sometimes massive, disfiguring, and bleeding profusely, are minor problems that can easily be controlled. They do not necessarily imply brain or skull injury and are a low priority item in management of the total head injury.

Skull

A blow to the head may result in a wide variety of skull fractures. These range from a simple linear fracture to a severe depressed fracture with bone fragments driven into the brain itself resulting in a cerebral laceration.

Skull fractures are of small importance in the total picture of head injuries. A fracture does not mean brain injury. However, the lack of a fracture does not imply less

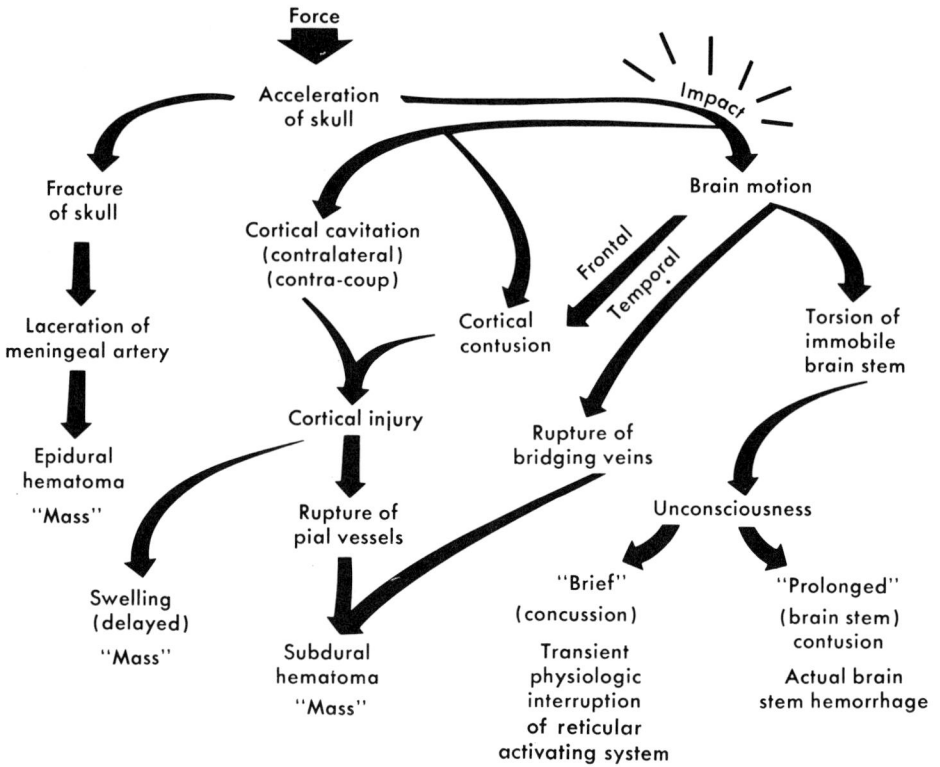

Fig. 20-1. Mechanisms in head injury.

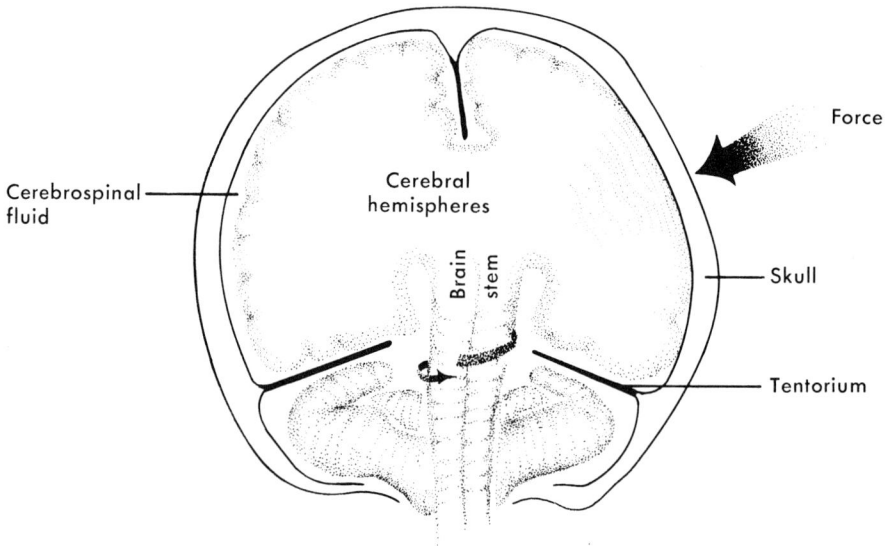

Fig. 20-2. Mechanisms of concussion and contusion.

brain damage. Fractures are immaterial in the face of the all-important brain injury. But since fractures and brain injury are frequently seen together in patients with head trauma and since the untrained person can more easily understand the concept of a fracture than a concussion, fractures have developed a reputation of unwarranted importance.

Brain (Fig. 20-1)

Brain damage and associated hemorrhage are the most important aspects of head injuries. An understanding of what can happen to the brain during trauma is mandatory. The semisolid brain is floating in spinal fluid and is free to move or swirl within the skull when the latter is suddenly accelerated by a blow. This swirling plus the direct transmission of force from the skull to the immediately underlying brain causes all the damage sustained by the brain in injuries (Fig. 20-2).

If the blow to the head is mild, then the predominant effect is brain motion. This most often results in nothing more than a headache, since the brain can tolerate limited motion. A moderate blow results in significant brain motion and clinical neurologic symptoms, because as the brain swirls more forcefully, it tends to twist or buckle the upper brain stem, an important junctional area between the cerebral hemispheres and the lower cerebellum and spinal cord. The brain stem is not as free to move and is twisted by the more freely movable and swirling hemispheres.

In moderate injuries this brain stem twist (Fig. 20-2) is not too severe and does not result in permanent damage. It does result in a temporary malfunctioning of the brain stem wherein it briefly ceases to carry nerve information. This cessation of function, particularly of an important net of nerve fibers called the reticular activating system, results in a loss of consciousness. In a moderate injury the brain stem rapidly recovers so that the unconsciousness lasts

only seconds or minutes to at most an hour, followed by rapid recovery. This is a brain stem concussion, or simply *concussion*.

Severe blows to the head result in remarkable brain stem twisting with actual tissue disruption and hemorrhage from which the brain stem may not recover. As expected, the loss of consciousness from such severe stem injury is prolonged, lasting many hours to days, weeks, months, or for as long as the patient lives. This is brain stem *contusion*.

Both moderate and severe injuries can cause surface bruises of the brain by forcing the floating cerebral hemispheres against the skull (Fig. 20-2). In addition, as the hemispheres are set into motion, they are raked over bony irregularities along the floor of the skull causing further bruises. These *cerebral contusions* do not result in a loss of consciousness (traumatic unconsciousness is always caused by *brain stem* injury) but can cause a varied array of neurologic abnormalities (see Diagnosis, cerebral contusion).

Concussion, brain stem contusion, and cerebral contusion all share one important common characteristic: they do not make a patient worse.* They affect the patient most severely at the moment of impact and remain stable or begin improving. This can best be emphasized by an example.

A patient reported by ambulance attendants to have been unconscious at the accident scene begins to arouse en route to the hospital, and when seen by the emergency department nurse on admission is awake but confused. Upon returning from x-ray an hour later, the patient cannot be aroused by voice or painful stimuli. The unconsciousness at that point is not a result of the obvious concussion sustained or any cerebral contusion. A deteriorating patient

---

*Cerebral contusion can lead to patient deterioration if swelling of the bruised area of brain occurs. This takes many hours to occur and is not an emergency department concern.

must be developing a new intracranial disease process. This distinction is crucial, because all intracranial disease processes leading to rapid neurologic deterioration demand immediate treatment, whereas concussion, cerebral contusion, and brain stem contusion do not.

The life-threatening posttraumatic disease process that leads to rapid deterioration and necessitates immediate therapy is *hemorrhage.*

The same forces that result in concussion and contusion also may cause vessel damage and hemorrhage. The cerebral hemisphere motion may tear bridging veins that travel from the surface of the brain to the overlying dura (see Fig. 20-1). Rupture of these vessels results in hemorrhage into the subdural space (subdural hematoma). A cerebral contusion may be accompanied by significant bleeding of vessels within the brain substance causing an intracerebral hematoma. Finally, if a skull fracture occurs with rupture of an underlying dural artery, the blood collects between the skull and dura (an epidural hematoma).

These hematomas tend to enlarge after the injury. This results in increased pressure and a forcing or shifting of the hemispheres away from the hematoma (Fig. 20-3). This shift forces the medial (deep) portion of the temporal lobe to extrude or herniate through the tentorial opening, a passageway connecting the vault occupied by the cerebral hemispheres and the posterior fossa in which lie the lower brain stem and cerebellum. This passageway is already occupied by the upper brain stem, the same structure that is injured by the twisting motion in concussion or brain stem contusion. When the temporal lobe herniates into the tentorial opening, it meets and puts pressure on the upper brain stem. This compression results in damage to the nerve systems of the brain stem and causes a series of clinical events that can be recognized and the presence of the hematoma and the herniation inferred.

The reticular activating system (consciousness) passes through the upper brain stem as do the corticospinal tracts, the latter controlling movement of the face, arm, and leg. In addition, the third cranial

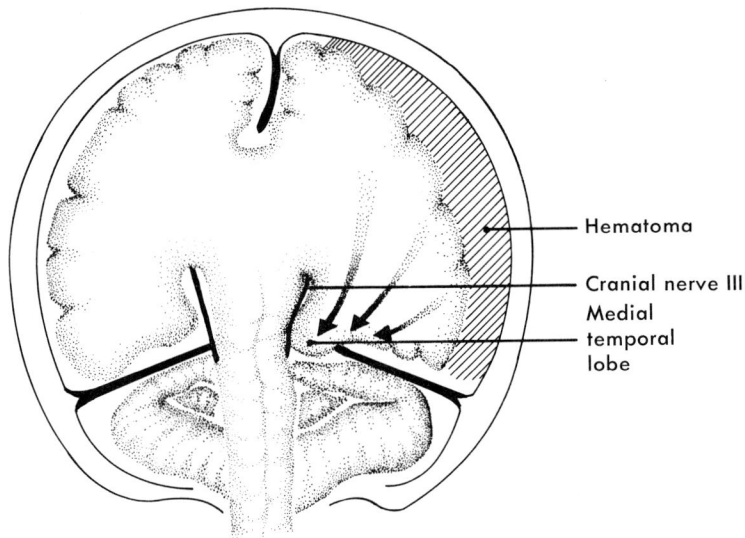

Fig. 20-3. Transtentorial herniation.

Hematoma

Cranial nerve III
Medial
temporal
lobe

nerves originate in the upper brain stem. These nerves control the size of the pupils. Thus, as the tentorial herniation proceeds, the patient can be expected to show deterioration in level of consciousness (reticular activating system), movements (corticospinal tracts), and in pupil size and reactivity (third cranial nerve).

Recognition of the events mentioned above is an important and necessary clinical skill if death and disability are to be averted in the patient with a hematoma.

NEUROLOGIC EVALUATION

If accurate diagnoses are to be made in the head injured patient, particularly those with hematomas, an immediate, brief, but thorough neurologic evaluation must be performed on admission to the emergency department. Such an evaluation includes a history and a neurologic examination.

The history can be crucial, and taking it is all too often perfunctory amid the bustle and excitement of the patient's arrival. The nurse or physician who fails to ascertain that a now unconscious patient had awakened at the accident scene only to lapse into coma has missed the best chance to diagnose an obvious hematoma.

Take a history from whomever you can. Do not be choosy. An ambulance attendant, a policeman, a friend, even a passerby may have important information regarding the injured, particularly when the patient arrives unconscious. If the patient will answer questions, this can be an excellent source of information—or lack of it, since a patient who is amnesic for events surrounding an injury probably has at least a concussion.

When interviewing the patient, try to determine what can be recalled of the accident. If the event cannot be recalled, what is the last recollection before the accident? Does the patient remember swerving, entering the freeway, starting up the ladder, getting into the car, eating his or her last meal, and so on?

What is the first recollection following the accident? Being moved? The policemen? The ambulance? Arriving in the emergency department? The severity of a concussion is usually proportional to the period of amnesia—the longer the lack of memory, the greater the injury to the brain.

Do not forget the patient's past medical history. Ask about any serious illness and if medications are taken. A diabetic who misses an insulin injection may lapse into unconsciousness in the emergency department; that patient needs the blood sugar lowered, not an operation.

If the patient is unconscious or cannot answer questions, the history must be obtained from others. Get the ambulance attendants, the police, or anyone who arrives to tell you about the patient. Was unconsciousness present for a while? Has unconsciousness always been present? Was the patient answering questions? Can the patient be consistently aroused? Was movement noted in both arms and legs or just one side? Was cyanosis or poor breathing noted for a while? Does the patient have any illnesses?

If the uncommunicative patient has any identification, examine it. A phone call can result in finding a relative or friend who may supply crucial medical information. Is there a card identifying a chronic disease (diabetes, seizures, etc.)? A physician's appointment slip?

Don't forget to look at bracelets; they may supply identification or medical information.

The neurologic examination should follow in rapid order. This includes five areas of concern: level of consciousness, pupil size and reactivity, respirations, movement, and examination of the head.

Level of consciousness

Establishing the level of consciousness is most important. An alert patient is awake and remains so when not disturbed. A lethargic patient, when not disturbed, will fall asleep but can easily be awakened by voice or a nudge, and once awake will answer questions. A stuporous patient is asleep but can be awakened for a short period of time by a loud voice or vigorous shaking. Once awake the patient will answer some questions but rapidly falls asleep again.

Orientation can be evaluated in alert, lethargic, or stuporous patients. A patient who knows his or her name, location, and the year, month, date, and day is considered normally oriented. Any mistakes in these answers should be noted.

Patients who cannot be aroused to speak or follow commands are in some form of coma. In response to painful stimuli (pinching), the patient may pull away or attempt to push the pinching hand away. This purposeful activity in response to pain is the hallmark of semicoma. If, in response to pain, there is either no movement at all or stereotyped posturing of the extremities, then the patient is in coma. This posturing should be recognized, because it means severe brain malfunction, though not necessarily permanent damage. Decerebrate posturing is characterized by marked straightening (extension) of all four extremities. Decorticate posturing is characterized by straightening of the legs but bending (flexion) of the arms at the elbows.

Pupil size and reactivity

Once the level of consciousness has been established, the pupils should be checked. Pupils are normally equal in size or within 1 mm of each other. They briskly constrict when a bright light is directed at them. It should be realized that very small pupils (1 to 2 mm) may not react to light because they are already as small as they can become. Small pupils are always reactive.

Respirations

Respirations should be carefully counted and the rhythm noted. Normal regular respirations (eupnea) suggest that the brain stem is not severely damaged, whereas periodic respirations (hyperventilation alternating with apnea), continuous hyperventilation, or irregular (ataxic) breathing implies significant brain stem injury. Irregular respirations are of added concern because they may not be adequately delivering oxygen and removing carbon dioxide.

Movement

Movement or strength is evaluated by having the cooperative patient hold both arms steadily in front of him or her, followed by lifting one leg at a time off the bed. Difficulty with leg lifting or a downward drifting of an arm should be noted. The uncooperative patient's movement is tested by the response to pain on either side (withdrawing, pushing your hand away). In the cooperative patient, test facial movement by tight eye closure and showing the teeth; in the uncooperative patient by symmetry of facial grimace to pinprick on forehead or cheek.

A patient who does not move one side of the body as well as the other, or who has unequal pupils, is said to be *lateralized*.

Head examination

The head should be examined carefully for lacerations and abrasions, which may be well hidden amid the hair. All lacerations should be probed with a sterile gloved finger for the presence of foreign bodies or a palpable depressed fracture in the skull. Blood issuing from the ears should be noted, and the skin over the mastoid examined for bruises.

Traumatized patients who arrive in the emergency department in coma or semicoma should undergo limited manipulation of the neck. These patients may have a cervical fracture but are unable to complain of neck pain. It is wise not to roll the patient's head from side to side or to flex the neck until a lateral cervical x-ray shows normal vertebral alignment.

The stress laid in this chapter on the

neurologic evaluation in no way precludes the basic emergency department procedures associated with the evaluation of other injuries. Principles stressed in other chapters must not be forgotten when dealing with the patient with multiple injuries.

DIAGNOSIS

It has been well established that therapy is most effective when appropriate to the diagnosis at hand. Diagnosis then becomes the first step to be taken if thoughtful aid is to be delivered. Being able to diagnose the patient's disease also changes the diagnoser from a pair of hands, however skilled, to a practitioner.

Scalp

Contusions (bruises), hematomas, and abrasions are relatively obvious and will not be dealt with further. It is only necessary to mention that in infants and small children whose total blood volume is small, significant blood loss may occur into a hematoma or from a laceration. This may precipitate these little patients into hypovolemic shock. This is not true in older children and adults, where a hematoma is never a cause of shock and a laceration very rarely so. A laceration must be searched for and when found probed with a sterile gloved finger. This is necessary to detect foreign bodies (glass, rocks, metal) as well as to determine the depth of the laceration. Deep lacerations that extend to the bone need one type of closure, while shallow cuts need another. Also, a depressed fracture may be suspected after palpation of the wound, and the radiologist alerted. A depressed fracture must be seen on x-ray to be confirmed.

Skull

As previously mentioned, skull fractures do not constitute an emergency in the sense of causing patient deterioration. In fact, only two kinds of fractures need any treatment at all: depressed fractures and

basilar fractures. Since it is as important to know what does not need therapy as what does, a brief discussion of all fractures follows.

Skull fractures fall into three main groups: linear, depressed, and basal.

Linear fractures are seen as thin, radiolucent lines on skull x-rays and do not involve any in-driven pieces of bone. These fractures do not need any treatment.

Depressed fractures are diagnosed by x-ray and seen as fragments of bone pressed in toward the brain. These fragments must be realigned or removed in the operating room. This, however, is not an immediate problem and can be handled within the first 24 hours of hospitalization. Depressed fractures are *not* a cause of coma or deterioration of the patient's condition.

Basilar skull fractures are rarely diagnosed by x-ray examination. These fractures occur along the base of the skull and usually cannot be seen on radiographs. Skull fractures of this type are detected by what results from them:

1. Aural bleeding or blood behind the eardrum (hemotympanum)
2. Periorbital ecchymoses (black eyes) without direct eye injury
3. Battle's sign (ecchymosis over mastoid area)
4. Rhinorrhea or otorrhea (cerebrospinal fluid running from nose or ear)

Rhinorrhea and otorrhea are frequently difficult to detect because of associated bleeding. A Uristix dipstick for urinary sugar detection will turn blue when wetted by blood and spinal fluid, but will usually not change in blood alone.

Basal skull fractures, even with spinal fluid leakage, are not necessarily associated with brain damage, are not the cause of coma or patient deterioration, and need only limited care.

Brain

The importance of recognizing brain injury rests in differentiating the three primary brain injuries (concussion, brain stem contusion, and cerebral contusion) from secondary hematomas. As will be stressed in the management section, treatment of the primary injuries differs markedly from that employed in hematomas.

Cerebral contusion

Cerebral contusion results in a lack of nerve function of the bruised portion of the cerebral hemispheres. Although the hemispheres have many functions, only a few systems are easily examined in the patient with head injury. Aphasia (difficulty with finding or saying the correct words or understanding commands) *in an alert patient* implies a frontal or temporal lobe contusion. Hemiparesis (weakness of the right or left arm, leg, and side of the face) *in an alert patient* also means frontal contusion. Numbness of one side of the body may mean parietal lobe contusion, but this is often an hysterical complaint. Finally, patients who are alert but are very confused, agitated, uncooperative, and frequently foul-mouthed, in the absence of heavy drinking, often are showing the effects of frontal or temporal lobe contusion.

It must be emphasized that in the emergency department, diagnosis of cerebral contusion can be made only in *alert* patients who cooperate enough to test cerebral function. Comatose and semicomatose patients may have a cerebral contusion, but they cannot be tested for it. Lethargic or stuporous patients who can cooperate enough to demonstrate some of the above findings may have a contusion, but these findings may just as well indicate a hematoma.

Concussion

The diagnosis of concussion is most frequently made by history when it is learned that a patient who is now alert was unconscious at the scene of the accident. Questioning the patient about the accident should demonstrate a lack of memory for the event itself and a variable period before and after. This patient may be disoriented but will show no other abnormal findings unless he or she also has a cerebral contusion (see above).

The neurologic examination in the patient with a concussion should not demonstrate any abnormalities in movement, strength, or sensation on one side of the body, and it should never reveal any pupillary inequality. Respirations should be regular. The patient may be disoriented but should not be aphasic.

If an alert patient who is known to have been briefly unconscious does have weakness or numbness or aphasia or general misbehavior, then cerebral contusion is the diagnosis—not hematoma. It is the alert state of the patient that rules out a hematoma.

If the patient arrives in a lethargic or stuporous state, one of two possible diagnoses exists. This may be a simple concussion with the patient in the process of waking up from it. The history will suggest whether this is true or not. If the patient was unconscious at the accident scene and has been progressively awakening, the likely diagnosis is concussion. If no alarming neurologic abnormalities are discovered on examination, then observation will probably be all that is necessary to make sure the patient continues to awaken.

However, if the patient was briefly unconscious, awoke at the accident scene, appeared fairly alert but became quiet in the ambulance and is found to be stuporous upon admission to the emergency department, concussion is not the cause. To repeat, the natural history of concussion is one of rapid improvement to an alert level of consciousness.

Two points should be reemphasized. First, the history is crucial and can be an invaluable aid in diagnosis. Second, the patient with a deteriorating level of consciousness does not meet the criteria for a diagnosis of concussion or brain stem contusion. Deterioration means possible hematoma.

Brain stem contusion

When it is recalled that brain stem contusion means hemorrhage into and significant damage to the upper brain stem, the historical course and neurologic findings in these patients are readily understood. Patients sustaining brain stem contusion are rendered comatose immediately and tend to remain so or, at best, to improve to semi-coma over a period of hours. Considering the transportation time from most accidents, this usually means that the patient will arrive in the emergency department in semicoma or coma.

Once again the history is extremely important. If the patient was found unconscious shortly after the accident and has remained so, brain stem contusion has occurred. A traumatic hematoma cannot collect fast enough to render a patient immediately comatose. This does not mean that a patient with brain stem contusion cannot also have a hematoma. It does mean that a patient immediately and persistently comatose after an injury cannot be given the diagnosis of hematoma based on the presence of the coma. We must look for other signs.

Lack of history also has an important bearing in these patients. If an injured person is found (in an alley, at the bottom of a cliff, in a home) and the time of injury is unknown, then it is not known if the patient was immediately rendered unconscious or was awake for a while and deteriorated to the present comatose state (a hematoma). Being unable to fix the time of injury and thus know the early post-traumatic history should immediately increase concern regarding possible hematoma.

The neurologic examination in brain stem contusion can detect a variety of abnormal findings. The level of unconsciousness is one of coma or semicoma during the first hours after the injury. Respirations can be normal, very rapid, periodic, or ataxic.

The reactions in patients with brain stem contusion are usually symmetric; that is, there is no pupillary inequality or a hemiparesis. The pupils are usually small, equal, and react to light. If the patient is semicomatose, then withdrawal from pain or attempts to push the painful stimulus away will be symmetric or equal on both sides. If the patient is comatose, then posturing (decerebration, decortication) will occur on *both sides* in the same manner. This symmetry in the examination reflects the symmetry of the usual brain stem contusion.

Occasionally, the brain stem is contused in an asymmetric manner. In such an instance, hemiparesis may be detected in the semicomatose patient, or one-sided decerebration or decortication may occur in the comatose patient. The contusion may involve one of the third cranial nerves, leading to unequal pupils. Thus lateralizing can be found in brain stem contusion. However, considering the serious depression in the patient's level of consciousness, *lateralization cannot be presumed to mean only brain stem contusion* (see Diagnosis, hematoma).

One point in favor of lateralization secondary to contusion and not hematoma is variability in the abnormal findings. First one side, then the other, then neither or both may posture in response to pain. One pupil may be large, then both large, then both small, then the other may dilate. This changeability of signs is characteristic of brain stem contusion.

It should be mentioned that shock is not caused by head injury or resulting brain damage. Any traumatized patient in shock must be presumed to have blood loss or cardiac embarrassment, and this should be vigorously investigated. Also, patients with intracranial hematomas never collect enough blood in the head to cause shock.

Shock in the traumatized patient means extremity, pelvic, abdominal, or thoracic hemorrhage, or tension pneumothorax, or cardiac embarrassment.

Hematoma

If the preceding sections have been read with care, the principles of diagnosis in hematoma should almost be obvious. When it is recalled that a hematoma gradually expands within the skull, putting increasing pressure on the brain and shifting the temporal lobe into the upper brain stem and reticular activating system, then the history of deteriorating level of consciousness is not difficult to understand.

In addition, as pressure is applied to the brain stem by a hematoma, the respiratory pattern usually changes. A patient initially eupneic who develops periodic or ataxic respirations is obviously deteriorating. Since the hematoma is most often on one side, it shifts one side of the brain into one side of the brain stem, leading to dysfunction of one of the third cranial nerves and one corticospinal tract; thus the frequent finding of lateralization (pupillary dilatation, hemiparesis) in patients with hematoma.

The history in traumatic hematoma may clearly indicate the presence of the mass lesion. A patient reported to have been more awake than when ultimately seen in the emergency department must be presumed to harbor a hematoma no matter what is detected by the rest of the neurologic examination. Close questioning of attendants arriving with the patient is always worthwhile. They may recall many aspects of the patient's behavior when quizzed, whereas little may be learned by a simple, "Has he been stable?" If a now comatose patient has mumbled his name, tried to roll over or sit up, moved both sides, or had equal pupils, that is a baseline against which to match the present examination.

Two complicated situations should be mentioned. Lack of any history, particularly in a patient found some unknown amount of time following an injury, places added weight on the examiner's training and experience and the results of the neurologic examination. Not knowing whether a patient's arrival level of consciousness is better or worse than an hour ago forces emergency department personnel to rely on signs of lateralization on admission, diagnostic tests, or the patient's course while in the emergency department (see below).

The effect of drugs can also complicate the issue. Not only can they be the cause of accidents, but the patient may be experiencing the maximum effect of the drug when he or she arrives in the emergency department. Deterioration in the level of consciousness may be the result of drug sedation and not head injury. Dig for a history of drug ingestion. This can raise the suspicion of drug effect and suggest a nasogastric sampling, a search for needle marks, and appropriate laboratory examination of blood specimens.

Regarding drugs, two points should be remembered: (1) drugs do not lead to lateralization of the neurologic examination and (2) a patient with head injury who has a deteriorating level of consciousness and is known to have taken drugs must be assumed to have a hematoma and treated as such. The treatment for hematoma is unlikely to hurt the patient if he or she does not have one, but withholding treatment may result in permanent disability or death if the patient has a hematoma.

Lateralized neurologic responses usually mean hematoma. As mentioned, an alert patient with hemiparesis does not have a hematoma but a cerebral contusion. A patient with any other admission level of consciousness in the absence of a history of rapid improvement must be presumed to have a hematoma if responses are lateralized. Any patient less than alert with pupillary inequality greater than 1 mm must always be presumed to have hematoma. Unequal pupils are always cause for considerable concern.

Continuing neurologic evaluation in the emergency department is a most important aid in diagnosis. As the treatment of any patient proceeds (IV, bladder catheter, venipuncture, x-rays, consultants), time must necessarily elapse. This presents an excellent opportunity for emergency department observations. Repeating the neurologic examination after the first 15 to 30 minutes in the emergency department may demonstrate improvement or deterioration of the patient's initial condition. If the patient is changing, then such information can be utilized to establish the diagnosis, particularly in those patients where initial history was sparse or lacking or in whom the examiner was unsure of the presence or absence of a particular finding (hemiparesis? pupils almost equal? really more sleepy than described at the accident scene?).

All too often patients considered to be "probably" stable or questionably lateralized are placed behind drawn curtains to await laboratory results or a consultation and are not checked again. The busy radiology department is an excellent place for a patient to lie totally unattended for an hour. If emergency department personnel do not recheck these patients, particularly those who are not alert, then a lethargic patient who is sent for skull films may become comatose in the x-ray department without anyone's being aware of the patient's deteriorating condition.

Some diagnostic tests may be employed in or near the emergency department because of their ease of performance and simplicity. These are skull films and echoencephalography.

Skull films are not needed immediately if taken just to see fractures. Films taken only for such reasons can be deferred for hours or not taken at all. Emergency skull films are justified in those patients in whom it is unclear whether they are deteriorating or who are probably stable but are lateralized. The goal of these films is to determine if the patient has a calcified pineal gland. This calcification is a normal finding, but its position on a skull film can confirm without doubt the presence of a hematoma.

Patients who are clearly and rapidly deteriorating do not need immediate skull films; they need immediate treatment for hematoma and preparations begun for surgery. In such a patient the neurosurgeon may wish to take enough time to obtain a single film but that decision should be left to the surgeon.

Alert patients never need emergency skull films, since their level of consciousness rules out hematoma.

Echoencephalography utilizes high-frequency waves to determine whether the brain has been shifted by a mass. It is easily performed in the emergency department by specially trained technicians or radiologists, but its reliability is not perfect. It is most useful in the depressed patient with no history and questionable stability or lateralization. If it indicates a significant shift (more than 2 mm of shift), the hematoma must be presumed, treatment begun, and either surgery undertaken or a more reliable test performed.

Like skull films, echoencephalography is not necessary in the alert patient, and is superfluous in the rapidly deteriorating one unless delay in surgery is unavoidable or the neurosurgeon wishes to invest the time necessary to conduct the test.

The most reliable nonoperative diagnostic tests utilized to establish or rule out traumatic intracranial hematoma are computerized axial tomography of the head (CAT scan) and angiography. CAT scanning is a 45-minute procedure that can detect the minute differences in density between normal brain and hematoma without the injection of contrast material into the cerebral arteries. Since absolute immobility of the head is required for the procedure, its usefulness in the frequently rambunctious, confused, head-injured patient remains to be demonstrated. Cerebral angiography involves injection of iodinated dye into the cerebral arteries so their position can be noted in relation to established normals and hematomas can be documented. It can be performed on less than cooperative patients but usually consumes one to two hours, a definite drawback in the deteriorating patient.

Lumbar puncture should not be performed on patients with head injury. It offers no diagnostic information about the injury. The only justification for a spinal tap in the emergency department is when meningitis is suspected, and even then it probably should not be done in the patient who also has a head injury until neurosurgical consultation has been obtained. Lumbar puncture should *never* be done when the head injury patient is lateralized or has pupillary inequality.

MANAGEMENT

Initial therapy must be aimed at problems that immediately threaten life. The patient's airway must be assured. If respirations are irregular, shallow, or lacking, an endotracheal tube should be inserted and artificial respiration begun. Major arterial hemorrhage from the extremities or neck must be stemmed and the blood pressure measured. A blood sample must be drawn and an intravenous line rapidly started.

All these issues have been mentioned in previous chapters, and details are available there.

Before commencing on a discussion of therapy for specific diagnoses, priority of head injury treatment should be mentioned. *Intracranial hematomas always require top treatment priority in head injury.* Bleeding scalp lacerations, obvious basilar skull fractures, and the question of cerebral contu-

sion all must take a subordinate position to the hematoma that is threatening the brain stem. In fact, the only traumatic diagnoses that take precedence over intracranial hematoma are respiratory failure and severe shock. Limb fractures, particularly when compound, look as though they need immediate treatment, but they do quite well if left immobile while the neurologic evaluation takes place or hematoma treatment is begun. It is hoped that well-trained emergency department personnel will avoid the serious error of starting therapy for obvious fractures, lacerations, and the like, while neglecting the neurologic evaluation and the opportunity to diagnose a hematoma and begin life-preserving therapy. The neurologic history can be taken while working over the patient, and the neurologic examination can be performed in less than two minutes.

Scalp

Contusions and hematomas need no treatment except for an ice pack, which may reduce discomfort. Abrasions should be gently washed with mild liquid soap diluted with saline and left unbandaged to dry and form a normal healing eschar (scab). Lacerations that are only mildly bleeding should initially be ignored while evaluation of the patient and other therapy is begun. Profusely bleeding lacerations should be covered with many sterile sponges, and a circumferential head wrap should be placed to force the sponges against the laceration and stop the bleeding by compression. Trying to place hemostats on bleeding points in a laceration is a waste of time. If the compression bandage does not at least reduce the hemorrhage to a tolerably slower rate, then the lacteration should be sutured. Closure of a laceration is the best way to stem hemorrhage.

Suture of lacerations must be done with some attention to detail. Improper laceration treatment often results in wound infection, which will prolong the patient's recovery and can be dangerous, since such infection can spread to the brain. After probing the laceration, preparation of the area for closure should be accomplished. This includes shaving the hair away from the edges of the laceration for a distance of 4 cm. This distance is necessary to adequately cleanse the scalp and keep adjacent hair from wandering into the operative field.

The wound should be irrigated within its depths with sterile saline followed by scrubbing of the scalp and the wound for five minutes with whatever soap solution is locally available. Paper or cloth drapes should then be applied to cover the hair while leaving the laceration clearly visible. Injection of the edges of the laceration with a local anesthetic containing epinephrine follows (epinephrine causes vasoconstriction and reduces bleeding).

If the laceration is completely through the scalp down to bone, then one type of closure is used, whereas if the laceration is shallow, a different plan is followed. It is beyond the scope of this volume to teach surgical technique.

Skull

Fracture treatment in the emergency department should be quite limited because of the generally unimportant nature of the lesions. As mentioned previously, linear fractures need no treatment and depressed fractures require nonemergency operations. That leaves basilar skull fractures for emergency department treatment consideration. In this regard, most neurosurgeons will begin antibiotic therapy in the hope of preventing meningitis. If the patient is actually leaking spinal fluid, observation should follow for a few days to see if leaking will stop spontaneously. Therefore, emergency department care for basilar skull fracture should be limited to diagnosis. Avoid ear irrigation or packing of either ear or nose if spinal fluid is detected.

Brain

Concussion needs no emergency department treatment. Many physicians will admit such patients to the ward for some hours of further observation, but the emergency department role in concussion is limited to diagnosis. Remember that the diagnosis of concussion cannot be made unless the patient is alert within one hour of the injury, thus ruling out a hematoma.

One rule that should always be observed in the emergency department regarding head injuries is that until the patient is transported to the ward, he or she remains the responsibility of the emergency department. From a neurologic point of view this means continued observation and repeated brief examinations. Often emergency department orders are not written, and monitoring the patient is at the discretion of the emergency department personnel. This responsibility holds for the alert patient waiting to go to the ward as well as for the semicomatose patient awaiting angiography.

Cerebral contusion needs no emergency department treatment as long as it is recalled that this diagnosis can only be made with assurance in an alert patient who has a hemiparesis, sensory loss, or aphasia. These patients are usually just observed, and steroids frequently are used to retard any edema from the contusion. This edema, however, takes days to develop and will not be manifest in the emergency department.

Brain stem contusion

These comatose and semicomatose patients need specific treatment and careful monitoring. If the possibility of hematoma seems unlikely, then therapy must be aimed at providing and maintaining an adequate oxygen supply, carbon dioxide removal, and blood pressure so that the brain stem contusion has the best environment in which to spontaneously improve—if it can. This means therapy should be aimed at maintaining an adequate airway and respirations and assuring that blood pressure is satisfactory.

The treatment scheme includes intubation, intravenous fluids, and control of gastric contents and urine output. An endotracheal tube should be inserted immediately to protect the patient's airway. Airway obstruction or poor respiratory drive with resultant hypoxia and hypercapnia only makes contusion worse. Once the tube is in place, rate and depth of respirations should be noted. If these seem adequate, proof of this is best obtained by an arterial blood sample. If the respiratory rate is below 10 per minute or the depth seems shallow, then artificial ventilation should be started. Supplementary oxygen should be supplied.

An intravenous line should be started in case fluids or drugs are needed. If the patient is not in shock, then large volumes of intravenous fluids are unwarranted and may aggravate the nervous system injuries.

A nasogastric tube should be inserted to remove the stomach contents and prevent vomiting and potential aspiration. A bladder catheter should be placed to ascertain the adequacy of renal perfusion.

Drugs are not helpful in brain stem contusion.

Once these procedures have been completed, appropriate x-ray films should be taken and the patient rapidly transferred to the intensive care unit where support will be provided while awaiting the hoped-for improvement in neurologic function.

Hematoma

These patients fall into two broad treatment categories. The first includes patients who are comatose and semicomatose on arrival and are lateralized, as well as those patients who arrive more awake (lethargy, stupor) but who are definitely deteriorating (dilation of a pupil, development of hemiparesis, becoming less responsive). The second group includes those patients who are *questionably* deteriorating but still have a relatively good level of consciousness (lethargy, light stupor) or who are stable in the lethargic and stuporous state but who are lateralized *without* pupillary inequality.

The first category indicates probable hematoma with active herniation, which is a neurosurgical emergency; the second suggests possible hematoma with relative stability. Patients in the first category need immediate therapy while those in the second may be watched closely while further investigations are carried out (echoencephalography, skull films, CAT scan, angiography).

Patients with probable hematoma are first treated much as for brain stem contusion; that is, intubation, intravenous line, nasogastric tube, and bladder catheter. In addition, three further steps are rapidly taken: hyperventilation, diuresis, and steroids (Fig. 20-4).

Artificial hyperventilation is used to lower the patient's carbon dioxide level. Reduction of carbon dioxide results in a decrease in intravascular blood volume within the skull, thus allowing more room for the hematoma, less shift of the brain, and reduction or retardation of brain stem compression.

Diuresis is accomplished using an osmotic diuretic such as Mannitol. This drug, when used in large quantities (1 g/kg of body weight), removes water from tissues. This water loss reduces the total bulk of the brain and thereby allows more room for the hematoma, less brain shift, and less brain stem compression.

Use of osmotic diuretics results in a large urine output as the water is evacuated from the body. The bladder catheter allows easy exit of this large urine flow.

Steroids, such as dexamethasone, are given in large quantities (10 mg IV). Although the efficacy of this drug is questioned, most who use it hope it will allow the brain vasculature to better withstand

Trauma

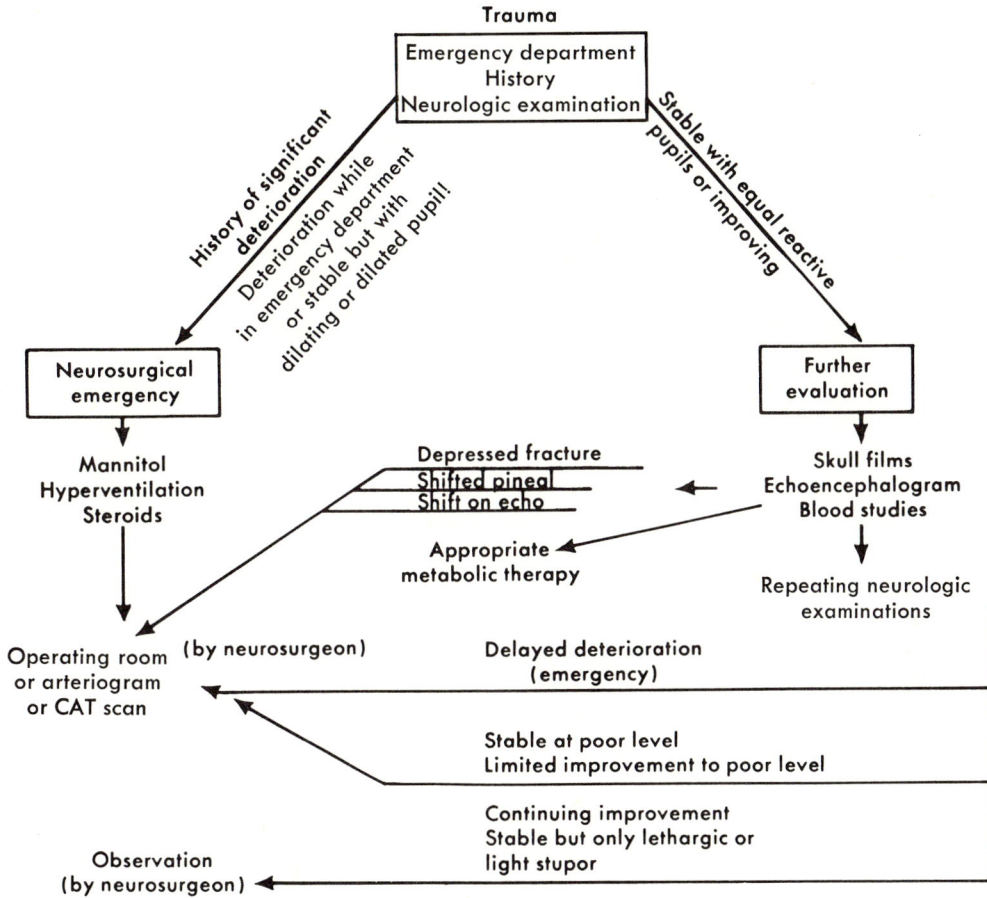

Fig. 20-4. Emergency department management of head injuries (see text).

compression by the hematoma and will reduce subsequent brain edema.

Once the above three steps are taken, nothing further can be done to help the patient short of surgery. This treatment will usually halt the patient's deterioration for an hour or so. This allows time to type and crossmatch the patient for whole blood, ready the operating room, and allow the neurosurgeon time to arrive, see the patient, and decide whether the diagnosis is sure. The neurosurgeon may wish to invest some precious time in further studies (echoencephalogram, angiogram, etc.) or go directly to the operating room. Emergency department medical hematoma

treatment will protect important brain functions while these decisions are made and implemented.

Patients with possible hematomas are managed somewhat differently. Usually their level of consciousness is too good to allow placement of an endotracheal tube. A nasogastric tube should be passed to avoid the complications of aspirated vomitus. The intravenous line should be started and the bladder catheter placed. These moves are in preparation for probable hematoma treatment if the patient should worsen.

Patients with possible hematomas usually undergo further diagnostic tests in an attempt to substantiate the presence or absence of hematoma. While these tests (echoencephalogram, skull films, CAT scan, angiography) are being conducted, emergency department personnel must continue to closely monitor these patients. The patient could start to deteriorate rapidly or a pupil may dilate at any time. If this happens (and it will not be detected unless the patient is closely watched), then probable hematoma therapy is begun (diuresis, steroids, intubation, and hyperventilation) and the operating room staff alerted.

Once the neurosurgeon has seen the patient, he or she may elect to continue the diagnostic tests, perform exploratory surgery, or simply admit the patient to the ward or intensive care unit for further observation.

By carrying out the above procedures emergency department personnel have been alerted to the possible diagnosis, have safeguarded the patient and the brain, and have given the neurosurgeon a viable patient and a reasonable opportunity to apply his skills.

SUMMARY

It should be obvious that the intent of this chapter is to encourage rapid, intelligent evaluation of head injury, to inculcate the ability to do so, and to suggest immediate therapy when it is absolutely necessary. When the continued existence of a patient as a sentient being hinges upon the rapid recognition and treatment of brain-threatening disease, it would seem specious to haggle over emergency department roles in the care of such a patient.

The nurse is the most constant presence in the emergency department. The nurse is the first to see the patient, the first to take the history, the first to conduct the examination, and the first to have the opportunity to begin therapy. Can the patient afford to have such a crucial member of the emergency department team merely take vital signs as a traumatic hematoma takes its toll of the brain stem? If you can answer "No" to that question, then mastery of the content of this chapter becomes mandatory.

REFERENCES

1. Queensburg, J. H., and Lembright, D:. Observations and care for patients with head injuries, Nurs. Clin. North Am. 4(2):237-247, 1969.
2. Youmans, Julian, R., editor: Neurological surgery, vol. 11, Philadelphia, 1973, W. B. Saunders Co., pp. 936-977.
3. Kahn, E. A., and others: Correlative neurosurgery, Springfield, Ill., 1969, Charles C Thomas, Publisher, pp. 533-596.
4. Finney, L. A., and Walker, A. E.: Transtentorial herniation, Springfield, Ill., 1962, Charles C Thomas, Publisher.
5. Evans, J. P.: Acute head injury, Springfield, Ill., 1963, Charles C Thomas, Publisher.

CHAPTER 21

Emergency management of facial injuries

Lawrence T. Moore, M.D.

The patient brought into the hospital emergency department with a facial injury elicits marked concern because of personal appearance. This appearance may not reflect the magnitude of the injury, but its apparent serious nature causes confusion.

In the United States 72% of all victims of automobile accidents have head and facial injuries. There are approximately 45,000 fatalities per year from automobile accidents, and for every death there are 116 injuries. Simple multiplication reveals 4.5 million injuries of which 72%, or 3.2 million, are facial injuries. Many of these are not serious enough to cause admission to a hospital, but their numbers reflect the frequency with which emergency department personnel are called upon to treat such injuries.

The watchword of the emergency treatment of acute facial injuries is "first things first." In decreasing order of importance, the following conditions should be evaluated immediately and treated with dispatch: airway, hemorrhage, shock, and associated injury.

AIRWAY

An adequate airway must be established. Any material can obstruct the upper air-

way of a patient following facial injury. Blood, broken dentures, fractured mandibular fragments, or foreign bodies are common obstructions. The patient may appear mildly agitated, wildly agitated, or comatose. Retrodisplacement of the tongue in a severely fractured mandible can effectively block the airway and result in rapid asphyxiation if this is not recognized. The patient should be immediately evaluated as to the patency of the airway, and if there is obstruction, immediate steps should be taken to determine the cause. The mouth and upper pharynx should be examined and all foreign material removed. Adequate lighting and suction apparatus are indispensable in attempting to clear the upper respiratory tract of foreign material. Hemorrhage may cause difficulty in breathing, and if the patient is conscious, he or she may assist in clearing the airway by coughing.

Tracheostomy, although an invaluable tool in the treatment of acute obstruction at or above the larynx, is usually not necessary. If there is a probability of severe edema within the larynx or if there is severe laryngeal trauma, tracheostomy should be done. This is more easily done in an emergency department with good lighting and good instruments than in a hospital bed under adverse conditions. Tracheostomy is reserved for those patients who have associated injuries, such as intracranial, chest, or high cord injuries. Tracheostomy may be required if there are multiple upper facial and mandibular fractures with marked instability of the mandible allowing excessive mobility of the tongue. As is often said regarding tracheostomy: "If you think of the possibility of needing one, do it now." Few people have died from an unnecessary tracheostomy; many have died because a tracheostomy was not done. A horizontal neck incision for the tracheostomy is best, can be done almost as rapidly as the old vertical incision, and leaves a much more cosmetic scar.[1]

CONTROL OF HEMORRHAGE

Hemorrhage in facial injuries can usually be controlled by pressure. Pressure may be applied externally or it may be necessary to utilize intracavitary packing. Nasal packing, palatal packing, or sinus packing may be done to control hemorrhage. If pharyngeal packing is necessary, of course a tracheostomy must be performed first. External carotid ligation is seldom necessary or helpful when evaluating the amount of bleeding. Remember the length of time that has passed since the injury; swallowed blood can exsanguinate a patient.

SHOCK

Acute shock is seldom seen in patients with uncomplicated facial injuries. If shock is evident when a patient is admitted to the emergency department, personnel should be immediately suspicious of concomitant problems such as intracranial injury, ruptured viscus or other intraabdominal injuries, intrathoracic trauma, or musculoskeletal disruption. A rapid physical examination can be done while the usual antishock measures are carried out. Following the examination a general impression is obtained and more complete studies are done as indicated.

ASSOCIATED INJURY

A complete examination of the patient and basic laboratory studies should be done as soon as possible. Urinalysis will assist in determining whether there is urologic injury; chest films will determine the extent of any intrathoracic damage or whether teeth or other foreign materials have been aspirated. The abdomen is examined to evaluate the conditon of the intraabdominal contents. Depending upon the patient's state of consciousness, a brief neurologic examination is done. In facial fractures with bleeding, the presence of blood behind the tympanic membrane does not necessarily mean basilar skull fracture. This can result from reflux through the eustachian tube. Of course, appropriate studies to rule out basilar skull fracture are necessary.

Because of the relative fragility of the facial bones and their "give" in the compression phase of blunt trauma, skull fractures are relatively uncommon when the force is applied from the facial side. This force is dissipated by the fracturing of the bones of the facial skeleton, thus more or less protecting the intracranial contents.[2]

Remember, associated injuries to the body should be cared for first. Facial lacerations can be closed immediately, but facial fractures can safely wait seven to ten days for definitive treatment.

Following initial evaluation, attention can be turned toward the local problem—that of treating the facial injury.

It is rare for facial injuries to require immediate surgery. An important exception is the occurrence of retroorbital hemorrhage. This requires immediate surgical intervention, and the appropriate specialist should be contacted without delay. Retrodisplacement of a fractured maxilla can rarely occur, severing the third portion of the internal maxillary artery. This also calls for immediate surgical intervention.

PLANNING EFFECTIVE MANAGEMENT
Observation

Accurate observation is of prime importance. It is helpful to divide the face into several areas, such as the upper third extending from the eyebrows to the hairline, the middle third extending from the eyebrows to and including the maxilla, and the lower third, the mandible. Examine the patient's facial injuries in a concise, predetermined manner. I have found it helpful to consider the soft tissue injuries first, regardless of the obvious appearance of associated bony injury. Wounds of the face should be cleansed appropriately to remove blood, dirt, and foreign material. Remember that road tattoos are permanent unless treated adequately. After the wounds have been adequately cleansed, it is surprising how thorough an examination can be done without the need for local anesthetic. For the most part, facial injuries are not painful. One may divide the face into the above three segments and examine these separately and concurrently, or the entire face can be examined as a unit as far as the soft tissue problem is concerned. Observation can be utilized to determine nerve deficit. If there are lacerations about the lateral side of the face over the course of the facial nerve, this will become immediately evident. Transections of ducts can be observed, although this is usually more difficult without anesthesia and deep exploration of the wound. Parotid duct severance can often be seen as well as lacerations of the tear ducts. Hematoma formation may be observed. If there is a rapidly forming hematoma, exploration should be done, usually through one of the lacerations, to determine the source of the bleeding. Small hemostats, fine suture material, and a set of small instruments should be present in all emergency departments to ensure availability of proper instruments for closing eyelid lacerations.

I. Simple lacerations
  A. Debridement—minimal
  B. Accurate closure with fine suture and without tension
  C. Compression dressing
II. Lacerations involving free borders
  A. Eyelids
    1. Close as soon as possible, beginning at free border with anchoring suture; rapid edema may make the border impossible to close if delayed
    2. Keep cornea protected
  B. Lips—close accurately so that vermillion border is intact and regular
  C. *Never* shave eyebrows
  D. Nose—accurate closure if alae involved (Remember that a two-surface scar at a free border contracts with resultant notching.)
III. Lacerations with apparent tissue loss
  A. Replace all viable tissue to evaluate possible tissue loss
  B. Excellent vascularity of facial tissue; if in doubt as to viability, save the tissue
  C. Actual tissue loss—wet dressings and request consultation

Palpation

Rapid edema that occurs with or without lacerations can mask the existence of many fractures of facial bones. However, there is usually at least one definite abnormality detected that makes x-ray studies of facial bones advisable. By visualizing the underlying bony structure of the face, palpation can be done using the following landmarks:

I. Frontal bone area
  A. Obvious fracture—frontal sinus involvement
  B. Sensory losses caused by crush injuries of the supraorbital nerves
  C. Motor injury to frontalis muscle
II. Periorbital examination
  A. Supraorbital area
    1. Crush injury
    2. Palpable fracture lines with or without displacement

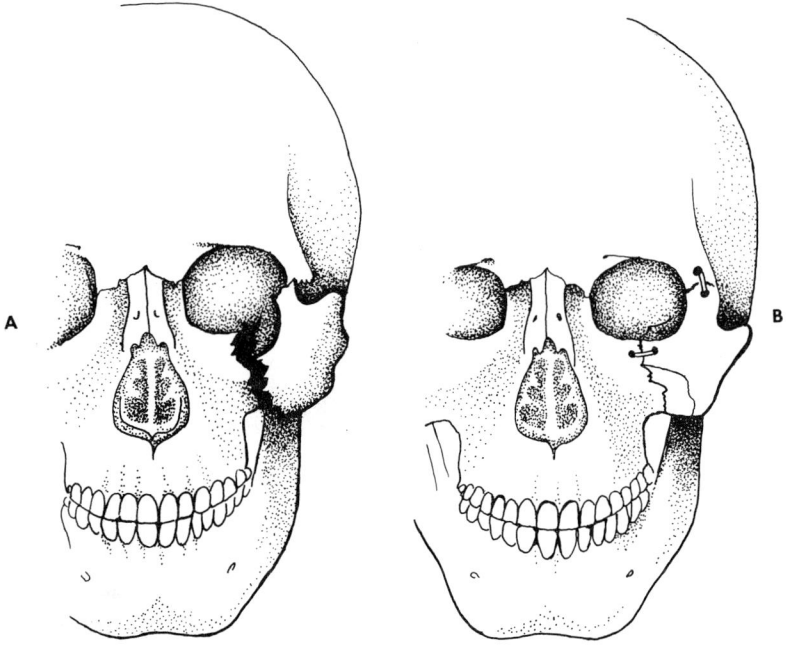

Fig. 21-1. A, Displacement of zygomatic compound. **B,** Internal wire fixation.

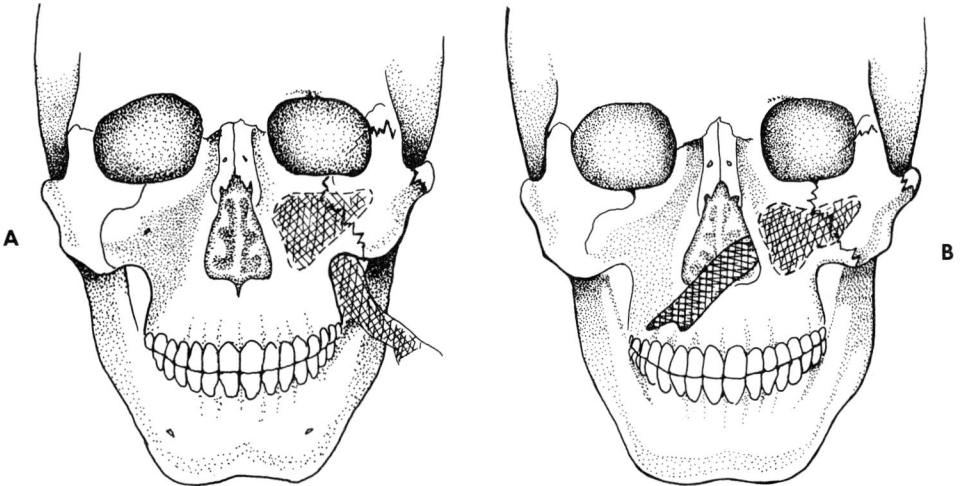

Fig. 21-2. Intraantral gauze stabilization for fracture zygomatic compound. **A,** Oral exit; **B,** nasal antrostomy exit.

3. Exophthalmos caused by depression of supraorbital ridge
B. Lateral orbital area
  1. Fracture lines with displacement; usually displaced medially or inferiorly and posteriorly
  2. Depression of the lateral canthus due to the fractured segment carrying the lateral canthal ligament
C. Malar complex and infraorbital area
This is actually a combination of a lateral and infraorbital injury. Treatment may be varied (Figs. 21-1 and 21-2).
  1. Visible depressions and crush as a unit compressing the zygomatic compound
  2. Diplopia
Remember that diplopia can be masked because of edema occurring between the time of injury and the time of examination. If this is not handled immediately and recognized when the edema subsides, marked visual disturbance will be evident.
  3. Anesthesia over the distribution of the infraorbital nerve because infraorbital foramen forms a path for a fracture
  4. Extraocular muscle entrapment
A missile striking the ocular area will cause a compression and then decompression of the floor of the orbit resulting in splintering of the small bones of the floor of the orbit. Entrapment of the inferior rectus muscle can occur upon decompression resulting in limitation of upward gaze. This must be tested before it can be recognized
  5. Enophthalmos
This occurs when the fracture of the floor of the orbit is severe and the retroorbital fat drops down into the sinus, thus giving a decrease in contents behind the globe and allowing it to drop back into the orbit
D. Medial orbital examination
  1. Fractures of the medial orbit wall with the attachment of the medial canthal ligament and lateral displacement of the eye
  2. Fractures into the ethmoidal cells
III. Nasal examinations
A. Displacement of nasal bones
B. Crush injury to the interorbital space
C. Cerebrospinal fluid rhinorrhea
D. Cartilage fractures with displacement
E. Intractable epistaxis
IV. Zygomatic arch examination
A. Visible or palpable depression of the zygomatic arch
B. Limitation of motion to mandibular excursion
This results from a compression of the zygomatic arch over the coronoid process of the mandible, which either prevents the mouth from opening if the fracture was sustained in a closed position, or causes limitation of motion to the mouth closing if the fracture occurred with the mouth open.
V. Maxilla
A. Malocclusion
  1. Caused by maxillary displacement or mandibular injury and fracture
  2. Open bite deformity with the anterior maxilla shoved superiorly
  3. Segmental malocclusion (Figs. 21-3 and 21-4)
B. Motion of maxilla—total or segmental
C. Disruption of maxillary unit with

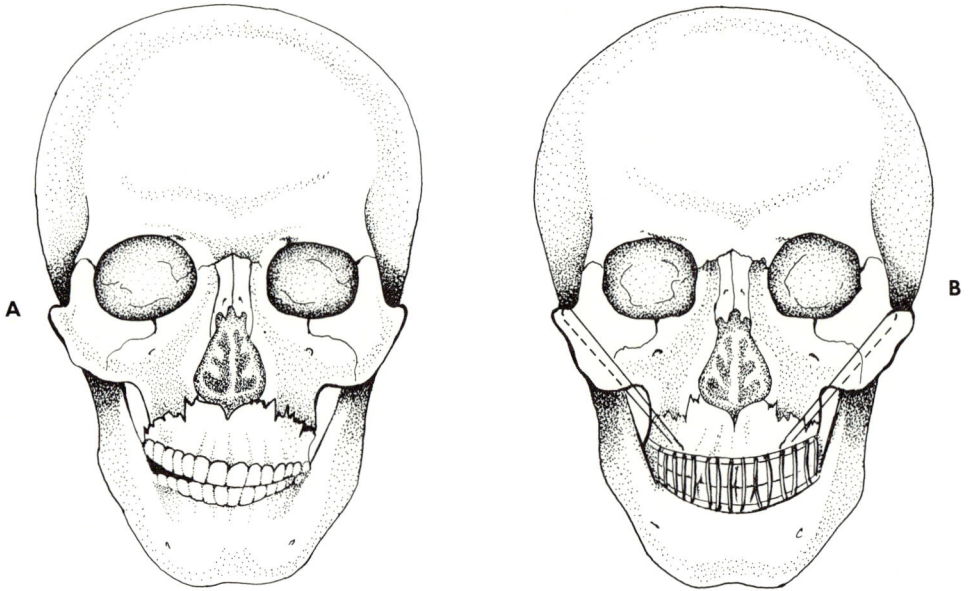

Fig. 21-3. A, Transverse maxillary fracture. B, Transverse fracture stabilization with circum-zygomatic wires to arch bar.

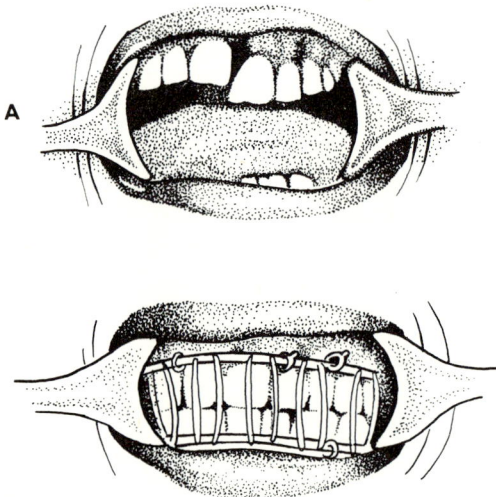

Fig. 21-4. A, Segmental displacement. B, Reduction by interdental wiring.

possible palatal fractures, that is, pyramidal fracture (Fig. 21-5)
  D. Cerebrospinal fluid rhinorrhea
  E. Dental fractures
VI. Mandible examination
  A. Malocclusion—complete or segmental
  B. Pain on palpation particularly around the condylar area
  C. Obvious fracture with free movement of segments
  D. Limitation of motion
  E. With fracture of the anterior mandible, concomitant condylar fracture(s) possible

X-ray examination

The majority of facial fractures can be diagnosed by observation and palpation; however, x-ray confirmation is essential. Fractures of the mandibular condyles can be missed because of their location. Although there are many views that can be utilized, in an emergency situation there

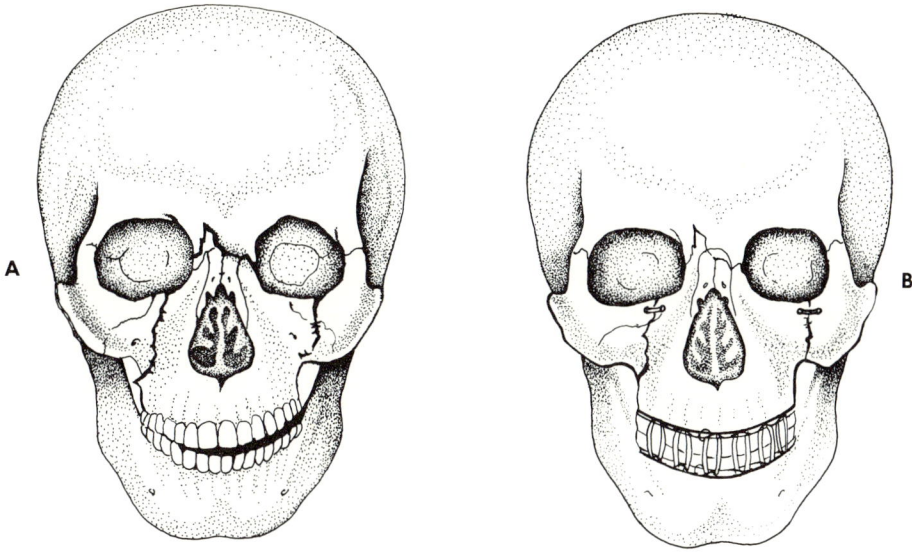

Fig. 21-5. A, Pyramidal fracture; **B,** with internal fixation and associated maxillary mandibular immobilization.

are a few that will acquaint the examiner with the major problems.

1. Waters' view
   a. The condition of the superior, lateral, and infraorbital walls can be ascertained plus the zygomatic compound and frontal and maxillary sinuses
   b. Many times the zygomatic arch condition is evident together with the nasal pyramid
2. Exaggerated Towne view
   a. Taken specifically for evaluation of the mandibular condyles
   b. Over 90% of fractures reveal medial displacement of the fractured superior segment of the condyle
3. Right and left oblique views of the mandible
4. Lateral nasal bone films

By mentioning the above necessary views, I do not mean to infer that other, more complete, diagnostic x-ray studies are not important. Sophisticated techniques, such as laminography, can often clarify a suspicion or corroborate an impression. In an emergency situation, however, it may be extremely difficult to obtain these films with any degree of accuracy. At a later time it would be advisable, if there is any further suspicion, to have x-ray films taken to more completely evaluate the problem. Following the emergency treatment and diagnosis the decision must be made as to whether emergency surgery in the operating suite is indicated, whether treatment in the emergency department is sufficient, or whether diligent observation in the hospital is mandatory because of the possibility of associated systemic injuries. It cannot be stressed too strongly that facial lacerations can be rapidly treated with a few key sutures and that fractures can wait until any other systemic injury is brought under control.

SUMMARY

In considering the emergency treatment of facial injuries, one need not consider the causative agent. Whether the trauma is the result of automobile accident, missile, or natural disaster is really of no consequence in the determination of the type of treatment to be given. Of course, the physician must use common sense; for instance, if the wound is contaminated with dirt, appropriate antitetanus measures must be utilized.

The facial burn is an entity unto itself and was purposely not considered in this discussion (see Chapter 16). Intraocular injuries have not been considered, since they constitute a specialized problem, and appropriate consultation should be requested immediately. The same pertains to intracranial injury and prolonged unconsciousness.

It is essential for the members of the emergency department team to request consultation of appropriate specialists as soon as the emergent problem has been evaluated and treatment begun. The plastic surgeon, the ophthalmologist, and the oral surgeon can work as a team in many instances to undertake the final care of the patient once the emergency is stabilized. Adopting a "first things first" attitude and logical treatment will give best results for the injured patient. This may obviate later extensive reconstructive procedures with less satisfactory results.

REFERENCES

1. Dingman, R. O., and Natvig, P.: Surgery of facial fractures, Philadelphia, 1964, W. B. Saunders Co., p. 105.
2. Pickering, P., and Moore, L.: Fractures of the middle third of the face, J. Int. Coll. Surg. 40(3):265-275, 1963.

CHAPTER 22

Ocular emergencies

Ralph D. Anderson, Jr., M.D.

Ocular injuries constitute a major source of blindness in the United States. This is in contrast to much of the rest of the world where a high incidence of blindness is the result of untreated eye disease such as trachoma, glaucoma, and cataract. In this country approximately half of all blindness in one eye and a fifth of blindness in both eyes is caused by trauma. Trauma is second only to amblyopia as the leading cause of blindness in children.

Eye injuries remain a significant factor in compensable industrial accidents. Safety measures in industry promoting less hazardous machinery and greater use of protective eyeglasses have done much to decrease the incidence of industrial blindness. The National Society for the Prevention of Blindness has stimulated the formation of Wise Owl Clubs. These groups are made up of employees who have had one or both eyes saved from a serious injury by the use of safety glasses.

In a fast moving, highly mechanized environment, eye injuries will continue to be emergency problems. Eye emergencies are seen almost daily in the office of every ophthalmologist. Thus virtually every emergency department can expect to encounter patients requiring eye care.

In the aftermath of injury, the loss of sight and fear of blindness are the most dreaded sequelae. This fear is rightfully based. The loss of no other sense can match the dysfunction of blindness.

It is well to have some assessment of the patient's vision prior to his or her appearance at the emergency department. This history should take into account the visual capability of *both* eyes and not just the injured eye. More than once an injured eye has been evaluated, treated, and patched before it was realized that the other eye was blind (or artificial!).

In determining the visual acuity, the emergency personnel should seek the best obtainable vision. If the patient wears glasses, this means measurement of the vision with glasses. If the patient's eyeglasses are not available, then distant and near acuity readings may be needed to obtain any meaningful value.

The patient's chief complaint and the account of any injury will do much to point toward the correct diagnosis. Usually there will be a precise awareness of the nature of the injury, such as a foreign body, chemical injury, or blunt blow. In fact, should there be no specific injury, attention would be diverted to the possibility of a medically diseased eye such as conjunctivitis, iritis, or acute glaucoma.[1]

In general, pain and visual loss are the symptoms that lead patients to seek emer-

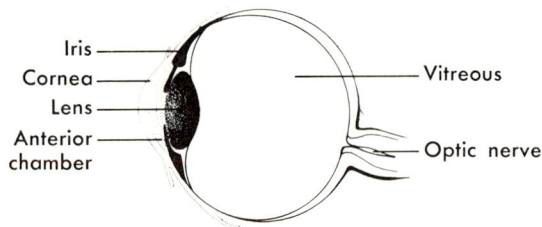

Fig. 22-1. Anatomy of the normal eye.

gency eye care. Familiarity with the anatomy of the normal eye will make assessment much easier (Fig. 22-1).

BASIC EQUIPMENT

The unique physical characteristics of the eye require special instrumentation and techniques for eye examination and treatment. The emergency department should have an ever ready "eye tray" containing an ample supply of ophthalmic preparations and medications.

Basic instruments include a reliable penlight, lid evertor, foreign body spud, cotton-tipped applicators, irrigating solution, ophthalmoscope, magnifying glasses, and a slit lamp. It seems hardly necessary to mention that such equipment requires diligence and attention to maintenance. It is distressing to note that the batteries of an instrument are dead, especially when the patient is suffering from a painful eye.

Magnification is the single most important aid in the examination of eye injuries. The Burton lamp is almost universally available and is commonly used in emergency departments. One disadvantage is that it is cumbersome. Better magnification and mobility are obtained with magnifying glasses, such as the Beebe loupe, or telescopic eyeglasses, such as those made by Zeiss and Keeler. The best magnification is obtained with the slit lamp. Truly capable and sophisticated emergency personnel will have a biomicroscope available and will be competent in the use of this instrument.

OPHTHALMIC MEDICATIONS

The supply of ophthalmic medications should be kept in an easily transportable eye tray. A basic supply of medications would include a miotic to constrict the pupil (pilocarpine), mydriatics to dilate the pupil such as 1% tropicamide (Mydriacyl), 1% cyclopentolate HCl (Cyclogyl), and 10% phenylephrine (Neo-Synephrine), and topical anesthetics, such as proparacaine (Ophthaine) and 0.5% tetracaine HCl (Pontocaine). Fluorescein strips, irrigating solutions, and an assortment of antibiotic eyedrops and ointments are also needed.

Adequate examination of the retina with the ophthalmoscope may require dilating the pupil with a mydriatic. The wrong choice of mydriatic agent could saddle the patient with prolonged blurred vision and photophobia. Tropicamide is preferable because it is a short-acting mydriatic. Pupillary dilation begins within a few minutes after instillation, and in a half hour the effect is beginning to wear off. Cyclopentolate produces the widest pupillary dilatation, especially if combined with phenylephrine. However, the duration is intermediate and may persist for over 24 hours. Because atropine eyedrops exert a mydriatic effect for days, there is little use for them in the emergency department.

Pilocarpine eyedrops will be needed in the immediate care of acute glaucoma. Common dosages are 1% to 4%. In the treatment of acute glaucoma frequent instillations of the pilocarpine drops are more important than the strength used.

Corneal anesthesia for foreign body removal requires the use of a topical anesthetic such as proparacaine (Ophthaine) or 0.5% tetracaine (Pontocaine). The sting of tetracaine is considerably greater than that of Ophthaine. However, tetracaine has the advantage in that its anesthesia is more profound. Repeated instillations of 0.5% tetracaine with 10% phenylephrine will effect the best anesthesia for foreign body removal.

FOREIGN BODIES
Symptoms

The most common cause of a foreign body sensation in the eye is something in the eye! However, this truism must be tempered by the awareness that a corneal abrasion feels exactly like a foreign body. Indeed, the abrasion may have been caused initially by a foreign body. In any event, the patient with a corneal abrasion will continue to complain that foreign material is present when, in truth, the abrasion is the reason for symptoms.

Loose foreign bodies may be washed out quickly with the profuse tearing that accompanies the discomfort. The apparent absence of an obvious foreign body will inspire diligent search by the examiner, particularly of the upper fornix. It is indeed embarrassing to learn that a foreign body was missed, only to have been discovered and removed at a later time by another examiner.

Inspection

Magnification is indispensable in searching for foreign bodies. The microscope of the slit lamp will afford the greatest assurance that all foreign particles have been revealed and removed. Again, inspection of the injured eye will be greatly aided by the comfort of topical anesthesia.

The lower fornix of the eye can be easily inspected by downward pressure on the lower eyelid. Any material then exposed can be easily irrigated from the eye or removed with a moistened cotton-tipped applicator.

Adequate inspection of the upper fornix is a different matter and requires eversion of the upper eyelid. The patient cooperates by diverting the gaze downward, the eyelid is gently pulled downward, and the lid is everted over a smooth instrument or cotton applicator stick. Very frequently an elusive foreign body will be discovered on the conjunctival surface of the upper eyelid.

Removal

A foreign body embedded in the cornea occurs frequently from grinding accidents, working under cars, and so on. If the foreign body is iron, it will rust quickly and the rust becomes bound very firmly to the corneal stroma. Such embedded rust is difficult to remove. Excellent anesthesia will be required in order to dislodge an embedded corneal foreign body. Also, removal of the particle should not be attempted without adequate visualization by means of magnification.

Steadiness is required by both the patient and the person removing the foreign body. The patient can keep the injured eye steady by fixating on an object with the uninvolved eye.

Needles or sharp-pointed spuds do not make good instruments for corneal foreign body removal and, therefore, should be avoided. A rounded "golf club" spud is preferable.

Sometimes the foreign body is easily dislodged and removed but a rust ring remains. Considerable digging at the rust ring may not be effective. Experience has shown that if the eye is patched for 24 hours, the stroma surrounding the rust ring becomes necrotic and soft. Then the rust ring can be easily "shelled out."

Very young children are not expected to be cooperative with attempts to remove ocular foreign bodies. In such a case, general anesthesia will be required to render the eye motionless.

Intraocular injury

A small foreign body striking the eye with high speed will penetrate the globe and come to rest within the eye. Such an intraocular foreign body injury may not exhibit signs commensurate with the seriousness of the situation. The usual history is that the injured individual was hammering, nailing, or chipping when he or she felt something strike the eye. Nevertheless, a 2 mm object traveling at a very high speed usually enters the eye so smoothly and quickly that immediate symptoms are very minimal. In addition, examination with the naked eye may fail to reveal this serious injury, and the nature of the accident goes undetected. This is a serious error because the courts have held that where an intraocular foreign body might logically exist, x-ray films are mandatory!

A small intraocular foreign body can wreak havoc to an eye. If the lens has been struck or pierced, a traumatic cataract will surely result. Intraocular bleeding is potentially blinding. And, finally, should the foreign body reach the posterior segment of the eye, the stage is set for a retinal detachment.

Definitive treatment of an intraocular foreign body is in the hands of the ophthalmologist. Sometimes an eye can retain an inert foreign substance amazingly well. On the other hand, organic matter, wood, copper, iron, and other such substances can eventually cause loss of the eye. The ophthalmic surgeon will weigh the hazards of leaving the intraocular foreign body alone against the potential damages of surgical intervention.

ABRASIONS

Abrasions of the cornea occur nearly as frequently as foreign bodies. The symptoms are identical.

The anatomy of the cornea is such that an ordinary superficial abrasion heals without scarring and without visual impairment. A severe abrasion or partial laceration of the cornea extending through the tough Bowman's membrane will always result in a whitish corneal scar, or leukoma. Again, a corneal abrasion will feel to the patient like there is something in the eye. Only after a thorough search will both the patient and the examiner feel secure that no such foreign body exists.[2]

Assessment

To detect a corneal abrasion a fluorescein strip is moistened and introduced into the lower fornix. With an ordinary white penlight, the dye will neatly stain and delineate any abrasion. A cobalt blue light greatly aids the visibility of the fluorescein dye. Every slit lamp has a cobalt blue light source.

One special type of corneal abrasion is frequently associated with the use of contact lenses. Typically, the contact lens wearer leaves the lenses in for a longer period than usual. Some hours later (usually at 2:00 A.M.) intense eye pain develops. There is profuse tearing, swollen lids, and the eyes cannot be opened. This is the "over-wearing syndrome," or *OWS!*

Treatment

Immediate pain relief will occur after the instillation of anesthetic eyedrops. It must be cautioned that it is unwise to dispense anesthetic medications for pain relief. Such self-medication by an injured person poses additional risks and dangers. For example, the anesthetic may mask increasing inflammation, further damage to the cornea may develop unnoticed, and drug reactions may occur. Industrial workers, particularly, may receive a gift tube of Butyn ointment for personal use after a corneal injury. Do not succumb to such bad habits.

Traditional treatment for a corneal abrasion consists of using an antibiotic medication (Pontocaine Ophthalmic Ointment) and patching the eye for 24 to 48 hours. Pain relief should be assured by oral medication. Be aware that a corneal abrasion is ordinarily quite painful. People primarily come to doctors for relief of pain, so be certain to provide adequate pain relief.

LACERATIONS

Frank laceration of the delicate eye is an injury of grave consequence and commonly leads to loss of useful vision. Magnification is not always necessary in this instance, since usually there is gross disruption in the normal architecture of the eye. This type of injury is seen most com-

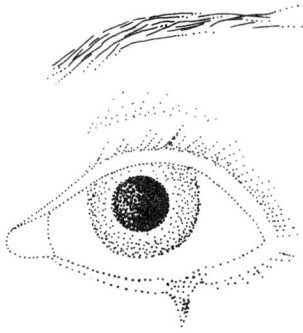

Fig. 22-2. Lower eyelid notch following inappropriate repair of laceration.

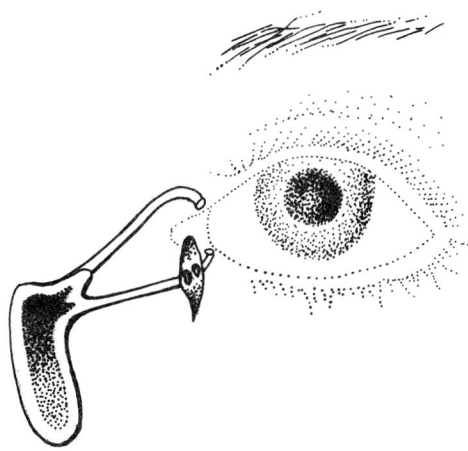

Fig. 22-3. Severed canaliculus with interruption of tear flow.

monly in automobile and motorcycle accidents. Usually, a considerable degree of damage has been suffered by the rest of the face.

The most important consideration here is not to inflict further damage to an already severely injured eye. The patient should be sedated, reassured, and restrained from excessive movement. In all cases, once the serious nature of this injury is apparent, further examination and treatment await the direction of the ophthalmologist.

Lacerations of the globe itself are usually accompanied by lacerations of the lids, lid margins, or structures of tear drainage (Fig. 22-2). The seriousness of laceration of tissues surrounding the eye varies greatly. A laceration of the skin of the eyelid not involving the margin is least serious. The lax skin of the eyelids generally affords easy approximation, and scarring after repair is minimal. Lid lacerations involving the margin are another matter. Inappropriate repair of such an injury will lead to a notch in the lid. This not only is quite disfiguring, but also a notch of the lower lid interferes with normal direction of tears to the tear ducts. Troublesome, persistent tearing (epiphora) results. Prevention of this complication is assured when the initial repair is managed by someone skilled in ophthalmic plastic repair.[3]

Immediate concern exists if the lower canaliculus has been severed. Any lower lid laceration involving the medial aspect should put one on alert to the possibility of a tear duct laceration. If this critical area of the periorbit *appears* to be involved, then it should be assumed that it *is* involved (Fig. 22-3). It is far better to prove that the tear drainage is intact than to assume so only to be forced to repair a severed canaliculus at a later date. Late repair of this injury is far more difficult than early repair because the ends of the severed canaliculus retract and become extremely difficult to find and to unite. The ophthalmologist will appreciate being called in early when a severed canaliculus is suspected.

BLUNT BLOWS

Contusion injuries form a unique group of ocular emergencies. It would be an unusual emergency department that did not see at least one contusion injury from a baseball during baseball season. Handballs, rocks, and fists inflict the major portion of these injuries. More than 12 million Americans play tennis. Ocular trauma from a speeding tennis ball may result in posterior vitreous detachment, retinal tears, and retinal detachments.[4] Racquetball is increasing greatly in popularity, and resultant eye injuries occur frequently. Any fall may result in a blunt blow to the face or eyes.

The eye is quite resistant to significant injury from blunt blows. The usual extent of damage consists of periorbital contusion and ecchymosis, the usual "black eye." Once serious injury has been ruled out, a black eye can be expected to clear without sequelae.

Blunt blows, abrasions, and foreign bodies of the conjunctiva may initiate a subconjunctival hemorrhage. The bright red blood contrasts sharply with the normal white of the sclera, and the appearance is more startling than serious. In fact, such hemorrhages frequently occur spontaneously and without any symptoms whatever. It is important to be absolutely certain that the subconjunctival hemorrhage is not associated with other, more serious eye problems.

Hyphema is the most common serious eye injury resulting from a blunt blow. There is no mistaking this bleeding, since the blood is readily visible in the anterior chamber through the transparent cornea. The blood ordinarily settles to the inferior aspect of the eye and forms into a pool below (Fig. 22-4).

In nine out of ten cases the hyphema clears spontaneously and the eye is no worse for the experience. However, 10% of these cases experience a secondary hemorrhage, generally occurring from the

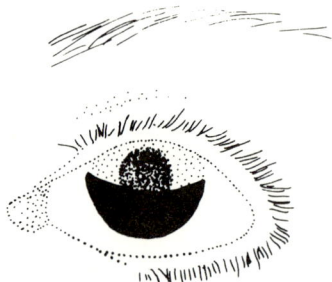

Fig. 22-4. Blood in the anterior chamber (hyphema).

second to the fifth day after injury. This secondary hemorrhage may be unrelenting and lead to further complications. Most authorities feel that excessive movement of the patient may hasten a secondary hemorrhage. Therefore, standard treatment involves bed rest and bilateral patching until it is assumed that no further bleeding will occur.

Despite the known resistance of the eye to serious consequence from blunt trauma, a significant blow may rupture the globe, dislocate the lens, cause vitreous hemorrhage, or a combination of these. Also, alterations in the aqueous dynamics may precipitate a type of contusion glaucoma that appears several months after the initial injury. The potential and hidden dangers of a black eye should not be minimized.

Blow-out fractures

Blunt blows to an eye are notorious for causing a specific type of orbital fracture. This so-called blow-out fracture of the orbital floor occurs when a blunt force to the front of the orbit raises the intraorbital pressure and then the weak inferior orbital wall gives way into the maxillary sinus (Fig. 22-5). The extent of the periorbital contusion and ecchymosis is quite variable. I have seen a beanball injury inflict a fracture of the floor of the orbit with *no* visible sign of external damage whatsoever.[5] If a blunt blow to an eye has occurred, one should automatically consider the possibility of a fractured orbit. In most cases, considerable swelling will be present. Sometimes the swelling is so marked that the eye is difficult to visualize.

This type of fracture has benefited in recent years from much exposure in the medical literature. Nevertheless, its presence still is frequently missed or if suspected, the signs and symptoms may be misleading. Remember that 15% of patients with orbital fracture also experience significant serious eye injury.

The tip-off leading to the diagnosis of

blow-out fracture may be the patient's complaints of double vision. This diplopia occurs when the inferior muscles of the eye become incarcerated in the fracture site. Consequently, there is anatomic restriction in the mobility of the involved eye. Commonly, the eye will not elevate properly. Nevertheless, the restriction of movement may occur in *any* direction.

Too much emphasis currently is placed upon x-ray findings in this type of fracture. Ideally, the classic case will demonstrate, on the Waters' view, a herniation of orbital contents into the maxillary sinus. Nevertheless, the x-ray studies may be falsely negative or falsely positive. The experienced examiner will place greater emphasis upon the clinical findings. The x-ray findings may not be confirmatory.[6]

The worst complication of untreated blow-out fracture is persistent diplopia.

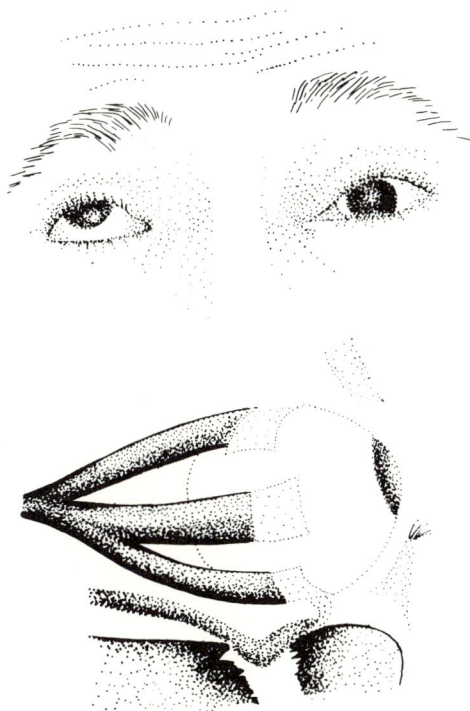

Fig. 22-5. Incarceration of inferior extraocular muscles in blowout fracture with restriction of upward gaze.

Surgical repair must be performed within a few days after such an injury to prevent this disability. The results of late repair of this injury are decidedly poor.

A second major complication of these cases is enophthalmos, or a sunken eye. Initially, orbital swelling may mask this feature. But, as the swelling subsides, the eye recedes more and more.

Th frequent occurrence of significant eye injury in orbital fractures would suggest that an ophthalmologist be called into consultation in almost every case. In like manner, the ophthalmologist should be mindful of the frequent simultaneous occurrence of other orbital and facial fractures when dealing with a blow-out fracture. The most common such associated fractures are of the inferior margin of the orbit and of the zygoma.[7,8]

CHEMICAL INJURIES

Industry continues to experience the occasional case of blindness from chemical accidents to the eyes. Also, children continue to spill toilet bowl cleaner into their eyes, and most big city hospitals have observed the devasting effect of alkalies used as weapons.

In general, alkalies are much more destructive to the eyes than are acids. The structure of the cornea is highly resistant to penetration by acids, whereas a strong alkali or basic substance can "eat" through the cornea in seconds. Not infrequently, newspaper accounts of supposed blindness from an acid accident are inexact in that the chemical in truth was an alkali.

Intervention

All chemical eye injuries should be approached as potentially blinding! Immediate and copious irrigation is indicated. Such treatment will be greatly facilitated by the instillation of a topical anesthetic. It is very difficult for the injured person to submit to the irrigation if the treatment itself renders pain.

No attention should be directed to specifically counteracting the type of chemical injury sustained. It is much more important not to delay the irrigation; the examiners should proceed promptly with ordering tap water or any of the numerous commercial irrigating solutions. Ask questions later.

Solid chemical matter lying in the fornices may not wash out readily. In these instances it is necessary to use a cotton-tipped applicator to adequately remove the substance.

Again when a chemical injury has been sustained by an eye, treatment is provided first and questions are asked later. The chemicals may continue to exert their destructive effect until physically removed from the eye.

RADIATION BURNS

The most common eye injury from radiation is the so-called welder's arc flash. This is a breakdown of the corneal surface caused by prolonged exposure to carbon arc lamps used in welding. The ultraviolet exposure causes damage to the surface epithelium of the cornea, cell destruction follows, and the employee experiences much pain. The breakdown of the cornea and the associated pain may occur some time after exposure. It should be noted that because of the nature of their work, welders also frequently sustain embedded foreign bodies in the cornea.

Pain relief is needed in cases of radiation keratitis, since the cornea always heals perfectly in a short period of time. The patient will request some relief of the eye pain. Severe radiation burns from welding may require patching for a day or less.

Less frequently, patients inflict radiation burns to their eyes from overexposure to sunlamps. Again, ocular pain is the most prominent feature along with redness and puffiness of the eyelid. Pain relief should be provided; convalescence will be benign and uneventful.

NONINJURY EMERGENCIES

The emergency department not infrequently will be called upon to manage acute ocular conditions that are not related to accident or injury. The typical problem is that of an acute red eye. The lack of a known injury does not necessarily mean that injury has not occurred. A red, painful, irritated eye from a foreign body can occur even if the patient was not aware that the foreign substance entered the eye.

Medical causes of red eye are classically grouped into acute conjunctivitis, acute glaucoma, and acute iritis. The differential diagnosis requires the usual attention to observable changes plus knowledgeable palpation of the eyes.

Acute conjunctivitis

Acute conjunctivitis is an infectious inflammation of the external surfaces of the eye. This excludes corneal infection such as corneal ulcer. The redness of conjunctivitis usually is most prominent in the fornices where a thick discharge is also found. This discharge will cause the patient to state that the eyelids are "stuck together" in the morning. Pain is not a prominent feature; however, there may be pain if the conjunctivitis is associated with an acute sty. These painful swellings of the lid are due to frank infection of one of the numerous glands in the eyelids.

In any event, emergency personnel would serve best by applying a patch and referring the individual to an ophthalmologist. Ordinarily, acute conjunctivitis caused by bacterial infection clears rapidly under antibiotic therapy. However, eye infections of viral origin are potentially much more serious and usually last much longer.

The virus of herpes simplex is the most common cause of infectious blindness in the United States. One should know prior to beginning treatment for acute conjunctivitis that the condition is truly a common "cold in the eye" and not herpes simplex conjunctivitis. Antibiotics will not help herpes, and the use of steroids may actually precipitate or aggravate herpes infections. Nonophthalmologists should not use steroid preparations in treating conjunctivitis.

Acute glaucoma

Acute glaucoma is extremely painful. The patient is in real agony from severe eye pain, which may radiate to the area around the eye. The globe is unmistakably rock-hard to palpation. The pupil is fixed and slightly dilated. The cornea lacks its usual luster and is described as steamy. Congestion of the globe is usually marked. However, the diagnosis is occasionally missed because the initial complaint was only severe headache, perhaps with nausea and vomiting. The gastrointestinal upset has been known to draw the examiner's attention away from the gravely sick eye.

Ophthalmologic management for acute glaucoma is urgent. Vision may be irreparably lost in a matter of hours. Also, a very early case of acute glaucoma may respond to medical treatment, and definitive surgery can then be deferred to a more favorable time. If medical measures fail, surgical intervention is imperative.

Acute iritis

Acute iritis is an internal inflammatory condition of the eye. It is noninfectious and might be likened to arthritis of the joints. The redness of iritis is classically circumcorneal; that is, it is most prominent surrounding the clear cornea. The spasm of the internal iris muscles causes the pupil to be smaller than usual. Exquisite tenderness to touch is a prominent sign of this acute condition. The patient will experience photophobia, or undue pain from light.

Iritis is not infectious and does not respond to antibiotics. The photophobia will require relief with sunglasses or patching. Initial treatment consisting of cortisone drops and mydriasis of the pupil will re-

quire follow-up surveillance by the ophthalmologist.

Loss of vision

Sudden loss of vision is a very frightening experience. Anxiety will be a prominent feature in any person who enters the emergency department with this complaint. The potential (if not real) possibility of permanent visual loss demands that ophthalmologic consultation be obtained.

In a young adult temporary loss of vision is usually caused by ophthalmic migraine. It is not necessary that headache coexist with the visual disturbance. The visual loss is usually a portion of the visual field, and it may be accompanied by flashing lights or zigzag lines. Commonly, a migraine history is obtained, either in the patient or in other members of the family.

Other causes of sudden loss of vision in a young person are much more rare. Sudden visual disturbance as a result of retinal vascular occlusion should be kept in mind as a severe complication in women taking oral contraceptives.[9]

In an older individual, retinal detachment and vascular accidents of the retina are frequent causes of sudden vision loss. Other than visual dysfunction, symptoms are minimal. Central vision as measured by visual acuity may be affected. Emergency personnel will greatly enhance the evaluation of this patient by assessing the state of the peripheral side vision. The procedure is simple. The patient directs a gaze at the examiner's nose while the examiner notes the ability of the patient to see a moving finger from each side, up and down. Retinal detachment usually is observable with the ophthalmoscope, and the treatment will be surgical.

SUMMARY

Visual loss and eye pain are common symptoms of ocular emergencies. Magnification will greatly aid the assessment of most emergencies. Treatment is aimed at relieving pain and assuring visual function. The unique and special characteristics of the eye will frequently require the services of an ophthalmologist.

REFERENCES

1. Stein, H. A., and Slatt, B. J.: The ophthalmic assistant: fundamentals and clinical practice, ed. 3, St. Louis, 1976, The C. V. Mosby Co.
2. Duke-Elder, S., and MacFaul, P. A.: System of ophthalmology: mechanical injuries, vol. 14, parts 1 and 2, St. Louis, 1972, The C. V. Mosby Co.
3. Mustarde, J. C.: Repair and reconstruction in the orbital region, Baltimore, 1967, The Williams & Wilkins Co.
4. Seelenfreund, M. H., and Freilich, D. B.: Rushing the net and retinal detachment, J.A.M.A. 235:25, 1976.
5. Anderson, R. D.: Blow-out fractures of the floor of the orbit: further concepts, Trans. Pac. Coast Otoophthalmol. Soc. 48:121-135, 1967.
6. Milauskas, A. L.: Fractures of the orbit: with clinical, radiological and surgical aspects, Springfield, Ill., 1969, Charles C Thomas, Publisher.
7. Smith, B., and Converse, J. M.: Plastic and reconstructive surgery of the eye and adnexa, St. Louis, 1967, The C. V. Mosby Co.
8. Converse, J. M.: Reconstructive plastic surgery, Philadelphia, 1964, W. B. Saunders Co.
9. Freidman, S., and Golan, S.: Acute ophthalmologic complications during use of oral contraceptives, Contraception 10:685-692, 1974.

CHAPTER 23

Ear, nose, and throat emergencies

Gordon R. Freeman, M.D.

In this day of specialization and medical litigation, it behooves personnel not only to care for all patients with diligence and concern, but also to avoid the pitfalls that may result in medical litigation. Competence in deciding what is an ear, nose, and throat emergency and deciding on proper referral or initiating primary care should be uppermost in the minds of all members of the emergency department team. Proper follow-up of any care provided is imperative.

As with any patient, an adequate history and physical examination are prerequisites to care of the patient in the emergency department. To properly perform a physical examination of the ear, nose, and throat, three important factors are required: (1) good illumination; (2) magnification, if needed; and (3) adequate physical control of the patient or proper sedation. Most of the personnel working with the emergency patient have had little practice using a head mirror and indirect illumination. Therefore, it is mandatory that all emergency departments have a head light to be utilized in performing examinations and caring for ear, nose, and throat emergencies. This leaves the operator with both hands free for care and examination. In many instances the small orifices under examination require magnification, and

therefore some optical equipment should be available for evaluating the patient.

Many ear, nose, and throat emergencies, particularly those related to foreign body, hemorrhage, or infection, create pain and discomfort prior to examination. During examination and emergency care the apprehensive patient, particularly a child, will commonly move or be uncooperative. This movement must be kept to a minimum either by sedation or mummification to prevent iatrogenic trauma.

Most emergency departments have the more commonly used ear, nose, and throat instruments. However, the instruments shown in Fig. 23-1 will help in providing better care for ear, nose, and throat emergencies. These instruments are small malleable wire curettes, various types of small dental or ear hooks, small and medium size alligator forceps, and large, curved tonsil hemostats or long right-angle clamps.

FOREIGN BODIES

Foreign bodies in the ear, nose, or throat are quite common, and they should be recognized as acute surgical emergencies. Foreign bodies may be animal, vegetable, or mineral; each of these types is managed differently when lodged in the various orifices of the human body. Because of this, some effort should be made to determine the nature of the foreign body and, if possible, its contour or shape. Animal or insect foreign bodies can produce a great deal of pain and destruction and frequently must be immobilized or destroyed prior to their removal. Vegetable foreign bodies are notoriously hydroscopic agents; as they absorb moisture, they enlarge and create increasing obstruction, which makes their removal more difficult. The more quickly a hydroscopic agent can be removed and the less exposure to water or humidification, the easier this type of

material can be recovered. Mineral foreign bodies cause the least tissue trauma and are usually radiopaque, but at times they can be the most difficult objects to remove because of slick surfaces, sharp points, edges, and the like.

Ear

The most common foreign body of the ear is cerumen. This, as well as many other types of foreign bodies, can readily be removed by proper irrigation with sterile solution. However, ears with known perforations or with bleeding or purulent dis-

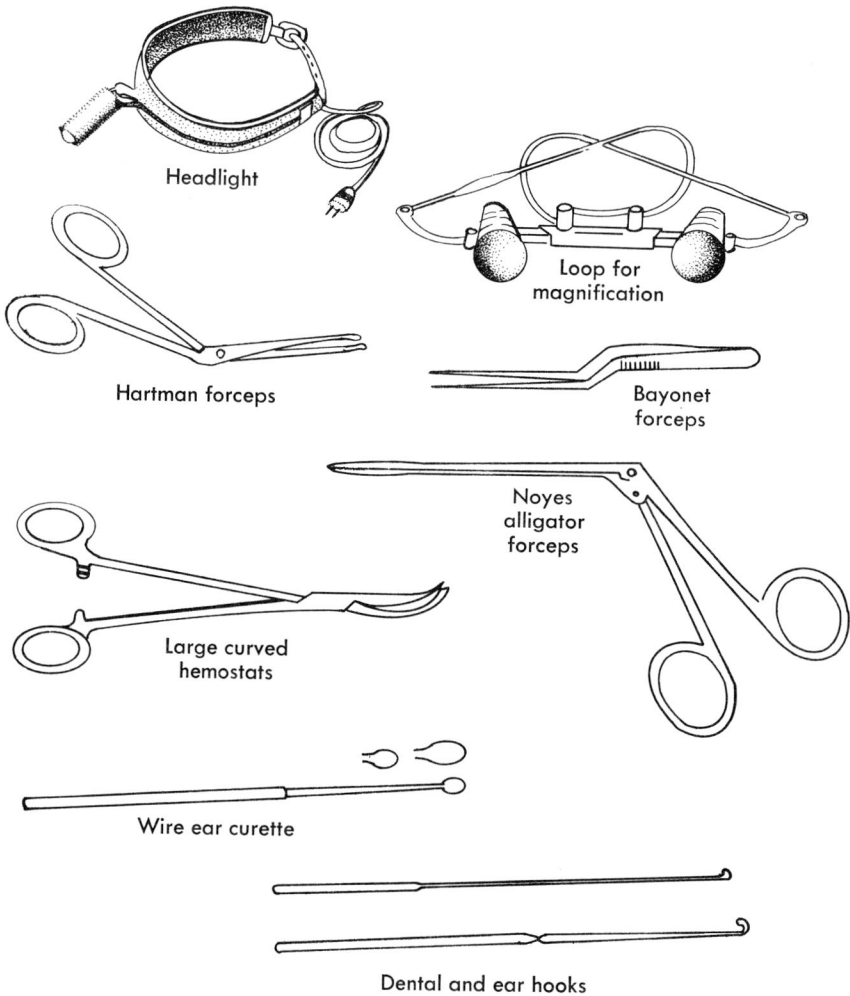

Fig. 23-1. Equipment for ear, nose, and throat examination.

charge should be evaluated properly and usually should not be irrigated. Hydroscopic foreign bodies should not be continually irrigated if initial irrigation fails to remove the agent with ease. Most foreign bodies of the ear, under adequate illumination and magnification and with complete control of the patient, can be removed using various small dental hooks (Fig. 23-1). Emergency department personnel unfamiliar with the removal of such foreign bodies should refer these patients to an otolaryngologist; care must be taken so that the tympanic membrane or middle ear is not damaged.

Nose

Foreign bodies of the nose not recognized immediately are usually characterized by unilateral purulent discharge. To adequately remove a nasal foreign body, the patient should be placed in a slight Trendelenburg position to reduce the possibility of aspiration. The nose should then be prepared by using a decongestant, such as phenylephrine (Neo-Synephrine), 0.5%, followed by a topical anesthetic, tetracaine (Pontocaine), 1%, or lidocaine (Xylocaine), 4%, to reduce the pain during manipulation and removal of the foreign body. The alligator forcep or a malleable ring curette bent at a 90-degree angle will remove most foreign bodies found within the nose. If the nasal foreign body is inadvertently pushed back into the nasopharynx, the patient should be retained in the Trendelenburg position and rolled over to face down position; the patient can usually spit out the object through the mouth. When there is doubt as to the location of a foreign body within the nose or if there has been the possibility of aspiration upon removal, chest x-ray examination is indicated prior to discharge of the patient.

Throat

The finding of a foreign body within the hypopharynx, or throat, is not com-

mon. However, it is quite common to have the patient feel that a foreign body is within the hypopharynx, when in reality the sensation is related to a scratch or irritation of the hypopharynx or cervical esophagus that occurred as the object was inadvertently swallowed. Because of possible complications, this patient should be cared for diligently to confirm the presence or absence of such a foreign body. Small bones, bristles, toothpicks, and the like are frequently found imbedded in the tonsillar areas, postlingual tonsil tissue, or within the piriform sinus. These objects will characteristically produce a sensation of pain or fullness upon swallowing. Adequate illumination with indirect laryngoscopy by the use of a mirror can usually locate such foreign bodies. With the use of topical anesthetics, the throat may be anesthetized and most of the foreign bodies above the larynx can readily be removed by a large curved hemostat. Patients with such foreign bodies deep within the piriform sinus or within the larynx per se usually are hospitalized, and direct laryngoscopy is necessary for removal of the foreign body. Large foreign bodies of the pharynx and hypopharynx can compromise the airway. A rapid search with a finger or a curved hemostat can frequently clear the airway in such an emergency. If the foreign body cannot be removed, passage of a small, firm bronchoscope beyond the foreign body will be necessary to provide an airway. If this is not possible, immediate emergency tracheostomy or cricothyreotomy is indicated. Any patient who has undergone foreign body removal or the traumatic introduction of an airway during such emergencies should be hospitalized and carefully observed for the possibility of posttraumatic laryngeal edema, which may later compromise the airway.

Esophagus

Foreign bodies of the esophagus are characterized by inability to swallow. Liquids and even saliva must constantly be expectorated as it is formed. Lower esophageal foreign bodies will frequently cause repeated vomiting of any material that has been swallowed. A chronic irritative cough is often present because of aspiration of the esophageal content. Esophageal foreign bodies are discovered by x-ray diagnosis. If the article is not completely radiopaque, small pieces of cotton soaked in barium can be used to denote the level of foreign body retention. Frequently, small strands of cotton will catch on a foreign body and will indicate the level or area of the retained material. Foreign bodies retained within the esophagus for a prolonged period of time compromise the blood supply of the mucous membrane and the esophageal wall, increasing the chance of spontaneous or iatrogenic perforation during endoscopy. When doubt exists as to the presence of a foreign body, the patient should be admitted and scheduled for endoscopy.

Esophageal burns by either acid or alkali constitute an acute surgical emergency requiring immediate emergency department care followed by admission and either immediate or delayed endoscopy depending on the patient's condition. The severity of burns within the mouth does not always indicate the amount of esophageal damage. The pH of the offending material should be ascertained, if at all possible, and immediate counter application of acid or alkali solutions should be done to neutralize the offending material. Dilute alkali solutions may be negated with large quantities of water or milk. More caustic alkali should be neutralized with weak (never strong!) acids such as diluted vinegar, lemon juice, or orange juice. Similarly, acids should be diluted and may be neutralized with weak bases such as magnesium oxide, milk of magnesia, calcium hydroxide, or aluminum hydroxide.[1] Severely burned patients will require treatment for shock and immediate antibiotic and steroid therapy.

Trachea and bronchi

Tracheal and bronchial foreign bodies are usually recognized by the severe episodes of coughing at the time of aspiration. Clinical examination will frequently reveal whistles or breath changes throughout the affected side of the thorax. X-ray studies to confirm the diagnosis should include inspiratory and expiratory phases of respiration to help in determining the site of foreign body obstruction. These patients require immediate hospitalization and diligent care because of the possibility of acute respiratory distress. Bronchoscopy is done as soon as possible. Foreign bodies of the respiratory and digestive tract are discussed in Chapters 26 and 29.

HEMORRHAGE

Hemorrhage of the ear, nose, or throat may be of minor importance or can be life threatening. Any patient with such an emergency must have a complete evaluation as to the cause of such hemorrhage. Factors such as systemic disease, anticoagulant therapy, blood dyscrasias, or various medications that induce bleeding must be discovered so that the underlying cause as well as the immediate hemorrhage can be treated.

Ear

Hemorrhage from the ear is usually traumatic in nature, but occasionally is related to infection. A bleeding ear should never be irrigated but may be evaluated by the use of suction and aspiration to determine the extent and area of bleeding. The more common causes of hemorrhage from the ear are external blows that damage either the canal or tympanic membrane, instrumentation in attempting to remove cerumen or a foreign body, and occasionally an insect. A frequent cause of hemorrhage from the canal and tympanic membrane is myringitis bullosa hemorrhagica or small blood blisters rupturing within the canal wall of tympanic membrane. Acute otitis media with spontaneous rupture of the tympanic membrane will frequently create spontaneous hemorrhage rather than purulent discharge from the ears.

Once the cause of the hemorrhage has been ascertained, it can usually be controlled by packing the ear canal with sterile cotton pledgets covered with antibiotic ointment and applying a sterile external dressing. Antibiotics should be prescribed, and proper follow-up by an otolaryngologist should be obtained as soon as possible. If, on examination, extensive damage to the tympanic membrane is determined, surgical apposition of the lacerated edges or grafting of the tympanic membrane should be done as soon as possible to ensure proper healing (Fig. 23-2).

The patient who has suffered a skull injury with the possibility of a basal skull fracture will often have bleeding or discharge from the ear, which may be a spinal otorrhea. The ears of such patients should not be investigated, cleaned, or manipulated, but a sterile dressing should be applied and antibiotics started; further neuro-otologic evaluation should be performed by competent personnel under sterile conditions.

A profusely bleeding ear in a patient who has recently had mastoid surgery or tympanoplasty is classified as a true emergency, since this may be related to the rupture of a major cranial artery or vein and profuse hemorrhage may result. Treatment consists of a sterile compression dressing and immediate consultation.

Nose

Nasal hemorrhage is quite common and at times life threatening. As with all excessive bleeding, hemorrhage needs to be controlled, and the cause of such bleeding must be determined and proper therapy initiated. Eighty-five percent of all nasal epistaxes occur in the anterior septal area or along the anterior floor of the nose. The remaining 15% to 20% of nasal hemorrhages are posterior and are usually more serious and profuse. Posterior epistaxis is related to the anteroposterior ethmoid artery or the internal maxillary artery, which is a branch of the external carotid. To properly control this nasal hemorrhage, anterior postnasal packing is mandatory. Most anterior bleeding points may be well controlled by soaking cotton pledgets with phenylephrine or epinephrine and placing them in the anterior vestibule of the nose. Once the immediate hemorrhage has been located and controlled, electrocauterization by the Bovie will usually be adequate to control anterior nasal bleeding. If there are signs of infection, crusting, or vestibulitis, anterior packing with cotton pledgets and antibiotic ointments will usually enhance healing and reduce the chance of repeated bleeding.

Postnasal bleeding

Postnasal bleeding can be life threatening, particularly in the hypertensive patient. To adequately control postnasal bleeding, the patient should be given some sedation, which not only will reduce anx-

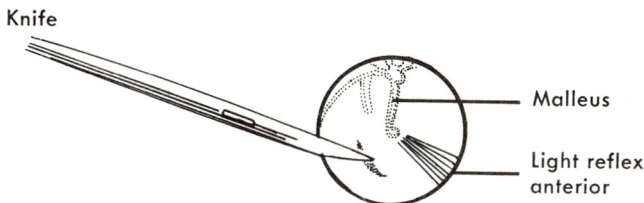

Fig. 23-2. Myringotomy; right eardrum; light reflex anterior; incision posterior, inferior quadrant.

iety but also the pain involved in controlling such hemorrhage. If time permits, a topical anesthetic placed within the nose by spray or cotton pledgets will reduce the pain related to the trauma of nasal packing. Postnasal packing can then be accomplished by one of two methods. Either a Foley catheter or a catheter specifically made for postnasal packing is passed through the nares. This is inflated and brought tightly against the posterior turbinates of the nose. The catheter is then fixed anteriorly by an umbilical cord pin or with adhesive.

A surer method of controlling postnasal bleeding is by the postnasal pack (Fig. 23-3). The postnasal pack is a roll or ball of gauze material to which three strings have been attached either by tying or suturing. Postnasal packing is then accomplished in the following method. A catheter is passed through the anterior nares to the nasopharynx and is then brought out through the mouth. Two of the strings attached to the postnasal pack are then tied to the catheter. The catheter is pulled back through the nares until the strings at the edge of the catheter can be obtained at

the anterior nares. The patient is then asked to relax and breathe rapidly through his or her open mouth as the two strings are pulled taut and the pack is brought up behind the palate and packed tightly with a finger into the nasopharynx. The third string is cut short enough so that it can be seen just below the palatal edge. This third string makes it easy to retrieve the postnasal packing when it is to be removed. The two anterior strings brought through the anterior nares are tied over a dental sponge or a roll of gauze to secure the pack. To properly control severe hypertensive nasal bleeding, an anterior pack consisting of 1.5 cm of Adaptic should be applied into both anterior nares. Most patients with anterior postnasal packing require hospitalization. They should always be placed on antibiotics with appropriate sedation and therapy for hypertension, or other systemic treatment of bleeding should be initiated.

Hemorrhage from the throat

Hemorrhage from the mouth and throat should always be differentiated from true hemoptysis and hematemesis. This differ-

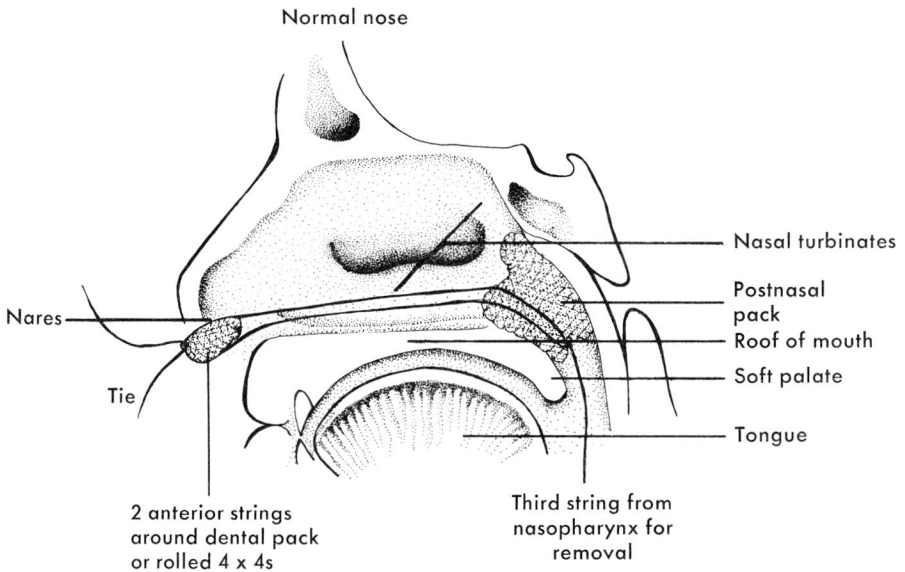

Fig. 23-3. Postnasal packing.

entiation is mandatory because hematemesis or hemoptysis is often a true surgical emergency requiring hospitalization and endoscopy. Bleeding from the mouth is usually related to various forms of gingivitis, pyorrhea, and other dental-related diseases.

A common cause of bleeding from the mouth, which at times can be profuse, is large venous varicosities of the nasopharynx, postlingual area, and beneath the tongue. This is much more common in the elderly patient. Hemorrhage from tonsils, adenoid tissue, and postlingual lymphoid tissue is not uncommon when infection increases the vascularity of such tissue. Hemorrhage is often related to pseudomembranes of tonsillitis that are denuded as the patient eats, clears the throat, and so on. Postsurgical hemorrhage related to dental extraction, tonsillectomy, or other surgical procedure in and about the nose, hypopharynx, or pharynx is a surgical emergency that may require hospitalization and surgical evaluation as to severity.

Hemorrhage from the larynx and hypopharynx is less common and most frequently is caused by a hemangioma or hemangiomatous polyp in those areas. In acute laryngotracheitis hemorrhage is related to the degree of cough and irritation present. This can usually be demonstrated by indirect laryngoscopy and the use of a mirror.

Any bleeding from the throat or mouth that cannot adequately be diagnosed or differentiated from hemoptysis or hematemesis will require prolonged emergency department observation and occasionally hospitalization or adequate referral. Hemorrhage of a traumatic nature, particularly in the pediatric patient, is quite common. This is usually caused by a foreign body that has lacerated the tongue, palate, or tonsillar fossa. Large lacerations of the tongue, palate, or tonsillar area will require adequate surgical closure of the wound to reduce the possibility of disfigurement and disability.

As previously mentioned, recent dental extractions can cause severe hemorrhage. If the patient is unable to locate dental attention, the hemorrhage can usually be controlled by packing a dental sponge into the socket and having the patient bite and hold the dental sponge in place for a prolonged period of time. Electrocoagulation will usually control bleeding of the pharynx, hypopharynx, and so on. However, as in any acute hemorrhage, the use of surgical ligature is the method of choice.

To reiterate, any hemorrhage that is difficult to control should be evaluated as to the possibility of a systemic, metabolic, or drug cause.

INFECTIONS

Acute infections of the ear, nose, and throat are the most common form of acute illness seen in the emergency department. Ocassionally, they represent acute emergencies that require hospitalization, but with proper diagnosis and care the patient can usually be returned home with relief of pain and the assurance that serious complications have been avoided.

Ear

Acute otitis externa. Acute otitis externa, an infection of the canal, is frequently more painful and appears to be more serious than acute otitis media. Occasionally, it is difficult to differentiate acute otitis media and mastoiditis from this entity. Acute otitis externa is characterized by marked swelling of the external auditory canal with cellulitis of the adjacent structures. The swelling and edema of the canal causes severe pain. The swelling at times is of such magnitude that it inhibits proper evaluation of the tympanic membrane.

Acute otitis externa should be evaluated as to a bacterial or mycotic infection. This diagnosis can frequently be made by placing some of the purulent material from within the canal on a glass slide and observing it under a microscope. Treatment consists of placing small cotton pledget wicks within the swollen ear canal and applying an antibiotic steroid ear drop to the cotton pledget at frequent intervals for 48 hours. The cotton may then be removed and the drops placed within the ear canal. Appropriate antibiotics and sedation should be prescribed for the patient's infection and pain. For a mycotic infection, appropriate acidified otic drops (acetic acid 2% in propylene glycol [Vosol]) should be used on the cotton wick rather than antibiotics. Any furnucle or area of cellulitis that appears to be organized and pointing should be incised and drained to shorten the patient's period of discomfort and to rapidly resolve the infectious process.

Acute otitis media. Acute otitis media is characterized by pain, a throbbing sensation or fullness within the ear, and frequently diminution in hearing. Rarely is the external auditory canal swollen, and the tympanic membrane is usually well visualized. There may be vascular redness in and about the anulus and malleus of the tympanic membrane; or a complete loss of contour and continuity may be noted, caused by the bulging of fluid or purulent material within the middle ear. Adequate care of otitis media includes antibiotics, decongestants, and pain medication; myringotomy is usually indicated also. This is performed by incising the posterior inferior quadrant of the tympanic membrane with a myringotomy scapel. Pain is usually relieved within a few hours, and the myringotomy will frequently avoid the following two complications of acute otitis media: (1) spontaneous rupture of the tympanic membrane, which frequently leaves a permanent perforation, and (2) subacute or acute mastoiditis if the infection continues and the tympanic membrane does not rupture. There is little excuse for sending a patient with acute otitis media home in severe pain when a myringotomy will alleviate the pain and promote rapid dissolution of the infection.

Acute mastoiditis. Acute mastoiditis is characterized by the findings of either acute otitis externa or otitis media. The patient usually has severe pain with a definite deafness and may complain of vertigo. X-ray studies of the mastoid will usually confirm the diagnosis. Consultation with an otolaryngologist is necessary for the patient with the above symptoms or with known otitis media with or without discharge from the middle ear and associated redness and swelling behind the auricle.

Nose

Acute infections of the nose, particularly cellulitis and furunculosis of the nose or face, not only are painful but also are potentially dangerous because of the possibility of intracranial complication from venous drainage. Furuncles and abscesses of the face should not be squeezed or manipulated. Prior to incision and drainage, these patients should be adequately protected with antibiotics to avoid the possibility of sepsis entering the cerebral venous circulation. Treatment should consist of warm soaks and heavy antibiotic therapy. The patient should be seen on a daily basis, and any questions of central nervous system symptoms require hospitalization for further observation.

Nasal septum abscess. Injury to the nasal septum is frequently followed by a septal abscess. The patient's symptoms are marked by acute nasal obstruction with a wide, serous-looking nasal septum that appears to be protruding through the vestibule of the nose. The patient usually complains of headache and may have a high fever. Treatment should consist of massive antibiotics as well as incision and drainage of the abscess. Because of the possibility of intracranial complications or the loss of cartilaginous structure by perichondritis, the patient should be referred to an otolaryngologist for initial and follow-up care.

Sinus

Almost every patient with frequent headaches has so-called "sinusitis" or "chronic sinus headaches." These headaches are usually related to tension or allergic disease. The patient with true sinusitis will usually have other symptoms and clinical findings as well as a headache. Adequate rhinoscopy with the use of decongestants will usually show inflammation of the turbinates with purulent material coming from the middle or superior meatus of the nose. Fever may be associated with sinus disease.

The patient manifesting clinical and physical findings of acute sinusitis with a severe headache persisting for more than 48 hours should have sinus x-ray films taken before being discharged from the emergency department. Acute sinusitis with orbital cellulitis or cellulitis of areas in and about the face or orbit is an acute emergency, and the patient should be hospitalized. This is a patient with potential central nervous system complications.

The usual care of acute sinusitis not requiring hospitalization includes the use of antibiotics, decongestants, and aspiration with a suction tip of the purulent material within the nasal sinus ostia. Antral irrigation will relieve the patient's discomfort as quickly as myringotomy relieves the pain of acute otitis media. Antral irrigations are performed by using a decongestant and then placing lidocaine (Xylocaine), 4%, on pledgets of cotton under the inferior meatus. These are left in place for five to ten minutes. Following this, an antral needle is used to penetrate the inferior lateral nasal wall under the inferior turbinates. The maxillary antrum is then irrigated with a sterile normal saline solution. Care should be exercised so that the lateral nasal wall is not penetrated too deeply. Never force irrigation solutions into an antrum where great resistance is met.

Throat

Tonsillitis and pharyngitis are relatively common infections and usually respond adequately to antibiotic therapy. However, a patient may complain of headache and sore throat associated with fever when the pharynx appears normal. This frequently represents acute nasopharyngitis and is almost as common as pharyngitis. Close inspection with a small mirror will indicate a purulent, inflamed nasopharynx when the pharynx appears normal. Treatment is the same as in pharyngitis or tonsillitis.

Acute paratonsillar abscess. This condition is characterized by acute tonsillitis with severe swelling and a change of speech. Those abscesses causing symptoms in 48 hours or less will often respond to warm saline gargles and large doses of antibiotics without incision and drainage. Those patients with severe pain and swelling who have had symptoms for 48 hours or longer usually have an organized abscess that will respond to incision and drainage.

The procedure for incision and drainage of a paratonsillar abscess is as follows. Infiltrate the upper pole of the tonsil or the enlarged area of the palate with lidocaine, 2%, with epinephrine. The areas of injection are at the uvula, the lateral pillar area, and the tonsillar edge. Then use a No. 12 curved blade to make a very fine incision just through the mucous membrane at the level of the upper pole and anterior pillar. Pass the tonsil hemostat through the incision and up over the upper pole of the tonsil, spreading gently as you proceed posteriorly until the organized purulent material is reached. Occasionally, in spite of marked swelling, no purulent material will be found. Do not overtraumatize or probe continually if an organized abscess cannot be found. When probing laterally maintain care not to injure the carotid compartment or spread infection through the various fascial compartments of the submaxillary triangle.

The acutely ill patient with high temperature and borderline airway often requires hospitalization for this incision and drainage procedure. Frequently a patient with acute pharyngitis, fever, and severe spasm of the strap muscles with stiffness of the neck and forward arching of the head will have a postpharyngeal or retropharyngeal abscess. Observation of the pharynx and indirect laryngoscopy with a mirror will demonstrate the swelling of these areas within the hypopharynx or posterior pharyngeal wall. Patients with postpharyngeal or retropharyngeal abscesses represent acute emergencies. These patients should be hospitalized, and any incision and drainage of these lesions should be performed within an operating room, frequently under general anesthesia.

Salivary gland

Infection or obstruction by stones can cause sudden enlargement of a secreting gland. Acute sialadenitis not only will cause swelling but also can be associated with pain and cellulitis in and about the gland area. Purulent material may be observed coming from the various salivary ducts. Acute infections of the salivary glands should be treated with antibiotics and copious amounts of fluids, and any medication that has a tendency to decrease salivation, such as antihistamines, atropinelike preparations, or other anticholinergic drugs, should be discontinued. Acute purulent parotitis, other than endemic mumps, can be a fulminating illness that requires hospitalization. This is particularly true in the geriatric patient. An acute swelling of a salivary gland caused by obstructing stones can frequently be diagnosed by x-ray examination. The removal of a salivary calculus is not an emergency procedure and should be performed by a skilled physician under optimal conditions.

Upper and lower airway

The assessment and care of acute infections of the epiglottis, larynx, and bronchi are well described in Chapter 32. Any patient with such an emergency should be cared for in an area of the emergency department or hospital where emergency endotracheal intubation or tracheostomy equipment is available at a moment's notice. Procedures such as direct laryngoscopy or bronchoscopy should be performed only by a competent endoscopist who is prepared to continue with a difficult intubation or tracheostomy. Prolonged use of an endotracheal tube in infections of the respiratory tract or in patients with severe anoxia or tissue toxicity is contraindicated; tracheostomy should be done as soon as the patient is stable. The judicious use of antibiotics, steroids, and racemic epinephrine as well as careful observation will frequently alleviate the necessity of intubation or tracheostomy in respiratory emergencies.

TRAUMA

Lacerations, contusions, abrasions, fractures, and burns, of the ear, nose, and throat and head and neck are common. Such injuries may be treated by emergency personnel or by specialists in otolaryngology, plastic surgery, general surgery, oral surgery, or orthopedic surgery. Although such emergencies usually require competent specialty referral, minor traumatic problems of the ear, nose, and throat and head and neck can be handled by emergency department personnel.

Ear

The most common injury to the external ear is laceration, which at times may almost completely sever the ear from the head. Suturing of any laceration of the ear should provide a repair that not only completely restores the continuity of the skin, but also ensures that the cartilage is well managed and completely covered. Cartilage is very prone to infection, which results in perichondritis and cartilage destruction. Severe contusions and abrasions of the ear can also initiate perichondritis. The early judicious use of antibiotics plus steroids will frequently inhibit this complication.

Pressure dressings should never be applied to the ear where the blood supply may be compromised creating pressure necrosis to the ear cartilage.

Severe burns or abrasions of the ear require loose fluff dressings so as not to compromise the blood supply to the injured epithelium. This type of injury requires hospitalization and early grafting.

As previously mentioned, any head trauma in which there is bleeding from the external auditory canal or middle ear requires a complete evaluation to rule out the possibility of skull fractures, lacerations of the tympanic membranes, or further inner ear injury. Sterile technique in this examination plus x-ray examination will provide a clue to the extent of injury of the external, middle, or inner ear.

Nose

The most common injury to the nose is nasal fracture, which often includes the septum. A cardinal rule is the sooner a nasal or septal fracture is reduced, the better cosmetic results can be obtained. The old adage, "let the swelling go down," is a poor excuse for not initiating immediate care of a nasal fracture. The practice of reducing the fracture simply by pushing the nose to one side or the other with thumb and finger is passé. Any injury that may result in poor cosmetic results should be referred to specialty care. Initial care should include x-ray films of the bony injury and an evaluation of the orbit and visual acuity, if orbital injury has occurred. If primary care is initiated within the emergency department, photographs should be obtained to substantiate the degree of injury. Further information concerning nasal and orbital fractures is found in Chapter 21.

Fractures of the maxilla and mandible

Fractures of the maxilla and mandible and other facial fractures are discussed in Chapter 21. Establishing the diagnosis of such injuries requires specific, close physical examination as to facial contour, soft tissue injury, and ocular examination as well as x-rays of the bony injury. The usual sinus series, particularly the Waters' view, will generally demonstrate fractures of the maxilla and orbit. Any fracture of the maxilla and mandible will require careful observation as to the state of dentition, particularly the occlusion of the patient. Close attention should be given to the gingival area and the palate for evidence of hematoma, crepitus, and open compound fractures. Fractures involving both the mandible and facial bones may be referred either to an otolaryngologist or a plastic surgeon with proper dental referral as required.

Larynx

Any crushing or direct injury to the neck that involves the larynx can be a surgical emergency. The patient who complains of vocal change or stridor should be carefully observed for the possibility of acute airway obstruction at a later date. This type of patient frequently requires tracheostomy, since it is not uncommon for acute injuries of the larynx to create airway obstruction as late as 24 hours after injury. Diagnosis of this injury should be made by careful observation and palpation of the external neck, including evaluation of the hyoid, larynx, and cricoid cartilages. Indirect laryngoscopy by mirror examination may reveal ecchymosis and edema with occasional hematoma. Soft tissue x-ray studies, including tomography, are often required to demonstrate fractures of the thyroid cartilage of the larynx. Injuries and fractures of the larynx require the use of antibiotics, steroids, and humidification to reduce the possibility of perichondritis and tracheal stenosis. If in doubt, hospitalize the patient.

MISCELLANEOUS INFORMATION
Allergy

Allergy is perhaps one of the commonest afflictions today. It is not within the realm of this chapter to discuss all the allergic manifestations related to the ear, nose, and throat and respiratory tract. The various skin and allergic manifestations that can affect the ear, nose, and throat or head and neck can usually be diagnosed by adequate history and evaluation of the symptoms presented. The usual treatment for acute allergic disease is to first eliminate the particular allergen if at all possible and then provide symptomatic treatment. This should consist of various antihistamines, mild and bland soaks, steroid ointments and creams, and the use of systemic steroids.

Anaphylactic shock

Anaphylactic shock may be caused by the venom of various insects or reptiles, exposure to noxious substances, or as is usually the case, by acute allergic response to medications taken systemically or orally by the patient. Acute anaphylaxis is usually an immediate response, but it may be delayed from 10 to 30 minutes. The symptoms include sudden anxiety and restlessness, often with a pounding or throbbing type of headache. This is followed by a feeling of suffocation or actual cough with bronchial asthma, which immediately proceeds to profound peripheral vascular collapse and respiratory failure. If treatment is not initiated promptly, death results.

The following are the specific steps to be taken in relation to anaphylactic shock.

1. Provision of an airway with an endotracheal tube in place and use of positive pressure resuscitation
2. Intravenous or intracardiac administration of 1 ml of epinephrine 1:1000
3. Immediate intravenous infusion of 5% glucose and water or 2.5% sodium bicarbonate
4. Intravenous administration of 100 mg of hydrocortisone (Solu-Cortef) immediately and again within 15 to 20 minutes; this dosage may be repeated every four to six hours.

5. From 50 to 150 mg diphenhydramine HCl (Benadryl) added to the infusion

The vasopressor levarterenol (Levophed) may be utilized intravenously to maintain blood pressure. If cardiac arrest occurs, closed chest cardiac massage should be instituted, and a defibrillator should be used if indicated. The patient should be hospitalized and placed in an intensive care unit with close observation and supportive therapy continuing for at least 24 hours before the patient can be considered out of danger.

Sudden deafness

Sudden deafness is an acute emergency. The etiology may be viral, infectious, or sudden vascular occlusion of the acoustic artery. Occasionally, it may be drug induced. A patient who describes sudden hearing loss whether unilateral or bilateral should have immediate otologic consultation. He or she should be hospitalized, and immediate care should be initiated. The patient with sudden deafness should never be returned home without otologic consultation.

Facial paralysis

Sudden facial paralysis related to head trauma is a surgical emergency. This usually represents a temporal bone fracture, and once the patient's condition is stable, decompression of the facial nerve is required for prompt recovery. Acute facial paralysis such as Bell's palsy, although not considered an acute emergency, does require urgent care, and the patient should have proper referral and follow-up.

SUMMARY

In discussing ear, nose, and throat emergencies, some omissions have been made because of the limited space available in an all-inclusive text. I have described and discussed the causes and treatments of the more common emergencies found in otolaryngology. I refer the reader to the Additional Readings at the end of this chapter for excellent detail and discussion of almost any subject related to otolaryngology. Every emergency department should have a small reference library that includes a good text related to ear, nose, and throat and head and neck disease. I must reiterate that to adequately treat such emergencies requires proper illumination and good specific instruments. Remember that most examining procedures and treatment of ear, nose, and throat emergencies can cause pain; thus, the use of sedation and proper control of the patient are imperative. By judicious care, emergency department personnel can provide treatment for most patients having the more common forms of emergencies related to the ear, nose, and throat and head and neck systems. However, once the emergency situation is under control, never be afraid to seek consultation for a patient with an emergency that can better be cared for by a specialist.

Appendix
ANTIBIOTIC THERAPY

Widespread use of antibiotics has shown that, although useful agents, they are not the trouble-free wonder drugs they were once thought to be. Anaphylaxis, sensitization, and various toxicities must caution our use of them. "Rules" to be considered when using antibiotics in the ear, nose, and throat patient include the following:

1. Avoid prophylaxis in the uninfected patient unless manipulation will probably initiate infection, causing serious complications if left untreated.
2. Select the appropriate antibiotic, considering organism sensitivities, route of administration, underlying disease, and patient sensitivity.
3. Administer the agent in the proper manner.
4. Be alert to recognize undesirable antibiotic reactions.

5. Use as specific an agent for the infection as possible.
6. Recognize and avoid the development of bacterial resistance when it appears.

Identification of the offending organism should not be replaced with guesswork. However, when time does not permit a culture and sensitivity, it is helpful to be aware of the probable pathogens.

The lists below identify the microorganisms isolated in descending frequency according to location.[2] (Organisms, of course, vary from one locale to another and from one time to another. Therefore, the clinician should also consider experiences in his or her local community.)

Paranasal sinuses
1. *Diplococcus pneumoniae*
2. *Streptococcus pyogenes* (group A)
3. *Hemophilus influenzae*
4. *Staphylococcus,* coagulase positive
5. *Klebsiella* or other gram-negative bacilli
6. *Mucor*

Mouth
1. Herpes viruses
2. *Candida albicans*
3. *Fusobacterium fusiforme* (Vincent's infection)
4. *Bacteroides*
5. *Treponema pallidum*
6. *Actinomyces*

Throat
1. Respiratory viruses
2. *Streptococcus pyogenes* (group A)
3. *Neisseria meningitidis* or *gonorrhoeae*
4. *Fusobacterium fusiforme* (Vincent's infection)
5. *Candida albicans*
6. *Corynebacterium diphtheriae*
7. *Bordetella pertussis*

Ears
Auditory canal
1. *Staphylococcus,* coagulase positive
2. *Streptococcus pyogenes* (group A)
3. *Diplococcus pneumoniae*
4. *Pseudomonas aeruginosa*
5. *Hamophilus influenzae* (in children)
6. Fungi
Middle ear
1. *Diplococcus pneumoniae*

2. *Hemophilus influenzae* (in children)
3. *Streptococcus pyogenes* (group A)
4. *Staphylococcus,* coagulase positive
5. *Streptococcus anaerobius*
6. *Bacteroides*

Larynx, trachea, and bronchi
1. Respiratory viruses
2. *Diplococcus pneumoniae*
3. *Hemophilus influenzae*
4. *Streptococcus pyogenes* (group A)
5. *Corynebacterium diphtheriae*
6. *Staphylococcus,* coagulase positive

Sensitization to topical antibiotics is of special importance to the ear, nose, and throat patient in whom the drug so frequently is in contact with mucous membranes. Because the sensitivity reaction may be severe and also may preclude the later systemic use of this drug, topical antibiotics are selected that are usually nonsensitizing and seldom used systemically.[3]

Low sensitization
  Bacitracin, gram-positive cocci
  Gentamicin, gram-negative organisms
  Polymyxin B, gram-negative organisms
Moderate sensitization
  Chloramphenicol, broad spectrum including *Staphylococcus aureus, Escherichia coli, Hemophilus influenzae, Streptococcus hemolyticus, Salmonella*
Potent contact sensitizer
  Neomycin, mostly gram-negative organisms (excluding *Pseudomonas, Serratia*) and a few gram positives

When systemic antibiotics are employed, identification of the causative organism becomes even more important. Because of the dominance of the gram-positive organisms in the ear, nose, and throat patient, penicillin is frequently the drug of choice. However, this is modified to ampicillin in the case of the pediatric otitis media patient to cover the possibility of *H influenzae.* Erythromycin is a viable choice in the penicillin-allergic patient.[4] Refer to the *American Hospital Formulary Service* for complete prescribing information.

DECONGESTANTS

Decongestants are sympathomimetic amines that effect blood vessel constriction and thereby reduce nasal mucosal edema. They may be applied locally by means of drops, sprays, or with a tipped applicator (epinephrine, 1:1000 or 1:10,000; ephedrine, 1% to 3%; oxymetazoline, 0.05% [Afrin]; phenylephrine, 0.25% [Neo-Synephrine]) or systemically (pseudoephedrine, 60 mg t.i.d.; ephedrine, 30 mg t.i.d.; phenylpropanolamine, 25 mg q.i.d.).

Sympathomimetic drugs must be used with caution in the hypertensive patient as they are likely to further increase blood pressure.

The time-honored method for intranasal decongestion and anesthesia is to apply a "cocaine mud." This is prepared by saturating cocaine flakes with a 1:1000 solution of epinephrine and applying it directly to the sphenopalatine ganglion and anterior ethmoidal nerve.[9]

EAR, NOSE, AND THROAT STEROIDS

Corticosteroids are used both topically and systemically to reduce inflammation and allergic diseases at almost any location in the body. They do not alter the cause of the disease but reduce the reaction of the tissues. Bacterial, fungal, or viral infections may be masked or enhanced by corticosteroids. Such infections should be treated with an appropriate antiinfective agent before corticosteroid therapy is initiated. If infection of any kind develops during corticosteroid therapy, the drug should be discontinued.[7]

A wide array of otic and intranasal corticosteroid preparations are available. Only minor differences in activity have been noted.[7]

REFERENCES
1. Gleason, M. N., Gasselin, R., Hodge, L., and Smithe, J.: Clinical toxicology of commercial products, ed. 3, Baltimore, 1969, The Williams & Wilkins Co.
2. Aaron, H.: Medical letter on drugs and thera-

peutics, New Rochelle, New York, 1974, Medical Letter, Inc.
3. Mawson, S. R.: Diseases of the ear, ed. 3, Baltimore, 1974, The Williams & Wilkins Co.
4. American Hospital Formulary Service, Washington, D. C., 1976, American Society of Hospital Pharmacists, Inc.
5. Modell, W.: Drugs of choice, 1976-1977, St. Louis, 1976, The C. V. Msoby Co.

ADDITIONAL READINGS

Ballantyne, J., and Groves, J.: Diseases of the ear, nose and throat, ed. 3, vols. 1 to 4, Philadelphia, 1971, J. B. Lippincott Co.
Coates, G .M., and Schench, H. P.: Otolaryngology, vols. 1 to 5, New York, 1972, Harper & Row, Publishers.
Krupp, M., and Chatton, M. J.: Current diagnosis and treatment, Los Angeles, 1973, Lange Medical Publishers.
Lederer, F.: Diseases of the ear, nose and throat, ed. 9, Philadelphia, 1961, F. A. Davis Co.
The Merck manual, ed. 12, Rahway, N.J., 1972, Merck and Co., Inc.

CHAPTER 24

Chest trauma

Richard M. Peters, M.D.

In this era of trauma by speed, violence, and industrial accident, no injury is more life threatening than one to the chest.

Though compliant to a greater degree than other skeletal structures, the chest cage is easily penetrated by missile or knife. Severe deforming forces result in destruction of functional integrity of the chest wall and compromise air exchange. Crushing injuries caused by sudden deceleration or heavy weights running over or falling on the chest may injure the heart, great vessels, tracheobronchial tubes, or lungs.

TREATMENT

Three general types of chest trauma are seen in the emergency department:

1. Closed blunt trauma to the chest with disruption of the integrity of the chest cage, bony framework, and injury to the lungs, heart, and great vessels
2. Penetrating injuries to the chest without significant disruption of the chest cage and with injury to the heart, lungs, and great vessels
3. Penetrating injuries to the chest with loss of chest wall substance leaving open communication into the chest cavity; possible injury to intrathoracic organs

Since total disruption of function of the circulation or respiration is tolerated for less than five minutes and partial disruption compromises function of all other organs and systems, prompt resuscitation is the primary concern. The presence of chest injury can be promptly ascertained by inspection and, if available, brief history. To evaluate the patient properly, the following facts about the injury comprise the emergency data base:

1. The time between injury and arrival at the emergency department
2. The type of injury, if blunt trauma; the injuring instrument, if penetrating trauma
3. Whether the patient has been unconscious; if unconscious on arrival, has this been true from time of injury

Immediate evaluation should include the following:

1. Is the upper airway patent?
2. Is the minute ventilation adequate? Is the respiratory rate excessive? Is there evidence of retraction? Does the patient complain of dyspnea?
3. Is the patient in shock? Blood loss is more often the cause of cardiopulmonary failure in chest injuries than is respiratory difficulty.
4. In penetrating wounds what are sites of entry and exit?
5. In blunt trauma where are contusions

over the chest? Are there areas of paradoxical motion? On palpation is there evidence of subcutaneous emphysema?

The following simple measures are adequate for immediate assessment of chest injuries. The management starts with the examination.

1. If the airway is obstructed, clear it immediately. Usually an oral airway is adequate (see Chapter 26).
2. Insert two catheters in peripheral veins and infuse Ringer's lactate.

Most patients with chest injuries have significant blood loss. If the heart or great vessels are injured, blood loss may be massive. Time from injury and degree of shock are the best indices of the severity of blood loss. Massive intrathoracic bleeding usually results from penetrating injuries to the chest that lacerate the heart or great vessels. If the patient enters profound shock less than 30 minutes after injury and blood loss is massive, an immediate operation may be essential even in the emergency department. Many of these patients die before reaching the emergency department.

More commonly, bleeding occurs at a slower rate. Since transportation times usually are greater than 30 minutes, even patients without massive injury can be in severe shock when brought to the emergency department. The metabolic acidosis associated with hypovolemic shock stimulates the patient to hyperventilate. The apparent shortness of breath soon after injury is more often a result of this metabolic acidosis than a direct consequence of the chest injury.

The lung reserve is large. Therefore, prior to fluid resuscitation the circulation will fail before the blood accumulating in the chest can displace enough lung to cause respiratory insufficiency. *On admission the first priority for the patient in shock with chest injury is to infuse fluid.* Once fluid replacement is initiated, definitive treatment of the chest injury to restore normal respiratory mechanics should be started.[1]

Chest x-ray examination

Chest x-ray examination is an important part of diagnosis and control of therapy for chest injuries but is not the first essential. If the patient is in any distress, the resuscitative steps of blood infusion, insertion of chest tubes, and endotracheal intubation and ventilation should be instituted prior to obtaining a chest x-ray film. Since a supine chest film can be misleading because of superimposition of air, lung, and fluid, an upright chest film is usually essential. However, it is imperative that before sitting the patient up the attendants ascertain that there is no cervical spine injury.

The x-ray film is used not for diagnosis of fractured ribs, but to assess the state of lungs, heart, and mediastinum. One looks for evidence of pneumothorax, hemothorax, lung collapse or infiltrate, and widening of the mediastinum. The latter raises the likelihood of a ruptured thoracic aorta and signifies the need for immediate aortography. Mediastinal emphysema suggests the possibility of a ruptured bronchus.

Pneumothorax

The most common cause of acute distress is the accumulation of air in the pleural cavity, which collapses the lung. When the lung is torn, during inspiration air is pulled out of the lung into the pleural cavity as the tear is opened up because the pressure within the lung is higher than in the chest cavity. During expiration, when the pressure in the pleural cavity exceeds that within the lung, the laceration will be sealed because the change in pressure differential pushes the edges of the laceration together. Therefore, air escapes into the pleural cavity on each inspiration but cannot escape during expiration. The air trapped in the confined pleural cavity fills the cavity and collapses the lung.

To correct this problem it is urgent to insert a closed chest drainage catheter and attach it to a chest drainage bottle. This prevents air from being sucked into the chest cavity through the chest wall during inspiration, but allows air to escape from the pleural cavity through the chest wall during times that pleural pressure exceeds atmospheric pressure.

Spontaneous pneumothorax

Pneumothorax can occur in the absence of injury of any kind. It results from rupture of a bleb or, when the patient is being ventilated with a respirator, rupture of alveoli. Rupture of blebs can occur in two major groups of patients: (1) those with chronic obstructive airway disease and bullous cysts and (2) otherwise normal young adults, 16 to 25 years old, who have small apical blebs that rupture spontaneously. Immediately after rupture the patient complains of acute pain in the chest, usually of pleuritic nature, although it may mimic the pain of coronary insufficiency. Patients with chronic obstructive pulmonary disease develop acute dyspnea. The younger patients, after a brief period of acute pain, may experience only dyspnea on exertion. Diagnosis depends on a good chest x-ray film. Treatment is insertion of a chest tube to reexpand the lung. Many of the patients have a previous history of such difficulty, and if the emergency department personnel will listen to the patient's complaint, they will usually be given the diagnosis by such patients.

Hemothorax

Blunt chest injury that fractures ribs usually results in intrathoracic bleeding. Penetrating injuries always result in some intrathoracic bleeding. Massive bleeding may occur from injuries to major vessels or the heart. The lungs are usually not a major source of bleeding since pressure in the pulmonary vessels is low. An immediate diagnostic and therapeutic step for the treatment of hemothorax is the insertion of a closed drainage catheter to evacuate the blood. The evacuation of blood serves to improve breathing mechanics and helps in the assessment of proper treatment. The amount that drains immediately from the chest bottle should be recorded and the additional drainage measured every 15 to 30 minutes. The significance of the amount of blood removed on insertion of the tube is determined by the time since injury. If 1,500 or more ml is drained and time since injury is less than 30 minutes, emergent thoracotomy is indicated. Less than this requires observation of the response to resuscitation and the amount of continued bleeding.[2]

A general guideline to the significance of blood loss through a closed chest drainage system is as follows: blood loss in excess of 200 ml per hour that shows little evidence of decreasing is a sign that urgent thoracotomy is required; blood loss of over 500 ml per hour after the first blood is evacuated indicates the need for *emergent exploration*. A total blood loss into the chest over a two-hour period greater than 4 liters usually indicates the need for urgent thoracotomy.

It is imperative to remember that chest drainage tubes, like all drainage tubes, can become blocked by clots. Therefore, if the patient requires more blood and fluids than is consistent with measured drainage, an immediate chest film should be taken to see if blood is accumulating in the chest. Also, careful assessment should be made to ascertain if there is another source of blood loss. Frequently, with chest injuries there is an associated injury to the spleen or liver. Positive findings in either case require urgent operation to control bleeding and to evacuate blood.

Open sucking chest wound

An uncommon civilian injury is one in which a significant hole is created in the chest wall so that air is sucked in and blown out of the chest during each breath. At first thought, it might seem that a hole in one chest cavity would not seriously compromise breathing since the patient can survive on only one lung. However, the mediastinum is so mobile that injury to one side affects ventilation of both lungs (Fig. 24-1). If any air is to be drawn through the trachea into the lungs, not just through the hole in the chest, the hole in the chest cage must be small enough that there is some resistance to air flow through it. If not, air will come in through the hole in the chest cage only and none will come in through the trachea.[3]

In an emergency, an open sucking chest wound should be immediately sealed with a dressing. Since most open chest wounds also result in injury to the lung, a closed chest drainage catheter should also be inserted to allow air and fluid to escape as in closed chest injuries. Patients with open chest wounds that have been sealed in the field are often in acute respiratory distress when first seen. This may be caused by a tension pneumothorax created by the dressing, which converts the open injury to a closed chest injury. In these cases the respiratory distress can be quickly relieved by briefly removing the chest dressing to decompress the tension.

The best treatment for pneumothorax in

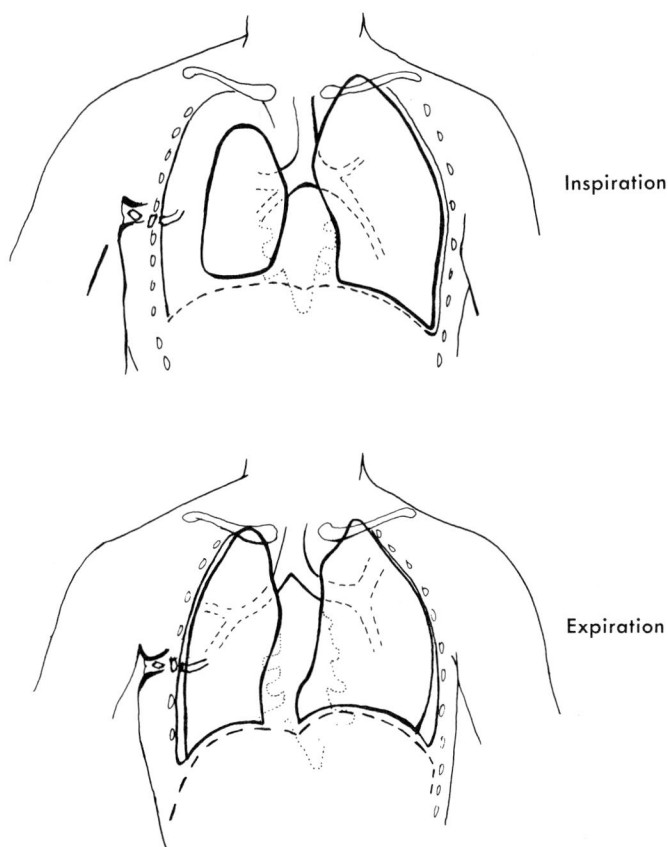

Fig. 24-1. During inspiration air comes in through the hole in the chest wall. During expiration it is partially pushed out. The mediastinum shifts away from the injured side during expiration and toward it during inspiration. The movement of air through the hole requires muscular effort but does not provide any exchange of gas with the blood.

patients with open chest wounds is intubation and continuous positive pressure breathing until the chest wall defect can be closed temporarily or repaired. A chest tube must be inserted to assure expansion of the lung if the wound is surgically sealed or sealed with a dressing.

Paradoxical motion of the chest cage—flail chest

A common type of injury following high-speed deceleration accidents is disruption of the chest cage as a result of blunt trauma. Blunt trauma may fracture a number of adjacent ribs in more than one place. These fractures disrupt the structural integrity of the chest cage so that the ribs no longer provide rigid support. Since inspiration of air into the lungs is accomplished by lowering the intrapleural pressure below atmospheric pressure, during inspiration the disrupted portion of the rib cage will be pushed in by the higher atmospheric pressure. During expiration the disrupted areas will be pushed out when the pleural pressure rises to near or above atmospheric pressure. The chest cage over th region of fractures moves in the wrong, or "paradoxical," direction—in during inspiration, out during expiration. This type of abnormal motion has also been named flail chest. Moving a portion of chest wall in a paradoxical manner makes ventilation of the lungs inefficient and, therefore, increases the effort required to breathe (Fig. 24-2).

Paradoxical respiration may be mild immediately after injury, but over the hours following injury the paradoxical motion increases. This increase results because the lungs become stiffer from the edema that accumulates in the contused portion, and the airway resistance rises due to failure to cough up blood and secretions. To ventilate the mechanically deranged lungs requires greater subatmospheric pleural pressures during inspiration, thus exaggerating the amount of chest motion.

The treatment of the patient with flail chest is to intubate and ventilate with a volume ventilator. Such patients have a more benign course if they are placed on a respirator early, before they become fatigued and the abnormal motion of the chest cage further injures the lung. For this reason it is important to predict immediately which patients are likely to have

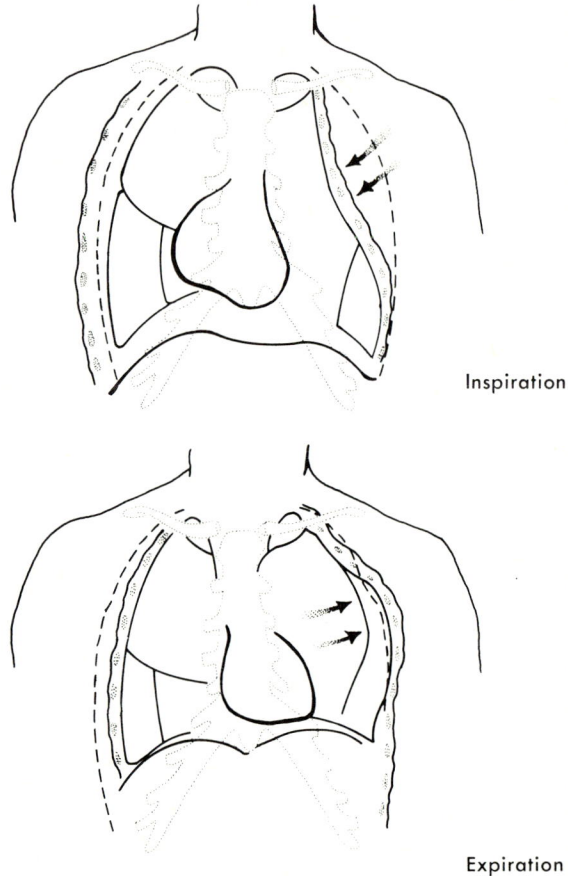

Inspiration

Expiration

Fig. 24-2. With a closed chest injury the crushed portion of the chest wall moves in during inspiration and results in shift of the mediastinum away from the side of injury. During expiration the injured chest wall moves out and the mediastinum shifts toward the injured side. This "flailing" of the fractured ribs is very painful and results in wasted muscular effort. The paradoxical motion becomes more marked when the lungs become stiff from the associated contusion.

significant paradox as a result of the late effects of the injury on lung function. A prediction can be made by observing the area of disrupted chest wall while having the patient cough or breathe deeply to exaggerate the swings in pleural pressure. In the unconscious patient, manual obstruction of the airway for one or two respiratory cycles will allow assessment of the seriousness of paradoxical motion. Whether or not paradoxical motion is apparent during quiet breathing, if a patient has significant paradoxical respiration with coughing or deep breathing, early intubation and continuous positive pressure ventilation are indicated.

Recent studies have shown that all patients with flail chests do not need respirator support if pain is controlled and pulmonary function maintained.[4,5] It is better in the emergency treatment to err in the direction of ventilating a patient who may not require it than not to ventilate a patient who needs support. Intermittent mandatory ventilation may be superior to continuous mandatory ventilation. If the arterial Po$_2$ is low, *first be certain the patient's blood volume is restored and cardiac output adequate.* If this has been achieved, continuous positive airway pressure, 5 cm H$_2$O, is indicated.

Ruptured bronchus

Blunt chest trauma can cause a blowout of one of the major bronchi or the trachea. These injuries usually result from accidents in which the upper chest is crushed momentarily by a strong force; for example, a car wheel running over a child's chest. These patients have acute respiratory difficulty, often massive subcutaneous emphysema, and pneumothorax. Their respiratory distress is not relieved by insertion of a chest tube or by positive pressure ventilation. Their only hope is that the admitting physician will be aware of this type of injury so that immediate evaluation and surgical repair can be undertaken.

These patients usually have very large leaks after the chest tube is inserted, so that a lot of air bubbles out through the tube on each breath. The leak is markedly increased by positive pressure ventilation, and there is no relief of the dyspnea.

These patients should be intubated with an endotracheal tube that is long enough to be inserted into one or the other mainstem bronchus. They usually require immediate operative repair of the lesion. If the patient's condition permits, bronchoscopy is indicated to assess the nature of the lesion.

Pericardial tamponade

When there is bleeding into the closed pericardial sac, the blood prevents filling of the heart and can lead to acute cardiac insufficiency. *After resuscitation from blood loss,* these patients have a low blood pressure, fast pulse, poor peripheral perfusion, evidence of low cardiac output, and a high venous pressure. In any patient with a penetrating injury to the chest or injury to the sternum, the index of suspicion concerning pericardial tamponade should be high.

If there is reason to suspect that hypotension and low cardiac output are caused by pericardial tamponade, the patient should have pericardiocentesis immediately to aspirate blood from the pericardial sac. At the same time, the patient should be prepared to be moved to the operating room for definitive operative treatment for the tamponade.

To perform a pericardiocentesis, a 14- to 16-gauge spinal (3 in) needle and a 20 to 30 ml syringe with stopcock are most suitable. The limb leads of an ECG should be attached to the patient, and the chest lead to the aspirating needle. (All emergency departments should have a short, sterile wire with alligator clips at each end for this purpose.) The needle is inserted slightly to the left of the xiphoid process at an angle of 45 degrees to the horizontal plane

Fig. 24-3. Pericardiocentesis.

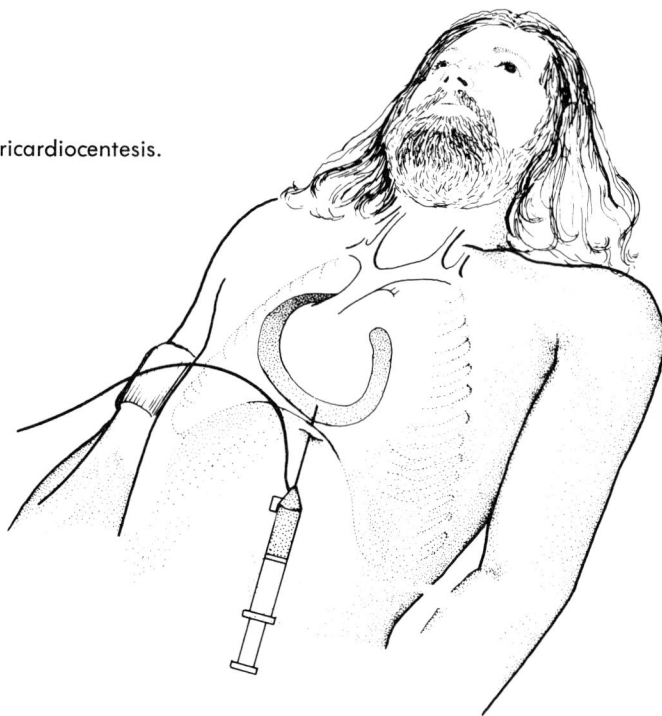

(Fig. 24-3). It is directed toward the right sternoclavicular joint. The needle usually needs to be inserted 4 to 8 cm. If there is an injury current recorded on the ECG (the voltage goes very high), the needle has made contact with the heart and should be withdrawn while continuously aspirating. Removal of as little as 20 ml may make a critical difference to the patient.

Most thoracic surgeons now consider the presence of pericardial blood to be a reason for immediate exploratory thoracotomy.[6]

Cardiac contusion

Patients who suffer direct trauma to the sternum may suffer a contusion of the myocardium. The manifestations may be similar to those of a coronary occlusion. Thus these patients have pain, conduction defects, and alterations in the electrocardiogram either immediately or later when the contussion causes the maximum degree of edema. The precautions taken for patients with coronary occlusion and an unstable conducting system apply to these patients also. These consist of continuous monitoring of ECG and introduction of a Swan-Ganz catheter to monitor wedge pressure. Hypovolemia is just as dangerous as hypervolemia in these patients. In the context of this discussion it is important to remember that a differential diagnosis may need to be made between a coronary occlusion and a contusion. Coronary occlusion can be the cause of a highway accident or result from the stress of the injuries.

Ruptured diaphragm

Rupture of the diaphragm occasionally results from crushing chest injuries. The common mechanism is a compressing force on the abdomen, such as a steering wheel or a high-riding seat belt driven into the abdomen. The patient may, at first, be relatively asymptomatic. When the stomach or bowel becomes distended, the patient may develop acute respiratory distress. The diagnosis is usually easily made if the physician thinks of this injury. Immediate treatment is to insert a nasogastric tube to decompress the distended stomach. The patient should have prompt repair. If respiratory distress is not manifest, repair may be postponed until resuscitation is complete.

Simple rib fractures

Simple fractures of the rib are common. They may follow a fall, severe exertion, or a severe cough. They are best diagnosed by physical examination. Gentle compression with both hands placed on the lateral surface of each side of the chest and pressure on the sternum are the first steps. If these maneuvers cause pain in a particular area, point tenderness over this area is evidence of fracture. Fractures are best treated by controlling pain either with intercostal nerve blocks or narcotics and encouraging the patient to cough, take deep breaths, and exercise the shoulder muscles. Strapping with adhesive tape or the use of a binder is contraindicated.

Elderly patients with chronic obstructive lung disease are at great risk of developing pneumonia and respiratory insufficiency following simple rib fractures. They may require hospital admission for such injuries.

Summary

The majority of patients with blunt or penetrating injury of the chest cage do not require open thoracotomy. They can be effectively treated by replacing lost blood, draining the pleural cavity with closed chest drainage, and ventilation with a positive pressure ventilator, if required.

A summary of procedures for handling chest trauma in the emergency department appears below.

CLOSED CHEST DRAINAGE

Closed chest drainage is a simple mechanical system designed to evacuate fluid and air from the chest cavities without creating an open sucking wound. It is highly effective when properly managed and ineffective to extremely dangerous when improperly managed. *Only trained, authorized individuals should be allowed to adjust or change the system in any way. This includes transporting such patients.*

The basic principles are to insert a catheter through the chest cage into the pleural cavity and connect it to the closed chest drainage system.

Insertion of chest drainage catheter

Insertion of a chest drainage catheter can be life saving, but if improperly done, it will be life threatening. The site chosen for introduction should be injected with lidocaine 1% and the anesthesia carried down to the pleura. The needle used for anesthesia or a thoracocentesis needle should be passed through the pleura; if air can be freely withdrawn, indicating that a pneumothorax is present, a catheter can be blindly inserted. The catheter can be inserted by developing a track with a hemostat and pushing the catheter in through the established track or by using a trocar. Disposable trocars, that fit in plastic thoracostomy tubes, are available. The catheter for an adult should be at least a No. 24 French; in children the catheter should be as large as feasible to insert between the ribs.

If no free air or fluid is aspirated, the catheter should not be introduced, since it may enter the lung and cause death from air embolus. Some experts prefer that the finger be introduced through the chest wall incision before inserting the chest tube to be certain the pleural space is free. I do not think this is usually necessary, but if no air or fluid can be withdrawn from the precise spot where the tube is to be inserted, it is essential. *Blind introduction of a chest catheter without prior aspiration of fluid or air or palpation to ascertain that the lung is not adherent to the pleura is very dangerous.*

Preferred drainage sites for pneumothorax are the second anterior interspace

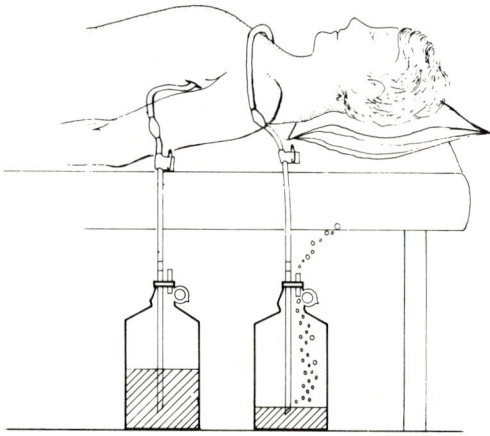

Fig. 24-4. The chest bottle acts as a one-way valve allowing air to bubble out of the vent tube as shown in the bottle on the right but preventing air entering through the tube because of the water trap. The bottle on the right has the proper amount of fluid. The tube is placed in the second anterior interspace to evacuate air. The tube on the left has drained blood from the posterior chest cavity. This bottle should be emptied of blood and refilled with enough fluid to just cover the tube going to the bottom of the bottle with 1 cm of water.

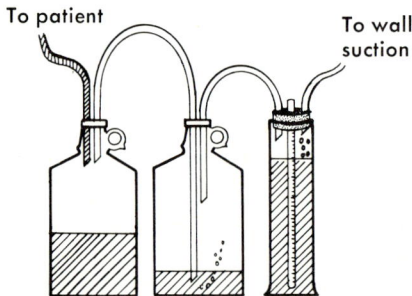

Fig. 24-5. The bottle on the left acts as a reservoir to store drained blood or fluid. The center bottle acts as the one-way valve as shown in Fig. 24-4. The bottle on the right is a suction pressure regulator. If suction pressure exceeds the height of column of water in the middle tube, air will bubble in through this tube. Likewise, if the suction should malfunction when intrapleural pressure exceeds this pressure, air or fluid can escape from the chest cage.

in the midclavicular line in the patient in acute distress; in less emergent situations and in small infants, we prefer the third or fourth interspace in the midaxillary line. The lateral scar is not visible, while a scar in the second anterior interspace is. In infants the apex of the chest is so small that catheters placed in the second anterior interspace do not function well.

For drainage of blood the fifth or sixth interspace in the posterior axillary line is the site of choice. If drainage is attempted lower than the sixth interspace there is great risk of perforating the diaphragm, since it frequently is at this level during quiet breathing, even in healthy subjects.

The closed chest drainage system

The closed chest drainage system consists of a bottle with two tubes passing through the cap. One of these tubes just passes through the cap; the other tube extends to the bottom of the bottle. This long tube is the one connected to the catheter inserted in the patient's chest. Approximately 1 cm of water should be added covering the tube that extends to the bottom of the bottle (Fig. 24-4).

Some institutions use a two-bottle system. In this system there is a second bottle between the patient and the bottle described above. This bottle has two short tubes going through its cap. One of these openings is attached to a tube that, in turn, is attached to the catheter in the patient's chest. The other end is attached to the long tube in the chest drainage bottle described above (Fig. 24-5). This system catches fluid draining from the chest in the first bottle, thereby preventing increasing amounts of fluid in the closed drainage bottle from raising the pressure necessary to force air out of the chest cavity. The complexity of this system leads to more errors and makes moving the patient more difficult. (There are commercial plastic containers that incorporate both these bottles in one molded unit. Unfortunately, they are expensive, and each type requires complete familiarity with its operation.)

When the chest bottle is connected to an intrapleural catheter and the bottle is placed below the level of the patient's chest, air can escape from the chest whenever intrapleural pressure exceeds atmospheric pressure plus the pressure necessary to displace the water covering the end of the chest tube (1 cm of water in a properly set up chest bottle). To pull air into the chest requires a subatmospheric pressure equal to the distance from the water in the chest bottle to the patient's chest. If the bottle is placed on the floor, this will be 80 to 100 cm of water, a pressure that exceeds the subatmospheric pressure an individual can create in the pleural cavity.

If the bottle is put in the patient's bed and maintained upright, a negative pressure equal to the height of the bottle will be required to pull air or fluid into the patient's chest. Except on deep breathing, pressures rarely exceed this level, but a deep inspiration prior to a cough will provide pressure in excess of that needed to pull air into the chest. For these reasons, bottles should always be 50 cm or more below the patient's back (see below for the single exception).

A common error in setting up chest drainage is to put too much sterile fluid in the chest drainage bottle. This requires the patient to create a positive pressure greater than the height of water in the bottle before air can escape (Fig. 24-4). In the single-bottle system, if both fluid and air are draining from the patient's chest, the bottle must be *emptied of the drainage fluid and the fluid replaced with the proper amount of sterile fluid whenever more than 5 cm of fluid accumulates in the bottle.*

Removal of air from chest cavity

For air to be removed from the chest cavity, the pressure within the chest must exceed atmospheric pressure plus a pressure equal to the distance between the bottom of the tube extending to the bottom of the bottle and the water level in the bottle.

Normally, during both inspiration and expiration, intrapleural pressure is subatmospheric when the patient is at rest. To raise the pressure above atmospheric, the patient must cough, strain, or use a blow bottle. Therefore, it is imperative to encourage the patient to be active so that intraplural pressure will be raised above atmospheric pressure at frequent intervals.

If the leak of air is large, the chest bottle may be connected to suction. This acts to keep the pressure in the bottle below atmospheric pressure so that air is continuously pushed out of the chest. Excessive suction can be harmful by sucking lung tissue against the catheter and occluding the catheter, by shifting the mediastinum in a patient with an inexpansible lung, and in case of suction failure, by blocking the outlet of the chest bottle. For these reasons a three-hole bottle is used as a pressure regulator (Fig. 24-5). If suction pressure exceeds the height of the water column in this bottle, air will bubble in through the open tube, thus limiting suction pressure. Likewise, if intrathoracic pressure exceeds the level in the regulator bottle, air will bubble out from the patient. The suction must be set high enough so that some air bubbles through the vent tube at all times; otherwise, the suction is less than that set on the regulator.

There are two major pitfalls to the use of this type regulator: the water in the bottle evaporates from air bubbling through it, and therefore the level must be checked at least every four hours to make sure suction is not decreasing; and the amount of suction (cm of water) applied to the regulator bottle is not the same as the amount of pressure (cm of water) at the end of the catheter in the chest. The resistance to flow through the narrow tubing connecting the chest bottle to the patient and suction apparatus is significant; consequently, there is a pressure drop down the tube. The closer the regulator bottle is to the chest bottle, the better. If the leak is large, resulting in a high flow rate, there will be a larger pressure drop. Therefore the pressure must be set at a higher level than is required within the chest, usually a minimum of 20 cm H_2O for a small leak and up to 40 cm or more for large leaks.

Pneumothorax and respirator

A common complication of continuous positive pressure ventilation is rupture of the lung. The development of such a bronchopleural fistula and pneumothorax in these patients with limited respiratory reserve can lead to acute decompensation and death. When such a complication occurs, these patients need immediate insertion of a large chest drainage catheter (No. 30 French or larger) connected to closed chest drainage.

In my opinion these patients are usually better treated without suction unless the leak of air from the lung is large. During the inspiratory cycle the respirator creates a positive intrapleural pressure that pushes air out of the pleural cavity during each cycle. If all the air cannot escape during inspiration with each cycle with one chest tube in place, a better alternative than suction is to place a second chest tube. The principle is that the cross-sectional area of the drain tubes should be large enough so that all the air is expelled during each inspiratory cycle when the pleural pressure exceeds the atmospheric pressure.

Evacuation of intrathoracic fluid

Pleural fluid that fills a chest tube provides a siphon to remove fluid from the chest. The sucking force exerted by the siphon is equal to the vertical distance from the chest bottle to the patient's chest. If the bottle is on the floor, this force is equivalent to 100 cm of water. In a patient whose lung has been totally collapsed for a number of days or weeks by blood or pleural fluid, it is dangerous to have the fluid removed in a few minutes because the lung will be unable to expand immediately to fill the space occupied by the blood or fluid. If the 100 cm suction is applied by the siphon, fluid will be removed very rapidly and the mediastinum will shift, causing cough, pain, and syncope. Therefore, in such patients the drainage bottle should not be placed on the floor but should be kept near the level of the patient to lessen the suction until the lung can expand. Expansion can usually be accomplished in a few hours unless the lung is entrapped in a pleural scar.

When draining blood following acute hemorrhage, no such precautions are required since prompt expansion of the lung can be expected.

SUMMARY
Immediate treatment

1. Ascertain that the upper airway is clear. If respiratory distress is severe despite a clear airway, provide positive pressure ventilation. Prepare to intubate the patient. Proceed immediately to evaluate the need for insertion of a chest tube (see Emergency treatment—chest tubes).

2. Institute procedure for hypovolemic shock therapy.

3. Ascertain the time from injury to admission. If less than 30 minutes and the patient is in profound shock, immediate thoracotomy may be necessary (see below).

Emergency diagnostic appraisal

1. Identify sites of entry and exit of penetrating injuries. Does the route of injuring agent suggest injury to the heart, great vessels, diaphragms, or esophagus?

2. Is there a sucking chest wound? Is it so large that air enters and exits freely? If so, seal it with a dressing, intubate the patient, and insert a chest tube on the side of injury.

3. Is there subcutaneous emphysema? If there is evidence of chest wall injury and the patient can cooperate, Valsalva's maneuver or cough may produce palpable subcutaneous emphysema that was not palpable prior to coughing.

4. Is there significant paradoxical movement of the chest cage? If paradoxical motion is not apparent during quiet breathing, ask the patient to take a deep breath to exaggerate motion.

5. Palpate the sternum gently to ascertain if there is abnormal motion or misalignment.

6. If none of the above are present, gently compress the sternum to see if this causes pain. Then place one hand on each side of the lower rib cage and compress gently. If pain is present, palpate the region of pain to elicit point tenderness. If point tenderness is present, rib fractures are present.

Emergency treatment—chest tubes

Do not insert chest tubes unless a thoracocentesis at the site proposed for insertion produces free air, fluid, or blood. Patients can be killed if a chest tube is inserted into the lung.

1. If subcutaneous emphysema is present, do a *thoracocentesis* in the second anterior interspace on the side or sides of the injury. *If, and only if, free air is aspirated,* insert a chest tube and connect it to water seal drainage. If no fluid or air is obtained on chest tap with evident subcutaneous emphysema or serious blood loss, obtain a stat chest film to ascertain if a pneumothorax or hemothorax is present or if the pleural cavity has been obliterated by previous pleurisy.

2. If there is evidence of clinically significant hemorrhage or significant amounts of blood coming out of the anterior chest tube, a thoracocentesis should be done in the fifth to sixth interspace in the posterior axillary line. If blood is obtained, insert another chest tube at this site.

3. If insertion of chest tubes does not relieve dyspnea, the patient should be intubated and placed on a volume-cycled respirator.

Chest x-ray examination

A chest x-ray examination should be obtained as soon as possible consistent with the need to resuscitate the patient. If there is no suspicion of a cervical spine injury, get an *upright* film. Check the following on the chest film:

1. Is the mediastinum widened; rupture of aorta?

2. Is there a pneumothorax or hemothorax? Have chest tubes been inserted? Are they positioned well?

3. In missile injuries what is the course of the missile?

4. Did the missile pass through the mediastinum or diaphragms? If so, what organs were in its course?

5. Is there evidence of the bowel or liver in the chest; ruptured diaphragms?

Ruptured bronchus

If insertion of a chest tube to evacuate air results in continued bubbling of air from the tube and does not relieve the patient's respiratory distress, a ruptured bronchus is likely. *The patient should be intubated with an endotracheal tube long enough to be placed in one or the other main-stem bronchus.* Bronchoscopy is indicated as soon as feasible, preferably with a fiberoptic scope through the endotracheal tube. These patients are among the most difficult to handle and usually require urgent operation.

Pericardial tamponade

Suspicion should be aroused if injury to the heart is likely, if the venous pressure is high with low systemic pressure, or if the patient has paradoxical pulse. If these findings suggest that circulatory insufficiency is the result of pericardial tamponade, a pericardiocentesis is mandatory.

1. Attach an ECG chest lead to a 14- to 16-gauge needle. Insert the needle through the skin over the left xiphocostal notch and direct it about ten degrees toward the right and at 30 to 45 degrees to the horizontal (Fig. 24-3).

2. Introduce the needle until the diaphragmatic pericardium is perforated. If the injury current occurs in the ECG lead, withdraw the needle until the injury current disappears. Blood can either be aspirated with the needle or a plastic catheter can be passed through the needle and left in place for continuous aspiration.

3. The patient with pericardial tamponade should be prepared for immediate surgery.

Thoracotomy

Judgment about the need for thoracotomy requires skill and experience. The majority of patients will be definitively treated by chest tube drainage, blood replacement, and if the chest cage is disrupted, respirator support.

The indications for emergency thoracotomy can be summarized as follows:

1. Continued or recurrent hemorrhage —blood loss in excess of 200 ml per hour that shows little evidence of decreasing: urgent exploration is required. Blood loss at a rate of over 500 ml per hour after the first blood is evacuated: *emergent exploration.* Total blood loss into the chest within two hours greater than 4 liters: thoracotomy probably required.

2. Widened mediastinum is an urgent indication for aortography. If disruption of the aorta is present, an urgent thoracotomy is needed to determine whether the thoracic aorta or branches are ruptured.

3. Pericardial tamponade requires an urgent thoracotomy.

4. A ruptured trachea or bronchus requires emergent or urgent thoracotomy, depending on the degree of respiratory distress.

5. A ruptured diaphragm requires urgent thoracotomy.

6. Thoracoabdominal wounds require urgent thoracoabdominal exploration.

7. Severe disruption of the chest cage or displaced sternal fractures can be helped by early operative repair of the crest cage.[7]

REFERENCES

1. Hughes, R. K.: Thoracic trauma: Collective reviews, Ann. Thorac. Surg. **1**:788, 1965.
2. Beall, A. C., Crawford, H. W., and DeBakey, M. E.: Considerations in the management of acute traumatic hemothorax, J. Thorac. Cardiovasc. Surg. **52**:351-357, 1966.
3. McNamara, J. J., Messersmith, J. K., Dunn, R. A., Molot, M. D., and Stremple, J. F.: Thoracic injuries in combat casualties in Vietnam, Ann. Thorac. Surg. **10**:389-401, 1970.
4. Shackford, S. R., Smith, D. E., Zarins, C. K., Rice, C. L., and Virgilio, R. W.: The management of flail chest. A comparison of ventilatory and nonventilatory treatment, Am. J. Surg. **132**(6):759-762, 1976.
5. Lewis, F., Jr., Thomas, A. N., and Schlobohm, R. M.: Control of respiratory therapy in flail chest, Ann. Thorac. Surg. **20**:170-176, 1975.
6. Beall, A. C., Gasior, R. M., and Bricker, D. L.: Gunshot wounds of the heart, Ann. Thorac. Surg. **11**:524-531, 1971.
7. Richardson, J. D., Grover, F. L., and Trinkle, J. K.: Early operative management of isolated sternal fractures, J. Trauma **15**:156-162, 1975.

CHAPTER **25**

Spinal disease

Randall W. Smith, M.D.

ACUTE SPINAL INJURY

The emergency department care of spinal injury is a combination of early recognition and appropriate modification of usual emergency department procedure in order to avoid further injury to the patient. "First, do no harm" has been suggested as a primary tenet for physicians, and nowhere is this more pertinent than in the care of those with spinal injury. The harm to be done in this kind of injury is to fail to appreciate that the injury has occurred or to mismanage the patient in the emergency department so as to increase the injury.

The problem in spinal trauma is that the spine may be fractured and because of that fracture may be unstable or movable to such an extent that the spinal cord and spinal nerves may be crushed. Even if the cord or nerves were damaged at the time the fracture occurred, their potential for recovery can be destroyed forever if the fracture site is handled inappropriately. It is therefore the task of emergency department personnel to recognize the possibility of spinal injury and to take action to protect the potentially vulnerable spinal cord and nerves. This protective care begins when the patient enters the emergency department.

Assessment

Arrival. Arrival can be the most crucial few minutes in the total care of the spine-injured patient. It is likely that ambulance attendants, paramedics, police, or firemen will alert emergency department personnel to the fact that the patient is complaining of neck or back pain following trauma. Once alerted, personnel must make the immediate decision regarding transfer of the patient from stretcher to emergency department gurney. This issue is simply resolved. Patients complaining of back pain can always be transferred by the "three-person lift" technique (Fig. 25-1). Those complaining of neck pain need additional attention. If the patient arrives on any of a variety of "scoop" or "break-away" stretchers, these can be placed on the gurney and removed while the head is held immobile. If, however, the patient arrives on the usual ambulance stretcher, movement of the patient should not occur until a portable lateral cross-table cervical spine radiograph is obtained. (During the wait for the radiology technician, vital signs should be determined and initial resuscitation begun.) For this neck film a cervical halter should be placed beneath the chin and occiput (Fig. 25-2) and traction gently

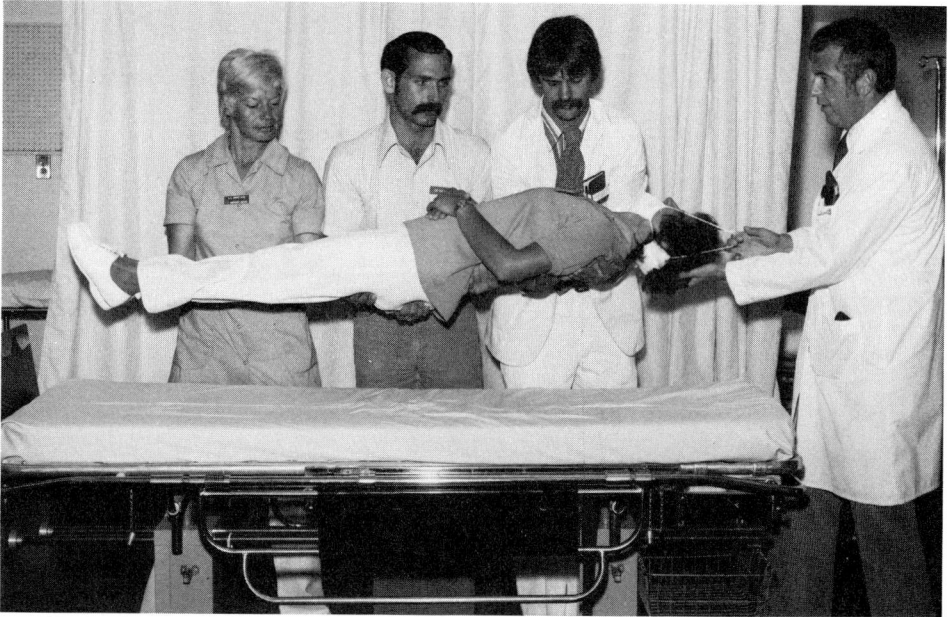

Fig. 25-1. Three-man lift technique including cervical support for movement of patients with suspected spinal fractures. For patients with thoracic or lumbar fracture, head support and traction are optional. Note position of each person's hands in relation to an even support of body weight and alignment of spine.

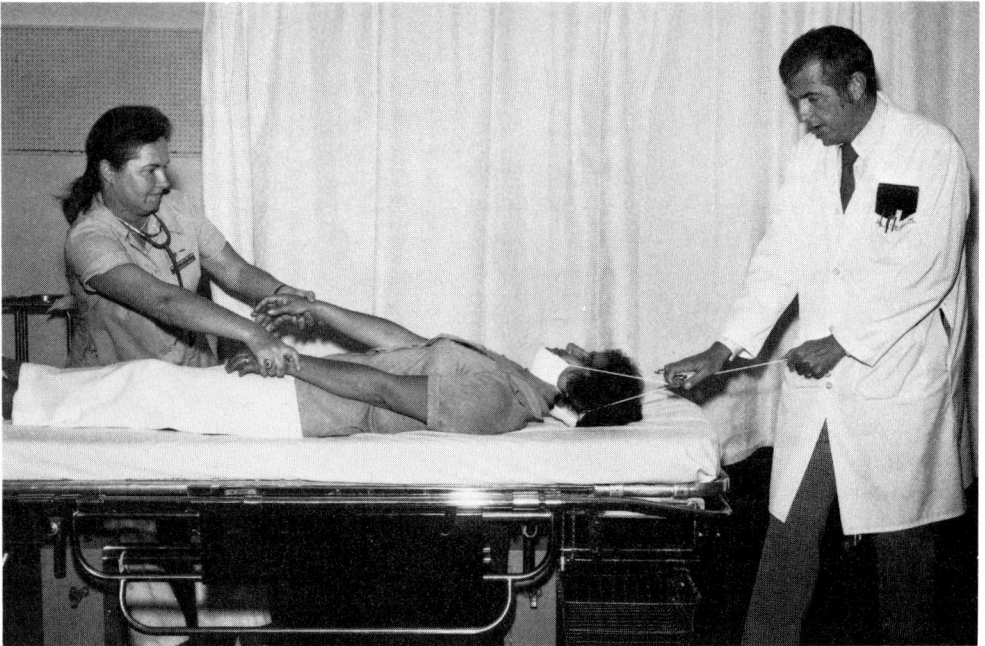

Fig. 25-2. Method of achieving adequate radiographic visualization of cervical spine. Note that downward pull on arms depresses shoulders so that neck, held stable by traction device, can be easily photographed using portable x-ray equipment.

applied while the patient's wrists are grasped and pulled toward the foot of the stretcher. This maneuver helps assure visualization of the entire cervical spine, a prerequisite in the evaluation of traumatic neck injury. If the films show normal alignment of all seven cervical vertebrae, then transfer to the emergency department gurney using the three-person technique with halter traction (Fig. 25-1) is safe.

If a fracture or misalignment of the cervical spine is detected on the initial film, then transfer to emergency department gurney or special fracture frame should occur under the guidance of those trained to safely accomplish this maneuver (neurologic or orthopedic surgeons, some emergency department physicians). If such talent is not available, then no transfer should occur, a 10-pound weight should be tied to the halter for traction and immobilization, and further assessment of the patient carried out on the ambulance stretcher. Once appropriate evaluation has occurred and the patient has stabilized, transfer to another facility should be accomplished on the same ambulance stretcher with the traction device in place and the head flanked by sandbags or rolled towels appropriately taped into position (Fig. 25-3).

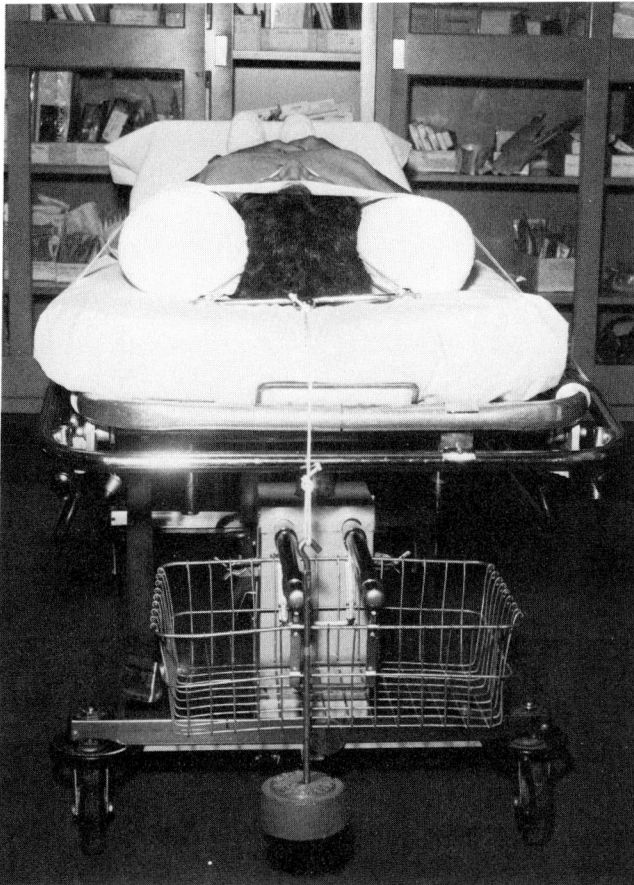

Fig. 25-3. Immobilization technique for patient transfer. Note rolled towels placed on either side of head to prevent neck from being turned. Note also that 2-inch tape is placed across forehead and rolls and secured to sides of stretcher to prevent lifting of head and to hold towels in place. Halter traction device is also pictured with weight suspended over edge of stretcher. The traction device is not mandatory for patient transfer.

History. A few simple rules serve well here. The most striking history is a total lack of one; that is, the patient is noncommunicative. When the traumatized patient is comatose it must be presumed that spinal injury is present until proven otherwise. The neck is most crucial here since subsequent evaluation of the patient's coma may well require the neck to be moved (emesis evacuation, airway manipulation, etc.). That is the reason for rule 1: *traumatized patients unable to deny neck pain need an immediate lateral cervical spine radiograph.* If the spine is well aligned (all seven vertebrae!) then the neck is discounted as a site of pathology in these severely ill comatose patients. Thoracic and lumbar radiographs should be taken some time in the care of these patients, but since the supine position is adequate immobilization of these areas, the films only need to be taken prior to assuming the sitting position. Thus, these films are not pertinent to emergency department activity.

One dilemma that frequently presents itself is "If a comatose patient arrives with an inadequate airway or poor respiratory drive, should intubation be accomplished prior to cervical spine evaluation for fracture? The concern, of course, is that head and neck movement attendant upon intubation may cause inappropriate motion of a fractured spine. The life-threatening nature of respiratory embarrassment cannot be forgotten, however, which is the reason for rule 2: *when respiratory inadequacy is reflected by cyanosis* (or arterial Po_2 less than 60 mm Hg) *it must be resolved immediately regardless of neck injury.* Mask oxygen should be applied but is frequently not successful in posttraumatic cyanosis. Certain maneuvers result in less neck motion (pharyngeal or nasopharyngeal airway placement plus AMBU bag assistance, "blind" nasotracheal intubation) but may be unsuccessful or ineffective. Cyanosis must be resolved.

The hyperextension of the upper cervical spine that occurs in standard endotracheal intubation using a laryngoscope is unlikely to result in further injury to the spine or spinal cord in most types of neck fractures. This type of intubation must be accomplished if all else fails to reverse the cyanosis. Maintenance of the cervical halter traction during the intubation procedure should be effective in preventing any further damage to the spinal cord.

The communicative patient is a fairly reliable indicator of spinal injury as very few spinal fractures occur without immediate pain. The discomfort need not be severe, however, which is the reason for rule 3: *any traumatized patient complaining of spinal pain must be managed as though an unstable fracture were present until proven otherwise.* The trick here is not to forget to ask. Traumatized patients frequently have multiple painful injuries and may not spontaneously complain of spinal pain even when a fracture is present. Any complaints of weakness, paralysis, or numbness must be elicited. These will assist in focusing the examination to follow. The history of a gunshot wound accompanied by complaints of spinal pain, weakness, or numbness requires the assumption of an unstable spinal fracture.

Examination. The vital signs can supply important clues in spinal injury. Spinal fracture without neurologic injury is not likely to be accompanied by shock. When shock is present it usually signifies spinal cord injury or blood loss in other areas. The hypotension due to spinal cord injury is rarely below 90 mm Hg systolic and is only seen in cervical or upper thoracic spinal injury when underlying spinal cord sympathetic systems are damaged. This leads to loss of peripheral vasomotor tone, vasodilatation, and a relatively inadequate circulating vascular volume.

Respirations are unaffected unless cervical or upper thoracic spinal cord injury has occurred. In such instances respirations are shallow and the chest cage will move minimally or not at all during deep inspiration. Rather, abdominal protrusion during inspiration is seen as the diaphragms compress the abdominal contents in the absence of intercostal muscle function and chest wall expansion.

Cyanosis should be carefully searched for (lips, nail beds) as this requires immediate supplemental oxygen by mask and preparation for ventilatory support. Cyanosis in the absence of thoracic cage injury usually implies upper cervical spinal cord damage.

A pertinent neurologic examination should be accomplished soon after admission. This examination includes the following.

Strength. Any patient who can forcibly flex both arms at the elbow and open and close both hands with ease and who can vigorously wiggle his or her toes and lift each leg off the gurney may be presumed to have no spinal cord injury. Patterns of weakness in spinal cord injury can vary (hands weak, legs strong; legs weak, hands strong; one arm and one leg weak) and suggest the location of the injury by their very pattern. In brief, arm and hand weakness always mean cervical injury, while leg weakness plus normal arms suggests attention be paid to the thoracic or lumbar spine.

Sensation. Although it may take a detailed neurologic evaluation to detect minor neural problems, any patient who manifests clear pain in response to pinprick testing (use a safety pin, not a venipuncture needle) across the entire dorsum of the hands, down the chest and abdomen and across the groin to the front of the thigh, the front of the calf, the lateral side of the foot, and over the buttock may be presumed to have no significant neural injury.

Diagnostic tests. Radiographs have already been mentioned. All initial lateral cervical radiographs should be taken porta-

bly. If normal alignment is present, then the awake patient can be safely transferred via the three-person, halter traction lift to the regular x-ray table for more complete views. If cervical spinal misalignment is noted, how many further films are needed and where they are taken should be left to the discretion of the neurologic or orthopedic surgeon.

All thoracic and lumbar spine films should be taken on the regular x-ray table as transfer of the patient there is safe using the three-person lift technique.

Arterial blood gases should be obtained on any spine-injured patient with arm or leg weakness. Routine blood chemistries and urinalysis are in order as well as blood for type and hold, in case surgery is contemplated.

Intervention

Immobilization of the cervical region on the ambulance stretcher using halter traction and sandbags or rolled towels has been described when patient transfer is anticipated. This type of immobilization is also indicated in the patient on the emergency department gurney once a fracture or misalignment has been identified. Skeletal traction using skull tongs will probably be applied by the orthopedic or neurologic surgeon for more permanent traction/immobilization.

The supine position on the gurney is adequate immobilization of the thoracic and lumbar spine. Traction is not effective in realigning these portions of the spinal column.

Respiratory assistance is not immediately required in spinal injury even when the cord has been damaged if cyanosis is not present. Supplemental mask oxygen is satisfactory until more detailed pulmonary evaluation can occur (arterial blood gases, pulmonary function studies). It may be anticipated that only spinal injuries which involve the cervical region and include cord damage with arm and leg weakness will require respiratory assistance, and then only if the patient's initial tidal volume is less than 600 cc.

An intravenous line should be started and Ringer's lactate begun at 100 ml per hour. This may be increased if the systolic pressure is below 95 mm Hg, but judgment is important here. In the young (less than 40 years old) and previously healthy patient a systolic pressure of 90 to 100 mm Hg, when there is evidence of definite neurologic injury as mentioned above, is due to vasoparalysis and need not be vigorously treated with large amounts of fluid. On the other hand, if the pressure is similarly low in a 60-year-old patient, when neurologic abnormalities are limited or absent, then vigorous therapy is in order as blood loss elsewhere is much more likely.

A urinary catheter should be placed in any patient in whom arm or leg weakness is found. Patients with documented fracture but without neurologic abnormalities need not be catheterized in the emergency department.

Drugs have a limited place in the treatment of spinal injury. Patients with leg or arm weakness should receive an intravenous bolus of steroids, 10 mg of dexamethasone being an appropriate amount in a convenient form. It is hoped that these steroids may assist the damaged spinal cord in recovery.

Analgesics such as pentazocine (Talwin) or narcotics may be used judiciously for spinal pain in the presence of fracture. Analgesics should be avoided when the blood pressure is low or when leg paralysis and arm weakness are present. A patient with cervical spinal cord injury and already limited respiratory capacity does not need further respiratory depression resulting from narcotics or barbiturates.

If spinal injury or paralysis is found following a gunshot wound, antibiotics (ampicillin, 1 g IV push) should be given.

In those patients in whom it has been radiographically established that no spinal fracture or dislocation is present, the options for further care are limited and simple. In the rare patient with frank weakness of more than one limb without fracture, the presumption must be contusion of the spinal cord. Treatment includes hospital admission, skilled nursing care, and steroids. When no fracture or dislocation has been established but there is weakness or numbness of one extremity, then acute nerve root injury by intravertebral disc rupture may be presumed. Treatment here consists of hospital admission, bed rest, and intermittent traction. The use of steroids is optional.

When no fracture or dislocation and no neurologic abnormalities are found, the diagnosis of spinal, muscular, or ligamentous strain is likely. This type of injury in the cervical region is frequently called whiplash, while in the thoracic or lumbar area it is commonly termed back strain. Initial treatment here includes analgesics (pentazocine, codeine compounds), sedatives/relaxants (Valium, SOMA, Robaxin), soft collars or corsets, and heat. These may be accomplished at home and the patient discharged, but the severity of pain plus other injuries often leads to brief hospitalization.

NONTRAUMATIC SPINAL PROBLEMS

Patients may come to the emergency department complaining of spinal pain (with or without neurologic abnormality) but without a history of trauma. Perhaps the onset of their pain followed rather mild injury (lifting an object, bending over, twisting, minor sports injury) such that the suspicion of fracture is low. In these patients the likelihood of an immedite threat to life or neurologic function is limited but must not be forgotten.

Assessment

Two important aspects of history must be clearly established in addition to ascertaining that the onset of pain followed little or no injury. The first is to elicit whether the pain extends into the arms or legs and whether it is accompanied by weakness, numbness, or urinary retention. The second is to ascertain the presence or absence of a history of tumor, particularly of the malignant lung, prostate, breast, or lymphatic variety.

Attention on the physical examination should be directed to detecting weakness in the extremities as well as determining whether sensation is intact, especially over the buttocks. Firm palpation of the spinous processes is important for detecting significant spinal discomfort, which may herald early involvement of the spine by tumor.

Diagnostic procedures include (1) films of the spine in the appropriate painful area unless they have been recently taken for the same pain and (2) urinary catheterization if there has been failure of micturition for more than eight hours.

Intervention

Spinal pain extending into one extremity with little or no weakness and no radiographic abnormalities other than arthritic changes suggests an intervertebral disc protrusion. Treatment here includes analgesics and bed rest or traction, which may be conducted at home or in the hospital.

Any radiograph that shows a fracture (usually of a vertebral body) or other changes consistent with involvement by a tumor is cause for concern. If pain is the only complaint and neurologic abnormalities are absent, bed rest or immobilization plus analgesics are satisfactory immediate treatment.

When any patient manifests urinary retention or weakness in both legs, the problem must be considered emergent. Patients with this constellation of signs and symptoms usually have compression of the spinal cord by tumor, although severe arthritis can present in this fashion. The spinal cord will not tolerate much compression, and steps must be taken to alleviate it. Emergency department personnel are to be lauded when they recognize this problem, for all too often it is not appreciated for what it portends. Lack of treatment results in permanent paraplegia. This syndrome of spinal cord compression is most frequently not appreciated when the patient's primary tumor is prostatic carcinoma. In these patients urinary retention is considered a manifestation of the urinary disease, the leg weakness is not appreciated, and the back pain is either not detected or ignored. Catheterization under these circumstances may be felt to be definitive treatment. This is not the case, as these patients should be treated immediately with intravenous steroids (dexamethasone, 10 mg IV push) and arrangements made for neurosurgical consultation and probably a myelogram.

Finally, spinal pain that does not extend into an extremity and is not accompanied by neurologic abnormalities or radiographic changes other than arthritis probably represents muscular, ligamentous, or arthritic disease. This can be safely handled by symptomatic treatment with analgesics, sedatives/relaxants, heat, and rest—usually at home.

SUMMARY

Once the most crucial goal in spinal injury and disease has been accomplished—recognition that it is or may be present—subsequent emergency department care should occur in an orderly fashion designed to identify the problems likely to severely damage the spinal cord or nerves. These severe problems, namely, spinal fracture in trauma or spinal cord compression by tumor, must be handled so that normal neurologic function is preserved or so that an already damaged nervous system is not injured further by routine emergency department procedures. The modifications of care necessary to safeguard the nervous system in these patients are neither difficult nor extensive. Failure to implement them, however, is indefensible.

ADDITIONAL READINGS

Dohn, D. F.: Hyperflexion injuries of the cervical spine. In Youmans, J. R., editor: Neurological surgery, Philadelphia, 1973, W. B. Saunders Co., vol. 2, pp. 1075-1084.

White, R. J., and Yashon, D.: Dorsal and lumbar spine injuries. In Youmans, J. R., editor: Neurological surgery, Philadelphia, 1973, W. B. Saunders Co., vol. 2, pp. 1085-1088.

White, R. J., and Yashon, D.: General care of cervical spine injuries. In Youmans, J. R., editor: Neurological surgery, Philadelphia, 1973, W. B. Saunders Co., vol. 2, pp. 1049-1074.

CHAPTER 26

Emergency respiratory care

Richard R. Uhl, M.D.

Patients often arrive in the emergency department with respiratory distress of varying magnitudes. We will discuss conditions requiring quick assessment to protect the airway from obstruction, preventing aspiration of foreign substances, and ventilation in cardiorespiratory failure. Consideration will first be directed to the causes of respiratory emergencies, particular concerns posed by them, and a description of the appropriate procedures. Included will be mask and mechanical ventilation, airway insertion, endotracheal intubation, and tracheostomy techniques.

AIRWAY PROBLEMS

Situations necessitating emergency airway management are listed in the following outline.

I. Unconsciousness
   A. Drugs
      1. Patient administration
      2. Physician administration
   B. Central nervous system
      1. Injury
      2. Hemorrhage
II. Obstruction
   A. Foreign body
   B. Burns
   C. Croup/epiglottitis
   D. Tumors
   E. Hemorrhage

III. Cardiorespiratory
   A. Respiratory failure
      1. Chronic lung disease
      2. Asthma
      3. Pneumonia
   B. Cardiopulmonary resuscitation
   C. Pulmonary edema
IV. Neurologic
   A. Myasthenia gravis
   B. Poliomyelitis
   C. Polyneuritis
   D. Poisoning
V. Trauma
   A. Crushed chest
   B. Quadriplegia
   C. Laryngeal laceration
   D. Drowning

The lung must be protected from aspiration of oropharyngeal and gastric contents. The former causes pneumonias; and aspiration of gastric contents, if the pH is less than 3.0, causes chemical pneumonitis[1] often resulting in lung abscess, empyema, sepsis, and death. Normally, the airway is protected by the gag reflex. Sensory afferent fibers of the glossopharyngeal (IX) and vagus (X) nerves supply the pharynx and larynx; motor efferent fibers via the vagus to the larynx cause the false cords to approximate, preventing aspiration. The epiglottis plays only a minor role.

Unconsciousness

When a patient has a depressed level of consciousness, protection of the airway must be questioned. Often this question regarding level of consciousness is answered during laryngoscopy. If the patient is rousable and responding appropriately, the airway is protected. If not, an endotracheal tube should be inserted. If the patient merely gags or coughs, the level of consciousness is too low to prevent aspiration. If purposeful movements are made to resist or to talk, the patient is probably competent enough to protect the airway. Unconsciousness may occur from drug ingestion or iatrogenic drug overdose, particularly in the treatment of status epilepticus, delirium tremens, nervous system injury, or hemorrhage.

Obstruction

Obstruction of the airway may occur in croup and in epiglottitis. Foreign bodies, tumors, and hemorrhage into the airway also cause obstruction. Facial burns result in rapidly progressive edema of the neck, tongue, and epiglottis and in obstruction. Patients with partial obstructions should be observed continuously for respiratory failure, which may occur catastrophically in seconds. Interpretations of arterial blood gas tension are often misleading, giving a false sense of security, and are not a substitute for patient observation.

Cardiorespiratory problems

When respiratory failure occurs in the patient with chronic lung disease or asthma, it should be treated with endotracheal intubation and mechanical ventilation. Cardiac arrest patients should be intubated even if they are quickly resuscitated and responding. A cardiac arrest may recur; or the patient may soon become unconscious or convulse because of poor cerebral perfusion, hypoxia, or the effects of resuscitation drugs (especially lidocaine). The patient needs mechanical ventilation to relieve an already damaged heart while in such a precarious state.

Pulmonary edema occurring from left ventricular failure, inhalation of irritants, drowning, or iatrogenic fluid overload is treated with positive pressure breathing because it increases alveolar pressure and, therefore, decreases the tendency to extravasate more fluid into the alveoli.

Neurologic disease

Patients with neurologic diseases such as myasthenia gravis, polyneuritis, and poliomyelitis and those with organic pesticide poisoning often develop diaphragmatic paralysis and must be ventilated.

Trauma

Trauma to the chest with rib fractures causes instability of the chest wall and paradoxical respiration. Normally, when the diaphragm descends, the chest expands. With paradoxical respiration the chest collapses on inspiration resulting in a rocking motion in which the chest goes in while the abdomen goes out; thus no air is exchanged (Fig. 26-1). Just as broken extremities require plaster stabilization, this condition requires intubation and approximately three weeks of mechanical ventilation to permit the fractures to heal and stabilize the chest wall. Cervical cord injuries also cause paradox. In this case the chest wall is unstable because of intercostal muscle paralysis. These patients also need mechanical ventilation for about three weeks.

Laryngeal and tracheal lacerations are splinted from within by an endotracheal tube, which is also necessary to facilitate removal of blood and clots and to maintain an airway.

Aspiration of water and gastric contents generally complicate near drowning, causing aspiration pneumonia and pulmonary edema. Both conditions cause hypoxia and require intubation and mechanical ventilation.

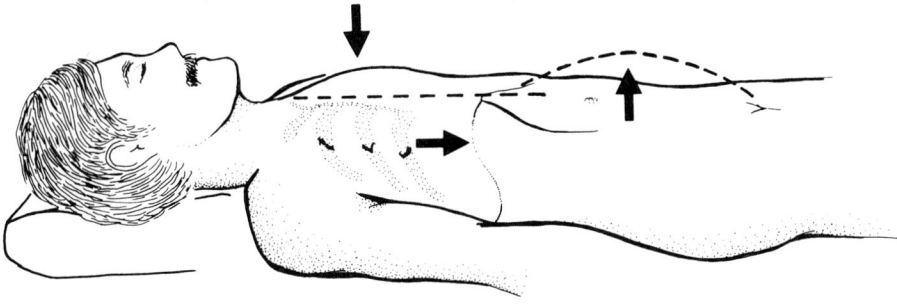

Fig. 26-1. Paradoxical respiration in presence of unstable chest wall from rib fracture or other causes. As diaphragm descends, stomach goes out, but chest is sucked in.

MANAGEMENT
Ventilation

It is imperative that the apneic patient be ventilated with high oxygen concentrations by the first person in attendance. This is done by mouth, bag and mask, or mechanically with a high pressure, 100% oxygen–delivering valve. It is desirable to use high oxygen concentrations as soon as possible. Most existent self-inflating resuscitation bags will give only 40% to 50%, but with modifications this can be raised to 65% to 85% (Table 26-1). The ability to fit a mask and ventilate the apneic patient is one of the most essential skills of all medical and paramedic personnel treating the acutely ill. A continuing in-service program of instruction must exist at all levels.

Nasopharyngeal intubation

The partially obstructed patient who is rousable and responding can be expected not to aspirate, and "snoring" ventilation may be improved by using an airway to relieve soft tissue obstruction. Oral airways are often poorly tolerated at this level of consciousness and cause retching. Nasopharyngeal airways are preferred. To avoid nose bleed the nasopharyngeal airway is inserted in such a way that the sharp, acute-angled tip passes medially, along the nasal septum, and the soft, obtuse-angled

Table 26-1. Percentage of oxygen delivered by resuscitation units with and without modifications*

Unit	Flow rate of oxygen added		
	5 L/min	10 L/min	15 L/min
Air-Viva	34.5	53.8	88.5
AMBU	29.8	36.8	44.6
Hope	29.8	32.6	39.1
PMR	28.5	34.9	41.0
Pulmonator	25.9	31.7	34.5
RFB	35.2	45.7	50.4
Modified AMBU	44.5	66.2	80.7
Modified Pulmonator	41.4	59.4	68.6
Modified Hope	43.9	57.6	65.0
Modified PMR†			80.0

*From Redick, L. F., Dunbar, R. W., MacDougall, D. C., and Merket, T. E.: An evaluation of hand-operated self-inflating resuscitation equipment, Anesth. Analg. 49(1):28-32, 1970.
†Modified by Respiratory Therapy Department, University Hospital, San Diego County, California.

bevel passes laterally, by the vascular nasal turbinates. Prior to insertion, a local analgesic/vasoconstrictor is applied topically to the nasal cavity. Phenylephrine 1%, 0.5 ml diluted to 2 ml with 4% lidocaine, or 2 ml of 5% cocaine is recommended. The latter raises blood pressure and may cause cerebral stimulation at this dosage. The tube is also lubricated with lidocaine jelly.

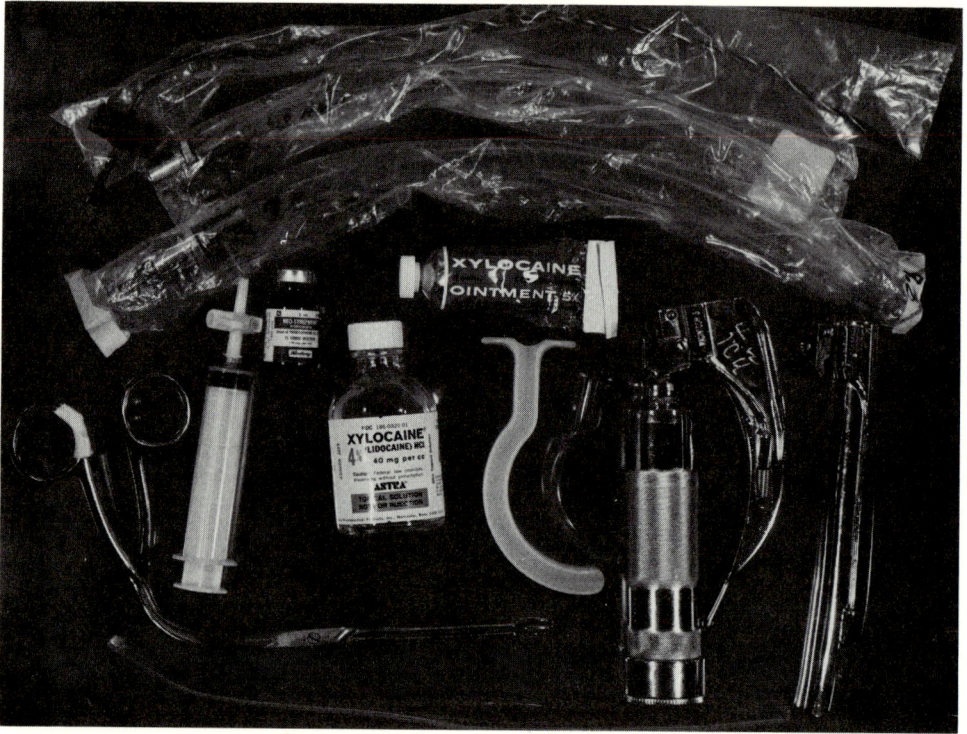

Fig. 26-2. *Above,* Endotracheal tubes and stylet. *Left to right:* Magill forceps; inflating syringe; phenylephrine; lidocaine; airways; laryngoscope with curved and straight blades. *Below,* Tonsillar suction.

Endotracheal intubation

Endotracheal intubation is a skill that should be known by all emergency department practitioners. A dummy* or cadaver may be used for initial instruction, followed by observation, and finally practice, ideally in the operating room. Equipment necessary for adults and children is shown in Figs. 26-2 and 26-3. The trachea may be intubated through the mouth or nose under direct vision or blindly through the nose.

In the emergency situation intubation requires *help!* It is impossible to intubate the trachea without assistants who can immobilize the patient, provide suction, and, finally, help ventilate the patient. Remember that *a*irway and *b*reathing are the first priorities in the ABC's of resuscitation and should receive primary attention.

Endotracheal intubation should be performed with the patient's head at midchest height of the operator, reducing the need to bend or lean over awkwardly. The patient's head and neck should be in the "sniffing" position with the head anteriorly displaced and hyperextended (Fig. 26-4). It is not necessary, and indeed is undesirable, to place pillows under the patient's shoulders.

Laryngoscopes facilitate intubation and have curved or straight blades. Intubation technique depends on the type of blade used. Most find the curved No. 3 Macintosh blade easiest to use. It is designed to keep the tongue entirely to the left of the blade and out of the way. When the patient's head is in the sniffing position, the lips and teeth are opened with the fingers. Four distinct motions will expose the larynx:

---

*Laerdal, Tuckahoe, New York.

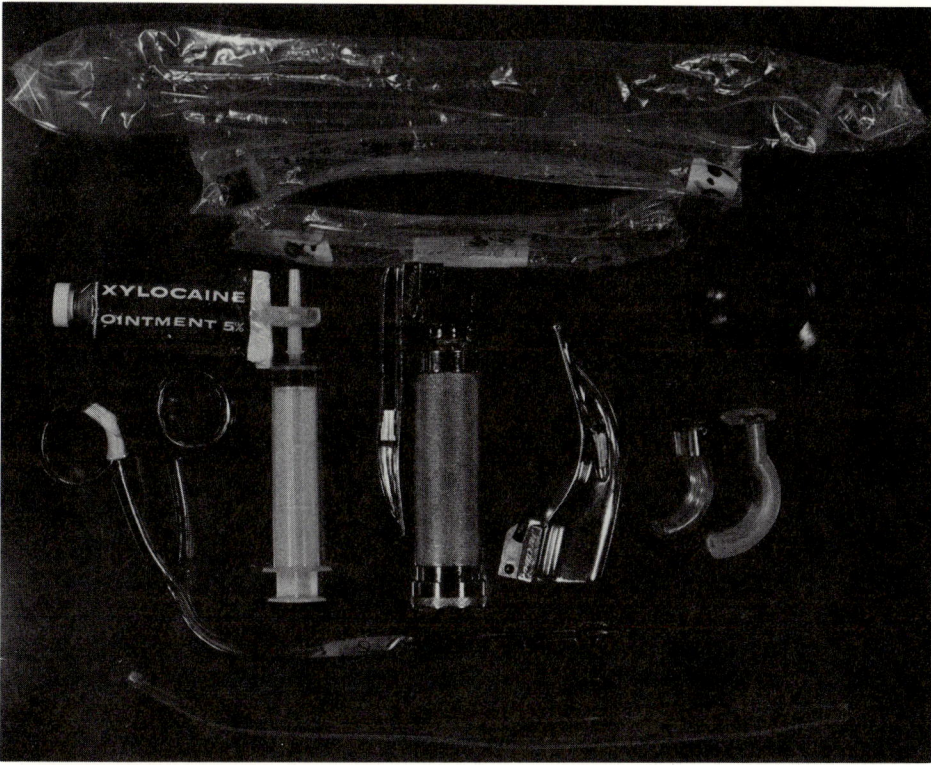

Fig. 26-3. *Above,* Pediatric endotracheal tube and stylet. *Left to right:* Magill forceps; lidocaine; inflating syringe; laryngoscope with straight and curved blades; airways; Rendell-Baker pediatric face mask. *Below,* Tonsillar suction.

1. The blade is directed toward the right anterior tonsillar pillar, and the tongue is thus displaced to the left by the blade.
2. The laryngoscope handle is then rotated toward the left, counterclockwise on the vertical axis, and the epiglottis is visualized.
3. The laryngoscope is advanced anteriorly and inferiorly so that the blade lies in the vallecula, the fossa between the tongue and epiglottis; thus the epiglottis lies *posterior* to the blade.
4. Moving the entire laryngoscope upward and toward the patient's feet in a 45-degree angle from the horizontal exposes the vocal cords.

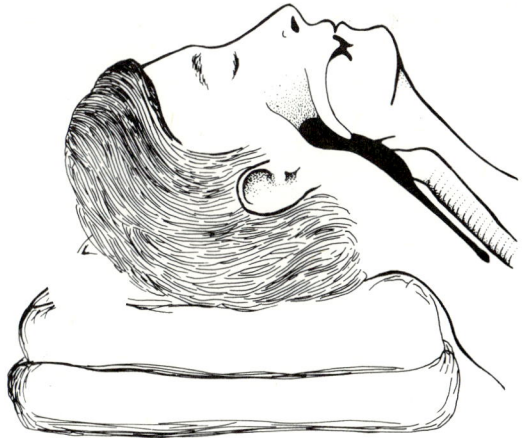

Fig. 26-4. The sniffing position. The head is anteriorly displaced and hyperextended.

The technique with a straight blade is essentially three movements:

1. The blade is advanced in the midline, without displacing the tongue to either side, until the epiglottis is seen.
2. The epiglottis is lifted anteriorly with the tip of the blade, thus lying *anterior* to the blade.
3. The entire laryngoscope is advanced anteriorly and toward the patient's feet in a 45-degree angle with the horizontal, and the cords are seen.

Care should be exercised to avoid breaking teeth and lacerating the lips. If a patient has a noticeably loose tooth, it should be purposefully removed during intubation lest it find its way into the trachea!

Nasotracheal intubation may be accomplished blindly in the breathing patient. Nose preparation was discussed in naso- pharyngeal airway insertion. The tube is well lubricated and gently advanced through the nare and nasal cavity into the nasopharynx where some resistance is met as the tube flexes into the oropharynx. Breath sounds can be heard at the tip of the tube. The tube is advanced "following" these breath sounds. As the tube enters the larynx, the patient often coughs. If the tube will not go in blindly or if the patient is apneic, the tube may be inserted nasally under direct vision. It is passed into the hypopharynx as before. A laryngoscopy is performed in the usual manner and Magill forceps are used to aim the tip of the tube into the glottis. Since it is usually difficult for the laryngoscopist to advance the slippery tube with forceps, an assistant pushes the tube into the trachea.

After either endotracheal method the

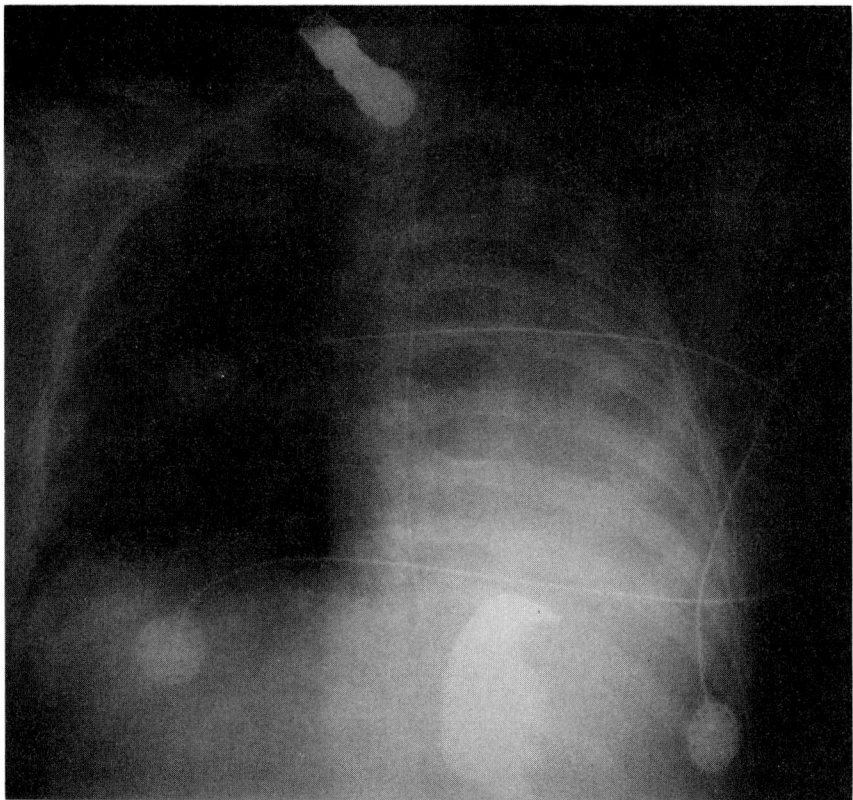

Fig. 26-5. Endobronchial intubation of right mainstem bronchus.

patient should breathe 100% oxygen spontaneously for several breaths, if breathing. The trachea should be suctioned to remove blood and secretions prior to applying positive pressure, lest the secretions be blown out into the lung.

Both lungs are then auscultated to rule out intubation of one bronchus (Fig. 26-5).

Types of tubes

Rubber, plastic, and silicone endotracheal and tracheostomy tubes are available. Rubber tubes are used only for brief intubation in the operating room. Plastic and silicone endotracheal and tracheostomy tubes, if cuffed, should exert as little pressure on the tracheal wall as possible to lessen the likelihood of tracheal injury and stenosis. This may be achieved by prestretching the cuff. To accomplish this the tube is immersed under sterile conditions in 90° to 95° C water, and the heated cuff is gently overinflated with 20 to 30 ml of air. Prestretching may also be done by gently injecting 30 ml of air into the cuff at room temperature and clamping the

pilot inflating tube for eight hours. In addition to inflatable cuffs, there are foam-filled cuffs and flanged tubes that will occlude the trachea and lessen the pressure on the tracheal wall.

Tube size and length are given for various ages in Table 26-2. Endotracheal tube size is in millimeters of internal diameter or French (external circumference):

Tube size (mm I.D.) × 4 = French size

Tracheostomy tube sizes are specified by number or by French size:

Number + 4 = External diameter
External diameter × 3.14 (pi) = French

As a rule of thumb for children over 2 years: 20 + age in years = French size.

A stylet is always used in plastic and silicone tubes. It is important to lubricate the stylet prior to insertion so that it is easily removed when the tube is in the trachea. It is embarrassing to have heroically intubated the trachea only to find that the stylet is "frozen" in the tube!

Immobilization of the tube is as im-

Table 26-2. Endotracheal tubes for infants and children*

Infants				Children				
Weight (kg)	Internal diameter (mm)	Length (cm) Oral	Nasal	Age	Weight (kg)	Internal diameter (mm)	Length (cm)	Type
0.5-1.0		7.0	8.0	6 mo	6	4.5	14	Plain
1 -1.4	3.0	7.5	8.5					(straight
1.4-1.9		8.0	9.0					sided)
1.9-2.2		8.5	9.5	1 yr	10	5.0	15	Plain
2.2-2.6		9.0	10.0	2 yr	12	5.5	16	Plain
2.6-3.0	3.5	9.5	10.5	3 yr	14	5.5	16	Plain
3.0-3.4		10.0	11.0	4 yr	16	6.0	17	Plain
3.4-3.7		10.5	11.5	5 yr	18	6.0	17	Plain
3.7-4.1		11.0	12.0	6 yr	23	6.5	18	Plain
4.1-4.5	4.0	11.5	12.5	8 yr	30	6.5	18	Plain
4.5-5.5		12.0	13.0	10 yr	36	7.0	20	Plain
				12 yr	45	7.0	20	Plain or cuffed
				14 yr	50	7.5	24	Plain or cuffed

*Modified from Smith, R. M.: Anesthesia for infants and children, ed. 3, St. Louis, 1968, The C. V. Mosby Co.

portant as insertion, for it prevents accidental or patient-induced decannulation. Tincture of benzoin or other suitable adherent is applied to the patient's face and to the tube, and waterproof tape is used liberally. The burned or bearded face poses a special problem. In these cases adhesive tape is applied around the benzoin-coated tube to form a raised "bump"; cotton twill hernia tape is placed around the patient's head above the ears and tied to the "bump."

Tracheostomy

In recent years more persons have been trained in endotracheal intubation. As a result the dramatic throat-cutting tracheostomy in the emergency department of past years is now seen more on television than in real life. Nevertheless, emergency tracheostomy is still needed in cases of supraglottic obstruction such as from tumor, foreign body, laryngeal edema and webs, and epiglottitis. For these reasons, emergency department personnel should still maintain tracheostomy capabilities.

Tracheostomy has become by and large an elective operative procedure and should be done in the operating room. Most surgeons prefer to perform tracheostomy over a previously placed endotracheal tube.

Mechanical ventilation

The emergency department is not the place for continuous mechanical ventilation. Nevertheless, patients do need to be ventilated temporarily while being resuscitated, prepared for surgery, or awaiting an available bed in the intensive care unit or transfer. Therefore, some basics need to be known.[2]

Mechanical ventilators in general use are classified as to the means by which they cycle off inspiration. *Pressure* cycled respirators initiate inspiration on a preset time basis and create increasing positive pressure across the airway; volume enters the patient until a preset maximum pressure

is reached, when the respirator cycles off. *Volume* cycled respirators cycle on by a similar time set, but cycle off when a preset volume is delivered. Because of these characteristics the performance of the two types differs, particularly in regard to leaks and changes in patient respiratory compliance ("stiffness").

When small leaks occur with a pressure cycled respirator, the respirator continues to deliver volume until the preset pressure is reached; thus in part the leak "compensates"; with large leaks or if the patient disconnects the respirator, however, it cycles on and stays on creating noise and hence an alarm of malfunction. The volume ventilator, on the other hand, is insensitive to leaks of any magnitude and will continue to methodically pump its bellows regardless of what is downstream. But with decreasing patient compliance, the volume ventilator has the advantage, for it will continue to deliver its volume even in the face of much downstream resistance, whereas the pressure ventilator will reach its preset pressure prematurely, causing the delivered volume to fall. Performance of individual ventilators is summarized in Table 26-3.

Respirator settings recommended initially are a tidal volume of 15 cc/kg body weight, frequency of 10 to 12 per minute,

Table 26-3. Characteristics of individual ventilators

Characteristics	Pressure cycled	Volume cycled
Compensates for	Leaks	Decreased compliance
Fails to compensate for	Decreased compliance	Leaks
Shortcomings	Oxygen control	Disconnect warning
Examples	Bird Mark 7 Bennett PR-2	Bennett MA-1 Emerson Engstrom Ohio 560

and 50% to 60% oxygen. If the patient has aspirated, arrested, or is in pulmonary edema, 100% oxygen is the initial setting. After 15 minutes on these settings arterial blood gases are obtained and the inspired oxygen percent is adjusted. Hypocapnia is treated by the addition of mechanical dead space rather than decreasing volumes. Patients require these high volumes to remain synchronous with the ventilator and to avoid the atelectasis that occurs with lower volume ventilation.[3]

There is another technique of mechanical ventilation, called intermittent mandatory ventilation (IMV).[4] By the use of a one-way valve the patient can take a spontaneous breath as he desires, rather than have his respiration controlled by the respirator. Periodically the respirator cycles on, closes the valve, and gives the patient a positive pressure breath. The mechanical rate is adjusted so that the combined patient ventilation plus mechanical ventilation is adequate to maintain pH = 7.40. When using IMV it is important to use only enough machine ventilation to hold pH at 7.40; do not overventilate. Modifications may be made to any respirator to make it supply IMV. In addition there are two specifically IMV devices, the Baby Bird and IMV Bird.*

PNEUMONIA

Pneumonia may be caused by bacteria (50%) or viruses or mycoplasma (10%), or it may be of indeterminant etiology (40%). Bacterial pneumonia has abrupt onset with shaking chills, fever, toxicity, and purulent sputum. Nonbacterial pneumonias have insidious onset, often preceded by upper respiratory complaints, myalgia, and headache. Diagnosis may be made in the emergency department by examination of sputum obtained from the airway, hopefully avoiding contamination

---

*bird Corp., Palm Springs, Calif.

by oral flora; this may be done by percutaneous transtracheal aspiration or, more recently, by fiberoptic bronchoscopy. Sputum in bacterial pneumonia contains polymorphonuclear cells and gram-positive cocci in 90% of cases, either pneumococci, occurring in encapsulated pairs, or staphylococci, occurring in clusters. Gram-negative organisms are usually *Klebsiella* species or other enteric organisms. The sputum in viral or mycoplasmal pneumonia contains few organisms, but large numbers of mononuclear cells. Mycoplasma may be identified by special staining techniques. Chest x-ray studies confirm the diagnosis.

Management

The emergency treatment of pneumococcal pneumonia is penicillin G, 600,000 units every 12 hours. Because penicillin-resistant staphylococci are so common in hospital-acquired infections, methicillin or one of the other penicillinase-resistant penicillins are preferred for staphylococcal pneumonia. Adult doses usually start at 1 g every 4 to 6 hours intravenously. Gram-negative pneumonia is treated with gentamicin, 1.7 mg/kg initially, repeated at eight-hour intervals dependent upon kidney function. Mycoplasmal pneumonia may be treated with erythromycin or tetracycline. There is no specific therapy for viral pneumonia.

Aspiration pneumonia

If a patient is unconscious and the airway cannot be protected, he or she will aspirate oral secretions and particulate material into the tracheobronchial tree and develop pneumonia. If regurgitation occurs, aspiration of stomach acid and particulate content will occur. If the stomach content is acid, chemical pneumonitis (Mendelson's syndrome),[1] in addition to bacterial pneumonia, will develop. This combination is notorious for abscess formation and empyema and is deadly. It is felt that this is most likely to occur if the pH of the aspirate is less than 3.0; however, this syndrome has developed even with alkaline aspiration. Nevertheless, if a patient is felt to have aspirated, the first tracheal suction should be tested for pH with indicator sticks. Although a neutral pH does not rule out chemical pneumonitis, an acid pH definitely confirms the diagnosis.

Management

Treatment of both types of aspiration pneumonitis involves suppressing the growth of bacteria aspirated. Aqueous penicillin G, 1,200,000 units every 6 hours, is the agent of choice to suppress upper airway flora, in particular, microaerophilic streptococci.[5]

If acid was aspirated, a massive inflammatory response will ensue with exudation of fluid, edema, hemorrhage, and, finally, pulmonary fibrosis. This response impairs pulmonary function and oxygenation, and for this reason the inflammatory response is suppressed with corticosteroids. One regimen advocates methylprednisolone, 30 mg/kg, as a stat dose.[6] Steroids are not administered topically to the trachea through the tube. Indication for bronchoscopy is unclear and depends heavily on the availability of a skilled endoscopist. Certainly,

all gross particulate material should be removed. Generally, this is possible through an endotracheal tube, but bronchoscopy may be necessary in a few cases. Fiberoptic bronchoscopy may be performed through an endotracheal tube by skilled operators. If acid aspiration is suspected, it is not wise to use sodium bicarbonate to neutralize the acid in the lung. The distribution of the acid in the tracheobronchial tree will not be the same as the injected bicarbonate, and iatrogenic alkaline aspiration will be induced in the normal lung and airway. Moreover, tissue may be burned by the heat of the neutralization reaction.

It is important that antibiotics and steroids, when used, are administered as soon as possible. Often there is some question as to whether the patient did aspirate. In these cases it is best to treat initially, pending further diagnosis. Diagnosis is confirmed by chest x-ray studies, blood gases, and the febrile course. Chest x-ray films usually become positive shortly after aspiration. Aspirated liquids gravitate to dependent portions of the lung. The lobes most frequently involved are the superior and medial-basal segments of the right lower lobe, and the superior and posterior

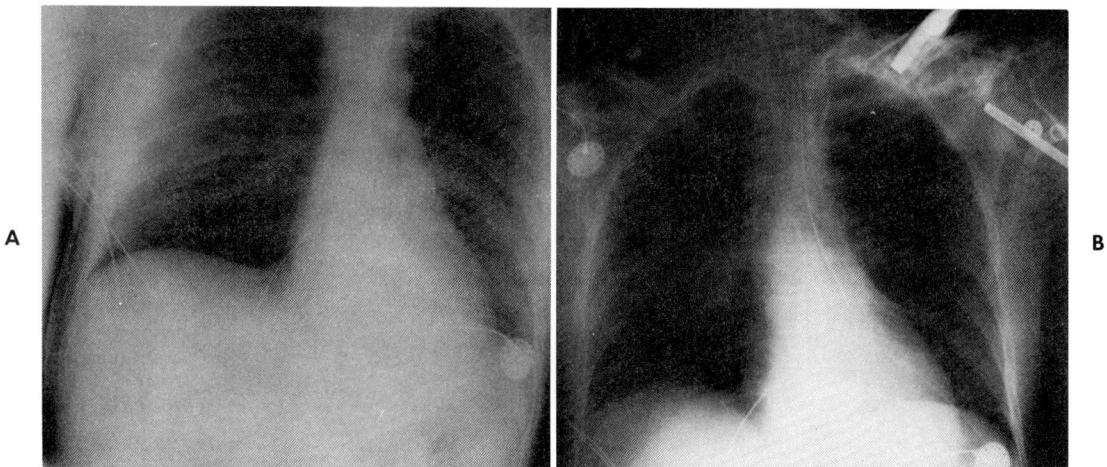

Fig. 26-6. A, Aspiration pneumonia. Loss of left diaphragmatic shadow. Loss of aortic shadow. **B,** One day after aspiration. Diaphragm and aortic shadows reappear.

segments of the left lower lobe. The latter two segments lie behind the heart contiguous with the aorta, and evidence of aspiration by examination is obscured. Aspiration into these lobes is often diagnosed by the presence of an air bronchogram behind the heart and the loss of the aortic shadow behind the heart, indicative of a radiopaque pneumonic area lying next to the aorta (Fig. 26-6). Diagnosis of aspiration may be aided by blood gas determinations that show hypoxia. The patient who has aspirated will become febrile early, often in the emergency department. Temperatures of 38° C (100° to 101° F) may be caused by atelectasis resulting from hypoventilation and may be corrected by hyperinflation and mechanical ventilation; temperatures over 38° C are generally associated with pneumonia unless caused by the primary disease.

PULMONARY EMBOLISM

Pulmonary embolism is not a disease per se, but a complication of thrombosis of the veins of the legs, pelvis, prostatic plexuses or the chambers of the right heart. Predisposing factors include varicose veins, obesity, pregnancy, chronic heart failure, cancer, and possibly oral contraceptives.

The patient seen in the emergency department with pulmonary thromboembolism will have an abrupt onset of tachypnea, anxiety, and chest pain, often radiating to the neck.

Sometimes hypotension and, occasionally, acute right heart dilatation and failure will occur. ECG changes show evidence of acute right heart strain, right bundle branch block, peaked P waves in leads II, III, and aV_F, and inverted T waves in V_{1-3}. The classic laboratory triad is elevated serum bilirubin and lactic dehydrogenase with normal glutamic-oxala-cetic transaminase. Chest x-ray studies may show no abnormality.

The diagnosis is often made on suspicion in the predisposed patient with acute symptoms, and it may remain obscure despite all diagnostic efforts. Radioactive lung scanning may confirm the diagnosis but is often equivocal.

Treatment consists initially of measures to support ventilation, oxygenation, and circulation. Once these are completed, heparin, 50 to 100 mg IV, is administered at four-hour intervals.

SUMMARY

Prompt action is necessary in extreme respiratory distress. Certain basic skills and critical judgment are needed to take care of these life-threatening emergencies. Airway equipment should be available and functioning. Most importantly, the emergency team must be prepared to provide emergency respiratory care.

REFERENCES

1. Mendelson, C. L.: The aspiration of stomach contents into the lungs during obstetric anesthesia, Am. J. Obstet. Gynecol. **52**:191-205, 1946.
2. Bendixen, H. H., Egbert, L. D., Hedley-Whyte, J., Laver, M. B., and Pontoppidan, H.: Respiratory care, St. Louis, 1965, The C. V. Mosby Co.
3. Pontoppidan, H., Geffin, B., and Lowenstein, E.: Acute respiratory failure in the adult, N. Engl. J. Med. **287**(14):690-698, **287**(15):743-751, **287**(16):799-806, 1972.
4. Downs, J. B., Klein, E. F., DeSautels, D., et al.: Intermittent mandatory ventilation: a new approach to weaning patients from mechanical ventilators, Chest **64**:331-335, 1973.
5. Bartlett, J. G., and Gorbach, S. L.: Treatment of aspiration pneumonia, J.A.M.A. **234**:935-937, 1975.
6. Wilson, J. W.: Treatment of pulmonary cellular damage with pharmacologic doses of corticosteroid, Surg. Gynecol. Obstet. **134**:675-681, 1972.

CHAPTER 27

Cardiac arrhythmias

John R. Morse, M.D.

A concise understanding of the clinical presentation, electrocardiographic diagnosis, and correct management of cardiac arrhythmias is fundamental to modern emergency department care. Many of the commonly seen cardiac arrhythmias will necessarily require hospitalization for further evaluation or therapy; however, many others may be adequately managed in the emergency department, thus avoiding more costly utilization of hospital facilities. Arrhythmia diagnosis remains the key to management, since appropriate forms of therapy are relatively limited once the rhythm disturbance has been identified.

Cardiac arrhythmias may be classified as follows:

I. Tachycardia (heart rate greater than 100 beats per minute)
   A. Supraventricular tachycardias
      1. Sinus tachycardia
      2. Paroxysmal atrial tachycardia (PAT)
      3. Atrial flutter
      4. Atrial fibrillation
      5. Paroxysmal atrial tachycardia with block
      6. Junctional tachycardia
   B. Subjunctional tachycardias
      1. Ventricular tachycardia
      2. Ventricular fibrillation
II. Bradycardia

A. Sinus bradycardia
B. Heart block
   1. Incomplete (first or second degree)
   2. Complete

The clinical picture accompanying an arrhythmia is dependent on the nature of the arrhythmia, the general condition and age of the patient, and, most importantly, on the absence or presence of underlying heart disease. Benign forms of paroxysmal supraventricular arrhythmias, characteristically found in healthy individuals without underlying cardiovascular disease, may cause no symptoms. Frequently, however, these patients report abrupt onset of palpitations, intermittent lightheadedness, or persistent nausea and fatigue. Conversely, in older patients with underlying heart disease, complicating arrhythmias may precipitate bouts of congestive heart failure or acute coronary insufficiency. The latter condition is by no means rare, and in fact a diagnosis of myocardial infarction must often be tempered in the elderly patient with known heart disease who has had a recent onset of tachyarrhythmia. Similarly, congestive heart failure with frank pulmonary edema may be seen in the previously compensated individual with valvular heart disease who suddenly develops a rapid supraventricular rhythm disturbance.

As with the tachycardias, bradycardia will manifest a clinical picture primarily dependent on the age and general condition of the patient, as well as the absence or presence of organic heart disease. Sinus bradycardia, often seen in young adults, is typically physiologic requiring no therapy. Sinus bradycardia in older patients, however, should cause some concern since this rhythm may represent disease of the sinus node mechanism. Although in elderly patients sinus bradycardia is often of no consequence, its presence may be one of many factors responsible for episodes of intermittent syncope or increasing degrees of congestive heart failure.

Bradycardia secondary to heart block usually implies organic disease of the cardiac conduction system. It is essential to recognize basic forms of heart block since correct diagnosis and appropriate management may be life saving. The clinical manifestations of heart block will be determined by the heart rate as well as by the patient's cardiac reserve. Older individuals with acute, intermittent heart block will often report distinct bouts of dizziness, light-headedness, or frank syncope with transient loss of consciousness. The term Adams-Stokes disease is applicable when such attacks are shown to have a cardiac basis. In chronic heart block where bradycardia has been sustained over weeks or months, congestive heart failure may be somewhat more frequent, especially in those individuals with compromised myocardial function.

The specific forms of heart block and their differential ECG diagnosis will be discussed in a later section. It is worth emphasizing, however, the importance of determining during the history whether the patient has been taking digitalis, quinidine, or related medications. Digitalis excess is probably the single most common iatrogenic cause of cardiac arrhythmias, especially those presenting as heart block. The knowledge of whether digitalis has been used is imperative if rational therapy is to be applied.

Finally, some general comments regarding ventricular arrhythmias, the seriousness of which cannot be overemphasized. Ventricular tachycardia and ventricular fibrillation should, without question, be considered medical emergencies requiring instant recognition and immediate therapy, usually in the form of electrical DC countershock. Diagnosis usually presents no major problem since these patients, if seen early, are typically quite ill, often without pulse, blood pressure, or spontaneous respirations. If doubt exists as to the diagnosis, direct current countershock should be administered.

Less dramatic forms of ventricular arrhythmias are equally common. Because of a slower rate or a more effective cardiac output, they may be tolerated considerably better. In such instances the differentiation from like forms of supraventricular arrhythmias with widened QRS complexes can be quite challenging, and cardiology consultation may be required for definitive diagnosis.

TACHYCARDIAS
Sinus tachycardia

Clinical presentation. Sinus tachycardia should never be considered a primary cardiac arrhythmia, since it is nearly always secondary to some other precipitating event. Typical examples include fever, electrolyte disturbance, severe anemia, acute blood loss, thyrotoxicosis, and overwhelming infection. A common setting for sinus tachycardia is seen with pulmonary disease where persistent hypoxemia with or without acidosis serves as a continual source of rate potentiation. Likewise, primary cardiac disorders such as acute myocardial infarction or congestive heart failure will often be accompanied by a marked degree of sinus tachycardia. Therapy should always be directed at the underlying cause of the tachycardia and never at the rhythm itself. In cases of chronic obstructive pulmonary disease, improved ventilation with correction of profound hypoxemia and acidosis will have a far more substantial effect on slowing the heart rate than will the inappropriate use of digitalis or other cardiotonic medications. This line of reasoning should be employed whatever the underlying source of the increased rate.

ECG recognition. Electrocardiographic diagnosis will be determined by the presence of P-waves that have a familiar sinus configuration and a 1:1 relationship with the QRS complexes (Fig. 27-1). In the absence of underlying heart block the PR interval should not be inordinately prolonged. The QRS complexes are of the supraventricular type, and the rate rarely exceeds 150 beats per minute. Vagal stimulation in the form of carotid sinus pressure should induce a gradual slowing of the sinus rate and, therefore, serve to differentiate this rhythm from more serious forms of ectopic tachycardia.

Paroxysmal atrial tachycardia (PAT)

Clinical presentation. Of the more common supraventricular arrhythmias requiring emergency department attention is a specific entity designated as paroxysmal atrial tachycardia (PAT). This arrhythmia is particularly prevalent in young, healthy individuals without organic heart disease; therefore, associated symptoms of chest pain or shortness of breath may be conspicuously absent. Characteristic of the history is the abrupt onset of rapid, regular palpitations, often of several hours' duration. As most of these attacks by definition are intermittent, their termination is likewise abrupt as the normal heart rate is suddenly resumed. Although PAT is commonly seen in the young individual without cardiac disease, it may also occur in older patients with underlying cardiac pathology. Ischemic chest pain as well as precipitation of congestive heart failure may complicate the clinical picture in such individuals.

Physical examination is usually not helpful except for the recording of a rapid,

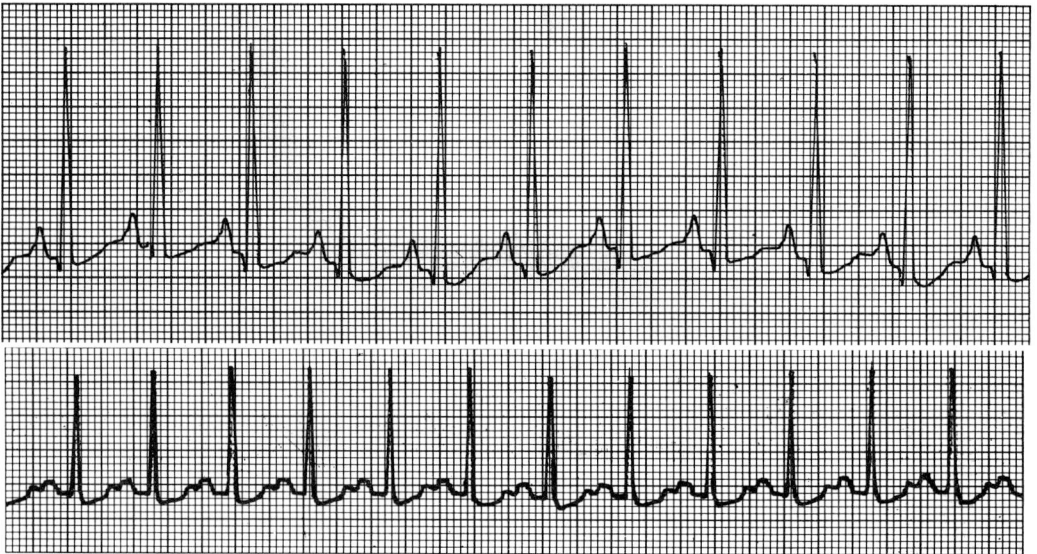

Fig. 27-1. Sinus tachycardia. (From Conover, M. H.: Cardiac arrhythmias: exercises in pattern interpretation, St. Louis, 1974, The C. V. Mosby Co.)

regular heart rate between 150 and 180 beats per minute and rarely as high as 200 beats per minute. The neck veins fail to show distinct flutter waves and the heart tones may demonstrate a peculiar "tic-toc" quality for which the term "embryonic heart sounds" has been coined.

ECG recognition. Definitive diagnosis of PAT is determined by careful analysis of the electrocardiogram. Characteristically, the rhythm is perfectly regular and the rate may vary between 150 and 200 beats per minute. The QRS complexes are of the supraventricular type (narrow, normal configuration) unless underlying conduction disease with bundle branch block is present. "Cherché le P" should now be the rule. Even a brief scan of the tracing will reveal a conspicuous absence of normally configured P waves previously seen with sinus tachycardia. Organized atrial deflections are indeed present; however, these are ectopic in origin and, therefore, are not easily identified. Furthermore, because of their rapid rate and the limited refractory period of the AV junctional tissue, they are more likely to reside in and be obscured by the T waves of the preceding QRS complexes (Fig. 27-2). A failure to demonstrate clear-cut P wave activity in the presence of a narrow complex tachycardia of greater than 150 beats per minute should strongly suggest a diagnosis of PAT.

Differential diagnosis is primarily one of distinguishing this rhythm disturbance from equally common forms of supraventricular tachycardia, namely sinus tachycardia, atrial flutter, and atrial fibrillation. Sinus tachycardia may be excluded on the basis of atrial rate (less than 150 beats per minute) and P wave configuration. Atrial flutter need not be confused with PAT if one remembers that in the former, atrial rate is usually twice that of the ventricular response (greater than 230 to 250 beats per minute) and the P waves are negatively directed. With PAT the atrial rate is always identical to the ventricular response and rarely exceeds 200 beats per minute. Atrial fibrillation can most often be differentiated by the basic irregularity of the QRS complexes as well as by the continual undulations of the isoelectric baseline.

One helpful aid allowing differentiation of any of the supraventricular arrhythmias is achieved by introduction of vagal tone in the form of carotid sinus pressure. Fortunately, the major categories of supraventricular rhythm disturbance all respond differently to carotid sinus pressure, and this distinction provides objective criteria by which a correct diagnosis can be made. Properly applied carotid massage will either abruptly interrupt a paroxysmal atrial tachycardia with immediate conversion to regular sinus rhythm or it will have no effect whatsoever. Conversely, sinus tachycardia should respond by a gradual slowing of the sinus rate with a similar gradual resumption of the previous rate on release

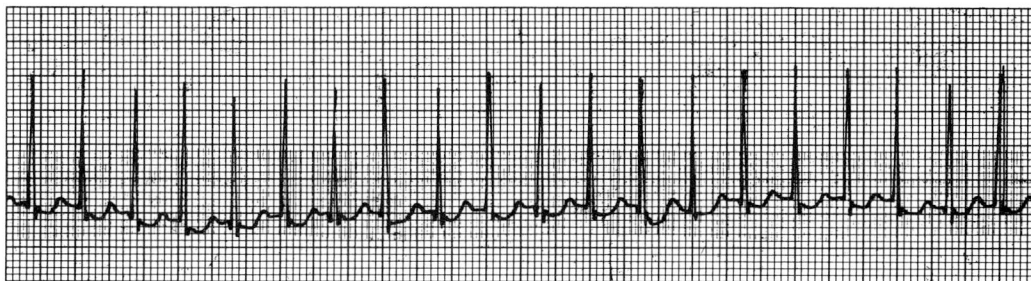

Fig. 27-2. PAT 1:1 conduction. (From Conover, M. H.: Cardiac arrhythmias: exercises in pattern interpretation, St. Louis, 1974, The C. V. Mosby Co.)

of carotid sinus pressure. Atrial flutter, atrial fibrillation, and paroxysmal atrial tachycardia with block respond in yet a different fashion by demonstrating a rather brisk augmentation of block at the AV node, thereby reducing the ventricular response without altering the basic atrial rate. This "dropping of ventricular beats" will often allow one to clearly recognize the presence of flutter or fibrillatory waves on the isoelectric baseline. A clear understanding of the effect of vagal maneuvers (carotid sinus pressure, intravenous administration of edrophonium) on the supraventricular mechanisms of the cardiac conduction system is essential to understanding the pathophysiology of these disorders. For a complete discussion of this matter the reader is referred to a standard text on the subject.[1,2]

In summary, the diagnosis of paroxysmal atrial tachycardia should be seriously considered in a previously healthy individual who presents with a regular tachycardia between 150 and 200 beats per minute that is of several hours' duration and reportedly of abrupt onset. The diagnosis may be confirmed on the electrocardiogram by noting the rate and regularity of normally conducted QRS complexes. Careful search will reveal no identifiable sinus P wave activity. Application of carotid sinus pressure will either immediately convert the rhythm to a regular sinus focus or, as is more often the case, will have no effect whatsoever. Carotid massage will help to distinguish this arrhythmia from other forms of supraventricular tachycardia.

Management. Once a diagnosis of PAT has been established, therapeutic alternatives follow routinely. The importance of considering the patient's resting blood pressure cannot be overemphasized. The large majority of patients with paroxysmal atrial tachycardia are relatively hypotensive; that is, the systolic pressure is less than 90 to 100 mm Hg. In this setting

carotid massage or any other vagal maneuver will usually be ineffective. One of the common errors in emergency department technique is attempting to apply carotid sinus pressure in the hypotensive patient. The anticipated response will most certainly be elusive, and the procedure will serve only to irritate the neck. Furthermore, related maneuvers such as pressing on eyeballs, induction of Valsalva's maneuver or, more seriously, the administration of intravenous digitalis, quinidine, barbiturate, or edrophonium (Tensilon) should not be attempted in the face of a low resting pressure.

A reliable and consistent means of treating PAT with hypotension may be instituted by stepwise, controlled elevation of the systolic pressure using metaraminol or norepinephrine in doses of 100 mg or 4 mg, respectively, per 1,000 ml. The rate of infusion is titrated against 10 mm increments of blood pressure elevation until a level of 140 to 160 mm Hg systolic is reached. The large majority of patients with benign PAT will spontaneously convert to a regular sinus focus on this regimen and many will achieve conversion well below the 150 mm systolic level. A few remaining individuals may require additional vagal tone in the form of carotid massage or intravenous administration of edrophonium, 10 mg slow IV push, or both, with careful ECG and blood pressure monitoring. The need for electric DC countershock should virtually be eliminated. If the diagnosis of PAT is correct, intravenous administration of digitalis is practically never necessary.

Unfortunately, this form of therapy is not universally applicable, especially in older patients with complicating cardiac or hypertensive disease. In these instances elevation of the blood pressure beyond the resting level may be hazardous and should not be done routinely. Intervention should be tailored individually, and conversion by electric means may be necessary. It is often advisable to admit such patients to the hospital for cardiac monitoring and definitive therapy.

Atrial flutter

Clinical presentation. Atrial flutter represents a form of supraventricular rhythm disturbance encompassing a somewhat wider group of disease entities than that seen with the more typical forms of paroxysmal atrial tachycardia. As with PAT, atrial flutter may rarely be seen in the young, healthy individual without underlying heart disease. In these instances, the presenting complaints may be indistinguishable from those of PAT. Precipitating causes often include indiscreet use of tobacco or alcohol, or undue physical or emotional strain. More often, no specific cause can be identified.

Far more commonly, atrial flutter is representative of some underlying cardiac condition. The patient's symptomatology and abnormal physical findings will more likely reflect the primary cardiac pathophysiology rather than the abnormal rhythm pattern. The therapeutic approach will, therefore, be tempered by both the presence and extent of cardiac disease.

Physical examination in those forms of atrial flutter without organic heart disease may disclose few clues of diagnostic significance. The pulse is usually rapid with a regularly irregular tempo. This irregularity is most often the result of some element of block at the AV node as the ventricles do not always respond in a regular fashion. A distinctive observation peculiar to atrial flutter is that of organized atrial flutter waves in the jugular venous pulse. A fair amount of expertise may be required, however, to properly interpret this sign. The remainder of the examination is usually nonspecific. Except for the presence of the tachycardia, one cannot differentiate atrial flutter from other forms of tachyarrhythmia.

ECG recognition. Definitive diagnosis of atrial flutter will be made upon careful analysis of the electrocardiogram. As with PAT, a brief scan of the tracing reveals an absence of familiar sinus P wave configuration. The QRS complexes are usually of the supraventricular type and of normal duration. In contrast to what is often believed, the ventricular rhythm in atrial flutter is not necessarily regular and may, in fact, be grossly irregular—the latter being determined by the level of block at the AV node.

Close attention should be directed toward analyzing atrial activity in all leads of a standard twelve lead electrocardiogram. Organized atrial deflections can usually be recognized at a rate of 220 to 300 beats per minute, and occasionally as high as 350. As opposed to the rhythm of the ventricular complexes, these atrial deflections are absolutely regular without even minor variations. It is helpful to observe the flutter waves in the inferior leads II, III, and aV$_F$. Their negative direction and rapid rate are responsible for the familiar "sawtooth" pattern that may help to distinguish atrial flutter from other forms of supraventricular tachycardia (Fig. 27-3).

The differential diagnosis depends upon separating flutter from two other major rhythm disturbances—atrial fibrillation and PAT with block. Again, carotid massage as a means of implementing vagal tone may produce a transient block at the AV node permitting one to observe the negatively directed flutter waves, their rate, and regularity. With atrial fibrillation a similar response to carotid sinus pressure should occur, allowing recognition of random atrial activity associated with an irregular ventricular response. The response of PAT with block to carotid sinus pressure will be similar to that seen with atrial flutter and fibrillation. If an appropriate block at the AV node occurs, the direction, rate, and configuration of the ectopic atrial waves may be easily differentiated from those seen in atrial flutter.

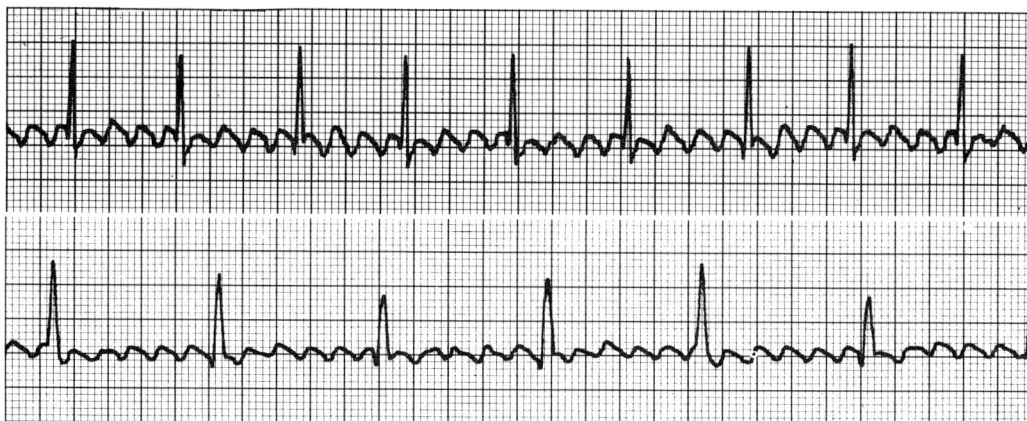

Fig. 27-3. Atrial flutter with sawtooth pattern. (From Conover, M. H.: Cardiac arrhythmias: exercises in pattern interpretation, St. Louis, 1974, The C. V. Mosby Co.)

Management. Therapy for atrial flutter, of course, depends upon the presence or absence of underlying heart disease. In the benign paroxysmal form with rapid ventricular rates treatment is directed at increasing block at the AV node, thereby reducing ventricular response. The most available means of achieving this is by intravenous use of one of the digitalis preparations, preferably digoxin, which has a more rapid onset of action. Occasionally, conversion to regular sinus rhythm will occur following digitalis administration. Far more typically, however, there follows an appropriate reduction in ventricular response resulting in a 3:1, or more commonly 4:1, atrioventricular block. Frequently following digitalis therapy atrial flutter will progress to atrial fibrillation, a condition easier to control. In any event, once the ventricular rate has been reduced to a physiologically tolerable level, additional means, either pharmacologic or electric, may be employed to restore sinus rhythm.

For reasons that are not entirely clear, there are some forms of atrial flutter usually associated with underlying rheumatic or coronary heart disease that are notoriously resistant to digitalis therapy. In these situations one should not hesitate to at-tempt electrocardioversion should moderate doses of parenteral digitalis fail to achieve a slowing of the ventricular response. Attention is also directed toward precipitating causes of atrial flutter such as hemorrhage, heart failure, fever, hypoxemia, and the like. As with any of the arrhythmias, these primary conditions must be corrected before any therapeutic benefit can be realized.

Atrial fibrillation

Clinical presentation. Much of what has been said regarding atrial flutter may also apply to atrial fibrillation, since the pathophysiology of these two conditions is quite similar. As with flutter, atrial fibrillation may also present as a benign paroxysmal disorder. The treatment is identical to that outlined for atrial flutter. Far more frequently, atrial fibrillation represents part of a total disease process in which the absence of organized atrial activity is secondary to some underlying cardiac disorder.

ECG recognition. Whatever the etiology, atrial fibrillation can be clearly recognized on the basis of specific electrocardiographic criteria. Although the physical examination may afford some clues, a definitive diagnosis should never be attempted without

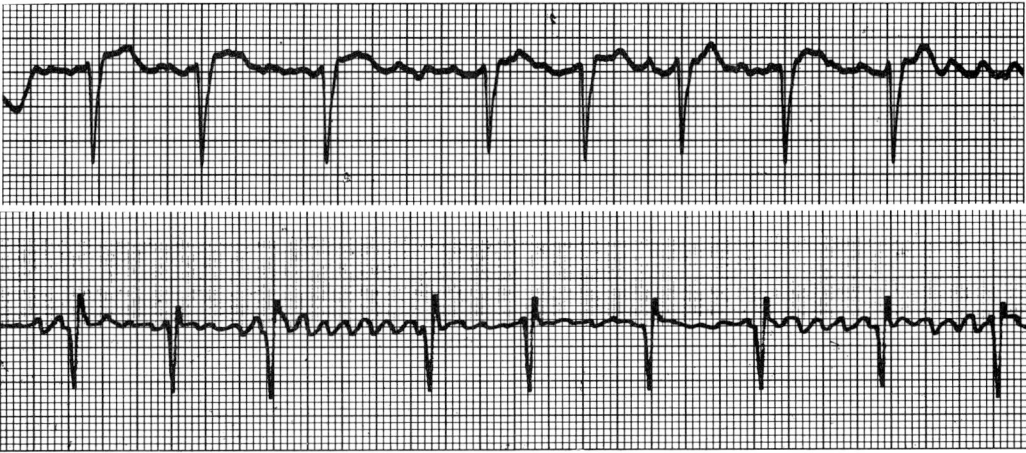

Fig. 27-4. Coarse atrial fibrillation. (From Conover, M. H.: Cardiac arrhythmias: exercises in pattern interpretation, St. Louis, 1974, The C. V. Mosby Co.)

ECG confirmation. The hallmarks of atrial fibrillation are easily recognized and need not be confused with other rhythm disturbances.

1. Organized atrial activity is distinctly absent on the ECG tracing, since by definition the atria are contracting at rates greater than 350 beats per minute. On occasion, large, coarse atrial waves may simulate those seen with atrial flutter. Careful measurement of the P-P interval, however, will always expose the basic irregularity of the atrial deflections (Fig. 27-4).

2. The ventricular response in atrial fibrillation is likewise irregular even at rapid heart rates. Because the atria are being depolarized at a rate far exceeding the conduction capacity of the AV junction, the ventricles are left to respond in a completely random fashion. Since the ventricular complexes represent only conducted beats through the AV junctional tissue, the basic irregular character of this rhythm is assured.

3. As with other supraventricular arrhythmias, the QRS complexes are narrow and of normal configuration unless underlying conduction disease is present. Even if right or left bundle branch block exists, however, a diagnosis of atrial fibrillation can usually be made because of the inherent irregularity of the rhythm as well as the presence of fibrillatory waves on the isoelectric segments.

The differential diagnosis of atrial fibrillation is usually not difficult, the most troublesome aspect being the distinction from that of atrial flutter. Careful measurement of the atrial rate as well as calibration of the atrial regularity will most often serve to separate the two. Carotid sinus pressure may be very helpful even though the anticipated response is identical in both conditions. Increasing the block at the AV node will "slow" the ventricular rate and allow one to recognize the fibrillatory atrial waves.

Management. Therapy is always directed at the underlying cardiac disease. Benign paroxysmal atrial fibrillation will usually respond to small increments of digitalis given intravenously with subsequent conversion to regular sinus rhythm. When underlying heart disease is associated with a rapid ventricular rate, digitalis still remains the drug of choice. The dosage and administration will, of course, be determined by the extent and severity of cardiac decompensation as well as the rapidity of the ventricular response. The mere presence of atrial fibrillation does not necessitate treatment especially if the ventricular response is "controlled." Except in the benign paroxysmal form, spontaneous conversion to regular sinus rhythm following digitalis administration virtually never occurs, and one must usually resort to cardioversion, either electrical or pharmacologic (quinidine), to restore sinus rhythm.

In summary, atrial fibrillation is probably the most common of the supraventricular rhythm disturbances spanning a wide range of disease entities but also including individuals without organic heart disease. Diagnosis rests primarily upon electrocardiographic interpretation where specific criteria have been established. Treatment, when indicated, is almost always in the form of digitalis therapy, and control of the ventricular rate remains the primary therapeutic objective. Benign paroxysmal atrial fibrillation will often spontaneously convert to regular sinus rhythm.

ARRHYTHMIAS RELATED TO DIGITALIS EXCESS

Any discussion of the supraventricular arrhythmias would be incomplete without mention of those abnormal patterns seen with digitalis excess. The relevance of this problem as it relates to emergency department care cannot be overemphasized. Although digitalis excess is capable of producing nearly any form of abnormal rhythm pattern, a few of these recur with enough frequency to require some familiarity with their recognition and management.

PAT with block

Clinical presentation. PAT with block describes a rhythm disturbance often associated with digitalis excess with or without relative hypokalemia. The descriptive name, PAT with block, is somewhat unfortunate, since this arrhythmia is often confused with the previously discussed PAT. Actually, the two have little in com-

mon; in fact, PAT with block is physiologically more closely allied with atrial flutter. Because PAT with block is so often seen as a manifestation of digitalis intoxication, its recognition and differentiation from other supraventricular arrhythmias (namely, atrial flutter) is of utmost importance. Continued administration of digitalis in the presence of PAT with block may prove extremely hazardous.

ECG recognition. The criteria for electrocardiographic diagnosis of PAT with block are the following:

1. A basic supraventricular mechanism with normally conducted QRS complexes is present, yet clear-cut sinus P waves with a 1:1 relationship to the QRS complexes are conspicuously absent.
2. Careful analysis and search for atrial activity will reveal atrial deflections of 150 to 200 beats per minute.
3. The relationship of these atrial deflections to the QRS complexes may be 1:1 with a prolonged AV conduction time (first degree block), or in the more advanced forms may demonstrate varying second degree heart block beginning with intermittent dropped beats of the Wenckebach variety progressing to a fixed form of 2:1 or even 3:1 AV block.

The differential diagnosis of PAT with block from benign PAT and atrial flutter depends primarily on the response to carotid sinus pressure. Following vagal stimulation, increased block at the AV node will reduce the ventricular response and unmask the basic atrial mechanism. Flutter may be easily differentiated on the basis of atrial rate and P wave configuration. On the other hand, benign PAT with 1:1 conduction will either spontaneously convert to regular sinus rhythm or will show no effect whatsoever. Increasing block at the AV node would not be expected.

Management. Treatment of PAT with block will depend upon (1) a positive history of digitalis administration and (2) the ventricular rate. If the latter is not excessive and the patient's general condition is otherwise acceptable, no specific therapy may be required. Obviously, close observation is mandatory in order to ensure the gradual return of a normal rhythm. In those forms of PAT with block where the ventricular response is more rapid (less severe degree of block), a controlled repletion of the serum potassium may be all that is needed. This can be achieved by intravenous administration of 30 to 40 mEq of potassium chloride diluted in 500 ml of 5% dextrose in water (D5W) given over a two- to four-hour period. If the arrhythmia is indeed the result of digitalis excess, a gratifying return to a sinus mechanism will often occur. Phenytoin (Dilantin) may be administered if potassium administration is unsuccessful or if hyperkalemia develops. Intravenous administration of 250 mg (not exceeding 50 mg/min) may restore the membrane potential of the myocardium if digitalis is responsible for the arrhythmia. If a high degree of AV block is present with an extremely slow ventricular response, intravenous administration of potassium chloride may be hazardous. In these circumstances observation and possible pacemaker insertion may be necessary.

Obviously, the continued use of digitalis is absolutely contraindicated in those cases where a history of prior digitalis administration has been obtained. This point again serves to emphasize the importance of differentiating this arrhythmia from atrial flutter where continued digitalis administration would be the treatment of choice.

SUBJUNCTIONAL TACHYCARDIA
Ventricular tachycardia and fibrillation

Clinical presentation. As stated previously, ventricular tachycardia and especially ventricular fibrillation are medical emergencies requiring immediate attention. These conditions are hardly ever seen as the primary cardiac disorder but are near-ly always related to some underlying pathologic process, such as acute myocardial infarction, pulmonary embolus, or severe congestive heart failure. Rarely, ventricular tachycardia may occur in healthy, young adults without associated heart disease; these instances are indeed uncommon. The clinical presentation of ventricular tachycardia or fibrillation is a dramatic event. These patients are most often unconscious, cyanotic, and without effective pulse or spontaneous respirations. In the case of ventricular fibrillation a full-blown cardiac arrest is clearly at hand, and in most cases of ventricular tachycardia, the clinical picture is no less critical. Despite the presence of organized electric ventricular complexes, little to no effective cardiac output is achieved. These malignant forms of ventricular tachycardia are no better tolerated than is ventricular fibrillation.

ECG recognition. A diagnosis of life-threatening ventricular arrhythmia in the setting of cardiac arrest should be fairly obvious. An example of ventricular fibrillation is shown in Fig. 27-5. The tracing is characterized by fine or occasionally coarse fibrillatory waves without identifiable QRS complexes. Recognition of these undulations is extremely important, since this condition must be differentiated from complete asystole of the heart, which may also be the source of a cardiac arrest.

Differential diagnosis. The more organized, less malignant forms of ventricular tachycardia may be somewhat difficult to differentiate from supraventricular tachycardia with wide QRS complexes. The latter condition exists when underlying disease of the conduction system, such as right or left bundle branch block, is present. Further, it may be tolerated to a remarkable degree despite the ominous appearance of the electrocardiographic pattern. Conversely, ventricular tachycardia is a far more critical event and is likely to require emergency cardiopulmonary

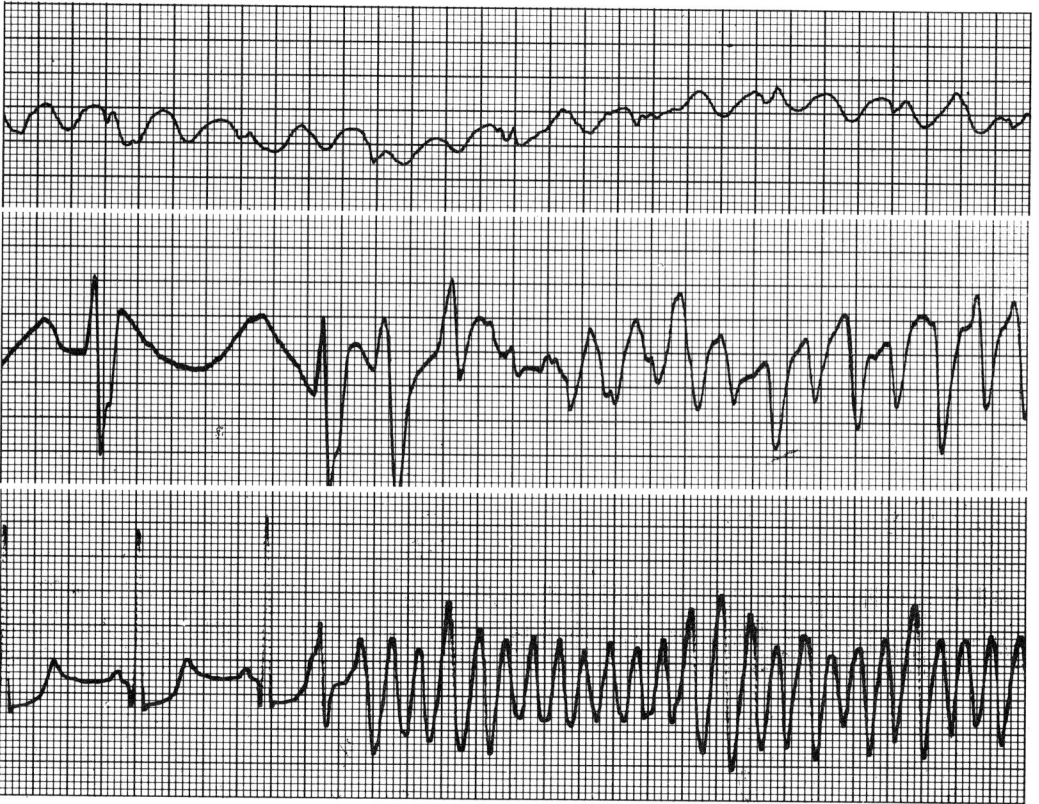

Fig. 27-5. Ventricular fibrillation. (From Conover, M. H.: Cardiac arrhythmias: exercises in pattern interpretation, St. Louis, 1974, The C. V. Mosby Co.)

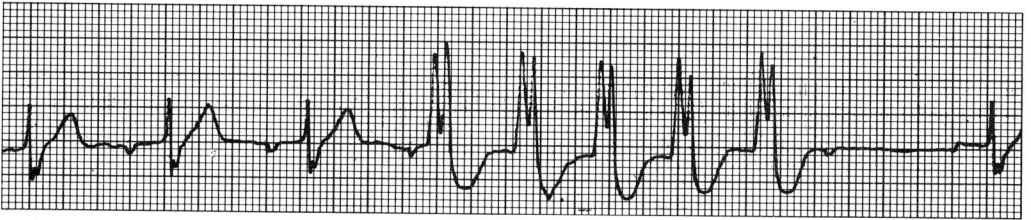

Fig. 27-6. Ventricular tachycardia with AV dissociation. (From Conover, M. H.: Cardiac arrhythmias: exercises in pattern interpretation, St. Louis, 1974, The C. V. Mosby Co.)

resuscitation. Although specific differentiation of these two arrhythmias may require some expertise, the following differential points are worth noting.

    1. In the case of ventricular tachycardia, there is often atrioventricular dissoci-

ation so that independent P waves (atrial rate) are seen superimposed on and often marching through the bizarre ventricular complexes (Fig. 27-6).

    2. Fusion beats (beats that are partially

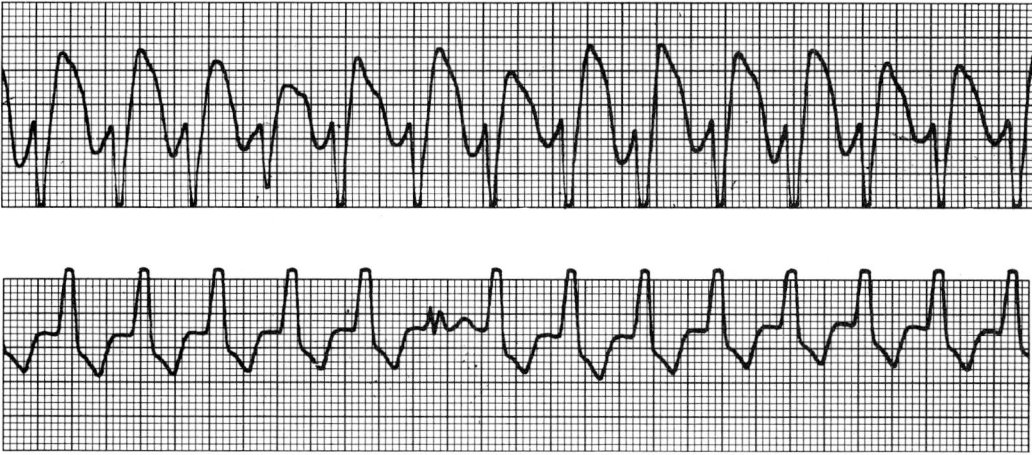

Fig. 27-7. Ventricular tachycardia with fusion beats. (From Conover, M. H.: Cardiac arrhythmias: exercises in pattern interpretation, St. Louis, 1974, The C. V. Mosby Co.)

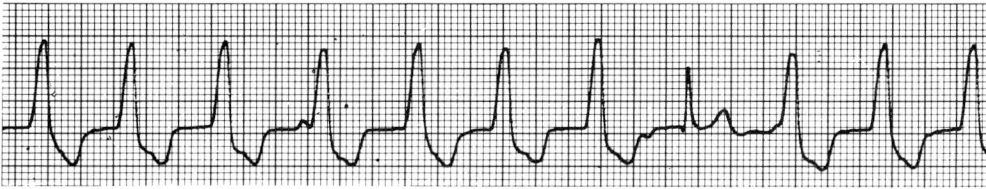

Fig. 27-8. Ventricular tachycardia with Dressler beats. (From Conover, M. H.: Cardiac arrhythmias: exercises in pattern interpretation, St. Louis, 1974, The C. V. Mosby Co.)

conducted and partially ectopic) may be observed with ventricular tachycardia (Fig. 27-7).

3. The fortuitous presence of captured beats with normal QRS duration should make the diagnosis of ventricular tachycardia reasonably secure, especially if these beats occur early in the cycle length (Fig. 27-8).

4. The availability of old electrocardiograms to confirm the premorbid QRS morphology is most helpful in differentiating ventricular tachycardia from supraventricular tachycardia with aberrant conduction.

Management. Emergency therapy for ventricular arrhythmia should be tempered somewhat by the clinical state of the patient. In the case of ventricular fibrillation, immediate defibrillation using 300 to 400 watt-seconds of direct current countershock across the left precordium should be administered as soon as possible. Simultaneous cardiopulmonary resuscitation should have already begun. If defibrillation has not been successful, 1 ml of epinephrine (1:1000) diluted to 10 ml is given intravenously as a bolus, and the countershock is repeated. Several attempts at defibrillation may be required to restore a supraventricular focus. The success or failure of this procedure will in large measure depend on the time elapsed prior to cardiopulmonary resuscitation as well as the level of hypoxemia and acidosis already incurred. The ability of emergency personnel to ventilate and perfuse the patient during the interval when no effective cardiac contractions are present will ultimately determine the outcome of attempted defibrillation.

Much of what has been said regarding ventricular fibrillation also applies to ventricular tachycardia. The situation here may be somewhat less critical, especially when a palpable pulse or blood pressure can be obtained. Frequently, however, the two conditions are indistinguishable. Immediate defibrillation should be performed on the unconscious patient. Lidocaine, 50 to 100 mg, or procainamide, 150 to 200 mg, may be given intravenously if time allows. As with ventricular fibrillation, repeated attempts at defibrillation may be necessary depending on the time elapsed and the level of acidosis. Intravenous administration of epinephrine is usually not helpful and may in fact be deleterious once ventricular tachycardia is established.

Not all individuals with ventricular tachycardia are in a state of cardiovascular collapse. Therapy may have to be tempered, since a normal level of consciousness may preclude immediate defibrillation. Intravenous administration of lidocaine, 50 to 100 mg given as a bolus, may abruptly abort the arrhythmia with conversion to a supraventricular focus. Similarly, procainamide, 150 to 250 mg IV, has proved to be extremely effective in terminating these arrhythmias; however, prolonged hypotension from procainamide may be a problem. Second line drugs such as phenytoin (Dilantin) or propranolol (Inderal) should be utilized only by experienced personnel familiar with their use. If none of these measures succeeds in restoring a more acceptable rhythm and the patient shows progressive signs of cardiac deterioration, elective cardioversion synchronizing the countershock to the patient's QRS complexes should be performed under light

intravenous analgesia. It is prudent to have an anesthesiologist available during this procedure. Some form of suppressant medication should be given prior to attempted countershock in order to stabilize the postconversion rhythm.

BRADYARRHYTHMIAS

The bradyarrhythmias represent a significant percentage of those rhythm disturbances requiring emergency care. Two major categories of bradyarrhythmia necessitate further clarification. The first, sinus bradycardia, is very common in young adults and under most circumstances should never be considered abnormal. Sinus bradycardia in older individuals, however, may represent disease of the sinus node and supraventricular conduction system often leading to intermittent syncopal episodes or, in the more chronic cases, to congestive heart failure.

Sinus bradycardia

ECG recognition. The diagnosis of sinus bradycardia is based on a sustained heart rate of less than 60 beats per minute. Distinct sinus P waves are present, which also maintain a 1:1 relationship with the QRS complexes. Often a phasic irregularity of the basic rhythm known as sinus arrhythmia may correlate with respirations. Occasionally, in the more chronic cases, "dropped beats" are seen with sinus bradycardia. This finding usually implicates some degree of sinus node dysfunction characterized either by exit block where an impulse fails to emerge from the sinus node or by complete sinus arrest where failure of sinus node depolarization occurs. In both instances a sinus P wave is not inscribed and "long pauses" are seen on the electrocardiographic tracing (Fig. 27-9).

Management. Long-term therapy for symptomatic sinus bradycardia is limited. Older patients with underlying cardiac and vascular disease usually do not tol-

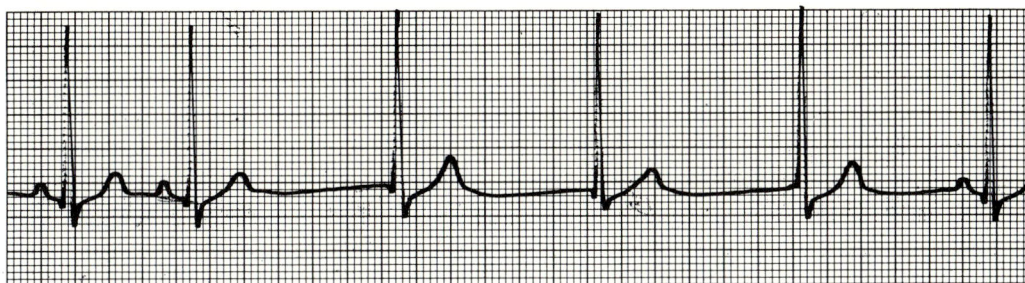

Fig. 27-9. Sinus bradycardia with sinus arrest. (From Conover, M. H.: Cardiac arrhythmias: exercises in pattern interpretation, St. Louis, 1974, The C. V. Mosby Co.)

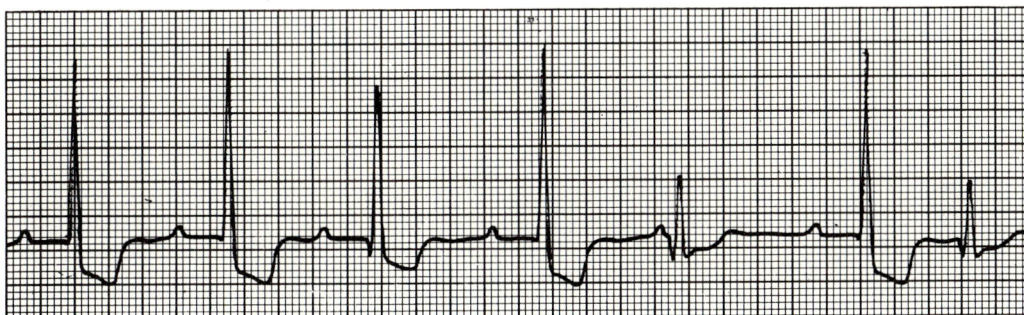

Fig. 27-10. First-degree heart block. (From Conover, M. H.: Cardiac arrhythmias: exercises in pattern interpretation, St. Louis, 1974, The C. V. Mosby Co.)

erate the slow rate for very long. Congestive failure, syncope, and frank Adams-Stokes attacks are common. Implantation of a permanent cardiac pacemaker remains the sole form of effective therapy over any extended period of time. Temporizing measures such as administration of atropine sulfate or sublingual administration of isoproterenol have not proved to be very helpful in the long run. Occasionally the disorder is nonprogressive, and these patients may be followed closely without specific therapy.

Heart block

Clinical presentation. The second category of bradyarrhythmia always implies some degree of abnormal function in the cardiac conduction system and is never seen in the absence of organic disease. The range of disorders manifesting as heart block is considerable, including myocardial infarction, myocarditis, myocardiopathy, infiltrative cardiovascular diseases, digitalis administration, and, most commonly, degenerative disease of the cardiac conduction system seen with advancing age. Heart block may be further broken down into the complete and incomplete forms.

Incomplete

ECG recognition. Most instances of incomplete heart block, although clinically significant, are not primarily responsible for the presenting symptom complex. The most benign form, "first degree block," is simple prolongation of the AV conduction time (PR interval), often seen with digitalis administration (Fig. 27-10). Progressive compromise of the AV conduction system may produce second-degree heart block, characterized by failure of conduction through the AV node of one or more ventricular complexes. All gradations of this form of block may be seen from an occasional dropped beat every four to five complexes to a fixed form of 2:1 or even 3:1 block (Fig. 27-11). As long as some conduction still exists, the term incomplete or second-degree heart block is applicable. Clinical symptoms depend entirely upon the effective cardiac rate.

Complete

Clinical presentation. Complete heart block is by far the most significant of the bradyarrhythmias, especially as it relates to emergency department care. In its acute form, complete block is likely to be seen as a sudden syncopal episode. In the more chronic cases, congestive heart failure with or without syncope is more typical. As with the incomplete forms of heart block, underlying heart disease is always present, and is usually severe. Digitalis intoxication, recurrent myocardial infarction, and degenerative disease of advancing age are probably the three most common causes of complete heart block. Clinical findings may range from none whatsoever to impending circulatory collapse. A characteristic clue on cardiac auscultation is the presence of a regular rhythm, which may

range from below 30 beats per minute to as high as 70 or 80 beats per minute. Typically, the first heart sound will vary in intensity despite the regularity of the rhythm, thus suggesting atrioventricular dissociation. A third and fourth heart sound may also be heard intermittently, again implying the presence of independent atrial contractions superimposed upon an otherwise regular ventricular rhythm.

ECG recognition. The definitive diagnosis of complete heart block is made on the electrocardiogram (Fig. 27-12). Definition stems from demonstration of ventricular complexes that are perfectly regular, having no temporal relationship to a superimposed, independent atrial rhythm. Since AV dissociation may be seen in other conditions (such as ventricular tachycardia), a failure of atrioventricular conduction must also be demonstrated. A helpful clue in distinguishing complete heart block from the incomplete form is noting the absolute regularity of the ventricular rhythm. If the latter appears to be even slightly irregular with occasional early beats, it is likely that intermittent AV conduction is taking place, inferring incomplete block with occasional captured beats.

The QRS complexes in the complete forms of heart block may be narrow or wide depending on level of block and location of the responsible pacemaker. Narrow

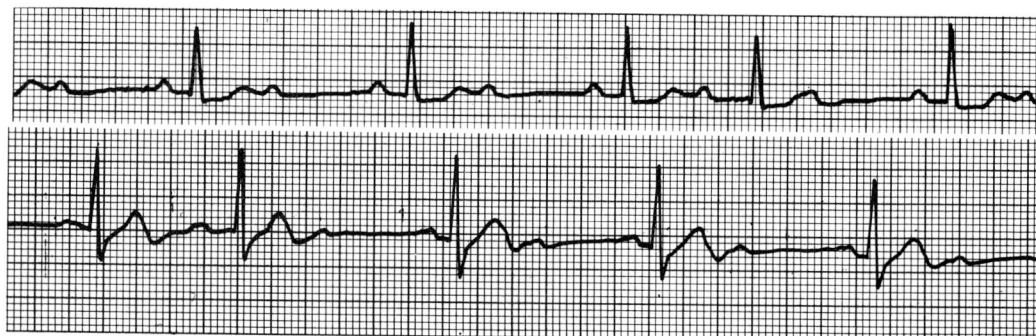

Fig. 27-11. Second-degree heart block with Wenckebach 3:2, 2:1. (From Conover, M. H.: Cardiac arrhythmias: exercises in pattern interpretation, St. Louis, 1974, The C. V. Mosby Co.)

complex block usually has a far better prognosis and suggests that the primary pacemaker is relatively high in the ventricular conduction system. Conversely, complete heart block with widened QRS complexes is extremely ominous and carries a poor prognosis despite aggressive therapeutic intervention.

Management. As with the incomplete forms of heart block, therapy will ultimately depend on the effective heart rate. Immediate implantation of a temporary transvenous pacemaker is preferable when a critically slow ventricular rate is accompanied by signs of cardiovascular embarrassment. This technique may be performed in the emergency department by experienced personnel; however, cardiac fluoroscopy should be available nearby. In those instances where emergency pacemaker facilities are not immediately available, 1 mg of isoproterenol (Isuprel) diluted in 500 ml of dextrose solution administered at a rate of 20 to 40 drops per minute may serve to transiently restore some level of AV conduction. Isoproterenol has also been shown to improve conduction and to increase the rate of any existing pacemaker. Therefore, the drug may be very effective in supporting the patient en route to the catheterization laboratory or x-ray suite where transvenous pacing can be properly performed.

In those forms of complete heart block with widened QRS complexes and significant hemodynamic compromise, it is likely that *permanent* transvenous or epicardial pacing will be required. In these instances the identical routine should be carried out as described above, and arrangements for permanent pacemaker therapy can be made on an elective basis.

SUMMARY

The clinical presentation, ECG recognition, and routine modes of management have been outlined for the more commonly seen cardiac arrhythmias likely to present for emergency department care. An attempt has been made to further classify these arrhythmias according to rate and site of origin. The tachycardias refer to those rhythm disturbances of greater than 100 beats per minute, while bradycardia includes any rhythm of less than 60 beats per minute. The terms supraventricular and ventricular are used to further pinpoint the site and nature of a tachycardia. Bradycardia is nearly always seen as a consequence of block or slowing at the AV or sinus node mechanism.

The key to arrhythmia management is always recognition. In most instances, this is done by careful analysis of the ECG tracing. Once a diagnosis is confirmed, therapeutic alternatives should follow routinely. Hopefully, through thoughtful analysis and judicious use of available therapies, emergency department personnel can treat many of the frequently seen cardiac dysrhythmias, thus avoiding more costly utilization of hospital facilities.

Since a complete discussion of the electrophysiology as well as recognition and

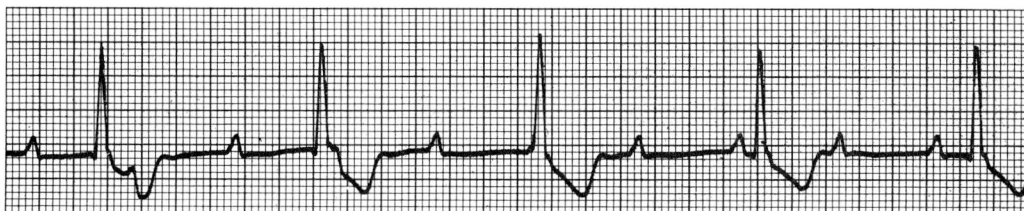

Fig. 27-12. Complete heart block. (From Conover, M. H.: Cardiac arrhythmias: exercises in pattern interpretation, St. Louis, 1974, The C. V. Mosby Co.)

treatment of the more subtle and difficult arrhythmias is beyond the scope of this presentation, the reader is referred to the several standard texts on the subject.

REFERENCES

1. Friedberg, C. K.: Diseases of the heart, Philadelphia, 1966, W. B. Saunders Co., pp. 483-628.
2. Hurst, J. W., and Logue, R. B.: The heart, arteries and veins, ed. 2, New York, 1974, Blakiston Co.

ADDITIONAL READINGS

Goodman, L. S., and Gilman, A.: Pharmacological basis of therapeutics, ed. 4, New York, 1970, Macmillan Publishing Co., chapter 21.

Kistin, A. D.: Problems in the differentiation of ventricular arrhythmias from supraventricular arrhythmia with abnormal QRS, Prog. Cardiovas. Dis. 9:1-66, 1966.

Dreifus, L. S., Watanabe, Y., Haiat, R., and Kimbiris, D.: Atrial ventricular block, Am. J. Cardiol. 28:371, 1971.

Marriott, H.: Practical electrocardiology, ed. 5, Baltimore, 1972, The Williams & Wilkins Co.

Clinical Aspects of Arrythmias—Symposium, Parts I and II, Prog. Cardiovasc. Dis. 16:439, 1975.

CHAPTER 28

Life support* in emergency departments

Mary Maude Winter, R.N.

Each year as a result of myocardial infarction, half a million Americans die suddenly. Sixty percent of these deaths occur before the patient can reach a hospital. Many of these deaths could have been prevented by initiating cardiopulmonary resuscitation (CPR). There are thousands of other victims of unexpected death resulting from automobile accidents, electrocutions, anaphylactic shock, and the like. With this huge toll of preventable "sudden death" victims it becomes imperative that every able-bodied person be trained in basic life support (CPR). When the victim arrives in the emergency department, he or she may be receiving basic life support or may succumb shortly after arrival. Emergency personnel of every acute hospital should be able to respond immediately and efficiently to these situations.

---

*"Life support" is the term preferred to describe the entire procedure of returning people from sudden death to responsible life. Cardiopulmonary resuscitation (CPR) is only one of the techniques involved in life support.

The information in the chapter is based on policies and procedures developed by the American Heart Association and the standards set forth by the 1973 National Conference on CPR of the American Heart Association and the American Red Cross and is consistent with the 1974 AHA guidelines.

There are two types of life support: basic and advanced. *Basic life support* is an emergency first aid procedure that incorporates the ability to recognize respiratory and cardiac arrest and to apply adequate cardiopulmonary resuscitation. Basic life support must be instituted within seconds to prevent biologic death.

Advanced life support includes basic life support plus cardiac monitoring, intravenous infusions, use of airway adjuncts, drug administration, defibrillation, and establishment of such postresuscitative care as is deemed necessary. Advanced life support requires medical direction and adequate facilities.

Although these life support measures only recently have been accepted as proper treatment of sudden death, the first successful resuscitation occurred in 1901. It was not until the inception of acute care units in 1961 that the ability to perform cardiopulmonary resuscitation became a requirement for all medical and hospital personnel and came into widespread use.

SUDDEN DEATH

Sudden death occurs abruptly and unexpectedly. There are two stages.

Clinical death. The cells of the brain

metabolize aerobically. Should delivery of oxygen to the brain cease for longer than four to six minutes in the adult, as in ventilatory or circulatory failure, the brain cells are irreversibly damaged. (The brain cells of infants and children are more resilient and may remain viable for up to 20 minutes in the absence of oxygen.) The four- to six-minute period following cessation of effective ventilation and circulation is called *clinical death*. The individual appears dead, yet reversal of all morbid symptoms is possible if delivery of oxygen is instituted before four to six minutes have elapsed. Clinical death is reversible.

Biologic death. The second stage of death is irreversible. It exists when such changes have taken place in the brain cells that their function cannot return. Other tissues in the body, such as heart, lungs, liver, and kidneys, can metabolize anaerobically for 15 minutes or longer after biologic death has occurred. With resuscitative efforts the heart and respiratory functions may return, but not conscious, voluntary cerebral function. Following biologic death the victim may survive for many days or months without hope of recovery.

The physiology of sudden death and its treatment may be better understood by considering the sequelae to ventilatory and circulatory failure.

Failure of ventilation

When respirations cease, there is no exchange of gases between the lungs and the bloodstream. Carbon dioxide accumulates, producing respiratory acidosis; oxygen is not supplied, the tissues become hypoxic, anaerobic metabolism commences, and lactic acidosis results. Response to this loss of vital function is immediate. There is strong activation of the nervous system, resulting in restlessness, increased pulse and respiration, and peripheral vascular constriction—all aimed at preserving the oxygen supply to the brain. When affected by hypoxia and acidosis, the heart is unable to function normally, resulting in arrhythmias, which reduce effective blood circulation. Initially, arrhythmias may simply impair the pumping action of the heart, but if these persist or are severe enough, they can cause total cessation of cardiac action. Thus the ultimate result of cessation of oxygen interchange in respiratory or ventilatory arrest is cardiac arrest.

Ventilatory failure often results from the depression of respiratory centers in the brain. Precipitating causes of respiratory center depression include anesthesia, sedation, drugs, electric shock, and inappropriate oxygen administration to individuals who have chronic lung disease.

Other factors that may interfere with the effective exchange of oxygen and carbon dioxide include airway obstruction caused by a foreign body in the tracheobronchial tree, airway obstruction by laryngospasm, which can be induced by many factors, and drowning and other causes of asphyxia.

Circulatory failure

Cessation of effective pumping action of the heart prevents adequate perfusion of the tissues since cardiac output is reduced. If there is disruption of the heart's rhythmic, electric activity (which precedes mechanical contraction) and a severe arrhythmia ensues, effective pumping action of the heart will be impaired or may cease entirely, resulting in cardiac arrest.

MECHANISMS OF CARDIAC ARREST

The three common mechanisms of cardiac arrest are ventricular standstill, ventricular fibrillation, and cardiovascular collapse.

Ventricular standstill

In ventricular standstill there is no electric activity and, hence, no mechanical contraction. This is seen on an ECG by the absence of all but a straight, undisturbed line.

Multiple factors may precipitate standstill, but there are three most commonly encountered (Fig. 28-1):

1. Parasympathetic activity: increased vagal activity precipitates suppression of the SA node, reducing heart rate. Excessive discharge from the vagus nerve can produce standstill if no subsidiary pacemaker takes over from the SA node. Vagal stimulation may proceed from irritation of the nasopharynx (perhaps with a nasogastric tube), compression of the carotid artery, or from deep pain.
2. Disease of the conduction system of the heart will produce slowing of transmission of the electric impulse, probably producing very slow rhythms, which may end in ventricular standstill.
3. Drug excess or electrolyte imbalance (e.g., hyperkalemia) may initiate standstill.

Ventricular fibrillation

In ventricular fibrillation (Fig. 28-2) the depolarization, or electric activity, in the ventricle is totally disorganized so that different areas of the ventricular myocardium are depolarized at different times. Therefore, the mechanical ability is disturbed and contractions of the heart cannot occur.

The following are some of the more common causes of this abnormality:

1. Heart disease, particularly acute myocardial infarction
2. Digitalis or quinidine intoxication
3. Hypoxia
4. Electrocution
5. Electrolyte disturbances such as hypokalemia (which may occur from excessive use of diuretics, particularly in conjunction with digitalis)

Cardiovascular collapse

Cardiovascular collapse (Fig. 28-3), which has been called "electromechanical dissociation," manifests itself as profound shock. Essentially, there is inadequate blood flow to perfuse the tissues. When blood flow decreases and the body is unable to compensate and so preserve the vital structures, the brain becomes hypoxic and death may result.

There are three main categories of disorders that may herald cardiovascular collapse.

The first is *cardiogenic shock*. Here, the

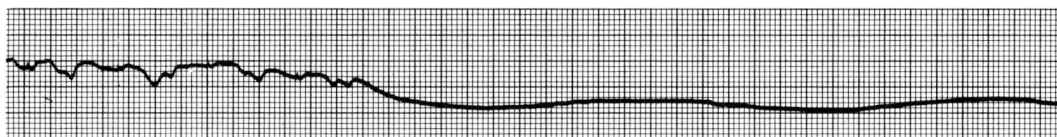

Fig. 28-1. Cardiovascular collapse going into ventricular standstill.

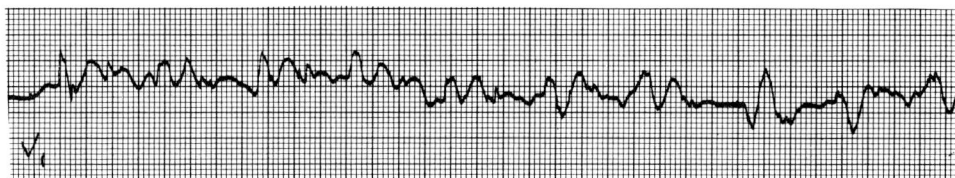

Fig. 28-2. Ventricular fibrillation.

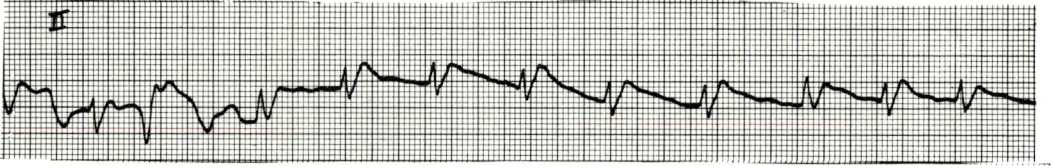

Fig. 28-3. Cardiovascular collapse, electromechanical dissociation. This rhythm is usually of low amplitude on ECG; it may have a different configuration from that shown above, but the carotid pulse inadequacy will verify diagnosis.

heart is diseased and cannot produce sufficient contractile force to pump effectively. The solution is to improve the heart's function.

The second is an *inadequate circulating blood volume.* This could be caused by hemorrhage, dehydration, vomiting, diarrhea, and the like. A perfusion pressure cannot be maintained, and hypovolemic shock results. The solution to this problem is to replace circulating blood volume.

The last category is *reduction of peripheral resistance.* The resistance, or tone, of the blood vessels diminishes, allowing pooling of blood in the periphery so that the volume of blood circulating is insufficient to create an adequate perfusion pressure. This has been called vasomotor collapse and, usually, is transient. However, occasionally gram-negative organisms elaborate an endotoxin that interferes with the resistance of the peripheral vessels and produces this phenomenon.

Prevention of arrest

Cardiac arrest rarely occurs unheralded. To prevent sudden death, medical personnel should follow these guidelines:

1. Become acquainted with the warning signs of impending myocardial infarction
2. Avoid excessive sedation
3. Watch carefully for signs of digitalis intoxication in patients taking digitalis and diuretics that may lead to hypokalemia
4. Promptly treat arrhythmias that predispose the patient to cardiac arrest

LIFE SUPPORT—MANAGEMENT OF ARREST

Some of the mechanisms that may produce failure of ventilation or circulation have been discussed. Although the reasons for the arrest may not be recognized immediately, it is essential that the initial diagnosis of cessation of vital function be made promptly. An estimated four to six minutes are available before biologic death occurs. It is necessary, therefore, in adults, to institute resuscitative measures within *three to four minutes;* otherwise, effective restoration to responsible life may not be possible. Children can sustain longer periods of deprivation of oxygen than can adults. Restoration of normal function can occur even when ten minutes have elapsed between the moment of the child's arrest and the commencement of resuscitation.

Diagnosis

Respiratory inadequacy may be caused by obstruction of the airway or respiratory failure. An obstructed airway can be recognized by noisy, labored breathing and excessive respiratory efforts. Respiratory failure is characterized by minimal or absent respiratory effort, failure of the chest to move, and inability to detect air movement through nose or mouth. If only breathing is inadequate or absent, rescue breathing may be all that is necessary to restore the patient.

Opening the airway and restoring breathing are the basic steps of artificial ventilation and should be applied initially in emergency resuscitation.

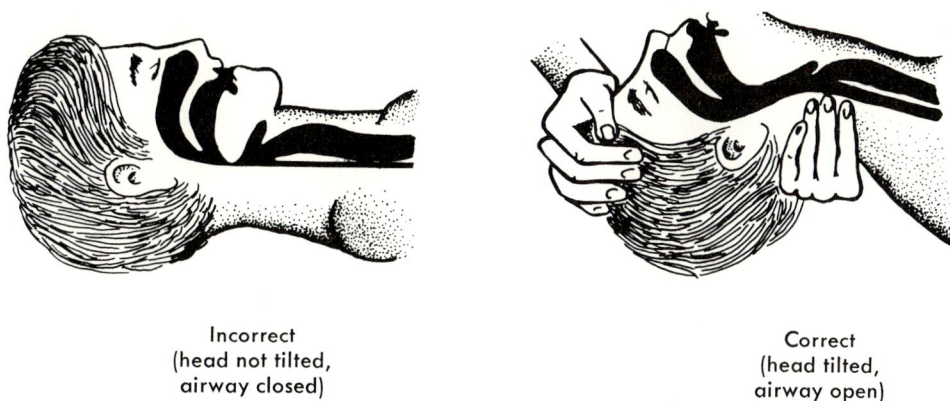

Incorrect
(head not tilted,
airway closed)

Correct
(head tilted,
airway open)

Fig. 28-4. Hyperextension of neck to open airway for successful resuscitation.

Airway

The first step in successsful resuscitation is to open the airway. This is done easily and quickly by hyperextending the head as far as possible. The person is positioned on his or her back and the rescuer places one hand under the neck and the other on the person's forehead. The rescuer then lifts the neck and tilts the head backward. This hyperextension of the neck (Fig. 28-4) lifts the tongue away from the back of the throat, thus relieving this anatomic obstruction. The head should be maintained in this position at all times. Should there be obvious foreign material in the throat, remove this immediately with the fingers. The first ventilatory effort will determine whether further obstruction exists. If maximum extension of the head fails to adequately open the airway, *forward displacement of the jaw* may achieve the necessary patency.

Breathing

If, after the airway has been opened, the person does not resume spontaneous breathing, begin artificial ventilation by mouth-to-mouth or mouth-to-nose resuscitation.

Mouth-to-mouth resuscitation. Mouth-to-mouth artificial ventilation is an effective means of providing needed oxygen. The body only extracts about a quarter of the oxygen inhaled from the ambient air, which leaves about 16% oxygen content in exhaled air. When performing artificial ventilation, the rescuer takes a deep breath and may provide the victim with as much as 18% oxygen. This concentration of oxygen is entirely adequate. Make no attempt to remove firmly fitting dentures; they will help to provide an airtight seal. If dentures are loose, remove them.

After achieving an airway with exaggerated neck extension, take a deep breath, make an *airtight seal* by pinching the victim's nose, place your mouth closely over the victim's mouth, and exhale deeply and quickly. If desired, a thin layer of gauze or a handkerchief may be used to cover the victim's mouth; this will not interfere with the oxygen input. Initially, give four deep breaths. In between breaths remove your mouth and allow the victim to exhale passively. After the initial four breaths, give *one* ventilation every five seconds—approximately 12 times per minute—until spontaneous breathing resumes.

Adequate ventilation is ensured by seeing the chest rise and fall, noting the resistance of the lungs as they expand, and hearing or feeling air escape during exhalation (Fig. 28-5, *A* and *B*).

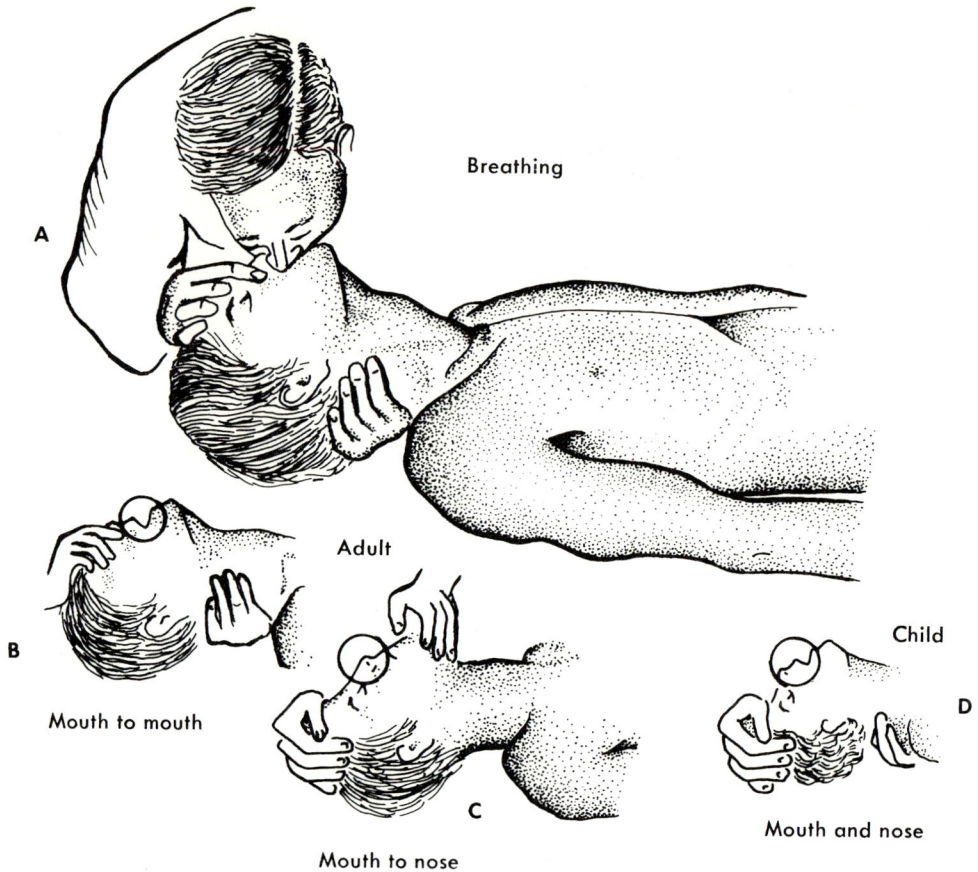

Fig. 28-5. Mouth-to-mouth and mouth-to-nose resuscitation. Note position of hands.

Mouth-to-nose ventilation. Mouth-to-nose ventilation may be used if it is impossible to open the mouth, if the mouth is seriously injured, if it is difficult to achieve a tight seal, or if for some other reason the rescuer prefers the nasal route. For this technique maintain the hyperextension of the neck by pressing one hand on the victim's forehead and using the other to lift the lower jaw and to seal the lips. The same method is used for breathing except that the rescuer's lips are sealed around the person's nose. It may be necessary to open the victim's mouth during exhalation to allow air to escape. Repeat this mouth-to-nose breathing cycle every three to five seconds (Fig. 28-5, *C*).

Foreign bodies. If adequate ventilation is not achieved in spite of hyperextension of the head and a good air seal around the nose or mouth, then persistent airway obstruction can be assumed. Roll the victim on his or her side toward you. Deliver sharp blows with the heel of your hand between the victim's shoulder blades. Then, again attempt to clear the mouth and upper airway with your fingers. The victim should be rolled back immediately and rescue breathing resumed. It may be necessary to repeat this maneuver several times. Endotracheal intubation may not be possible if there is upper airway obstruction.

The Heimlich procedure. Another maneuver that may be used in the event of inhaled foreign bodies is the Heimlich procedure.[1] If food or other inhaled material blocks the larynx or trachea, the victim becomes unable to speak or to breathe and, unless the obstruction is relieved, will die in a few minutes. Each year in the United States several thousand deaths are attributed to choking. The Heimlich procedure, named after its originator, was introduced in 1974 as a way to relieve sudden obstruction of the airway caused by inhaling foreign material. The principle involved is simple. A sudden increase in intrathoracic pressure is created by upward pressure on the diaphragm; the increase in pressure tends to expel the inhaled material.

The procedure may be performed standing or with the victim supine. When standing, the attendant, with his arms around the victim's waist from behind, grasps one fist with the other hand and makes a quick, upward and inward thrust into the epigastrium. With the victim supine, the attendant kneels astride the victim's hips, and with both hands presses into the epigastrium. The objects expelled into the mouth have included a variety of foods, pills, and other articles. According to a recent report, this procedure has been remarkably successful. It cannot, however, be recommended as a method of resuscitation. The limitation in all manual methods of resuscitation is the difficulty of maintaining a clear airway and in ensuring adequate ventilation of the lungs. In the absence of equipment, expired air resuscitation remains the procedure of choice.[2]

Near drowning. These patients rarely have water in the lungs, but frequently it is present in the stomach. Should the rescuer see water coming from the person's mouth at any time, firm but gentle pressure should be instituted over the epigastrium with the patient's head turned to the side.

Stomach distension. Rescue breathing can cause stomach distension. This is frequently seen in children but is not unusual in adults. It occurs most often when ex-

cessive pressures are used for inflation or if the airway is obstructed. Stomach distension can be dangerous because it may reduce lung volume by elevating the diaphragm, promote regurgitation, and cause vagal tone that may result in bradyarrhythmias after resuscitation. Institute the same technique for relief of distension as for near drowning. In a hospital an endotracheal or nasogastric tube may be inserted depending on the patient's condition and the duration of arrest.

Circulation

When an airway has been established and four breaths delivered the next approach is to check circulation and heart action. This can be done by palpating for the carotid pulse. With the tips of the index and middle fingers of one hand, gently locate the patient's trachea and slide your fingers laterally into the groove between the trachea and the muscles at the side of the neck. If present, the carotid will be felt. The pulse area should be "felt" rather than compressed.

The carotid is the pulse to be checked for several reasons. The peripheral circulation may not be adequate to produce a radial pulse, and except in hospital situations the femoral pulse is often inaccessible, as the person is dressed. The neck area of the carotid pulse is immediately accessible. The carotids are the first arteries to arise from the aorta, and therefore they are more central and frequently will persist when other pulses are no longer palpable. The absence or questionable presence of a carotid pulse is an indication for starting external cardiac compression.

Precordial thump. This maneuver is recommended only in arrest of a monitored patient, or when the arrest is *witnessed* in an unmonitored patient. It is not recommended for children. It is not useful for the anoxic heart, for standstill, or for established ventricular fibrillation.

When an arrest is witnessed in either the

monitored or unmonitored patient, a *single,* quick precordial thump is delivered by raising the fist 6 to 10 inches and delivering a blow to the midsternum. This may restore an effective rhythm in cases of heart block, ventricular tachycardia, or ventricular fibrillation of *recent* onset, that is, within the first 30 to 60 seconds of cardiac arrest.

In the resuscitative procedure the time of delivery of the thump varies. In the monitored patient it is the *initial* maneuver of life support; that is, it is delivered immediately when arrest is diagnosed. In the witnessed arrest of an unmonitored patient an airway is established, breathing commenced, and absence of pulse determined, and then the precordial thump is delivered.

No time should be lost assessing the effect of the precordial thump or in delivering repeated thumps. One is all that is recommended.

External cardiac compression. External cardiac compression *must always* be accompanied by artificial ventilation. For external compression to be effective, the patient must be on a firm surface. The aim is to depress the sternum 1½ to 2 inches so that the heart is compressed between the sternum and the spine. If the patient is in bed, a wide board should be inserted under the chest, but compression should not be delayed while waiting for such a board.

Position yourself to one side of the patient in close contact. Place the long axis of the heel of one hand parallel to and over the long axis of the lower half of the sternum. Great care must be taken not to place the hand over the tip of the sternum. Place the other hand on top of the first with the fingers interlaced. Then moving forward so that the shoulders are directly above the patient's sternum and keeping your arms straight, exert pressure vertically downward to move the lower sternum 1½ to 2 inches in the adult. The compressions should be regular, smooth, and uninter-

rupted, with the moments of relaxation and compression being of equal duration. The hands should not be lifted from the chest during relaxation. The present preferred compression rate is *60 per minute,* which maintains blood flow and allows cardiac refill. With two rescuers, breaths should be interposed every five seconds without any interruption of the rhythm of compression. *The ratio is five compressions to one breath.*

Nothing should interrupt external cardiac compression for longer than five seconds with two exceptions: (1) Endotracheal intubation should *never require interruptions of longer than 15 seconds.* (2) Interruptions of up to 15 seconds may be absolutely necessary when transporting the patient.

A single rescuer must perform both artificial ventilation and compression using a 15:2 ratio. This consists of two very quick lung inflations after every 15 compressions. Because of these interruptions to ventilate the patient, the rescuer must compress at a faster rate—at least 80 compressions per minute—to achieve the actual compression rate of 60 per minute.

Pupils. Pupils should be checked every five minutes during cardiopulmonary resuscitation, since they can indicate that oxygenated blood is reaching the patient's brain. Change in pupil size indicates adequate oxygenation. If pupils remain fixed (do not react to light) and are either constricted or dilated, serious brain damage may have occurred or may be imminent. Age or use of drugs can change normal pupillary reaction; for example, morphine can cause constriction, and atropine dilation, of the pupils.

Checking pulses. The carotid pulse should be palpated periodically during compression to check effectiveness of compression. A pulse should be felt with each compression. Compression should be stopped very briefly after one minute to ascertain if spontaneous effective heartbeat has returned. This should be checked every five minutes after commencing compression.

Complications. Complications can occur from improperly performed external cardiac compression. Even with correct technique, it is inevitable that rib fractures will occur in some patients. Other complications include fracture of the sternum, pneumothorax, hemothorax, lung contusions, laceration of the liver, and fat emboli. However, complications can be minimized by careful observance of correct technique. Remember the following:

1. Never interrupt external cardiac compression for longer than five seconds, except for endotracheal insertion and transportation, as mentioned earlier.
2. Never compress over the xiphoid process, since this can cause laceration of the liver.
3. The heel of the hand should remain in constant contact with the lower half of the sternum, and the rescuer's fingers should never touch the patient's ribs when compressing.
4. Never use sudden or jerky movements to compress the chest.
5. Never compress the abdomen and chest simultaneously.

A maximum sense of urgency should continue throughout the procedure. In arrest the most important aspect in diagnosis is time. Delay in commencing resuscitation is the single most disastrous factor. Arrest of vital function is an *emergency with a time limit of approximately three minutes* in which to commence resuscitation. Results are poor if the full six minutes have elapsed before beginning. Interruptions should be eliminated unless essential to resuscitation. This feeling of urgency should possess the rescuer until spontaneous breathing and a strong palpable pulse have been restored.

There are some circumstances in which external cardiac compression may not be effective. Internal thoracic injuries, cardiac tamponade, or severe emphysema with enlargement and fixation of the rib cage may require measures other than external cardiac massage. In a hospital where necessary skill, equipment, and facilities are available, the physician should open the chest and perform internal cardiac massage while ventilation is being administered. Flail chest may require only mouth-to-mouth resuscitation. If external compression is indicated in a patient with flail chest, it should be instituted with full recognition that further internal injuries may be caused by this maneuver but that it represents the only alternative to sudden death.

Basic life support should be continued until the patient recovers or can be transferred to a hospital and into the care of qualified personnel, or until the pupils have been fixed and dilated for 15 to 30 minutes and the victim has remained deeply unconscious with absence of spontaneous respiration and heart beat.

ADVANCED LIFE SUPPORT

It is essential that the emergency department defibrillator be constantly available and in perfect working order. Personnel should be entirely familiar with the machine. They should check it daily for function and to be certain that the necessary adjunctive equipment is present. Defibrillators that register "stored" energy should be checked at regular and frequent intervals with suitable test equipment to determine the delivered energy.

Upon admission of a patient in cardiac arrest, the first action should be to defibrillate.

If a patient is brought in by ambulance, CPR will have been instituted and continued until defibrillation.

If the patient arrests in the emergency department and two rescuers are available, one obtains an airway and the other prepares to defibrillate immediately. The rationale: 75% of those who arrest are in ventricular fibrillation rather than standstill. The speed with which ventricular fibrillation is terminated has a distinct bearing upon the outcome. A prompt application of electric shock to the fibrillating ventricle can return the patient to normal heartbeat within seconds, often precluding the need for any other cardiopulmonary resuscitative measures.

Precordial shock

There are four common methods of delivering precordial shock:
1. A blow to the chest with closed fist
2. Artificial pacemaker devices
3. Cardioversion
4. Defibrillation

There are two types of machines used for defibrillation: the DC and the AC machine. The DC machine is preferred for the following reasons:

1. It delivers the charge in approximately 0.005 second, thus making it possible to avoid the vulnerable period (cardioversion), whereas the AC machine delivers the charge in 0.25 second, and therefore there is danger of a lag into the vulnerable upsweep of the T wave. *(AC machines cannot be used safely for cardioversion.)*

2. It works with standard cables, whereas the AC requires special cables and can blow fuses.

3. It has low amperage so that myocardium is not as likely to be damaged as with an AC machine with its high amperage.

Cardioversion and defibrillation are not synonymous, and the terms should not be used interchangeably.

Defibrillation

Defibrillation is the treatment for ventricular fibrillation. When electrodes are correctly placed on the chest and the machine is activated, there is an instantaneous discharge of a dense field of current through the heart. This momentarily stops all electric activity in the heart. One hopes that when it starts again, a more acceptable

pacemaker will be in control. Most tachyarrhythmias are believed to be self-perpetuating; thus, interruption of their action stops them.

Procedure

1. The diagnosis selects the patient—an unconscious patient without a palpable pulse or with a picture of ventricular fibrillation on the monitor.

2. The machine should not be synchronized since there is no R wave. Hence, the synchronizer switch must be *off;* otherwise, there will be no delivery of current.

3. Defibrillation should be carried out within 30 seconds, if possible, and before two minutes have lapsed in estimated arrest time.

4. Upon diagnosis, turn on the machine and charge it to 400 watt-seconds while moving to the patient's bedside. Position the defibrillator comfortably close to the patient.

5. If electrode paste is used, prepare paddles by covering the face of them completely with a thin layer. It is not recommended to place paste on the chest since this can be messy or inadequate.

If saline pads are used, be sure they are only damp, not dripping, as this can provide an excellent conductor of electricity; if the chest is made wet, it can dissipate the charge across the outside rather than through the heart. Ready-prepared pads are also on the market, which are merely placed on the patient's chest and the electrodes applied over them.

6. Clean the patient's chest to remove any perspiration.

7. The position of saline pads or electrodes on the chest should be such that the heart is encompassed. The usual position for anterior paddles is just below the right clavicle to the right of the sternum and below the apex of the heart to the left of the midclavicular line.

With anteroposterior paddles the posterior paddle is positioned under the patient's back below the heart, and the anterior paddle is on top of the chest over the heart.

8. A firm pressure on the paddles must be used so that the skin is smoothed out, and skin burning and dissipation of electric current avoided. Once correct position is achieved, pause a moment to see that all is as it should be.

9. *"Everyone stand away from the bed."* This instruction should be given by the person delivering the charge, who should also take care not to touch the bed.

Properly functioning equipment and a complete supply of drugs must be available in the emergency department at all times. This must be checked frequently. The fundamentals of CPR must be thoroughly understood by all personnel. If the first "shock" does not convert the ventricular fibrillation, repeat twice; then go immediately to CPR.

A frequent cause of failure to defibrillate, if the machinery is functioning, is acidosis. It is not possible, as a rule, to convert the acidotic patient (see above).

Cardiac monitoring

The patient, if not already attached to a cardiac monitor, should have electrocardiographic monitoring established as soon as possible. The patient who arrests is particularly vulnerable to cardiac electric instability for several hours following arrest. Personnel performing advanced life support should have received instruction in arrhythmia recognition and treatment, and should have demonstrated their proficiency. It is important that lethal or potentially lethal arrhythmias be terminated quickly. The recognition and treatment of the early warning signs of such arrhythmias can prevent their occurrence.

Cardiac monitoring is so desirable in the arrested person that a monitor-defibrillator with ECG electrode–defibrillator paddles is recommended, since immediately upon contact with the chest, the paddles will detect the cardiac rhythm.

Intravenous therapy

An intravenous route for administration of drugs should be established. This should be accomplished as soon as possible and must be a routine part of the procedure. The intravenous equipment should be firmly taped and capable of withstanding the other arrest procedures (e.g., defibrillation) and not become dislodged from the vein. Consequently, indwelling catheters are much preferred to needles for these infusions. The solution recommended is 5% dextrose and water, which is infused at a rate sufficient to keep the vein patent. All medications to be infused should be hung in tandem to this main line and controlled scrupulously.

Essential drugs

Certain drugs are considered important in an emergency. Some are regarded as useful; others are thought to be essential. The essential drugs include oxygen (see Airway adjuncts), sodium bicarbonate, epinephrine, atropine sulfate, lidocaine, morphine sulfate, and calcium chloride or calcium gluconate.

Sodium bicarbonate. Metabolic acidosis is the first problem demanding correction, and sodium bicarbonate should be given first. In the presence of acidosis the myocardium responds poorly to catecholamines. The early and regular administration of sodium bicarbonate can return the pH to normal and enable the myocardium to respond to the circulating and administered catecholamines. The recommended dosage is as follows: sodium bicarbonate, 1 mEq/kg, from syringes containing 50 ml of an 8.4% solution (50 mEq), should be given immediately. This should be repeated in ten minutes if the patient remains unresponsive. (Example: The patient who weighs 70 kg will receive approximately 70 ml of the above solution initially *and again in 10 minutes.*) In another 10 minutes give *half* the initial dose if patient is still unresponsive.

After these three doses have been given, arterial blood should be drawn for determination of blood pH and base deficit. Metabolic alkalosis from excessive sodium bicarbonate administration should be avoided. If laboratory facilities are not available and the patient remains arrested *after the first two doses* of sodium bicarbonate, half the initial dose should be given every ten minutes until the patient responds.

Epinephrine. Although epinephrine can produce lethal ventricular arrhythmias, it has been shown to be effective in enhancing ventricular fibrillation and thus effectiveness of defibrillation, restoring electric activity in standstill, and improving contractility in electromechanical dissociation.

Epinephrine exerts a strongly positive inotropic effect on the heart, improves automaticity, and elevates perfusion pressure.[3] Because of its dramatic effects, it should be handled with caution. A 1:1,000 solution is available in a 1 ml ampule, and a 1:10,000 solution is available in a ready-to-use syringe. Either 0.5 ml of a 1:1000 or 5.0 ml of a 1:10,000 strength should be given by direct intravenous injection every five minutes during resuscitation. The intracardiac approach is not recommended; it is fraught with danger and, even if efficiently accomplished, is of questionable value.

Atropine sulfate. One of the most valuable drugs available for treating slow rhythms or heart block, particularly when hypotension is present, is atropine. Slow rhythms are often caused by stimulation of the vagus nerve, as mentioned earlier in this chapter. Atropine blocks the action of the vagus nerve and acetylcholine at the cell level, thereby allowing greater sympathetic control and thus increasing the heart rate. A dose of 0.5 mg is given at five-minute intervals to a total dose of 2 mg. If preferred, the entire 2 mg may be given initially. In cardiac arrest it is used to treat standstill and is given directly intravenously. Atropine is relatively contraindicated in the presence of either glaucoma or benign prostatic hypertrophy.

Lidocaine. Lidocaine is a valuable antiarrhythmic agent, which reduces the automaticity of the ventricle by increasing the stimulation threshold of the ventricle. Its effect is immediate and of short duration. When given in therapeutic doses, it neither affects myocardial contractility nor produces hypotension to the same extent as other antiarrhythmic drugs. But it can cause central nervous system irritability and convulsions and may cause hypotension in large doses. Lidocaine is particularly effective in controlling multifocal, premature, ventricular ectopic beats and ventricular tachycardia. It is of no value in standstill and should probably not be used if this catastrophe threatens. It is very useful when repeated successful defibrillation reverts to ventricular fibrillation. Because of its short duration, lidocaine is usually given intravenously as a bolus of 1 to 1.5 mg/kg. This should be followed immediately by intravenous infusion (2 g/500 ml yields 4 mg/ml) of up to 4 mg per minute while ventricular arrhythmias persist. A second bolus of 0.5 to 1.0 mg/kg may be given if the infusion does not sufficiently suppress the arrhythmia. The infusion dosage is then reduced to 1 to 2 mg per minute for the 24 hours following arrest from ventricular fibrillation to prevent further ventricular irritability.

Morphine sulfate. Morphine is not indicated in the cardiopulmonary emergency, but is of the first magnitude in treating pulmonary edema. It is also important for patients with myocardial infarction for the relief of pain. Morphine reduces venous return by vasodilation and reduces anxiety and respiratory rate, all desirable in the patient with pulmonary edema. As little as 2 mg intravenously may dramatically reduce blood pressure and therefore should be the first amount given to test patient response.

Calcium chloride (calcium gluconate).

Calcium increases myocardial contractility, prolongs systole, and increases ventricular automaticity. It is worth noting that sinus impulse formation can be suppressed and sudden death can occur in the fully digitalized patient following intravenous administration of calcium. In profound cardiovascular collapse and in standstill, it is useful. Calcium must not be administered together with sodium bicarbonate, since this mixture results in the precipitation of calcium carbonate. Large doses of calcium, when repeated, may produce dangerous blood levels. Recommended doses are 5 ml of 10% calcium chloride (6.8 mEq calcium) or 10 ml of 10% calcium gluconate (4.5 mEq calcium) intravenously at ten-minute intervals during standstill in the nondigitalized patient.

As with levarterenol (Levophed), care must be taken that calcium does not extravasate since tissue sloughing will result.

Drugs that may be useful are described below.

Levarterenol (Levophed, norepinephrine). This catecholamine is chiefly alpha adrenergic and has been widely used (probably inadvisedly) in all types of shock. It is a potent vasoconstrictor. There are problems with reduced cerebral, cardiac, and renal blood flow with the use of this drug. If it is used, it should be only on a short-term basis because of vasoconstriction and its tendency to sequester plasma in the abdominal organs. Vasodilators and fluid challenge are now preferred in the treatment of many types of shock other than cardiogenic, about which there is no agreement as to treatment.

Dopamine (Intropin). This precursor of norepinephrine stimulates both alpha- and beta-adrenergic sites. In addition, it dilates the renal and mesenteric vasculature via "dopaminergic" (nonadrenergic) receptors. Cardiac output, contractility, and stroke volume are increased with moderate dosage (5 to 30 μg/kg/min). Urine output is increased as a result of increased renal blood flow at dosages up to 30 μg/kg/min. At dosages above 30 μg/kg/min, alpha-adrenergic activity becomes more prominent and may lead to a decrease in renal blood flow and urine formation. Initial dosages of 2 to 5 μg/kg/min are recommended before increasing the dose. Solutions ranging in concentration from 800 to 1600 μg/ml (400 to 800 mg in 500 ml of IV solution) are recommended with close observation for patient response.

Isoproterenol (Isuprel). This beta-adrenergic drug, when given intravenously, is a strong cardiotonic that increases the force of contraction and heart rate dramatically. It is also a vasodilator, but its hypotensive possibilities are offset mostly by its effect on cardiac function. This drug is used in the presence of ventricular standstill and complete heart block. Caution should also be used because it can greatly increase ventricular irritability; in a patient with a tendency to ventricular tachyarrhythmias, isoproterenol probably should not be used. There is some evidence that its use in patients with myocardial infarct is suspect; it can extend the infarct since it significantly increases myocardial oxygen consumption. In conjunction with levarterenol it may be useful in maintaining perfusion of vital organs since it mitigates some of the constrictive effects of levarterenol. Dosages range from 1 to 5 mg/1,000 ml D5W in a microdrip administration set, which must be meticulously monitored, according to heart rate.

Propranolol (Inderal). An antiarrhythmic agent with beta-adrenergic blocking action, this drug is useful in repetitive ventricular arrhythmias where lidocaine is not effective or cannot be used. It is particularly useful when digitalis toxicity is the cause of the ventricular tachyarrhythmia. This drug is relatively contraindicated in heart failure (unless the tachycardia is the cause of heart failure) because of its negative effect on contractility and heart rate. It is also contraindicated in bronchial asthma and in the presence of heart block. Both isoproterenol and glucagon counteract its effects to some extent and can be used if needed. Dosage for propranolol is 1 mg intravenously, but it must be given slowly. *It can be lethal when given intravenously.* The patient must be closely monitored. Repeated doses, if necessary, may be given slowly every five to ten minutes under constant cardiac monitor.

Corticosteroids. Corticosteroids are useful for postresuscitation problems of shock-lung and cerebral edema.

Airway adjuncts

When arrest continues for longer than a few minutes and airway adjuncts are available, they may be used by technicians skilled in their use. Airway adjuncts are not essential for cardiopulmonary resuscitation (Fig. 28-6).

Oxygen. Supplemental oxygen should be used as soon as it becomes available. Be-

cause of the intrapulmonary shunting and ventilation-perfusion abnormalities associated with low cardiac output, marked divergence occurs between alveolar and arterial oxygen tension; hypoxemia and thus metabolic acidosis ensue. These two conditions make resuscitation difficult, if not impossible.

Oropharyngeal airway. An oropharyngeal airway should be inserted whenever a bag-valve-mask or automatic breathing device is used. These airways should be available in all sizes and should be carefully inserted to avoid pushing the tongue back and occluding the airway.

Masks. Masks should be well fitting, transparent, have an inflatable cuff, and be available in one average size for adults and additional sizes for infants and children. Oxygen may be attached if the patient is breathing spontaneously, or mouth-to-tube ventilation can be performed effectively with this device. An

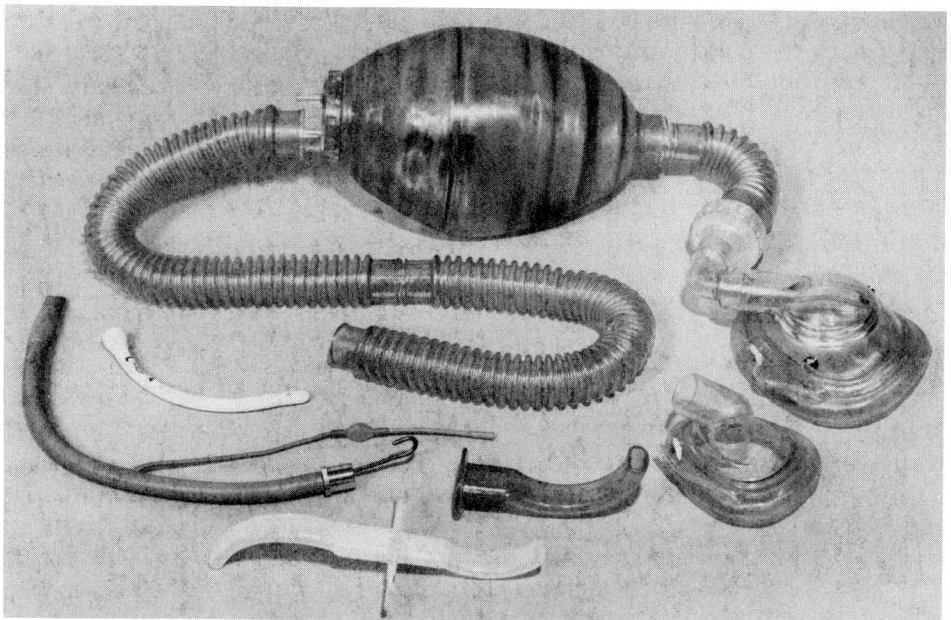

Fig. 28-6. *Top,* Bag-valve-mask device (note transparent plastic). *Left to right,* Endotracheal tube with stylet; nasal airway; oropharyngeal airway with internal metal piece; child's face mask with tube for inflating cuff; S tube oropharyngeal airway.

oropharyngeal airway should be used in conjunction (Fig. 28-7).

Bag-valve-masks. The bag-valve-mask should be used by physicians, nurses, and paramedic personnel who have specific training. This apparatus is difficult to use satisfactorily (deliver adequate ventilatory volumes) by any but highly competent personnel. The bag-valve-mask should be self-refilling and of transparent plastic with an inflatable, contoured, resilient cuff around the mask. It should contain no sponge rubber because of difficulty in cleaning, disinfecting, eliminating ethylene oxide, and fragmentation. It should be available in adult and child sizes. The bag-valve-mask should deliver high concentrations of oxygen via the ancillary oxygen inlet at the back of the bag. *The bag-valve-mask should not be used without oxygen.* The valve should be a true, nonbreathing valve, not a pop-off valve, except in pediatric models.

Endotracheal intubation. Oxgenation via exhaled-air methods or by mask *must always* precede attempts at tracheal intubation.

Gastric distension is associated with high inflation pressures. This distension, by elevating the diaphragm, can impede the ventilatory efforts and can cause regurgitation of gastric contents, leading to aspiration pneumonia. An endotracheal tube can prevent this aspiration and should be inserted by trained personnel as soon as practical. Remember, no more than 15 seconds should interrupt external cardiac compression (ECC) to insert the endotracheal tube. Only this and essential transportation (15 seconds) should interrupt ECC for longer than five seconds. Should the efforts to intubate the trachea continue beyond 15 seconds, the purpose of resuscitation is being defeated. Successful tracheal intubation isolates the airway, keeps it patent, prevents aspiration, and assures delivery of a high concentration of oxygen. Endotracheal tubes should be cuffed, of various sizes, have standard 15 mm fittings, and be provided with a stylet. The endotracheal tube can be conveniently used in conjunction with the bag-valve-mask device. Portable or installed suction equipment or both should be available. There should be multiple sterile suction catheters of various sizes available for advanced life support.

Oxygen-powered mechanical breathing devices. Pressure-cycled automatic resuscitators or IPPB respirators *should not* be used in conjunction with external cardiac compression. The compression triggers termination of the inflation cycle prematurely, and the lungs are never adequately ventilated.

Oxygen-powered, manually triggered (time-cycled) ventilation devices are acceptable if they provide instantaneous flow rates of 100 liters per minute or more for adults. Ideally, these ventilation devices should permit the use of 100% oxygen and manual triggering while the head, jaw, and neck are supported with both hands.

Nasogastric tube. A nasogastric tube should be inserted when gastric distension is a problem, preferably after endotracheal intubation has isolated the airway. Cardiac compression should *not* be interrupted during insertion of a nasogastric tube.

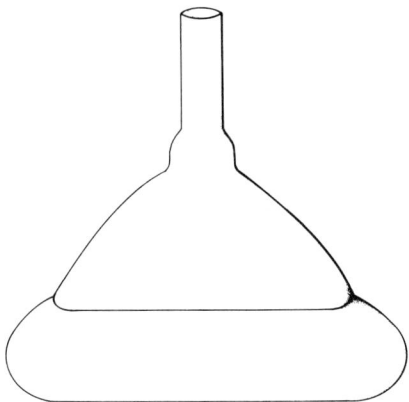

Fig. 28-7. Mask with tube for mouth-to-tube resuscitation (must be used with an oropharyngeal airway).

Bellows-type airway devices. Caution should be exercised with this type of airway adjunct. They are widely advertised but are not satisfactory for delivery of oxygen and, in some instances, are dangerous since they tend to cause the operator to occlude the patient's airway.

VARIATIONS IN CARDIOPULMONARY RESUSCITATION FOR CHILDREN

The ABC's of resuscitation are followed as for an adult:
A. Airway
B. Breathe for patient
C. Compress chest
The technique in each step differs slightly from that used for adults.

Airway

1. Infants and young children should be suctioned, and if a foreign object is lodged in the throat, a finger should be inserted quickly to dislodge and remove it.
2. An oral airway can be helpful because infants are nose breathers, and therefore distress could result from an obstructed septum. The airway also minimizes dead space and provides for easier air exchange by increasing passage.
3. Do not overhyperextend the head since this can obstruct the pliable trachea of an infant.

Breathing

1. Place mouth over both the mouth and nose of the infant (because of the infant's small face) (Fig. 28-5, *D*). Lower inflation pressures must be used for infants and children.
2. *An airtight seal is not necessary;* the breaths should be administered in gentle puffs from rescuer's cheeks.
3. If possible, insert an oxygen tube into the *rescuer's* mouth; enriched air will be of benefit.
4. Watch rise and fall of chest; as in all

ventilatory effort, it should move with each breath.
5. Watch for distension of the abdomen, which is common.
6. Check femoral or carotid pulse.

Chest compression

1. The pressure point in small children and infants is the midsternum; the ventricles are anatomically higher in the chest because of the child's relatively large liver.
2. Use only the fingertips for infants.
3. Use the heel of one hand for young children.
4. A firm surface is necessary.
5. The rescuer may encircle the chest of the infant with the hands and compress with the thumbs.

Rates, pressures, and ratios

Respirations:
   Infants: 25 to 30 breaths per minute.
   Small children: 20 to 30 breaths per minute.
Compression:
   Rate: 120 per minute for infants.
   Force: Compress chest wall ½ to ¾ inch in infants (10 to 15 lbs of pressure); compress ¾ to 1 inch in children up to 6 years (20 to 25 lbs of pressure). Pressure should be just sufficient to palpate a femoral pulse.
With one rescuer:
   Generally, the infant can be cradled in one arm while ventilation and compression at a ratio of 1 ventilation to 5 compressions are performed.
With two rescuers (for children, not infants):
   Five compressions to one breath. Do not do both simultaneously since this can result in pneumothorax.

Other points

In children resuscitative efforts should be continued for a longer time than in adults since recovery has been witnessed after prolonged unconsciousness (up to three hours).

If a foreign body is suspected of occluding the child's airway, use the following procedure:

1. Turn the child upside down over your forearm and deliver a blow between the shoulder blades and quickly resume ventilation.
2. Slip your finger down the child's throat to remove object if a blow on back is unsuccessful.
3. If unable to remove the object, continue to ventilate anyway! Anoxia will cause the larynx to relax, and the foreign body may be removed.

The best position for resuscitation is supine, although a semi-Fowler's position may be tried if the lungs are not inflating. However, the infant should be returned to the supine position as quickly as possible.

SUMMARY
Basic life support: ABC's of resuscitation

1. Diagnose cessation of ventilation.
2. Open and maintain airway by hyperextension of head and neck.
3. Ventilate with four quick, deep breaths.
4. Feel for carotid pulse.
5. If pulse is absent give one quick, precordial thump with the fleshy part of closed fist.
6. Check carotid pulse.
7. If pulse remains absent commence external cardiac compression. Find correct pressure point (lower half of sternum) and place heel of hand on long axis of sternum. Do not lift hands during compression. Do not allow fingers to touch victim's chest. Give 60 compressions per minute: ratio with two rescuers, 5 compressions to 1 breath; with one rescuer, 15 compressions to 2 breaths. Rate of compression: two rescuers, 1 compression per second; with one rescuer, 80 compressions per minute to allow for time lost during ventilation.
8. Check pupils for reaction.
9. *Do not interrupt* external cardiac compression for longer than five seconds.
10. Check carotid pulse regularly for effectiveness.

In hospital—advanced life support

1. Defibrillate as soon as possible.
2. Attach to cardiac monitor.
3. If defibrillation fails continue CPR (basic life support).
4. Obtain an intravenous lifeline.
5. Give sodium bicarbonate and epinephrine (separately, flushing between).
6. Check carotid pulse, monitor, and pupils.
7. Defibrillate.
8. Continue drug administration as indicated to correct acidosis and maintain adequate cardiac rhythm.
9. Continue to evaluate effectiveness by pupil and pulse checks until patient is restored.
10. Use airway devices as indicated.

Post resuscitation

Cerebral edema usually persists for some hours following cardiac arrest. The patient will need careful support and observation to prevent another arrest, to diagnose the cause of the initial arrest, and to determine any complications resulting from resuscitation measures. Intravenous administration of lidocaine to control ventricular arrhythmias and ventilatory support may be required.

Emergency personnel should continually monitor any patient after an arrest:

1. Oxygen administration
2. Pain relief with morphine
3. Atropine for slow rhythms
4. Pulse and blood pressure checks
5. Careful observation for shock (confusion, pallor, sweating, cold skin, oliguria or anuria)

When to stop life support

Basic and advanced life support should be continued until the patient is restored to responsible life or until cerebral death is evidenced by the following:

1. Deep unconsciousness
2. Widely dilated and fixed pupils for a period of 30 minutes
3. Absence of spontaneous ventilation
4. Myocardial death as evidenced by progressive widening and slowing of the QRS complex

Life support *should not be begun* if the patient is in the terminal stages of incurable disease or if he or she cannot be restored to meaningful life. Nor should it be begun if it is known for certain that arrest has been present for more than 10 minutes (except in cases of drowning or in the very young).

NOTE: Any person who enters the emergency department with a history compatible with acute myocardial infarction should not be discharged on the basis of a "normal ECG." Also, enzyme changes may take several hours, and thus initial normal enzyme values cannot rule out an infarct.

REFERENCES

1. Heimlich, H. J., Hoffmann, K. A., and Canestri, F. R.: Food-choking and drowning deaths prevented by external subdiaphragmatic compression, Ann. Thorac. Surg. 20:188-195, 1975.
2. Colebatch, H. J. H.: Personal communication.
3. Meyers, F. H., et al.: Review of Medical Pharmacology, ed. 3, Los Altos, Calif., 1972, Lange Medical Publications.

CHAPTER 29

The acute abdomen

Ronald L. Bouterie, M.D.

Acute abdomen is a frequent diagnosis, yet difficult to define precisely. One can consider this condition in terms of broad categories with various subheadings and divisions that must be painstakingly evaluated. In a diagnostic review by Meng,[1] over 170 clinical entities were listed. Dr. Francis Moore's definition, that the acute abdomen is one that requires an acute decision, is valid. It should go a step further, however, for this complex problem also requires acute judgment.

The examiner who sees such a patient must distinguish those conditions that require surgery from those that do not. It is more important to determine whether or not surgery is necessary than to specifically identify the disease process. This does not mean that efforts should not be made to make the correct diagnosis, since certain entities require very different modes of therapy. When an individual is acutely ill, precious time can be lost with needless and exhaustive special studies that do not add to the ultimate management of the patient. For example, if an individual has right lower quadrant pain very well localized in McBurney's point, with nausea, anorexia, a low-grade temperature, and marked peritoneal irritation, there is very little need for anything more than a very thorough history, physical examination, routine lab-

oratory examination, and appropriate x-ray studies to make the diagnosis of an acute abdomen, most likely appendicitis. The need for further evaluation, such as by a barium enema, is unwarranted and contraindicated if appendicitis is present. However, acute diverticulitis may cause right lower quadrant pain, and acute cholecystitis, pelvic inflammatory disease, and ruptured ovarian cysts have been found when appendicitis was suspected. There are no surgical emergencies that require immediate surgery without an adequate evaluation of the patient, but thoughtless, prolonged diagnostic studies only lead to costly and dangerous procrastination.

The conscientious examiner will listen to the patient's complaints, ask pertinent questions, and will evaluate the entire patient—not just the abdomen. The clues obtained from this firsthand contact will lead to requests for proper laboratory tests and x-ray and special studies that will help the examiner make an "acute decision."

Patients who need surgery have either an inflammatory, obstructing, vascular, or hemorrhagic condition that causes the acute abdominal problem. Trauma may be another cause. The pathologic processes listed above frequently overlap, and traumatic injuries may cause any of the above; similarly, inflammatory diseases obstruct,

431

and obstructing lesions become ischemic and may perforate. Because of this a separate general discussion on symptoms and signs seems appropriate.

SYMPTOMS
Abdominal pain

The pain experienced in the abdomen arises from somatic and visceral pathways. In general, visceral stimuli are produced by an exaggeration of normal reflexes. The more sudden or acute the distension of a viscus, the more severe the pain. Stretching of the capsules of solid organs can cause pain very similar to that of the hollow viscus. These visceral pains are poorly localized, and several organs may produce pain in the same location (Fig. 29-1). Midline abdominal pain is characteristic of intra-abdominal organs, whereas lateral pain is more likely caused by retroperitoneal structures. Duodenal and gallbladder pains are characteristically localized in the epigastrium. Intestinal pain is experienced periumbilically, and large bowel pain, which is not as well localized, is usually experienced in the hypogastrium. When the pain arises from the sigmoid, the patient may

experience suprapubic or presacral discomfort.

The character of visceral pain is cramping and colicky. If colic is present, one must distinguish between biliary, ureteral, and intestinal involvement. The specific workup for each will be discussed later in the chapter.

Somatic pain is caused by stimulation of afferent spinal nerve fibers. These arise from the parietal peritoneum and mesentery and spread along T_6 to L_1 dermatomes. This is sharper and more localized pain. It is related to the position of the inflamed or diseased part. With peritonitis the pain is proportionate to the amount of muscular rigidity present.

Referred pain is a third type of pain experienced in the abdomen. Conditions that are not inflammatory rarely give rise to this type of pain. Typically, it appears in areas that are distant from the primary disease process. The most notable example is irritation of peritoneum underlying the diaphragm causing a spread of pain through the phrenic innervation to produce shoulder pain.

Several generalizations of surgical signifi-

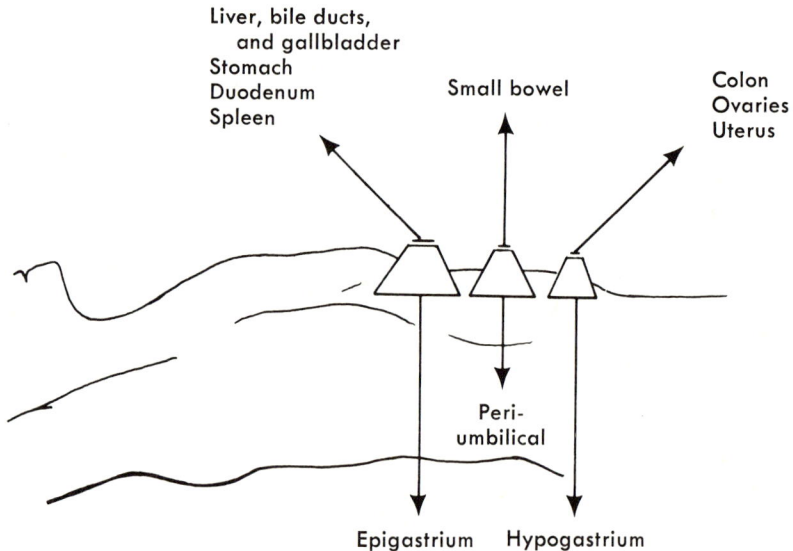

Fig. 29-1. Visceral transmission from large intraabdominal areas to one specific location.

cance can be made. It is rare for abdominal pain to be strictly constant, but if it does persist for six hours or more, the patient has a surgical entity. If pain arises from the distension of a hollow, smooth muscle organ, it tends to be intermittent, whereas pain in relationship to inflammation is more constant. If it awakens the patient from sleep, it most likely has an organic basis.

Anorexia

Anorexia is a vague symptom seen in various organic diseases. Loss of appetite is produced by inflammatory conditions, cancer, hepatitis, uremia, and certain endocrine disorders. But of all the symptoms that have been described for acute appendicitis, anorexia stands out as the most consistent.

Vomiting

Vomiting is associated with central nervous system lesions, visceral stimulation, and direct irritation to the stomach. It frequently is accompanied by autonomic stimulation. The patient appears cold, clammy, and pale and may have an irregular pulse. In general, vomiting without nausea suggests an intracranial lesion; such vomiting is projectile, sudden, and unexpected. Vomiting immediately after eating occurs with uremia or high intestinal obstruction. Therefore, the time of onset of vomiting is very important to elicit. The earlier it occurs in intestinal obstruction, the higher the lesion. Pain precedes vomiting by several hours in acute appendicitis. Severe colic causes vomiting from pain and its intense visceral stimulation as well. The examiner should determine how long the patient has been vomiting and the frequency. Marked losses will cause metabolic derangements and dehydration.

The absence of bile in the vomitus indicates pyloric obstruction. Fecal vomiting is associated with gastrocolic fistulae or long-standing, neglected, intestinal obstruction.

Blood may be present in the vomitus.

Generally, blood is an irritant to the stomach, and its presence causes vomiting. When blood is present in the vomitus, the lesion is usually in the upper gastrointestinal tract, not lower than the duodenojejunal junction. The higher the lesion, however, the more spontaneous the vomiting. For example, a large volume of bright red blood is rapidly regurgitated with esophageal variceal bleeding, whereas blood will accumulate in the stomach from duodenal bleeding long enough for it to be reduced by acids. The characteristic coffee-ground material is then vomited.

Lower bowel function

Constipation can be defined as a delay that is abnormal to the patient's own bowel habits. The stool is usually of insufficient quantity. It is hard and dry because of its abnormal retention with extraction of fluid. Poor bowel habits, lack of bulky foods, and decreased abdominal wall muscular power are frequent causes. However, intrinsic lesions, such as tumors or neurologic defects as with Hirschsprung's disease, are also causes of constipation. For example, a large tumor exerting pressure upon the lower bowel wall will cause constipation. Obstipation is the absence of lower bowel function. No flatus or feces are passed, and obstruction is strongly suspected.

Diarrhea refers to the consistency of the stool and not necessarily the frequency. Intrinsic bowel lesions, such as villous adenomas, produce large amounts of mucus and fluid. Partial obstructions and inflammatory conditions of the bowel can cause diarrhea. Regional enteritis may be suspected with protracted diarrhea and abdominal cramps. Frequent small, bloody stools are seen with ulcerative colitis; bulky, frequent, and very foul stools lead one to suspect malabsorption, either primarily intestinal or pancreatic in origin. Pathogens, notably *Salmonella* and *Shigella*, frequently cause diarrhea; amebiasis and staphylococcal enterocolitis are common causes also.

Melena refers to the black, sticky stools

indicative of an upper gastrointestinal source of bleeding. Blood reduced by acids gives the stool its character. On the other hand, bright red rectal bleeding (hematochezia) is usually from the lower intestinal tract. Nevertheless, blood may be transported rapidly from the stomach and passed per rectum as bright red blood. Small amounts of blood on the surface of the stool or after a normal stool has passed suggest anal origin.

EXAMINATION

As the entire patient is examined, the facial expression, respiratory rate, and vital signs are carefully appraised. If peritonitis is present, a slow, full pulse indicates an early process, but a rapid, thready pulse warns that it is advanced. An elevated temperature indicates an inflammatory condition. In acute appendicitis the temperature is rarely over 38° C (100° F). When it is higher, one should either doubt the diagnosis or consider the possibility that the appendix has ruptured. A subnormal temperature is recorded in patients in shock or shocklike states that are produced by acute blood loss or a marked reduction in blood volume, as in acute pancreatitis.

Inspection

The examiner notes if the patient lies still with the legs flexed as in an acute inflammatory condition or if he or she is perspiring and pale with an anguished expression and is moving about constantly, seeking a position of comfort as with colic. If distension is present, it is best seen in the reclining patient by observing the level of the umbilicus to an imaginary line drawn from the xiphoid to the pubis. If the umbilicus is above that line, distension is present. This is constant even in obese patients (Fig. 29-2).

In thin or cachectic individuals with mechanical obstruction sometimes peristalsis will be seen like the arching of a cat's back. Masses must be sought in all patients with an acute abdomen. Hernias have been missed because drapes were not turned down far enough.

The umbilicus may protrude when fluid is present, and discolorations in the flank (Grey Turner's sign) or umbilicus (Cullen's sign) indicate retroperitoneal bleeding as in acute hemorrhagic pancreatitis.

Palpation

Palpation demands gentleness and concern. It is said that the rough hand will find tenderness where there is none and the cold hand will find rigidity or muscle spasm where there is none. It is helpful to ask the patient to identify the precise spot where the pain is present or to cough and locate it this way. That area is avoided until the remainder of the abdomen is examined. Gentle palpation using the pads of the fingers is vital to appreciate the location of tenderness and to evaluate the presence of rigidity and muscle spasm. If the patient is asked to take a deep breath and

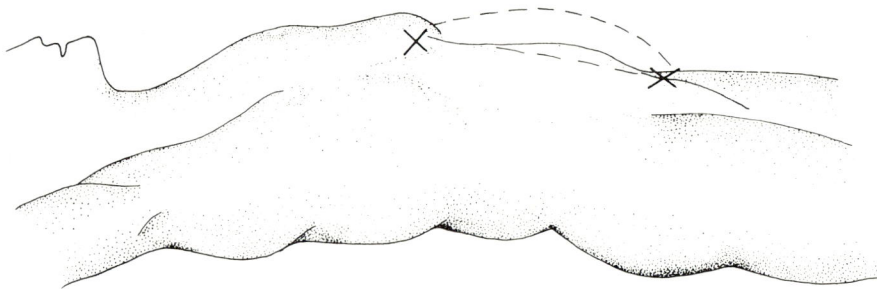

Fig. 29-2. Abdominal distension in reclining patient.

exhale, voluntary spasm of the rectus muscle will disappear on exhalation, but involuntary spasm will persist. Spasm of the rectus muscle is well localized to the area of complaint. It is reflex in nature and can also arise from acute renal pain as in pyelonephritis or obstructive uropathy.

In an acute inflammatory process the tenderness may be so localized that a fingertip may find the point of maximum tenderness. Rebound tenderness will be elicited, when present, by pressing gently and slowly, but deeply, and releasing the pressure rapidly. With obvious peritonitis, there is no need to perform this painful maneuver.

Special examinations are helpful in localizing the disease process. If a patient flexes his or her thigh against pressure from the examiner's hand, pain is experienced when an inflammatory process irritates the psoas muscle (iliopsoas test). Similarly, if the thigh is flexed to 90 degrees and rotated externally and internally, pain is elicited when the obturator internus muscle is irritated by an inflammatory mass (obturator test). The sign of contralateral tenderness means that pressure on one side of the abdomen causes pain on the opposite side (Rovsing's sign); this is an excellent way to distinguish intraabdominal from intrathoracic processes that cause abdominal pain. No pain will be found in the opposite side of the abdomen if the disease process arises in the thorax.

If a pain is experienced on inspiration with palpation in the right upper quadrant, it is usually because an inflamed gallbladder is striking the examining hand (Murphy's sign). Fist percussion in the lower thoracic wall will elicit pain with cholecystitis or hepatitis, but usually no inflammatory process is present in the upper abdomen if there is no pain.

When efforts are made to relax the patient, gentle, soft palpation may find a mass. Mild sedatives help, and certainly examination under anesthesia can be very rewarding. The mass may be intraabdominal or within the abdominal wall. If the patient extends and raises both legs, the tensing of the abdominal muscles will more clearly define abdominal wall masses, but may totally obscure intraabdominal masses (Fothergil's test). It is also helpful in distinguishing intraabdominal tenderness from abdominal wall injury.

Intraabdominal masses are usually mobile with respiration, whereas retroperitoneal masses tend to be fixed and unchanging with deep respiration. Local heat is sometimes present in an acute inflammatory process localized to the area of the disease, and because of the acute excitation of the somatic impulses the area may be hyperesthetic.

Percussion of the abdomen affords the same information as rebound tenderness. Light percussion over an area of involvement elicits rather acute tenderness. Percussion gives the examiner clues to intraabdominal masses that cannot be palpated. A hypertympanitic abdomen is seen in intestinal obstruction or in a perforated viscus. The progressive loss of liver dullness is classically described with free peritoneal air. This condition can exist even with the absence of air under the diaphragm.

No patient is ever completely examined for an acute abdomen without a pelvic or rectal examination or both. Lesions discovered within the cul-de-sac or masses in the adnexa or tenderness elicited on cervical movement may prevent a needless operation. A rectal examination may reveal masses in the pelvis, tenderness on either side, or tumors within the rectum. It should be done carefully, but it must also be done gently. A well-lubricated finger should enter the anal sphincter with gentle pressure (a rough examination will cause pain). The right and left anterior walls of the rectum can be gently palpated. The finger is rotated completely and placed into the rectal ampulla; masses can be missed if this simple maneuver is not performed.

Auscultation

One should listen for bowel sounds for at least five full minutes before it can be said that they are not present. The quality of bowel sounds is carefully appraised. Fairly constant and loud borborygmi that have no definite pattern and vary in intensity occur in gastroenteritis or functional gastrointestinal diseases. They are not associated with abdominal discomfort. The regular, rhythmic contractions seen in acute mechanical obstruction must be distinguished from the above. There is an interval of silence between these contractions, and the borborygmi are heard with gradually increasing intensity when a mechanical obstruction exists. The high-pitched tinkles of dilated, fluid-filled loops of bowel give one the impression of an intestinal obstruction. Abdominal bruits may or may not be significant when detected.

NONSURGICAL ENTITIES
Intraabdominal conditions

Fecal impaction may occur with the chief complaint being abdominal pain. Constipation and even diarrhea may be present with this troublesome condition. The diagnosis is simply made by a rectal examination, and treatment sometimes begins as the examining finger makes the diagnosis.

Primary peritonitis more commonly occurs in young nephrotic children. Pneumococci and streptococci are the usual causative organisms.

Pelvic inflammatory disease is often mistaken for conditions such as appendicitis, and acute peritonitis can occur with gonococcal infection of the salpinx. Unlike patients with other types of bacterial peritonitis, the patient with gonococcal infection will appear to be in good spirits; she will be warm and not acutely ill, despite the presence of diffuse abdominal tenderness (see Chapter 30).

Ruptured ovarian follicles occur in every woman, but secondary bleeding may be so severe that there is considerable tenderness in the lower abdomen. A culdocentesis is sometimes positive for blood.

Hepatitis causes right upper quadrant pain that can be distinguished from acute cholecystitis by determination of the hepatic enzymes.

Extraperitoneal conditions

Extraperitoneal conditions that can simulate an acute abdomen include acute abdominal wall injury, such as hemorrhage into the rectus muscle, renal colic, urinary bladder distension, and the very treacherous acute pancreatitis, which can prostrate an individual, causing a shocklike state with a high hematocrit and high hemoglobin levels. Severe abdominal pain localized in the epigastrium and boring into the back is typical. The presence of pleural effusions from the irritation of pancreatic fluid in the lesser sac and the elevated amylase or urinary diastase levels help to distinguish this condition from acute intraabdominal entities that require urgent surgery.

General medical diseases

Pneumonia, notably right lower lobe pneumonia, may cause abdominal pain. Porphyria, although quite rare, must be considered when other conditions cannot be determined. Mumps, hemolytic disease, metabolic conditions such as hyperthyroidism, Addison's disease, and even myocardial infarction can cause acute abdominal pain. Patients with lymphomas, purpura, or hemolytic conditions may have acute localized tenderness. Patients with hyperparathyroid crisis, cystic fibrosis, or hyperthyroidism sometimes present with abdominal pain, diarrhea, and malabsorption.

Toxins

Acute poisoning from ingestion of lead, insecticides, toxic mushrooms, arsenicals, and the like may cause severe abdominal pain and vomiting. These patients could undergo unnecessary surgery unless a careful history is taken. The bite of a black widow spider may involve generalized muscle spasms of the abdomen that manifest as nontender muscle rigidity. Noticing a small wheal of local erythema on an extremity may prevent needless surgery (refer to Chapter 18).

Drugs

Porphyria secondary to chloroquine or barbiturate ingestion can cause abdominal pain. Retroperitoneal bleeding from poorly controlled anticoagulation therapy may produce shocklike states and, occasionally, intestinal obstruction by bowel wall hematoma. Ileus can be caused by ganglionic blocking agents. Antibiotics can cause colitis with pain and distension, and a bloody diarrhea may occur later. With the ever-increasing drug problem, narcotic withdrawal must be kept in mind. The addict with withdrawal symptoms may have such intense abdominal pain that surgery could be considered. Therefore, a drug history should be taken. In addition to the above, it is important to know if the patient has been taking significant quantities of aspirin or nonsteroidal antiinflammatories such as indomethocin (Indocin).

Conditions affecting dermatomes T_6 to L_1

Pain from herpes zoster may be present two weeks before the characteristic vesicular rash appears. Fractures of the vertebrae, herniated disks, and arthritis are known to cause acute abdominal pain, just as does neuritis from long-standing diabetes.

SURGICAL ENTITIES
Inflammatory conditions

Appendicitis. The patient who has an inflammatory condition of the abdomen experiences both visceral and somatic pain. For example, in acute appendicitis the initial complaint is periumbilical discomfort that localizes to the right lower quadrant later and becomes sharper in character. It is followed by nausea and vomiting (Fig. 29-3). Typical signs of localized peritoneal irritation then occur. Laboratory examination usually shows a leukocytosis with a shift to the left depending on the severity of the inflammatory process. Mesenteric adenitis may be distinguished from appendicitis; the blood count is characteristically low as in viral conditions, with predominance of lymphocytosis and pain located along the route of the mesentery. The urine of the patient with appendicitis

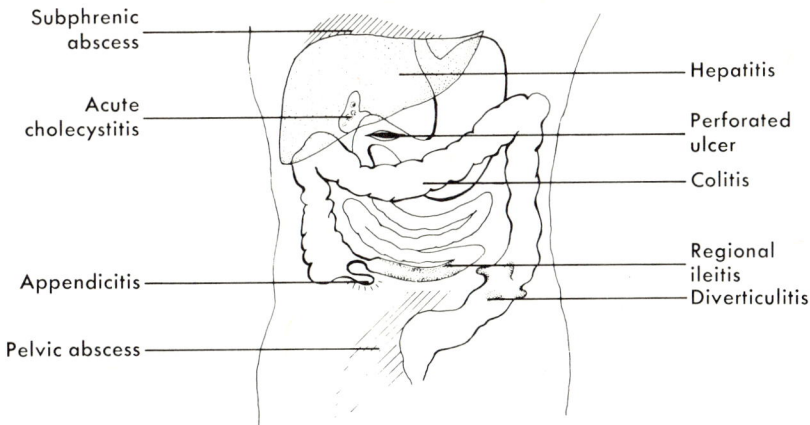

Fig. 29-3. Acute inflammatory conditions.

may have a high specific gravity, and acetone may be present. Blood cells may be present on microscopic examination. A fecalith, when seen on the flat plate of the abdomen, is always fortuitous in making the diagnosis of acute appendicitis. This condition can be very difficult to diagnose at times since many of the classic symptoms may not be present. If the diagnosis is in doubt, it is far better to explore the patient and remove a normal appendix than to send the patient home with acute appendicitis.

Acute cholecystitis. In acute cholecystitis, obstruction of the cystic duct is nearly always present, and it may produce progressive gangrene and perforation. A history of fatty food intolerance is frequently elicited. The pain begins in the epigastrium and localizes to the right upper quadrant of the abdomen with radiation to the back and the tip of the scapula. The blood count may be elevated, although it is not as consistently elevated as in acute appendicitis.

Examination of the urine may reveal the presence of bile and an absence of urobilinogen if common duct obstruction is present. Elevation of the bilirubin and alkaline phosphatase levels, with the absence of elevated hepatic enzymes, leaves little doubt as to the diagnosis. The flat plate of the abdomen may show a distended gallbladder, and infrequently, calcified stones will be present. Confirmation of this diagnosis is made with an oral or intravenous cholecystogram. The evaluation of such a patient should include frequent examinations, since worsening of the condition and increasing severity of signs warrant urgent surgery.

Regional enteritis. Regional enteritis may cause acute abdominal pain with localized findings that are indistinguishable from acute appendicitis. The history of chronic debility, weight loss, abdominal cramps and diarrhea may make one doubt the diagnosis of acute appendicitis. A gastrointestinal series with a small bowel study could reveal the telltale string sign in the distal ileum. Nevertheless, exploration for appendicitis more often makes the diagnosis.

Meckel's diverticulitis is an extremely difficult diagnosis to make preoperatively, but its signs and symptoms specifically indicate a surgical entity.

Acute diverticulitis. Acute diverticulitis with abscess formation usually occurs in the left lower quadrant, but there may be right lower quadrant findings. A mass is sometimes palpable. The usual patient is beyond the age of 40, and the inciting pathologic process is localized abscess formation. Diverticula tend to perforate within the epiploic appendages of the colon. Free perforation occurs in only 1% of cases, but when it does, air under the diaphragm, an absence of liver dullness, and spreading peritonitis make surgery urgent. Perforated intestinal lesions give a similar picture with marked boardlike rigidity. Air under the diaphragm is noted on the upright x-ray of the abdomen in two thirds of these patients. Foreign bodies and carcinoma that perforate the bowel cause diffuse bacterial peritonitis. The more common perforated duodenal ulcer will give rise to an initial chemical peritonitis, but within six to eight hours bacterial peritonitis ensues.

Nonintestinal inflammatory conditions

Liver abscess. A pyogenic liver abscess is commonly the result of acute cholangitis or appendicitis. The temperature is elevated, spiking in character, and associated with chills. The patient may be jaundiced with an elevated alkaline phosphatase level and a high white blood cell count. The diaphragm may not move on fluoroscopy and appears elevated. A liver scan frequently localizes the process precisely.

Secondary intraabdominal abscesses. Other intraabdominal abscesses localize in the subphrenic spaces, the pelvis, or in multiple locations (20% of cases). Because pelvic abscesses are not as dangerous and are more readily drained, one should be familiar with the abdominal watershed in septic intraabdominal conditions. A reclining patient tends to have infected material gravitate to the subphrenic spaces, whereas an upright position promotes drainage into the pelvis (Fig. 29-4).

Fever in a typical swinging pattern is the most common presenting finding. Antibiotics have altered this picture, and indeed in some patients there is no fever at all. Pain, tenderness, and a mass are fortuitous findings, but unfortunately they are not always present. Extraperitoneal and lesser sac abscesses are difficult to diagnose and, therefore, are more dangerous. A leukocytosis and anemia in long-stand-

ing cases may make the diagnosis suspected, but laboratory findings otherwise are not specific.

X-ray examination may reveal an elevation of the diaphragm, air-fluid levels, or even tiny bubbles of gas if anaerobic gas-forming organisms are present. Chest findings such as atelectasis, pneumonitis, or pleural effusions are present in most patients. The liver-lung scan is most helpful in making the diagnosis. Ordinarily simultaneous scanning of the lung and liver reveals no separation. When a subphrenic abscess is present, a distinct space is detected between the lung and liver on a combined scan. In a septic patient, gallium-67 scan has been most useful in localizing collections of pus that would have otherwise gone undetected. Another newer

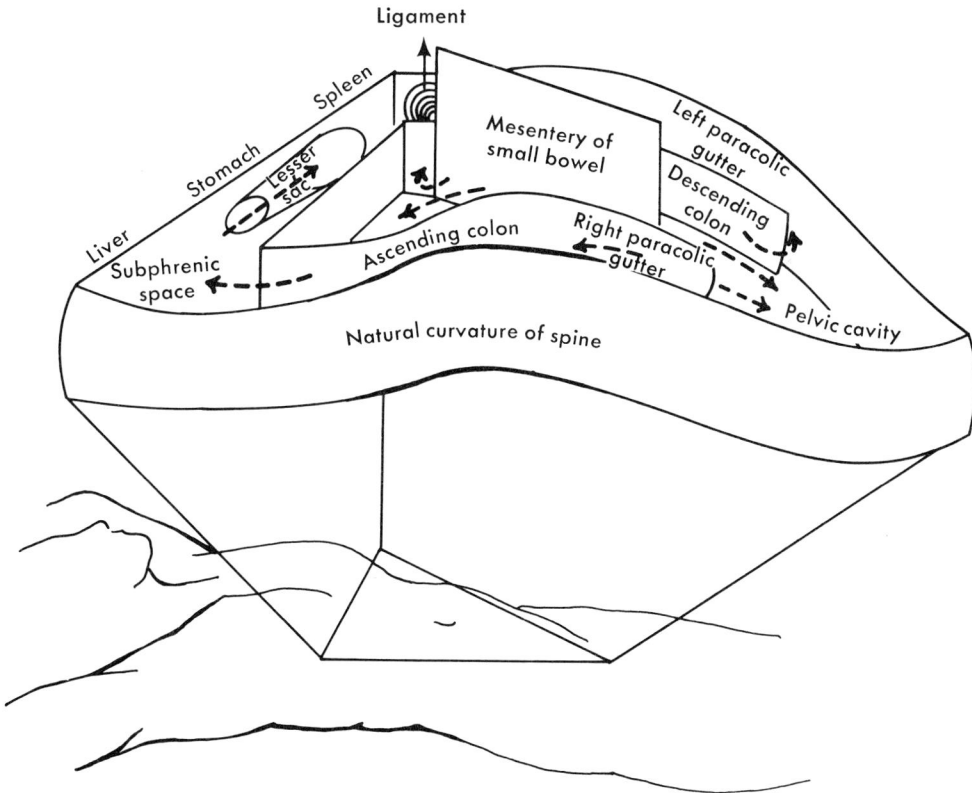

Fig. 29-4. The abdominal watershed.

diagnostic study of considerable use is ultrasonic scanning of the abdomen. Masses obscured by tenderness or undetected by size or location can be found, and it can be determined whether they are fluid filled or solid.

In general, an intraabdominal abscess is associated with abdominal findings. Local heat and edema of the skin (Krukow's sign) may be present, but more often abdominal distension, hypoactive bowel sounds, and abdominal tenderness occur. The mortality rate of untreated subphrenic abscesses is 50% or greater.

VASCULAR CONDITIONS

A ruptured aneurysm of the abdominal aorta or splenic artery is such a catastrophe that it is included in this category rather than in the broader spectrum of hemorrhagic conditions (Fig. 29-5).

Midline back pain, constant and boring in character, is unlike any back pain the patient has previously experienced. The abdominal pain is usually encircling, girth pain. A tender, pulsatile mass with syncope or frank shock alerts the examiner to the diagnosis. It is one of the few conditions that demands immediate surgery. A large majority rupture retroperitoneally and are temporarily tamponaded until surgery can be performed; even so, over 50% of these patients die.

Ischemic conditions of the bowel usually occur secondarily to advanced closed loop obstructions. In elderly patients with cardiac disorders, primary mesenteric infarcts may take place from thrombosis, embolism, atherosclerosis, or low cardiac output with no demonstrable vessel obstruction. Occasionally, premonitory signs occur, such as vague abdominal cramps, nausea, and anorexia. With infarction the abdominal pain is so severe that narcotics may not relieve it. Diarrhea and rectal bleeding may also occur.

There are signs of low cardiac output or a peculiar mottled cyanosis of the abdomen. Bowel sounds at first are hyperactive, and distension is present. When tenderness is found, the bowel sounds are absent.

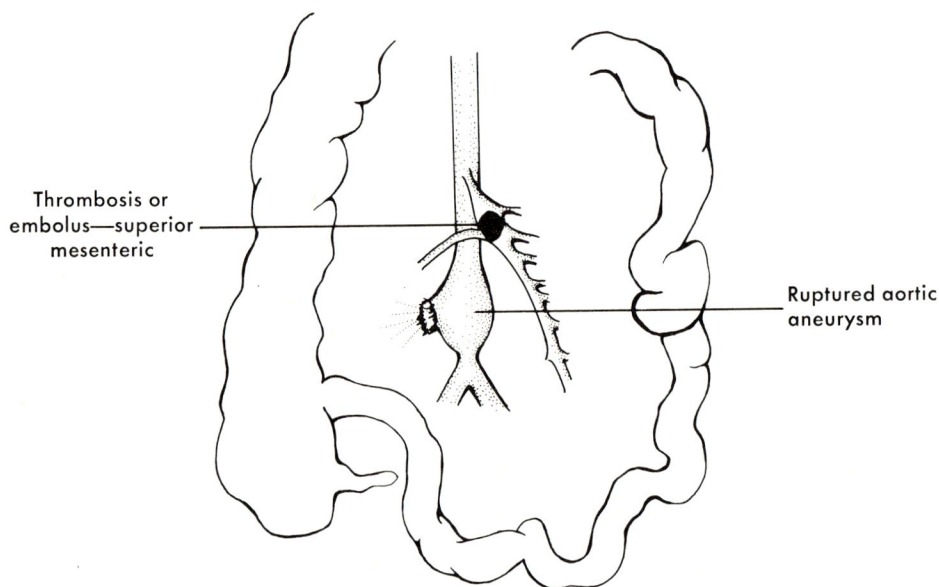

Thrombosis or embolus—superior mesenteric

Ruptured aortic aneurysm

Fig. 29-5. Vascular conditions.

The white blood cell count is very high (above 20,000) in most cases. X-ray films may show air within the loops of bowel, and should a paracentesis be performed, a characteristic foul, dark, hemorrhagic fluid is obtained.

When the pain is progressive, irreversible damage has already taken place, and sepsis is likely. The mortality rate is high, and early recognition and treatment are the only hope for survival. Those who survive the massive resection that is sometimes required may be alimentary cripples.

HEMORRHAGE

Intraabdominal hemorrhage can take place from either a ruptured ovarian cyst, ectopic pregnancy, or a ruptured spleen, liver, or kidney. When blood is present in the abdomen, the abdomen becomes diffusely tender. When the patient reclines, the blood irritates the undersurface of the diaphragm and causes shoulder pain (Kehr's sign). Another very excellent sign of intraabdominal bleeding is syncope with a fall in blood pressure and an increase in pulse when the patient changes position rapidly from a reclining to a sitting position. Often the patient appears to be pale and diaphoretic and may have a very rapid pulse. The physical findings demonstrate a type of doughy rigidity and tenderness. A flat plate of the abdomen reveals obscured psoas shadows or a ground-glass-like appearance. An ectopic pregnancy is considered in a woman who has missed a menstrual period and who has a sharp, sudden pain in either lower quadrant of the abdomen. Rapid laboratory studies are now available to indicate pregnancy.

Intraluminal hemorrhagic conditions

Upper gastrointestinal hemorrhage (Fig. 29-6). From 50% to 70% of upper gastrointestinal tract hemorrhages are the result of peptic ulceration. About two thirds of these are from duodenal ulcers. Esophageal varices may be responsible for 10% to 15%. Causes of lesser frequency are gastritis, Mallory-Weiss syndrome, hemangioma,

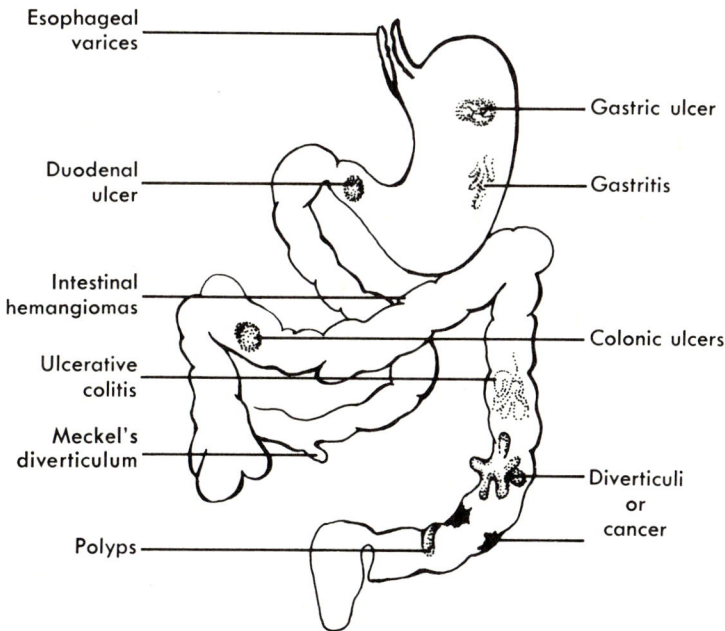

Fig. 29-6. Intraluminal hemorrhage.

prolapsing gastric mucosa, and other uncommon conditions. With intraluminal hemorrhage, surgery is not considered unless the patient requires more than 6 to 8 units of blood in the first 24 hours. Massive gastrointestinal hemorrhage occurs if more than 500 ml of blood is required in less than eight hours to maintain a stable circulation. An early recurrence of a bleeding episode within a matter of days requires urgent surgery, since mortality is high. Team efforts of medical and surgical personnel are necessary for any patient with upper gastrointestinal hemorrhage.

Emergency endoscopy has become the accepted initial diagnostic study by most institutions. A large Ewald tube is passed through the mouth, and ice water is lavaged through this tube with a Toomey bladder syringe until the return is clear. Successful endoscopy can then be performed with a much higher yield than with an emergency gastrointestinal series. Arteriograms may be helpful but only in active bleeding. The source can be located if there is at least 0.5 ml of blood loss per minute. In the high-risk patient this method could be therapeutic as well as diagnostic. Vasopressin (Pitressin) has been successfully infused into the affected artery at a rate of 0.02 to 0.04 units per minute via a pump apparatus, and hemorrhage was controlled.

Lower bowel hemorrhage. Lower gastrointestinal hemorrhage, when severe, is most often caused by diverticulosis and, in order of frequency, cancer, ulcerative colitis, colonic ulcers, and polyps. The same criteria are employed for lower gastrointestinal hemorrhage as for upper gastrointestinal hemorrhage when considering surgery. A barium enema may be therapeutic as well as diagnostic. The intraluminal pressure of the barium administration has been shown to cause cessation of bleeding in diverticular disease. This should be considered at the earliest possible time.

OBSTRUCTIVE CONDITIONS
Nonintestinal obstructions

Twisted ovarian tumors or cysts or any other mass that has a pedicle within the abdominal cavity will cause severe abdominal pain if the blood supply is obstructed by twisting. Unless a mass is present, the diagnosis can be difficult.

Bile duct obstruction. Obstructions of the biliary tract produce coliclike pain in the right upper quadrant of the abdomen. Acute cholangitis is suspected when there is a spiking fever and chills, jaundice, and colic (Charcot's triad). Early decompression will prevent septicemia and hepatic abscesses.

Urinary tract obstruction. Acute urinary obstructions do not always require surgery, but the colic experienced is severe and characteristic. The pain is in the flank and typically radiates downward into the groin or scrotum. If repeated pyelograms and persistent symptoms indicate failure of the progression of the stone, surgery will be required.

Intestinal obstructions

The patient with the classic triad of abdominal pain, distension, and vomiting is considered to have intestinal obstruction. The examiner determines what type of obstruction is present—one that is secondary to an inflammatory process or primarily of a mechanical nature. If it is a mechanical obstruction, at what level is the intestine obstructed? The danger of intestinal obstruction is that it not only produces volume depletion but also compromises the bowel leading to strangulation and possible perforation (Fig. 29-7).

The workup of the patient is done in conjunction with the therapy directed to the above conditions. If obstruction is secondary to an inflammatory process, the patient may have a silent but distended abdomen. The bowel sounds are disorganized, high-pitched, and with occasional tinkles, and the x-ray examination will demonstrate air-fluid levels in an orderly fashion. The bowel walls may be thickened, and fluid may be seen between loops. Clinically, the picture of peritonitis is present.

With mechanical obstruction the examiner first of all seeks any external hernias where incarceration of bowel may exist. Pain and organized borborygmi with intervals of silence are diagnostic. In late obstructions the abdomen is silent, distended, and diffusely tender. Signs of peritoneal irritation indicate a possible compromise of the circulation of the bowel. On x-ray examination, which includes a flat plate and upright film of the abdomen or lateral decubitus, air-fluid levels are without an orderly pattern and frequently change location with subsequent films. The amount of distension seen on the x-ray film indicates the level of the obstruction.

Some generalizations can be made about mechanical obstruction. There is a gradual diminution in the sensitivity of the gastrointestinal tract the farther the lesion is from the external orifices. The pain is more a function of how fast tissue damage is taking place than of how much or how great the damage is. For example, pain that is elicited from inflammatory processes is not as great as colic pain from acute distension of a hollow viscus. The further down the intestinal tract, the more insidious is the presentation of symptoms. Patients with high obstructions will vomit early but will have less distension. Patients with large bowel obstructions will vomit late. If the ileocecal valve is incompetent, the distension will be massive. Obstipation is present in most cases of complete obstruction, and one must never be deluded by the presence of diarrhea or evacuation of gas following an enema. This does not rule out the diagnosis of intestinal obstruction. The more common causes of small bowel obstruction are adhesions, hernias, and tumors in that order, whereas carcinoma, diverticulitis, and volvulus are the usual causes of large bowel obstruction. The causes of mechanical obstruction are listed in the following outline:

I. Lesions of the bowel
   A. Regional enteritis
   B. Strictures (radiation or potassium)
   C. Extrinsic masses or abscesses

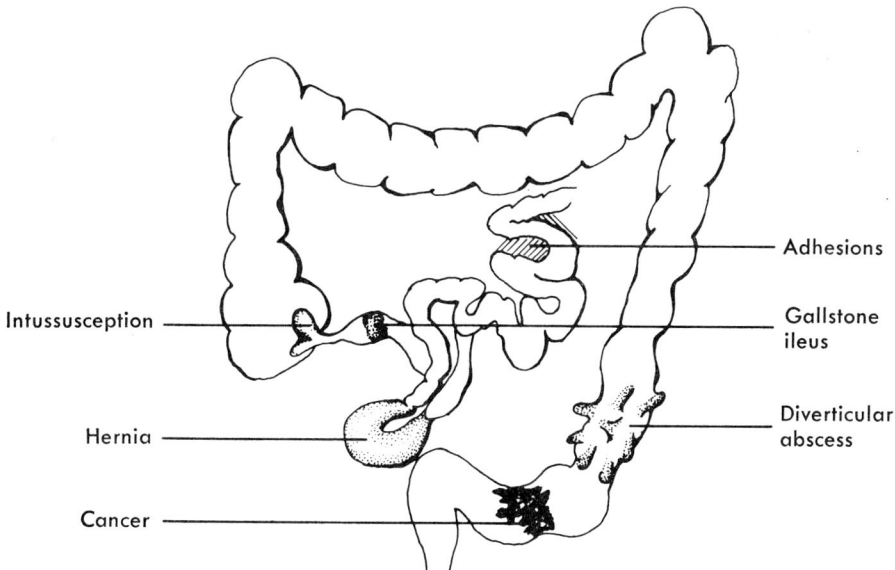

Fig. 29-7. Obstructive conditions.

D. Atresia, diaphragmostenosis
E. Hematoma
II. Extraluminal causes
   A. Adhesions
   B. Hernias
   C. Extrinsic masses or abscesses
III. Intraluminal causes
   A. Impactions
   B. Gallstones and foreign bodies
   C. Intussusception
   D. Neoplasms
IV. Volvulus

Colonic obstruction with a competent ileocecal valve is a closed loop obstruction. The pressure is evenly distributed from the point of obstruction, but the cecum with the greatest diameter is vulnerable to maximal distension and perforation (Laplace's law). Generally, if the cecum is greater than 10 cm in diameter, perforation is imminent. When cramping is occurring continuously or at very short intervals, strangulation is threatening.

The laboratory evaluation of a patient with intestinal obstruction should include electrolyte determinations in addition to the blood count and urinalysis. Preparation for surgery includes replacement of any deficits, nasogastric decompression, and antibiotics if strangulation is feared. There are few indications for nonsurgical management with long tubes. This only leads to costly delay and dangerous consequences.

TRAUMA

An individual with blunt injury to the abdomen from an automobile or motorcycle accident or a fall or blow of any type may show signs of an acute abdomen. One may have a penetrating wound to the abdomen from a missile or a stab wound. In either case, trauma to the abdomen demands careful evaluation (Fig. 29-8).

Blunt trauma

Solid viscus injury. Blunt trauma to the abdomen is by far more dangerous than penetrating wounds. This is largely due to

the fact that during the evaluation of the patient, the greatest difficulty in management is diagnosis. By and large, the organ most commonly injured is the spleen.

The patient will have evidence of intraabdominal hemorrhage. A large venous route for rapid fluid administration, such as Ringer's lactate, should be established, and a blood type and crossmatch should be obtained. Once this is accomplished, further evaluation can continue.

Laboratory findings will not necessarily show a drop in hematocrit despite an obvious blood loss, but an elevated white blood cell count is commonly seen in patients with ruptured solid organs. X-ray studies of the abdomen will sometimes show a loss of the psoas shadow or the ground-glass appearance, as previously described, when blood is present. The displacement of the stomach or a large mass in the left upper quadrant indicates a ruptured spleen, and approximately one third of the patients will have associated rib fractures in the left lower thorax. Blood in the urine alerts one to the possibility of kidney injury, and

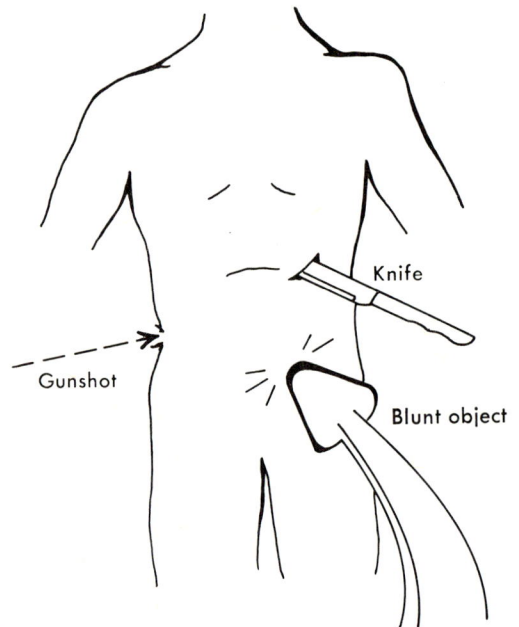

Fig. 29-8. Trauma to abdomen.

no patient with blunt abdominal trauma should be operated on without first having an intravenous pyelogram.

When the diagnosis is uncertain but intraabdominal injury is suspected, a four-quadrant abdominal tap may be done. The recovery of unclotted blood is indicative of intraabdominal bleeding, but the test is meaningful only if it is positive. The diagnostic peritoneal lavage is thought to be more useful. For an adult, 1 liter of normal saline is introduced into the peritoneal cavity, and the patient is turned to a lateral decubitus position if the condition permits. The returned fluid is analyzed for leukocyte count, red blood cell count, and amylase determination. This is a simple and accurate test. In a five-year study Root[2] found false-positive results in only 1% of the tests and false-negative results in 3%.

Arteriography is extremely helpful.[3] When radiologists are familiar with this technique, they will be able to determine the presence of even the most insidious subcapsular hematoma. This procedure has saved patients from extensive observation and needless explorations.

Hollow viscus injury. Blunt injury to the bowel is unusual because the small bowel is in a collapsed state most of the time. When it does occur, it is in the area of the ligament of Treitz, which fixes at the duodenojejunal junction. The bowel distal to this point is freely movable, and tears are sustained in this vicinity. The duodenum, on the other hand, is fixed across the spine, which makes it susceptible to injury either by compressing against this bony column or from sudden deceleration.

Physical findings are usually indicative of peritonitis, and early surgery is indicated. Retroperitoneal air bubbles seen on x-ray films of the abdomen indicate duodenal involvement. Air under the diaphragm is seen with rupture of an intraperitoneal hollow viscus.

Penetrating wounds of the abdomen.

Patients who have penetrating wounds of the abdomen are explored in most institutions. No one disputes the fact that missile wounds to the abdomen demand exploration, but in some hospitals stab wounds are so frequently seen that there is a recent trend in programs of nonsurgical management. Smithwich and co-workers[4] have utilized the technique of injecting a large bolus of radiopaque material into a catheter that is placed into the stab wound and secured tightly with a purse-string suture. X-ray films are taken, and the dye is sought in the peritoneal cavity. If it is found intraabdominally, exploration is undertaken. The authors report a high degree of accuracy, but false-positive and false-negative results have been reported by others. Considerable experience is necessary to interpret the findings.

McClelland and co-workers[5] recommend local exploration of stab wounds to see if the peritoneal cavity has been entered. Nance[6] has recommended close observation and frequent examination to determine changes in the patient's condition. In a study of over 600 stab wounds at Charity Hospital in New Orleans, he reported no increase in mortality, and only 40% of these patients observed required ultimate exploration.

Regardless of the method, all patients are worked up in a stepwise fashion, and if there are signs of peritoneal irritation, if peritoneal lavage or arteriogram is positive, or if there is x-ray evidence of intraabdominal organ injury, urgent surgery is required.

Mass casualties

Although the term "mass casualties" implies multiple injuries, abdominal trauma is very much a part of this concept. Several cases of abdominal trauma simultaneously admitted to the emergency department will tax the personnel, the facility, and the reserve supplies to the fullest. Furthermore, with the increasing incidence of civil disorder as well as natural disasters such as earthquakes and floods, multiple trauma patients will be admitted, and emergency department personnel should be familiar with mechanisms of managing mass casualties. They must constantly train and drill together as a team until they master their plan thoroughly. Only by thorough familiarization and organization of coordinated endeavors will they be an invaluable unit for their community. Mobilization of additional personnel—medical, paramedic, and nonmedical—is required. Triage stations and resuscitation rooms should be predesignated. Reserve supplies should be kept up to date and readily available. Adequate facilities for the care of mass casualties have been demonstrated to be as effective in reducing mortality as the intensive care units have been in effectively altering the mortality rate in cardiac emergencies.

SUMMARY

It should be said again that it is more important to determine if the patient requires surgery than to pinpoint the exact diagnosis.

It is beyond our scope to dwell on definitive surgical management or basic principles of surgery as they pertain to the acute abdomen. If all of the nearly 200 entities were presented in detail, several volumes would be required. The careful appraisal of the patient will lead to early surgical treatment or prevent needless surgical operations. The following outline summarizes acute abdominal conditions:

I. Nonsurgical entities
  A. Intraabdominal conditions
  B. Extraperitoneal conditions
  C. General medical diseases
  D. Toxins
  E. Drug complications
  F. Conditions related to dermatomes of T_6 to L_1
II. Surgical entities
  A. Inflammatory conditions
    1. Septic
      a. Perforating
      b. Nonperforating

    2. Chemical
      a. Gastric
      b. Bile
  B. Vascular conditions
    1. Rupture of major vessel
    2. Ischemia
      a. Primary
      b. Secondary
  C. Hemorrhage
    1. Intraabdominal (see B-1 and E-1)
    2. Intraluminal
      a. Upper gastrointestinal
      b. Lower intestinal
  D. Obstructions
    1. Nonintestinal
    2. Intestinal
      a. Upper gastrointestinal
      b. Lower intestinal
  E. Trauma
    1. Blunt
    2. Penetrating
      a. Stab wound
      b. Missile

REFERENCES

1. Meng, G. R.: The acute abdomen: a diagnostic review, J. Military Med. **137:**50, 1972.
2. Root, H. D., Hauser, C. W., McKinley, C. R., LaFave, J. W., and Mendiole, R. P., Jr.: Diagnostic peritoneal lavage, Surgery **57:**633, 1965.
3. Freeark, R. J., Love, L., and Baker, R. J.: An active diagnostic approach to blunt abdominal trauma, Surg. Clin. North Am. **48:**97, 1968.
4. Smithwick, W., Gertner, H. R., Jr., and Zuidema, G. D.: Injection of Hypaque (sodium diatrizoate) in the management of abdominal stab wounds, Surg. Gynecol. Obstet. **127:**1215, 1968.
5. McClelland, R. N., Jones, C., Shires, G. T., and Perry, M. O.: Trauma to the abdomen. In Shires, G. T., editor: Care of the trauma patient, New York, 1966, McGraw-Hill Book Co., pp. 354-409.
6. Nance, F.: Surgical judgment in the management of stab wounds of the abdomen: a retrospective and prospective analysis based on a study of 600 stab patients, Ann. Surg. **170:**569, 1969.

ADDITIONAL READINGS
Signs and symptoms

Botsford, T. W., and Wilson, R. E.: The acute abdomen, Philadelphia, 1969, W. B. Saunders Co.

Byrne, J. J.: Recent advances in diagnosis and treatment of the acute abdomen, Surg. Clin. North Am. **39**:1337, 1959.

Clain, A., editor: Bailey's demonstrations of physical signs in clinical surgery, Baltimore, 1967, The Williams & Wilkins Co., pp. 487-552.

Dunphy, J. E., and Botsford, T. W.: Physical examination of the surgical patient, ed. 3, Philadelphia, 1964, W. B. Saunders Co.

Menaker, G. J.: The physiology and mechanism of acute abdominal pain, Surg. Clin. North Am. **42**:241, 1962.

Schwartz, S. I.: Principles of surgery, New York, 1969, McGraw-Hill Book Co., pp. 830-867.

Yao, S. T., Vanecko, R. M., Freeark, R. J., and Shoemaker, W. C.: Unusual causes of acute abdomen, Arch. Surg. **69**:296, 1968.

Inflammatory conditions

Brown, D. W.: Combined lung-liver radioisotope scan in the diagnosis of subphrenic abscess, Am. J. Surg. **109**:521, 1965.

Farmer, R. G., Hawk, W. A., and Turnbull, R. B., Jr.: Regional enteritis of the colon: clinical and pathological comparison with ulcerative colitis, Am. J. Dig. Dis. **13**:501, 1968.

Halliday, P., and Loewenthal, J.: Subphrenic abscess, Aust. N. Z. J. Surg. **33**:260, 1964.

Holm, H. H., Kristensen, J. K., Rasmussen, S. N., et al.: Indications for ultrasonic scanning in abdominal diagnostics, J. Clin. Ultrasound **2**:5, 1974.

Kanvolinka, C. W., and Olearczyk, A.: Subphrenic abscess: current problems in surgery, Chicago, 1972, Year Book Medical Publishers, Inc.

Kazarian, K.: Decreasing mortality and increasing morbidity from acute appendicitis, Am. J. Surg. **119**:681, 1970.

Littenberg, R. L., Taketa, R. M., Alazrahi, N. P., Halpern, S. E., and Ashburn, W. L.: Gallium-67 for localization of septic lesions, Ann. Intern. Med. **79**:403-406, 1973.

Magilligan, D. S., Jr.: Suprahepatic abscess, Ann. Surg. **96**:14, 1968.

Wheelock, F. C., and Warren, R.: Ulcerative colitis, N. Engl. J. Med. **252**:421, 1955.

Vascular conditions

Darling, R.: Ruptured arteriosclerotic abdominal aortic aneurysms: a pathologic and clinical study, Am. J. Surg. **119**:397, 1970.

Davis, J. E.: Reversible vascular occlusion of the colon, Ann. Surg. **171**:789, 1970.

Hardy, J. D., and Turrinis, H. H.: Abdominal aortic aneurysms: special problems, Ann. Surg. **173**:945, 1971.

Ming, S. C., and Levitan, R.: Acute hemorrhagic necrosis of the gastrointestinal tract, N. Engl. J. Med. **263**:59, 1960.

Pierce, G. E., and Brockenhough, E. C.: The spectrum of mesenteric infarction, Am. J. Surg. **119**:233, 1970.

Hemorrhagic conditions

Baum, S., and Nusbaum, M.: The control of gastrointestinal hemorrhage by selective mesenteric arterial infusion of vasopressin, Radiology **98**:497-505, 1971.

Ferguson, L. K.: The diagnosis and management of bleeding from the lower intestine, Surgery **45**:352, 1959.

Finsterer, H.: Operative treatment of severe gastric hemorrhage of ulcer origin: reply to critics, Lancet **2**:303, 1936.

Nusbaum, M., Baum, S., Blakemore, W. S., and Tumen, H.: Clinical experience with selective intra-arterial infusion of vasopressin in the control of gastrointestinal bleeding from arterial sources, Am. J. Surg. **123**:165-172, 1972.

Palmer, E. B.: The vigorous diagnostic approach to upper gastrointestinal tract hemorrhage: a 23-year prospective study of 1400 patients, J.A.M.A. **207**:1477-1480, 1969.

Wagstaff, J. K.: Clinical diagnosis in gastrointestinal hemorrhage, Gastroenterology **36**:26, 1959.

Obstructive conditions

Cohn, J., Jr.: Strangulation obstruction: collective review, Surg. Gynecol. Obstet. **103**:105, 1956.

Vest, B., and Margulis, A. R.: The roentgen diagnosis of postoperative ileus-obstruction, Surg. Gynecol. Obstet. **115**:421, 1962.

Welch, C. E.: Intestinal obstruction, Chicago, 1958, Year Book Medical Publishers, Inc.

Traumatic conditions

Aakhus, T., and Enge, I.: Angiography in traumatic rupture of the spleen, Br. J. Radiol. **49**:855, 1967.

Bouterie, R. L.: Abdominal trauma, Compr. Ther. **2**:43-52, 1976.

Bouterie, R. L.: Medical support for the amphibious ready group in Vietnam, J. Military Med. **136**:242, 1971.

Drapanas, T., and McDonald, J.: Peritoneal tap in abdominal trauma, Surgery **100**:22, 1960.

Perry, J., Jr.: Diagnostic peritoneal lavage in blunt abdominal trauma, Surg. Gynecol. Obstet. **131**:742, 1970.

Wilcox, G. L.: Nonpenetrating injuries of the abdomen causing rupture of the spleen: report of 100 cases, Arch. Surg. **90**:498, 1965.

CHAPTER 30

Emergencies in obstetrics and gynecology

Robert T. Gordon, M.D.

Emergency department staff are called upon to assess and care for various obstetric and gynecologic problems. There are minor but severely annoying conditions, such as vaginitis, side effects of the pill or intrauterine devices (IUDs), and acute life-threatening conditions presenting as pain, vaginal bleeding, and shock. Complications of pregnancy are especially challenging because two lives are involved.

The most common obstetric and gynecologic emergencies are bleeding, pain, complication of pregnancy, and trauma.

VAGINAL BLEEDING

To assess the severity of vaginal bleeding, one should compare the number of sanitary napkins or tampons used with the amount normally used during menstruation. Use of more than one pad every two hours should be viewed with concern. An accurate menstrual history is essential in differentiating the cause of bleeding. The type of contraceptive the patient is using should be known, since some oral contraceptives have a higher incidence of breakthrough bleeding than others. Also, IUDs are associated with heavier periods and a greater chance of a pregnancy's being ectopic.[1]

If profuse bleeding has been a recurrent problem with an IUD, it should be removed.

A speculum examination of the vagina and cervix may reveal local causes for the bleeding (Fig. 30-1). A biopsy of any suspicious area should be done. After eliminating an anatomic cause, dysfunctional uterine bleeding is treated with progesterone, 100 mg IM, or medroxyprogesterone (Provera), 10 mg PO for five days. Bleeding will be controlled in 24 to 36 hours but will recur in two to six days. This "hormonal curettage" will correct bleeding in a majority of patients. If not, or if bleeding has been massive, hemostasis is best achieved by dilatation and curettage (D & C). Estrogens are best avoided because they set up a vicious recurrent cycle.

Excessive menstrual flow and intermenstrual bleeding are not normal at the menopause; bleeding that occurs six months after the last period should also be viewed with suspicion. The only way to exclude malignancy as the cause of bleeding is by a D & C.

The most common cause of severe vaginal hemorrhage is a disturbance of pregnancy. Asking a patient is she is pregnant

Hydatidiform mole
or choriocarcinoma

Ectopic pregnancy

Abortion

Fibroid
polyp

Carcinoma
of cervix

Cervical polyp

Vaginal
ulceration

Cervicitis

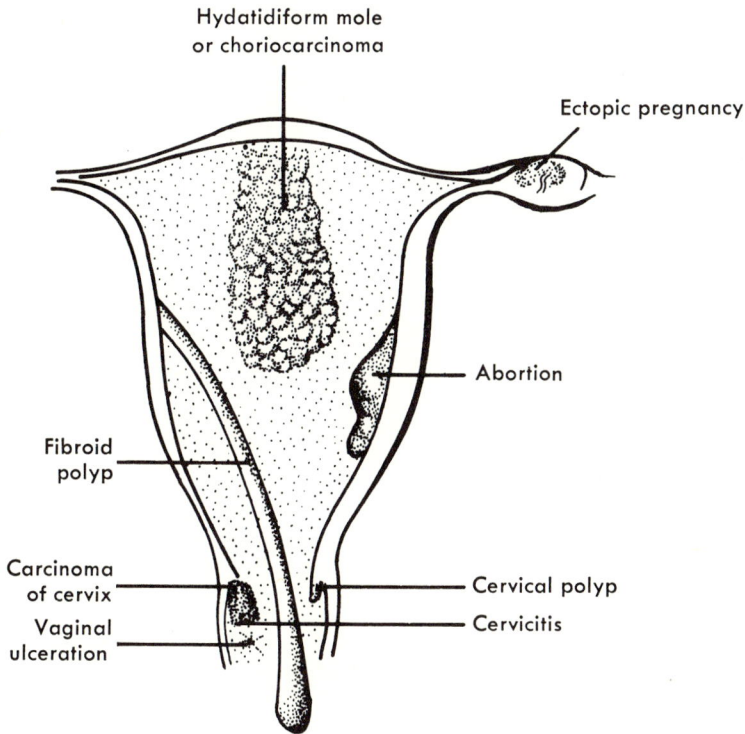

Fig. 30-1. Causes of vaginal bleeding.

can be informative. Few women can forget the secondary symptoms of pregnancy: amenorrhea, nausea and vomiting, breast tenderness, and urinary frequency.

Abortion

Abortion is the most common emergency in early pregnancy. It is the termination of a gestation before the fetus becomes viable (in most states, before the twentieth week from the last period). Intentionally occurring abortions are termed "therapeutic" if legal, and "criminal" if not. "Habitual" abortion is the occurrence of three or more consecutive spontaneous abortions. If accompanied by infection, they are termed "septic." In this type fetal death usually precedes the clinical signs by two or three weeks. Various types of abortions are assessed in Table 30-1.[2,3]

The possibility of an ectopic pregnancy should always be considered.

Clinical presentation. The pregnancy test is only of value when negative; it reflects the status of the placental tissue and not of the fetus.

Management. In threatened abortions the outcome is uncertain. It should be explained to the patient that with a normal pregnancy, symptoms will subside and the pregnancy will continue. If the conceptus is abnormal, abortion will occur. Management includes bed rest, sedation, and avoidance of coitus. Except with a habitual aborter, hormonal or other type therapy has not proved to be effective, and such therapy has been implicated in producing a missed abortion.

Inevitable and incomplete abortions are similarly managed, since the former cannot

Table 30-1. Assessing abortion

Type of abortion	Amount of bleeding	Uterine cramping	Passage of tissue	Tissue in vagina	Internal cervical os	Size of uterus
Threatened	Slight	Mild	No	No	Closed	Agrees with length of pregnancy
Inevitable	Moderate	Moderate	No	No	Open	Agrees with length of pregnancy
Incomplete	Heavy	Severe	Yes	Possible	Open with tissue in cervix	Smaller than expected for length of pregnancy
Complete	Slight	Mild	Yes	Possible	Closed	Smaller than expected for length of pregnancy
Septic	Varies, usually malodorous; fever present	Varies; fever present	Varies; fever present	Varies; fever present	Usually open; fever present	Any of the above with tenderness
Missed	Slight	No	No	No	Closed	Smaller than expected for length of pregnancy

be salvaged. Upon initial evaluation tissue found in the vagina or cervix is removed. An intravenous infusion with 20 units of oxytocin (Pitocin) in 1 liter of Ringer's lactate should be started. Antishock therapy including oxygen and blood replacement is used as needed. In all cases curettage is performed.

With *complete* abortion, curettage is not necessary. However, approximately 20% of these patients will require a subsequent D & C resulting from a placental polyp or chronic endometritis producing irregular bleeding. If there is any doubt regarding the completeness of the abortion, a D & C is indicated.[2-4]

All Rh-negative eligible women who abort should receive Rho(D) immunoglobulin (RhoGam).[5]

Septic abortion

An abortion is septic when complicated by infection. Most result from instrumentation of, or introduction of chemicals into, the uterus to induce abortion. Septicemia and endotoxic shock are the major causes of death. *E coli* is the most common organism in endotoxic shock. However, infection with *Pseudomonas* is the most lethal.

Clinical presentation. Fever, chills, and constant lower abdominal pain complicate an abortion. Decreased voiding, dark urine, and jaundice are found in the more severe cases. Upon examination there is abdominal distension, hypoactive bowel sounds, and lower abdominal tenderness with rebound. Vaginal examinations disclose a malodorous discharge. Rarely, gas bubbles suggesting clostridial infection are seen. Movement of the cervix produces pain. The uterus is soft, tender, and there is parametrial tenderness. A tender adnexal mass is indicative of tubo-ovarian abscess, or that a pyosalpinx may be present.

Anaerobic and aerobic cultures and sensitivities of the endocervix are obtained along with gram-stained smears. The latter provide guidelines for antibiotic therapy.

The complete blood count will usually reveal a marked leukocytosis. A leukopenia is associated with a poor prognosis.

The BUN and creatinine levels provide a gross evaluation and baseline of renal function.

Platelets, serum fibrinogen, and clotting time assess the possibility of a clotting disorder.

Whole blood should be typed and cross-matched.

An upright abdominal x-ray may reveal the presence of a foreign body within the uterus or intraperitoneal cavity. Free air under the diaphragm is indicative of uterine perforation. Rarely will gas-forming organisms produce air in the uterine cavity.[2-4]

Management. An aggressive policy is indicated if complications are to be minimized. Any tissue in the vagina and endocervix should be cultured and removed with ring forceps. A liter of Ringer's lactate with 20 units of oxytocin should be administered. Oxygen and whole blood are given as needed to combat shock.

Antibiotic therapy is begun. Initially, penicillin, 20 million units per day IV, plus kanamycin, 0.5 g IM every 12 hours (in patients with normal renal function), or penicillin plus gentamicin, 1 to 1.5 mg/kg every eight hours, may be used until the sensitivity studies enable a more specific approach to therapy.

Tetanus toxoid, 0.5 ml IM, is given if instrumentation is suspected. Bed rest in semi-Fowler's position helps prevent intraperitoneal spread of infection. Urinary output should be recorded hourly using an indwelling catheter.

Monitoring of the central venous pressure is most helpful in replacing fluids and preventing circulatory overloading. Oral intake should be restricted.

Within six to eight hours after antibiotic therapy is begun, curettage should be performed to remove the focus of infection. If the patient's condition does not respond to this and specific antibiotic therapy, hysterectomy is indicated. The latter may be the only life-saving treatment in the case of clostridial infection.[6]

Complications. Endotoxic shock will develop in 2% to 4% of these patients (see Chapter 7).

Renal failure is not rare and is more common when toxic materials are used to induce an abortion.

Pelvic thrombophlebitis develops as a result of advancing parametritis and pelvic cellulitis. The diagnosis is often one of exclusion. Embolism, when it occurs, results in showers of small amounts of septic material as opposed to the type of emboli orginating in the legs. Heparin is the treatment of choice; however, inferior vena caval and ovarian vein ligation are indicated when medical measures fail.

Missed abortion

A missed abortion occurs when the conceptus, dead at least four weeks, has not been expelled. Abortion usually occurs spontaneously before problems arise; however, a patient may present as an emergency because of unexplained ecchymosis or bleeding caused by an intravascular consumption coagulopathy.

Clinical presentation. The signs and symptoms of pregnancy have regressed, fetal heart tones are absent, and the uterus is small for the length of pregnancy. The pregnancy test is negative. A hematocrit should be obtained to assess the amount of bleeding. Platelets and fibronogen should also be drawn to assess the presence of a consumption coagulopathy.

Management. In the asymptomatic patient who has a normal fibrinogen level when fetal death is initially diagnosed, spontaneous abortion may be awaited. Most women abort within five weeks. Weekly fibrinogen levels are obtained, and the patient is observed closely.

With a fibrinogen level between 150 and 200 mg/100 ml, the pregnancy should be terminated by oxytocin infusion and amniotomy.

If the level is less than 150 mg/100 ml and the patient is not in labor, 5,000 units of heparin should be given intravenously every four hours. Serial fibrinogen levels are obtained and the pregnancy is ended by oxytocin infusion as soon as the fibrinogen level is above 200 mg/100 ml. Heparin is continued until delivery.

If the patient is initially hypofibrinogenemic and in labor, or is bleeding, fibrinogen, 2 to 10 g IV, is given. *Fresh* whole blood can be given as needed. Oxytocin infusion is used to empty the uterus.[7]

Curettage is usually necessary after delivery. All Rh-negative eligible women should receive Rho(D) immunoglobulin.

Complications. The major complication of missed abortion is bleeding resulting from a consumption coagulopathy. The management is explained above.

Ectopic pregnancy

Gestations outside the uterine cavity are one of the most serious emergencies, accounting for 6% of maternal mortality. Over 95% occur in the fallopian tube, but they can also occur in the ovary, abdomen, or the cornua of the uterus. Etiologic factors include preexisting pelvic inflammatory disease, tuboplasty, endometriosis, and the use of an IUD. A woman who becomes pregnant with an IUD in place has a 1 in 25 chance of the pregnancy's being ectopic.

Clinical presentation. Pain is present in over 90% of patients. It may be cramping and mild or sharp and excruciating, as associated with tubal rupture. Usually the pain is lateral. With the subdiaphragmatic collection of blood, reflex shoulder pain will occur. In some, the sudden onset of abdominal pain is associated with syncope. The pain has no constant relationship to associated vaginal bleeding.

Vaginal bleeding, present in 75% of patients, is usually an intermittent, slight, brownish spotting, frequently occurring after a missed period. Profuse bleeding occurs in only 5% of the patients.

The majority of patients have periods of amenorrhea lasting 6 to 12 weeks in duration. However, any type of menstrual irregularity may occur.

A tender adnexal mass is felt in 60% of conscious and 90% of anesthetized patients. It must be remembered that repeated examinations can lead to rupture of a mass

with resulting hemorrhage and shock.

Rectal pressure and the urge to defecate may be present as a result of blood collecting in the cul-de-sac. Nausea and vomiting may also be a complaint.

Pregnancy tests, positive in 50% of cases, are not diagnostically important since they do not reflect the location of placental tissue, only its viability.

The hematocrit will reflect the extent and progression of intraperitoneal bleeding.

Assessment. The temperature is usually less than 38° C (100° F). With cervical movement sharp localized pelvic pain is elicited. During the first six to eight weeks the uterus may be compatible with the stage of gestation. An adnexal mass may be felt. Clinical shock and collapse, seen in 10% of patients and often occurring after a pelvic examination, is indicative of extreme intraperitoneal bleeding. Discoloration of the umbilicus is a rare sign indicative of hemoperitoneum.

Culdocentesis may clarify difficult cases (Fig. 30-2). The patient is placed in the lithotomy position, feet in the stirrups with the upper torso elevated 30 degrees. A vaginal speculum is inserted, and the cervix and posterior fornix are cleaned with an antiseptic solution. The posterior lip of the cervix is grasped with a long, single-tooth tenaculum. An 18-gauge spinal needle, best attached to a Luer-Lok syringe, is inserted in the midline through the posterior fornix approximately 2 cm behind the junction of the cervical and vaginal mucosa. The needle should be inserted 2 cm with a quick motion. Aspiration is accomplished as the needle is withdrawn. The return of nonclotting blood is indicative of intra-abdominal bleeding. A nonproductive tap is not a negative tap and should be repeated, as should a tap productive of fresh blood that clots.

Management. Hemorrhage and shock are treated with intravenous fluids, oxygen, and blood replacement as soon as available.

An unruptured ectopic pregnancy may still be present in the absence of a hemoperitoneum and negative culdocentesis. An examination under anesthesia and a repeat culdocentesis are necessary. If the diagnosis is still not definite, laparoscopy or culdoscopy should be employed to clarify the situation. The latter procedures are not indicated when hemoperitoneum has been proved by culdocentesis. In such a case an exploratory laparotomy is recommended. A salpingectomy or salpingo-oophorectomy should be performed.

All Rh-negative eligible women should receive Rho(D) immunoglobulin.[8]

Complications. The major complications are hemorrhage and shock, usually the result of a delay in recognition. Long-term problems include infertility; only one third of these patients ever deliver a live child.

Corpus luteum cyst

Differentiation of a bleeding corpus luteum cyst from an ectopic pregnancy can be made only at laparoscopy or laparotomy.

Hydatidiform mole

This entity results from the hydropic degeneration of the chorionic villi, producing grapelike vesicles.

Clinical presentation. Hydatidiform mole should be suspected in cases of recurrent bleeding during the first half of pregnancy especially if prolonged nausea, vomiting, unexplained hypertension, or toxemia exists. In half the cases the uterus is larger than normal for the presumed phase of pregnancy. Enlarged theca-lutein cysts may be felt in the adnexa. Fetal heart tones are absent. Sometimes the passage of "grapes" has occurred, making the diagnosis obvious. Serious bleeding with resultant shock can be a presenting problem.[3]

The pregnancy test is positive; however, chorionic gonadotropin titers are not necessarily diagnostic because high values are also consistent with multiple gestations. Anemia is usually found.

Sonography can be diagnostic even in the first trimester. There is absence of the fetal skeleton on abdominal x-ray films after 18 weeks of gestation. Chest x-ray examination is obtained to exclude metastasis.

Obtaining clear vesicles is diagnostic. Otherwise, the clinical picture and suggested studies should confirm the diagnosis.

Management. Hypovolemic shock should be treated immediately with oxygen, intravenous fluids, and whole blood. If there is heavy bleeding, evacuation of the uterus must be accomplished as soon as possible. An infusion of 1 liter of Ringer's lactate with 30 units of oxytocin is begun. Uterine perforation is an extreme danger during

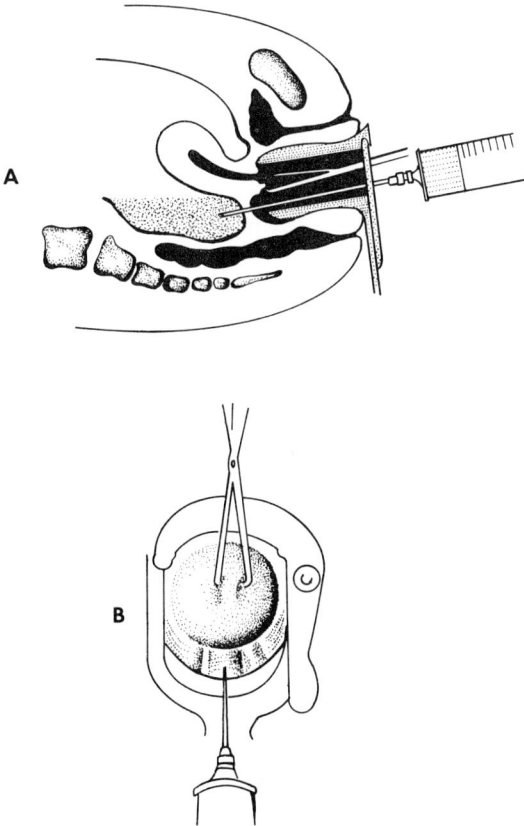

Fig. 30-2. Culdocentesis. **A,** Lateral view; **B,** front view.

curettage, and a suction curet should be employed if available.

If the diagnosis is made before bleeding produces an emergency condition, the use of prophylactic chemotherapy with methotrexate or actinomycin D should be considered before the uterus is emptied if adequate follow-up is uncertain. Any anemia is corrected with blood replacement before chemotherapy is begun.[9]

Hysterectomy is sometimes indicated if medical methods are unsuccessful or if the patient has completed childbearing.

From 5% to 10% of these patients develop choriocarcinoma.

Follow-up management. Weekly gonadotropin levels, by HCG titer initially and then by serum assay when the former becomes negative, are indicated for the first eight weeks. Thereafter, if the levels are normal, monthly tests are sufficient for six months and then every three months for one year. Serial chest x-ray films should also be obtained. Oral contraceptives are used to prevent pregnancy for one year so that any gonadotropin level present can be interpreted correctly. Any recurrences require aggressive management to assure complete cure.[3,9]

PELVIC PAIN

The likely causes of pelvic pain associated with vaginal bleeding are abortion, ectopic pregnancy, or dysmenorrhea. The latter usually can be diagnosed by history of its absence during the initial years of menstruation, its later cyclic recurrences, the gradual development of symptoms, and the absence of abdominal rigidity. The treatment is symptomatic with analgesics.

Midcycle or ovulatory pain (mittelschmerz) results from rupture of the graafian follicle. The discomfort is usually lateral. Diagnosis is suggested by the absence of pelvic findings, history of similar prior episodes, and characteristic time in the cycle. Reassurance and analgesics are all that are needed. Patients who use an

IUD may experience severe pelvic cramping as a result of excessive uterine irritability. Examination shows no abnormalities. The IUD should be removed, analgesia be given, and another form of contraceptive provided.

Pelvic inflammatory disease

Since the usual case of "acute salpingitis" is more extensive than inflammation of the fallopian tubes, the term pelvic inflammatory disease (PID) more accurately describes the condition. The ovaries and pelvic peritoneum are involved, although the fallopian tubes bear the primary insult. The majority of infections are of gonorrheal origin, but secondary pathogens frequently complicate the picture. Predisposing factors include promiscuity, previous infections, and use of an IUD. The attack may be the initial one or an exacerbation of a chronic problem.[9]

Clinical presentation. The most common symptom is bilateral, nonradiating pelvic pain, frequently beginning just after the menses have ended. A dull ache initially, it becomes progressively more severe making coitus and even walking uncomfortable. Fever as high as 39° C (103° F) and chills are present, as is occasional vomiting; however, bowel disturbances are unusual. There may be vaginal spotting. On examination there is bilateral lower abdominal tenderness with guarding and rebound. There may be urethral or Bartholin's gland discharge. The cervix may be acutely inflamed and draining purulent material. Pain is produced by cervical manipulation. The bimanual examination is often unsatisfactory because of the severe discomfort and abdominal rigidity; however, when felt, the uterus is normal in size. In the first attack no pelvic masses are palpable; however, in chronic cases, masses due to pyosalpinx or tubo-ovarian abscess may be palpated on rectovaginal examination.

Leukocytosis as high as 30,000 and an elevated sedimentation rate are present.

Gram-stain smear may reveal the *Gonococcus*. Cultures and sensitivities will demonstrate the causative organism so that antibiotic changes can be made on follow-up.

PID is often confused with appendicitis. The major feature of PID is its bilaterality, whereas appendicitis localizes to the right lower quadrant and is associated with gastrointestinal disturbances.

Management. If the patient is only mildly ill and can be cared for as an outpatient, bed rest, warm baths and douches, analgesics, and interdiction of coitus are recommended. Ampicillin, 500 mg four times a day for seven days, is given.

If the patient is severely ill with a high fever and severe peritonitis, hospitalization is indicated. Ampicillin, 1 g IV every four hours, or aqueous penicillin, 12 million units per day, may be given in addition to the above measures while cultures are pending. Surgery is not indicated in uncomplicated cases. If the diagnosis is in doubt regarding appendicitis, laparotomy is indicated. If uncomplicated salpingitis is found, the tubes should not be removed or incised.

During the acute phase, an IUD should not be removed unless the patient wants to change her form of contraception.

Tubo-ovarian abscesses may develop if initial therapy is inadequate. Cul-de-sac abscesses unresponsive to medical management may require drainage via a colpotomy. A leaking or ruptured abscess may occur and requires immediate surgery and aggressive medical therapy.

Follow-up management. Pelvic examinations are unnecessary for one week after the attack as long as the patient is improving. After this time examination, including cultures, should be done to evaluate the need for further care. The patient's sexual contacts must be evaluated for care.

Torsion of pelvic structures

An ovarian cyst is the most common pelvic structure to undergo torsion. A similar clinical picture may be produced by torsion of a paraovarian cyst, a pedunculated subserous fibroid, or by twisting of a normal or abnormal fallopian tube. With right side involvement, this condition can be confused with appendicitis.

Clinical presentation. There is usually acute, one-sided pelvic pain associated with nausea and vomiting. Pain of the inner thigh may also be present. Sometimes with a rapid torsion there is associated syncope. Abdominal guarding, tenderness, and rebound are present. A tender adnexal mass is sometimes palpated. Occasionally, the onset of symptoms is more gradual or the pain may subside only to recur.

Laboratory studies. A white blood cell count will reveal leukocytosis with a shift to the left. Many times the exact cause of the symptom complex cannot be determined. However, appreciation of the acute condition makes only one therapeutic course applicable.

Management. Intravenous fluids and analgesics are given in preparation for exploratory laparotomy. Treatment is excision of the involved tube and ovary without previously unwinding the pedicle.

Bartholin's gland abscess

The Bartholin gland and duct are often the site of gonorrheal and other types of infection with resultant obstruction of the secretions. With an acute infection of the gland or of a preexisting cyst, an exquisitely tender, erythematous, fluctuant fullness of the inferior labium minorum develops making walking painful.

Management. With an abscess a local anesthetic is not used. After the area is cleansed, a small incision is made in the mucosa of the vestibule just distal to the hymenal ring. There is marked relief with the escape of the malodorous pus. Cultures are obtained. A Word catheter is inserted, and the bulb is inflated with 2 to 5 ml of water. It is left in place for four to six weeks until a sinus track develops.

Drainage occurs around the stem. After the catheter is removed, the gland resumes its normal function. Coitus and other activities are not affected by the catheter.

If a catheter is not available, the abscess cavity is packed with iodoform gauze for 24 hours, and a new pack is inserted twice a week for four to six weeks.

Hot sitz baths and antibiotics are used until the acute phase subsides.[10]

Vulvovaginal infections

Rarely, vaginal infections produce a copious discharge resulting in severe itching and burning. Frequently, there is associated acute vulvitis or the vulva may be the primary site of an infection.

Trichomonas vaginitis typically produces a frothy, yellow-green, fetid discharge. Petechiae of the cervix or vagina are characteristic. The appearance of motile, oval flagellates is diagnostic when a drop of discharge is mixed with a drop of warm normal saline and examined microscopically. The vagina and vulva may be cleansed of the irritating discharge with aqueous benzalkonium (Zephiran). Metronidazole (Flagyl), 500 mg, may be given twice daily for five days, or if poor compliance is suspected, 2.0 g given in one dose may be used with similar success and is specific curative therapy. Alcohol should not be consumed while on metronidazole because of a possible Antabuse reaction. The patient's consort should be treated simultaneously.

In patients with severe candidal vulvovaginitis the labia are markedly red and edematous. A whitish, curdlike vaginal discharge is found. Diagnosis may be made by microscopic identification of budding mycelia on a wet smear of the exudate. A culture may be made on Nickersen's medium. Patients on combined oral contraceptive and antibiotic therapy or who are diabetic are at greater risk. Nystatin (Mycostatin) suppositories inserted into the vagina twice a day with cream applied to the vulva for two weeks, or miconazole nitrate (Monistat) used daily until the tube

is finished, is specific treatment. Sitz baths are also helpful.

If *Trichomonas* and *Candida* are excluded as the causative agents of vaginitis, the causative organism is *Haemophilus vaginalis* or a mixture including normal flora plus various strains of *Streptococcus, Staphylococcus,* and colon bacilli. Oral ampicillin, 500 mg four times a day for five days, is the treatment of choice.[9]

Herpes simplex virus infection of the genital area is now a commonplace venereal disease. Initially, the lesions appear as vesicles but later rupture to produce shallow, very painful ulcers. Urination is often difficult because of herpetic lesions in the bladder or urethra and also because the urine stream contacts the vulvar lesions. Urinary retention can occur because of the severe dysuria. Although there is not a treatment of choice, the use of heterotricylic dyes has been found to relieve discomfort and to promote more rapid healing. Vesicles should be ruptured and the lesions painted with 1% neutral red or 0.1% proflavin and followed by exposure to any artificial light for 15 minutes. General measures include sitz baths and oral analgesics. Some patients may require indwelling catheters. Screening for other venereal diseases should be done.

COMPLICATIONS OF PREGNANCY

Emergencies occurring during pregnancy include bleeding, pain, and convulsions or coma. Acute surgical emergencies such as appendicitis and twisted adnexal cysts may occur in the gravid female. In an evaluation of such patients the distortion of the intraabdominal contents by the enlarging uterus must be borne in mind (for example, the appendix rising in the abdomen). Surgical intervention should not be delayed once a diagnosis is made.

Placenta previa

The various types of placenta previa are determined by the placenta's relationship to the internal cervical os: (1) total, os completely covered; (2) partial, os partially covered; (3) marginal, the placenta extends to the edge of the os; and (4) low lying, the placenta is in the lower uterine segment.

Predisposing factors include increasing age, increasing parity, and previous cesarean sections. A significant negative in the history is the absence of hypertension or toxemia.

Clinical presentation. Painless vaginal bleeding, usually bright red, appears suddenly and without cause. Frequently, the patient will awaken at night in a pool of blood. Unless she is in labor, there is no abdominal discomfort. The uterus has normal tone and is nontender. Malpresentations and delayed engagements are often found.

The hematocrit may reveal the extent of the bleeding. When available, ultrasound is the method of choice for placental localization. Soft-tissue radiography is less accurate before 32 weeks. Two lateral views (supine and standing) are needed to identify the placenta.

Radioactive isotope localization is less accurate before 32 weeks and in recognizing posterior implants.

In term pregnancy or when the bleeding is excessive, little is gained by localizing the placenta by indirect means, and many times indicated termination of the pregnancy is delayed. There is little danger that a gentle speculum examination to rule out local causes of bleeding will precipitate hemorrhage. At this time a sample of blood should be obtained to rule out fetal bleeding. If these causes and abruptio placentae are excluded, further evaluation and management depend upon the extent and persistence of the bleeding and the maturity and condition of the fetus.

Management. Hemorrhage and shock are treated with intravenous fluids, oxygen, and blood replacement.

Digital examination should not be initiated if the fetus is premature because initial bleeding, in the absence of such manipulation, usually subsides. In each case, indirect methods are used to localize the placenta. Expectant care should be utilized in such cases until fetal maturity is reached.

If the bleeding is heavy, an immediate cesarean section is indicated regardless of fetal maturity.

If the bleeding is slight and the fetus mature, a double set-up examination is done. A cesarean section is indicated with a complete previa, a partial previa in a nullipara, or a posterior partial previa in a multipara. In a stable multiparous patient the membranes should be ruptured with marginal or partial placenta previa with the cervix dilated at least 5 cm. Oxytocin (Pitocin), 10 units in 1 liter of 5% dextrose, is carefully infused to induce labor. If effective labor is not obtained or if fetal distress or recurrent bleeding occurs, cesarean section should be done.

With a dead fetus a cesarean section is indicated if bleeding is a threat to the mother.

Complications. Postpartum hemorrhage may occur because of the inability of the lower uterine segment to contract adequately or because of lacerations in the friable lower segment.

Infection potential is greater because of the close proximity of the placental site to the vagina.

Placenta accreta occurs because of the poorly developed decidua in the lower uterine segment. Many times hysterectomy is the only form of therapy.

Perinatal mortality is about 20% and is mainly due to prematurity and intrauterine anoxia secondary to blood loss and cord prolapse.[2-4,11]

Abruptio placentae

All degrees of premature separation of the normally implanted placenta occur, thus accounting for the varying signs and symptoms. In the majority of cases there is external vaginal bleeding. When the bleeding is concealed, the patient may demonstrate signs of blood loss that are not expected since the extent of bleeding is not appreciated. Predisposing factors include toxemia of pregnancy, chronic hypertension, increased parity, and a history of a previous abruption.

Clinical presentation. Abdominal pain is usually associated with vaginal bleeding. The uterus is rigid (the most reliable sign), tender, and gradually enlarging. Fetal palpation is difficult, fetal heart tones may be inaudible, and the amniotic fluid is port-wine colored. There may be variable evidence of hypovolemia.

Hematocrit is needed to evaluate blood loss. Blood is also drawn for fibrinogen level and for a clot observation test. The latter is done as follows and should be repeated hourly. Ten milliliters of whole blood is drawn in a test tube:

1. If no clot forms, the fibrinogen level is less than 60 mg/100 ml.
2. If a clot forms but fragments within one-half hour, the fibrinogen level is less than 150 mg/100 ml.
3. If a clot forms and remains intact, the fibrinogen level is greater than 150 mg/100 ml.

With marked signs and symptoms the diagnosis is obvious; however, painless vaginal bleeding without uterine tenderness does not exclude the diagnosis. In the latter case a double set-up is used to exclude the other possibilities. Care is influenced by the concept that some complications are time related; their development and severity depend upon the duration as well as the magnitude of the separation.

Management. Hemorrhagic shock is treated with intravenous fluids, oxygen, and whole blood transfusion.

An amniotomy must be done regardless of the condition of the cervix or of the level of the presenting part. Port wine–colored fluid will be seen. This not only confirms the diagnosis but helps immobilize the detached portion of the placenta and reduces the extravasation of blood into the myometrium.

Oxytocin, 10 units in 1 liter of Ringer's lactate at a rate of 20 drops per minute, is started to stimulate contractions.

If fibrinogen is less than 150 mg/100 ml or if there is generalized bleeding, 2 g of fibrinogen is given intravenously. The amount required to control bleeding may vary from 2 to 20 g.

If the fetus is alive and delivery is not expected in the time it would take to do a cesarean section, the latter should be done.

With a dead fetus greater effort is made to effect a vaginal delivery. However, if the patient is not responding to antishock therapy and the labor is not progressing, cesarean section is performed to control the bleeding by emptying the uterus.

Complications. Coagulation defects result from clotting retroplacentally and intravascularly with consumption of the clotting factors, especially fibrinogen.

Acute renal failure, usually acute tubular necrosis, results primarily from blood loss and hypovolemic shock.

Couvelaire uterus results from bleeding between the muscle bundles of the uterus. Rarely this causes uterine atony and bleeding that is unresponsive to administration of oxytocin necessitating a hysterectomy.

Fetal mortality may approach 100% depending upon the length of gestation and extent of abruption.[2-4,11,12]

Vasa praevia

Vasa praevia exists when there is a velamentous insertion of the umbilical vessels and these vessels are in advance of the presenting part. It is a rare but extremely lethal condition for the fetus. The isolated perinatal mortality rate is higher than for either placenta previa or abruptio placentae, with which it is most often confused. The mother is not affected by the condition. However, the fetus is endangered by exsanguination from a torn fetal vessel or by asphyxia resulting from occlusion of vessels by the presenting part.[4]

A high index of suspicion is needed whenever vaginal bleeding occurs during the last trimester or during labor. Rarely, the vessels can be palpated by digital examination. Determination of the fetal origin of the blood in the vagina may be accomplished by the Kleihauer acid elution technique for fetal hemoglobin, the Apt test, or by examining a smear for nucleated red blood cells.

Management. Once the diagnosis is made, delivery is accomplished by cesarean section unless delivery is imminent. However, in the absence of fetal heart tones, cesarean section is not necessary because the mother is in no danger. Infants are usually anemic at birth and require transfusions; therefore, O-negative settled cells should be available for the infant.

Hypertension

A pregnant patient beyond 24 weeks' gestation having hypertension and proteinuria constitutes the serious complication of preeclampsia. She might come to the emergency department complaining of headaches, blurring or double vision, or epigastric pain. It is considered severe preeclampsia if the blood pressure is above 160/110 mm Hg, if proteinuria is greater than 3+, or if oliguria or pulmonary edema is present. Preeclampsia, one of the major causes of maternal and perinatal mortality, may be seen before 24 weeks when associated with molar pregnancies. The patient is hyper-reflexic, and the eyegrounds frequently demonstrate retinal sheen and segmental arteriolar spasm.[3,13,14]

The patient should be admitted to the hospital and managed as outlined under eclampsia regarding laboratory studies, urinary output, use of magnesium sulfate, and correction of hypertension.

If the infant is mature, delivery should be accomplished when the patient is adequately covered with anticonvulsant therapy. If the infant is premature, the acute episode is managed with anticonvulsants, a low-salt, high-protein diet, and rest.

Diuretics have been shown to be of no benefit. The patient is then observed closely until the fetus is mature, at which time the pregnancy is terminated.

Complications associated with preeclampsia include eclampsia, abruptio placentae, hemolytic anemia, and prematurity.

Convulsions or coma (eclampsia)

A woman in the latter half of pregnancy with convulsions or coma should be considered eclamptic until proved otherwise. Eclampsia is a rare complication of pregnancy that may arise after a short period of toxemia that may have been overlooked.

Clinical presentation. The patient may be convulsing, in a coma, stuporous, or have regained consciousness. The majority note the convulsions to be heralded by frontal or occipital headaches and visual disturbances. Epigastric pain and vomiting may also occur. Oliguria, if present, is an ominous sign. Hypertension, albuminuria, and edema are invariably found; however, the latter may be insignificant.

Urinalysis reveals proteinuria but is otherwise normal. Blood count may reveal anemia, hemoconcentration, or helmet cells, and there may be a decreased platelet count associated with microangiopathic thrombocytopenic hemolytic anemia. BUN and creatinine determinations provide a gross evaluation of the renal status. Creatinine clearance later gives more detailed information about kidney function.

When hypertension, albuminuria, and edema are present, the diagnosis is eclampsia. If they are not present, other causes of convulsions should be evaluated: cerebral vascular accident, hypertensive encephalopathy, epilepsy, intracranial injury, drug intoxication, or diabetic complications. An accurate history is extremely helpful.[2,3]

Management. Airway patency should be assured; oxygen is given by mask. An indwelling urinary catheter to gravity drainage is inserted and the output measured hourly.

To control actively occurring convulsions, diazepam (Valium), 5 to 10 mg IV, is given, and this dose repeated in two to four hours, if necessary.

When urinary output is assured, magnesium sulfate, 4 g IV initially and 1 g hourly thereafter, is administered. Caution must be exercised in the presence of oliguria because magnesium is excreted in the urine. The magnesium level may be followed by the patella reflex, which should be present but not brisk. Calcium gluconate should be available in case magnesium sulfate toxicity (respiratory paralysis) develops.

As long as the fetus is alive, the blood pressure should not be lowered below a diastolic pressure of 100 mm Hg. Arbitrarily lowering the pressure to a "normal" value may compromise placental perfusion and the fetus. A titrated infusion of hydralazine HCl (Apresoline), 20 mg in 1 liter of 5% dextrose, is used to "control" the hypertension. The blood pressure must be taken every five minutes to monitor the effect of the infusion.[3]

A padded tongue blade to insert between the teeth is kept available to prevent injury to the tongue in the event of a convulsion.

No rigid time rule should be applied as to when the patient should be delivered after being seen. However, regardless of the stage of gestation, after adequate anticonvulsant therapy has been administered the pregnancy should be terminated—vaginally if delivery is imminent, by cesarean section otherwise. General anesthesia is best employed.

Complications of eclampsia include cerebral vascular accidents, circulatory collapse, renal failure, and coagulation defects.

Postmortem cesarean section

Fetal salvage from a postmortem cesarean section is greater the longer the duration of pregnancy and when the mother dies suddenly rather than after a lingering illness. The chances of fetal survival are diminished greatly after maternal death over five minutes. An attempt should be made in all cases after 28 weeks, and every effort should be made to obtain the husband's consent.

Amniotic fluid embolism and uterine rupture

Amniotic fluid embolism and uterine rupture are rare complications of pregnancy. The former is manifested by vascular collapse, dyspnea, and cyanosis following a rapid delivery which may have occurred at home. If the patient survives the first few hours, bleeding from a consumption coagulopathy may develop. Care for acute cor pulmonale and pulmonary edema should be given as well as heparin, 1,500 units every hour.

Uterine rupture most often occurs in those patients with a history of cesarean section. The history is that of a woman in the latter part of pregnancy or in labor who develops sudden abdominal pain with nausea and vomiting. Subsequently, shock ensues. There may be vaginal bleeding, or if the rupture occurs during labor, contractions cease. Examination reveals a patient in shock, generalized abdominal tenderness, fetal parts easily felt, usually absent fetal heart tones, and a high presenting part. Management consists of care of hemorrhagic shock and immediate laparotomy. Whether or not hysterectomy is necessary depends upon the extent of the rupture.[2-4]

Postpartum hemorrhage

To make the correct diagnosis of postpartum hemorrhage, knowing the interval since delivery is important. During the first 24 hours after birth the major causes are uterine atony, vaginal and cervical lacerations, and retained placental fragments. After initial evaluation, an oxytocin solution should be infused intravenously and antishock measures begun if needed.

Further evaluation to eliminate the other causes should be done in the operating room.

Delayed uterine bleeding is usually due to retained products of conception or sub-involution of the placental site. After preparation to stabilize the patient, including intravenous fluids containing oxytocin, a D & C should be done.[2-4]

Delivery

On occasion a pregnant patient will be seen in the emergency department with delivery imminent, and no time to transfer her to the delivery room. Efforts to delay delivery by holding the presenting part in the vagina or forcing the legs together should be condemned. Asepsis should be maintained as much as possible with sterile sheets placed between the legs. At this stage the woman needs only assistance—not interference.

As the head distends the perineum and vulva, its delivery is controlled by pressure applied laterally beneath the symphysis. Delivery should not be hastened once the head delivers. The mouth and nostrils should be gently suctioned with a bulb syringe. The remainder of the body should be delivered gradually with the head kept lower than the torso. The cord should be doubly clamped and cut at least 7.5 cm from the infant.

Paramount in caring for the infant is (1) cleaning the airway of material with gentle bulb suction, (2) maintaining the infant in a gentle head-down position, and (3) keeping the infant warm by wrapping it in a blanket.

Efforts to extract the placenta by traction on the cord or squeezing the fundus should be avoided. Normally, placental separation will occur after five to eight firm postpartum contractions. Indications of this are the following: (1) the uterus becomes globular and firmer, (2) there is a sudden gush of blood, and (3) the uterus rises in the abdomen and the cord advances farther out of the vagina. The placenta then is either expelled or expressed into the vagina for delivery.

If there is excessive bleeding from uterine atony, 20 units of oxytocin in 1 liter of Ringer's lactate should be rapidly infused intravenously until there is uterine response. An alternate method is to give ergonovine (Ergotrate) maleate or methylergonovine maleate (Methergine), the dose of each being 0.2 mg IM.

If the placenta does not deliver or if lacerations of the perineum and vagina are found, the patient should be transferred to the delivery room for definitive care.

It is important to have the mother's Rh status evaluated, so that if she is Rh-negative and eligible, Rho(D) immunoglobulin can be given. Women who are not going to nurse should be given a lactation suppressant such as Deladumone OB.

HISTORY OF TRAUMA

Injuries to the pelvic area may result from coitus, rape, falls, abortion attempts, and other trauma. Pain may be severe because of the rich nerve supply and bleeding profuse because of the equally rich vascularization.

Small lacerations of the vulva may be repaired under a local anesthetic. More extensive lacerations and hematomas, especially those extending into the vagina, will require general anesthesia for evaluation and repair.

Hymenal lacerations following coitus rarely result in bleeding requiring suturing. This generally can be controlled by pressure to the bleeding point; however, in rare cases ligation is required.

Lacerations of the vagina usually require general anesthesia for adequate evaluation and repair.

Chemical burns of the vulva and vagina may occur from the injudicious use of vaginal medications or douch solutions. Rarely, potassium permanganate ulcerations are seen following abortion attempts. Care is supportive with cleansing and use of antibiotic creams (Sultrin, AVC) to overcome secondary infections.

A small child may introduce a foreign body into the vagina. The parents may be unsuspecting and alarmed by an ensuing discharge. The foreign body may be felt on rectal examination or visualized on gentle vaginal examination with the use of a nasal speculum. If this is unsuccessful, examination under anesthesia is indicated. The object can then be removed with a blunt hemostat.[15]

Sexual assault

An alleged rape victim requires special understanding and attention. Written witnessed consent for examination, collection of specimens, and release of information to proper authorities should be obtained.[16,17]

History. The history should be in the patient's words and should include pertinent negatives. Stating whether the patient was raped should be avoided; use phrases such as "alleged" or "suspected" rape. The patient's menstrual history, type of contraception used, and last coital experience will provide for an evaluation of the risk of pregnancy.

Examination. The examination should include the patient's general appearance, that of her clothing, and her emotional status. A general examination is necessary to find injuries remote from the genital area. The pelvic area is evaluated for secretions, bruises, and lacerations. The wide variability of the hymen should be appreciated. The vagina, fornices, and cervix are inspected for trauma with a nonlubricated, but water-moistened, speculum. A common finding after recent coitus is erythema of the posterior fornix. With forced, prolonged, or repeated coitus, this area may be superficially abraded. Allegations of anal or oral contact will direct a search of these areas.

Clinical presentation. A microscopic examination of the washings of any dried secretions from the perineum and thighs and of a specimen from the vaginal pool and cervical mucus is made for sperm. Specimens for acid phosphatase and blood group antigen are also obtained. These are important if the male is oligo- or azoospermic. Cultures for *Neisseria* are made from the cervix in appropriate media. Baseline serology is done as is a pregnancy test if the possibility of an early gestation exists. Specimens are obtained in the presence of a witness, clearly labeled, and *not* sent for analysis in the *routine* manner; unless they can be positively identified, the reports may not be submitted as evidence.[16,17]

Management. Prophylaxis against venereal disease is recommended. Procaine penicillin G, 4.8 million units, is given intramuscularly. With penicillin allergy, erythromycin, 500 mg qid, is given for ten days.

For the prevention of pregnancy the following is used (however, the patient is cautioned in writing that the drug is not guaranteed to be effective and that side effects may occur): Stilbestrol (DES), 25 mg bid PO, or Premarin, 10 mg tid PO, for five days. If the patient does not have a period within one week after the last pill is taken, a D & C should be done.[18,19]

Therapeutic abortion is indicated for a pregnancy that results from rape or where DES therapy has been ineffective in preventing the pregnancy.[18]

If the victim of a sexual assault is a child, the evaluation is kept as normal as possible. The parents should be warned to avoid terms such as "ruined" or "dirty" so as to prevent guilt feelings in the child. A small, prewarmed instrument is used. Repair of lacerations should be done under general anesthesia, using small needles and fine, absorbable suture material.

Follow-up management. Arrangements for follow-up care should be made to assure that serology and gonorrhea cultures remain negative, that the patient has not become pregnant, and to give psychologic support as needed.[16,17] (See Chapter 31.)

SUMMARY

Treating women with gynecologic complaints or obstetric complications requires patience and an understanding of the potential difficulties. If the problems are handled in a systematic manner, the subtleties differentiating emergencies from nonemergencies will be more obvious and the care rendered correct.

REFERENCES

1. FDA Drug Bulletin: Intrauterine devices, Aug. 1973.
2. Cavanagh, D.: Obstetrical emergencies, Springfield, Ill., 1961, Charles C Thomas, Publisher.
3. Reid, D., Ryan, K., and Benirschke, K.: Principles and management of human reproduction, Philadelphia, 1972, W. B. Saunders Co.
4. Pritchard, J., and MacDonald, P.: Williams obstetrics, ed. 15, New York, 1976, Appleton-Century-Crofts.
5. Goldman, J. A., and Eckerling, B.: Prevention of Rh immunization after abortion with Anti-Rh(D)-immunoglobulin, Obstet. Gynecol. 40:366, 1972.
6. Keith, L. G., and Poma-Herrera, P.: Aggressive treatment of septic abortion, Am. Fam. Phys. 3:99, 1971.
7. Lerner, R., Margolin, M., Slate, W., and Rosenfeld, H.: Heparin in the treatment of hypofibrinogenemia complicating fetal death in utero, Am. J. Obstet. Gynecol. 97:373, 1967.
8. Katz, J., and Marcus, R. G.: The risk of Rh isoimmunization in ruptured tubal pregnancy, Br. Med. J. 3:667, 1972.
9. Lee, L., and Schmale, J. D.: Ampicillin therapy for Corynebacterium vaginale *(Haemophilus vaginalis)* vaginitis, Am. J. Obstet. Gynecol. 115:786, 1973.
10. Goldberg, J.: Simplified treatment for diseases of Bartholin's gland, Obstet. Gynecol. 35:109, 1969.
11. Hibbard, L.: Placenta previa, Am. J. Obstet. Gynecol. 104:172, 1969.
12. Hammond, H.: Death from obstetrical hemorrhage, Calif. Med. 117:16, 1972.
13. Haynes, D.: Medical complications during pregnancy, New York, 1969, McGraw-Hill Book Co.
14. Schewitz, L.: Hypertension and renal disease in pregnancy, Med. Clin. North Am. 55:47, 1971.
15. Buchsbaum, H.: Accidental injury complicating pregnancy, Am. J. Obstet. Gynecol. 102:752, 1968.
16. Evrard, J. R.: Rape: The medical, social and legal implications, Am. J. Obstet. Gynecol. 111:197, 1971.
17. ACOG Technical Bulletin: Suspected rape, No. 14, July 1970.
18. FDA Drug Bulletin: Postcoital diethylstilbestrol, May 1973.
19. Blye, R.: The use of estrogens as postcoital contraceptive agents, Am. J. Obstet. Gynecol. 116:1044, 1973.

CHAPTER 31

Emergency management of sexual assault*

Theresa L. Crenshaw, M.D.

Roger T. Crenshaw, M.D.

In 1976, according to FBI figures, there were 56,730 forcible rapes in the United States: approximately 53 out of every 100,000 females in the country were raped. In 1976, within the San Diego city limits alone there were 255 rapes and 215 children were sexually molested. These figures reflect reported rapes only. It is estimated that one out of ten rapes that occur is reported to the authorities. In children, an even smaller percentage is reported. Comparison of the statistics of recent years shows that the incidence of reported rape continues to increase.

There are several reasons women do not report the crime. The three most frequently mentioned are the manner and behavior of the police, the trauma of the courtroom experience, and the nature of the emergency management.

Until recently, emergency departments have had the reputation of being indifferent, inadequate, and additionally traumatic to the victim. Efforts are being made across the nation to change this image through education, improved services, sexual assault crisis intervention teams, and community action groups.

DEFINITIONS

Rape. Two elements are necessary to constitute rape: (1) sexual intercourse (carnal knowledge) and (2) commission of the act forcibly and without consent. The slightest penetration by the male organ constitutes carnal knowledge; neither complete penetration nor ejaculation is required. Force may be defined as the use of actual physical force to overcome the victim's resistance, or the use of threats that result in victim acquiescence because of fear of death or grave bodily harm (Hilberman, *The Rape Victim*).

Types of rape. The types of rape include female rape, child rape, date rape, gang rape, homosexual rape, and married rape. To date, however, no law protects a woman from being raped by her huband.

Child sexual abuse. Unfortunately there is no precise meaning that is uniformly used in the law and literature. Generally the term includes the crimes of child molestation and incest and excludes forcible rape and other forms of physical child abuse (California Penal Code).

Sexual assault. Sexual assault is a more general term referring to any sexual act imposed by one or more individuals on another who is unwilling to participate or under the age of legal consent.

RAPE VICTIMS

Women are usually the victims of rape. However, homosexual rape occurs not infrequently. This behavior is especially prevalent in prison populations. There have been rare reports of women raping men, but the fear of ridicule probably prevents men from reporting such occurrences. It is thus impossible to assess the incidence or significance of this behavior. Among children, while females are the most common target, preadolescent males are also molested. There is a significant incidence of homosexual molestation of young males as well. Women do molest or rape other women; however, it is rarely reported. For convenience, the sexual assault victim will be referred to as "she," but it is understood that males are included where appropriate.

There are many myths and misconceptions concerning the rape victim. These myths are well described in *The Rape Victim* by Elaine Hilberman and *Against Our Will* by Susan Brownmiller. Among the most destructive are the statements that a woman cannot be raped unless she wants to be, and conversely, that if a woman does get raped, she provoked it in some way.

Every female is vulnerable to rape. Statistics show that women belonging to all economic and social classes are raped. Women of all ages are raped, whether prostitutes or virgins, married or single. Some rapists prefer to rape military wives since they are so often alone. Others rape only prostitutes, knowing that they have little chance in court. There is no typical rape victim, and commonly held stereotypes are not valid.

The circumstances under which the sexual assault victim seeks emergency care are highly diverse. She usually comes to the hospital for help shortly after the incident has occurred. Sometimes she is accompanied by the police, sometimes by family or friends. Some victims prefer to come alone, hoping that family and authorities will not become involved. The victim may arrive in the emergency department within an hour of the assault, or not until several hours have passed. This time is usually spent debating the wisest course of action, contending with hysteria, and regaining some composure. Some women do not seek medical attention until several days or weeks after the assault when fear of pregnancy or venereal disease forces them to do so.

PHYSICAL INJURY AND TRAUMA

The physical condition of the rape victim varies tremendously. She may be physically unharmed or brutally traumatized. Many have reflexively bathed or changed clothing since the assault. In many cases of sexual assault there is no physical injury requiring medical attention; that is, the victim is threatened with a weapon, raped, and released. If force or violence has been used, there may be injuries, such as bruises, bleeding, broken bones, and knife wounds. However, the victim should be asked if she was hurt even if there are no apparent physical signs of injury. Bruises can take a day or more to become evident. Some rapists learn methods of torturing and injuring victims without leaving marks.

In the genital area, hymenal tears, vaginal tears, and lacerations may be present. Bleeding and pain may occur. More serious injuries such as perforation of the vagina or rectum must be ruled out. If foreign objects have been forced into the vagina or rectum or if a gang rape was involved, the damage may require pelvic exploration and repair under anesthesia.

In the child victim there may be trauma

with bleeding and lacerations, or little evidence at all depending on whether the male attempted to insert the entire penis, a finger, or simply rubbed against the vulva, ejaculating externally.

CHILD MOLESTATION

Child molestation is far more common than society would like to believe. One study published by J. T. Landis interviewed college students and found that approximately one third of his study population had been molested in childhood. Of the third that were molested, 54% of females were exposed to exhibitionists and 27% were fondled by adults. The majority of females experienced heterosexual approaches. Of the males who were molested, 84% of the assaults were homosexual in nature and 16% were heterosexual.

Our society attempts to protect itself from the reality of child molestation in the following ways. The FBI collects and reports statistics on crime in the United States. However, they do not record child molestation or child sexual abuse. The main issue is credibility. "Who will believe the child?" "What about the seductive child, the imaginative child?" "All children lie," and "Children cannot tell the difference between fact and fantasy." With these misconceptions, uncomfortable situations can be avoided. However, until these attitudes are changed, adequate care and treatment of the molested child cannot be effected.

Charged and ambivalent emotions surround the event to an even greater extent than for adult rape. The reasons are not difficult to understand. The child molester is usually not a stranger, but someone *known* to the family. Since he is usually a family friend, mother's boyfriend, grandfather, father, stepfather, brother, or neighbor, the parents may not believe the child. If the story were true, the family structure might be challenged or destroyed.

Parents respond in unexpected ways. They may express frank disbelief: "Your uncle would never do a thing like that." They may be punitive rather than supportive: "I told you not to talk to strangers." Their reactions may be overreactions due to feelings of guilt for failing to protect their child. If the assailant is a family member or a friend, they are additionally concerned about complications and consequences of acknowledging the event.

Confusion still clouds the issue of how to best care for the sexually assaulted child. Little research has been done to answer questions regarding the child's credibility. Few protocols exist and those that do exist are incomplete. A great deal more energy and research needs to be devoted to this area before there can be security that sexually abused children are receiving the best possible psychological, medical, and legal care.

From evaluating adults who have been sexually molested as children, it is known that the experience can have severe sexual and social consequences. However, with proper medical and psychological management *at the time* serious consequences can usually be avoided.

The way parents and authority figures deal with the incident has a great deal to do with the child's immediate and later adjustment. Children tend to mimic the gravity they see reflected in the attitudes of the adults around them. If they are scolded, they will feel guilty. If they are closely guarded thereafter, they will feel fearful. If the incident is treated with disgust, hysteria, and despair, they will feel damaged. If they are not believed, they will feel betrayed.

Perspective is often lacking. Regaining that perspective is extremely important. If a child has been genitally fondled but not harmed, deal with it as a significant but minor incident. If she has been raped or injured, react with the same concern that an auto accident of equal magnitude would warrant.

A pelvic examination is indicated whenever there is genital discomfort or bleeding, or if it is suspected that vaginal penetration has occurred. If the examination is treated by the physician in the same manner that a rectal exam performed to evaluate appendicitis would be handled, it will be no more traumatic, either physically or psychologically.

Observe the total person as well: emotional character, demeanor, brambles in the hair, marks, bruises, and torn clothing. Was she hit or dragged? Make careful notes on all findings. Take photographs if possible. A case can be won or lost on these points alone.

The greatest assistance the physician can be, medically and legally, is to take time and care assessing the history and veracity of the child's experience and documenting these impressions on paper. Education and counseling of the child's parents should be considered. Providing guidance to the parents can be as significant as providing direct care for the child. The parents often need direct help themselves.

ASSESSMENT

Rape is a criminal act and a legal term, to be proved or disproved in the courts. The responsibility of the emergency personnel is to determine what occurred as objectively and as completely as possible. What did the victim say? What was her mental state? Was there evidence of force, evidence of penetration of the penis into the vagina, or evidence of ejaculation? Did intercourse occur? Was it possible? Can it be ruled out?

The thoroughness of the physician, the completeness of the written record, and the proper collection of evidence will often determine whether the accused rapist is convicted or not. If there is a missing link, the accused may be freed on a technicality.

Rape victims will present with a wide spectrum of emotional and physical conditions. Usually, the physical injury will be minimal and the emotional trauma insidious. Occasionally both the physical and emotional components will be severe and obvious immediately. This wide variation of emotional settings and medical needs challenges the expertise of any emergency facility.

*Rape protocol**

The purpose of this protocol is to provide guidelines for the management and care of the sexual assault victim. The objectives of care are as follows:
1. To reduce or eliminate trauma to the patient before, during, and after the physical examination.
2. To care for the immediate medical and psychological needs.
3. To collect evidence systematically, efficiently, and effectively.
4. To provide competent counseling and treatment for possible pregnancy and venereal disease.

5. To suggest appropriate follow-up care for medical and psychological needs.

This protocol was designed to be flexible, so that it can conform to any size emergency facility. For example, the persons to whom tasks are assigned can be varied. If there is no triage nurse, the emergency department nurse takes over from the emergency department clerk. The small or understaffed emergency department can follow the rest of the procedures by relying more heavily on family, friends, or advocates to stay with the victim. A nurse practitioner or other established sexual assault team member can take over from the clerk and complete the examination, evaluation, and treatment if such personnel are available.

The protocol is designed so that the emergency department physician's time commitment to the procedure is minimized without sacrificing quality of care. In this way, waiting time will be reduced and the busy physician will be less likely to transfer sexual assault victims or otherwise defer caring for them promptly.

PART I: PROCEDURES PRIOR TO MEDICAL EXAMINATION
General

1. Treat patient with courtesy and respect.
2. Be natural and caring.
3. If there is a delay, explain it to her; let her know that she has not been forgotten.
4. Consider the needs of friends and relatives.

Before the physician sees the patient

A. Emergency department clerk or secretary:
1. As soon as you learn it is rape, quickly and discretely record name, address, and minimal necessary check-in data.
2. Immediately notify triage nurse* that you have a "code X" (rape).
3. Bring patient to private waiting room.
4. Assess manner of family and friends.
5. Inform them that the nurse will be with them soon.
6. Ask if the patient has any pain, or if she is bleeding; if so, tell triage nurse promptly.
7. Inquire if she has children, how they are being cared for, and so on.
8. Offer to call an advocate if she would like (Explain advocate).†
9. Inform police as required by law, if they did not bring in the victim.
10. Provide a sexual assault information packet and explain its purpose.‡
B. Triage nurse:
1. Respond to secretary's coded call immediately.

---

*Nurse who screens patients regarding priority of emergency needs and directs them accordingly.

†An advocate is usually a female member of the community dedicated to the emergency and follow-up care of the rape victim. She will respond to a call for help and will remain with the victim until she is no longer needed.

‡Some emergency departments have available a prepared packet or brochure with information on pregnancy, venereal disease, treatment options, and counseling resources. This printed material is not only timesaving and useful to the patient, it also ensures that all patients receive uniform and complete information, regardless of who treats them or when they are seen.

2. Consult with patient regarding whom she prefers to have stay with her: nurse, family, or friends.
3. Offer to call family or friend to stay with her in emergency department, or to provide assistance with children.
4. Assign nurse to stay with her or to check on her frequently.
5. *Do not leave her alone* unless she insists on it.
6. Assess the usefulness of family and friends. If they are visibly distraught or upset, they are not in a condition to help and probably need help themselves. Alternatives:
   a. Call a counselor (from hospital or community) to spend time with them while the rape victim is being cared for.
   b. Speak with them alone for a few moments. Explain to them that the patient needs them to be calm, supportive, and empathetic. Ask them if they are able to help in that manner. Often, with some guidance, they will be able to draw on their resources and be of assistance.
   c. If they are irate, irrational, or overtly angry, separate them from the patient. Be gentle but firm, and have physician or counselor evaluate them with regard to their most appropriate care.
   d. If they use terms such as ruined, violated, dirtied, or loss of innocence, explain the harm these attitudes can do the patient. Ask them to refrain from using such expressions.
   e. Send them for a clean change of clothing, toothpaste, and the like.
   f. Provide counseling or sedation if indicated.
C. Nurse assigned to patient:
   1. Make patient feel safe and comfortable.
   2. Offer to listen if she feels like talking.
   3. Evaluate her immediate needs to determine order of patient care.
      a. Assess need for possible blood work, x-ray and laboratory studies, acuteness of medical and psychiatric needs, and call physician's attention to these problems so that procedures can begin as soon as possible.
      b. Assess her condition to tolerate a pelvic examination. If she is extremely upset, it would be best to have a counselor spend time with her before the examination to help prepare her for it. Is sedation indicated?
      c. Accompany patient to x-ray department, laboratory, counselor's office, and so on.
   4. Prepare her in advance for people (i.e., counselor, physician, police) and events (i.e., examination) that she will encounter in the emergency department.
   5. Encourage her to ask questions if there is anything she does not understand.
   6. Take history of incident and record in the chart. Taping may be used as an alternative (with a signed consent).
   7. Prepare examining room.
   8. Place evidence collection kit in examination room.
   9. Disrobe patient and examine closely for bruises, scratches, and other injuries. Record legibly in chart.

10. Collect clothing and other items of evidence as indicated (fingernail scrapings, etc.).
11. Provide hospital gown or operating room gown.
12. Ask if she has ever had a pelvic or rectal examination before. Explain them if she has not.
13. Explain consent forms and have her sign them.
14. Let victim know the following:
    a. What is expected of her during physical examination.
    b. What the physician will do.
    c. Why the procedures are necessary.
    d. That it is necessary to collect evidence even if she is uncertain whether or not prosecution will be pursued.
15. Explain the financial arrangement with the county or state.

PART II: THE MEDICAL EXAMINATION: HISTORY AND PHYSICAL
Nurse

During and after the physician's examination.
1. Inform physician when patient is ready to be examined. *Do not set her up in stirrups until physician is there.* (Have her sitting on the edge of the table draped and ready.)
2. Have a working knowledge of the specimens to be obtained.
3. Assist the physician as well as the victim during the examination.
4. Administer medications for prevention of pregnancy and venereal disease if ordered and explain possible side effects.
5. Explain possible consequences of rape, emotionally and physically, and encourage questions.
6. Provide measures for cleanliness after the examination (shower, toothbrush, etc.).
7. Provide change of clothing (operating room gowns and disposable paper dresses have been used).
8. Provide access to a telephone.
9. Give follow-up wound care instructions.
10. Recommend follow-up counseling.
11. Make return appointments and referrals in cooperation with the hospital's social service department.
12. Help in obtaining transportation from hospital.
13. Supply victim with "Sexual Assault Follow-up and Information Packet" or other printed material if available.
14. Keep patient under observation for 20 minutes following an injection before releasing from emergency department.

Physician

1. *Respond promptly.*
2. Obtain history of assault. (Use History of Sexual Assault form if available.)
   a. What happened, how long ago, how many individuals involved, where it occurred, and so on.
   b. Inquire into sexual events: oral sex, anal sex, vaginal penetration, the use of foreign objects, by what means he ejaculated, did he use a con-

dom or other possible contraceptive measure (i.e., withdrawal or a vasectomy—rapists sometimes volunteer this information).

    c. Ask if there was any other violence or injury. Were threats made, verbally or nonverbally?

3. Obtain directed medical history.

    a. Specifically ask about menstrual, contraceptive, coital, and venereal disease history, and activity post assault (changes of clothing, bathing, douching, etc.). Is she pregnant, on birth control pills, IUD, hysterectomy, tubal ligation?

    b. If she is taking birth control pills, determine how long she has been taking them. Has she missed any doses during the present cycle?

4. Obtain social history.

    a. Has she ever had intercourse, at what age, date of last intercourse, marital status, current sexual relationship(s).

5. *Perform physical examination* with female hospital employee as standby.

    a. Tell the patient what you are going to do before you do it. Allow time for her to relax. Should pain occur, momentarily interrupt the examination until she is ready to proceed.

6. Special treatment and consideration is necessary for children, virgins, and elderly women, that is, nasal or pediatric speculum. Do not assume the victim has or has not been having sexual relationships with men—ask.

Discussing sex with a stranger is difficult for most people to do under any circumstances. It is especially difficult when upset or under stress. It is important not to rush the patient. If the interviewer expresses a sense of comfort in asking the questions, it increases the patient's comfort, and the interview usually progresses well.

PART III: EVIDENCE COLLECTION
Methods of collecting legal evidence

1. For the victim's comfort and for legal purposes use a speculum that has been warmed and lubricated with *water or saline only*.

2. Obtain specimens for semen analysis from all body orifices indicated by history (mouth, oral pharynx, vagina, and rectum).
   Wet mount preparation: Drop of secretions plus a drop of saline. This should be examined for five minutes under a high-power field.
   Document presence or absence and the number of motile/nonmotile sperm per high-power field. This may be done by calling a laboratory technician to the emergency department. Do not send the specimen to the laboratory, where it may stand and dry out.

3. Collect specimens for acid phosphatase determination from areas suspected to contain sperm or seminal fluid. Place aspirated or scraped specimen in capped, labeled tube.

4. Obtain permanent smear of secretions from involved areas. Pap smear is best, but methylene blue or gram stain may be used. Ask pathologist to document presence or absence of sperm.

5. Police should not be present during physical examination. It is upsetting to the victim and is *not* necessary to maintain the chain of evidence.

6. Comb for foreign pubic hairs (let patient do combing if she prefers).

Ask her to remove a few of her own pubic hairs for comparison purposes. Place in labeled vials.

7. Further tests to document identity of offender are the following: scrapings from beneath fingernails; secretions for ABO antigens; collection of dust, dirt, and debris for neutron activation analysis.
8. Obtain photographs as indicated with prior consent and explanation.
9. Clothing: all clothing should be saved to be analyzed for semen and bloodstains. Circle suspected areas with a laundry marker. Save underwear and torn clothing. Take care to preserve them carefully. *Do not crumple or place in plastic bags* where bacterial action would alter the evidence. Wrap in paper or place in paper bags.

PART IV: MEDICAL PROCEDURES
Medical tests

1. Culture body orifices involved for gonorrhea: vaginal vault, endocervix, mouth, throat, and rectum.
2. Baseline test for syphilis.
3. Pregnancy test on any female past menarche.
4. Urine or blood sample for drug screen. Blood alcohol level if patient appears intoxicated or gives history of drinking.

Treatment

1. *Venereal disease prophylaxis:* prophylactic treatment should be recommended if there are no contraindications. Gram stain will not rule out exposure to gonorrhea; the culture may be falsely negative, or the patient may have bathed or douched before examination.
   Inform patient fully of the fallibility of the tests and inform her of the possible danger to her sexual partner(s). Explain to the victim that venereal disease is transmitted through all mucous membranes (i.e., oral-genital). Sex is unsafe—
   a. Unless she receives prophylactic treatment, or
   b. Until it is determined whether she has contracted venereal disease and, if so, has completed treatment.
2. Inform her of other possible venereal diseases besides gonorrhea and syphilis (i.e., crabs, trichomonas, monilia, herpes, condyloma, etc.).
3. *Medications and recommended dosages:*
   a. *For both gonorrhea and syphilis—prophylactic:* 1 g aqueous procaine penicillin G, 4.8 million units IM in two doses given in two sites. Probenecid, 1 g PO, is administered orally one half-hour prior to the injections.
   b. *Syphilis—treatment:*
      (1) Benzathine penicillin G, 2.4 million units total by IM injection at a single session, is the drug of choice in the treatment of primary, secondary, or latent syphilis of less than one year's duration, according to the 1976 treatment schedule recommended by the Venereal Disease Control Advisory Committee of the Center for Disease Control in Atlanta.
      (2) For patients allergic to penicillin, give tetracycline hydrochloride, 500 mg four times a day PO for 15 days.

(3) Or, erythromycin, 500 mg four times a day PO for 15 days.
  c. *Gonorrhea—treatment:*
    (1) Aqueous procaine penicillin G, 4.8 million units IM in two divided doses given simultaneously in two sites; probenecid, 1 g PO, to be given one-half hour prior to injections.
    (2) Ampicillin, 3.5 g PO, preceded by probenecid, 1 g PO.
    (3) Tetracycline hydrochloride, 1.5 g PO, followed by 0.5 g PO qid for four days (total dose 9.5 g) (contraindicated during pregnancy).
    (4) Erythromycin, 1.5 g PO, followed by 0.5 g PO qid for four days (total dose 9.5 g).
    (5) Spectinomycin hydrochloride, 2 g IM (single dose), for gonorrhea only.
4. Pregnancy prophylaxis. The "morning-after pill" or "DES" should be explained if victim is menarchial and is using no secure form of contraception. A large dose of synthetic estrogen prevents implantation of the fertilized egg in the wall of the uterus. A full course of 25 mg taken two times a day for five days must be initiated beginning within 24 hours of the sexual assault if it is to be effective.
Hormonal therapy:
  a. Ethinyl estradiol (Estinyl), 2.5 mg bid for five days, or
  b. Diethylstilbesterol (DES), 25 mg bid for five days.
    DES (or other similar estrogen compounds) should be explained as a preventative measure. It should be given only after an informed consent has been obtained. The choice to take DES should be the victim's. Risks and possible side effects should be thoroughly explained. Some possible side effects include the following:
  c. Danger to the fetus if the victim is already pregnant at the time of the sexual assault. (She may not be aware of an early pregnancy.)
  d. Danger to the fetus if she remains pregnant as a result of the sexual assault (DES failure).
  e. Nausea and vomiting, possible vaginal spotting, breast tenderness, insomnia, and rash during the course of treatment.
Antinauseant therapy:
  f. Bendectin, 1 tablet tid as needed for nausea and vomiting, or
  g. Prochlorperazine (Compazine), 10 mg PO, or 25 mg PO, every six hours prn.
  h. DES has been linked to a rare form of vaginal cancer in daughters of women who took DES from 1945-1970 as an antimiscarriage drug during their pregnancy with those daughters. However, the mothers did not develop cancer, and there is no evidence to suggest that there is any risk to them.
Victim should be informed that taking estrogens may result in increased risk to fetus if pregnancy follows and should be asked to sign a consent that if she misses a menstrual period in spite of therapy or fails to have withdrawal bleeding from estrogens, menstrual extraction or abortion will be performed. Treatment, if no menses occurs in four weeks:
  i. Menstrual extraction or D & C.
  j. Adoption counseling, if indicated.

5. Tissue trauma.
   a. Wound care, suture lacerations, prophylactic antibiotics, if contaminated.
   b. Tetanus toxoid, if indicated.
   c. Treat areas of trauma appropriately.
   d. Follow-up, as indicated.
6. Psychological trauma. Every sexual assault victim, adult or child, should receive at least one hour of follow-up consultation with hospital social service personnel, other trained counselor, or therapist
   a. To determine if further treatment is necessary.
   b. To provide assistance and guidelines to prepare parents or victim for possible consequences of the sexual assault.
   c. To alert them to symptoms that may require counseling should they occur.

Follow-up

1. Appointment with gynecologist or family physician in two weeks to check for venereal disease and pregnancy.
2. Repeat gonorrhea cultures at follow-up visit; further tests and treatment as indicated.
3. Repeat VDRL in eight weeks.
4. The follow-up counseling visit should be scheduled as soon as possible following the assault, preferably within the first week. Prophylactic counseling can be a minimum of one hour. An average of six to eight hours is found effective in preventing the major psychosocial sequelae of sexual assault in most cases.

SUMMARY

Rape is not a medical diagnosis but an issue of consent that will be determined by the legal process. However, whether penetration has occurred, and whether there has been intercourse or ejaculation can often be determined by a thorough physical examination and history.

Steps to follow in dealing with rape victim

1. Record brief but complete history of the alleged sexual assault in patient's own words.
2. Collect and identify with appropriate labels all evidence collected.
3. Make specific diagnosis of trauma, contusions, lacerations, emotional status, affect, and so on.
4. Explain procedures and treatment options to patient.
5. Provide appropriate treatment as indicated for venereal disease, pregnancy, psychological trauma, and the like.
6. Do not neglect family and friends; they frequently need counseling and assistance too.
7. Maintain complete and legible written records at all times.

LABORATORY SPECIMEN CHART

Evidence collection

Label all specimens. Stamp all labels with addressograph plate. Indicate the exact source of the sample.

____ Combing of loose pubic hair.

____ Victim's pubic hair (with roots).

____ One wet mount.

____ One slide for Pap smear or gram stain.

____ Four vaginal swabs (two deep and two shallow), or vaginal aspirate: irrigate with 10 ml sterile saline, place in container.

____ Fingernail scrapings or clippings.

____ Saliva sample on paper disk.

____ Two blood samples: one purple top, and one red top.

____ Collect all clothing, dirt, or debris.

Medical tests

____ Transgrow cultures for gonococcus: vaginal vault, endocervix, mouth, and rectum.

____ Baseline VDRL.

____ Baseline pregnancy test for any female past menarche.

____ Appropriate urine or blood samples for drug screen.

____ Blood alcohol level if indicated.

SUMMARY

A woman who has been sexually assaulted experiences consequences that require both professional expertise and family support to deal with effectively.

Three distinct variables will affect her eventual recovery: (1) the sexual trauma itself, (2) the quality of emergency management, and (3) the reactions of family and friends.

1. The most prominent effect of sexual assault is due to the personal and sustained experience of fear of death. Whether overtly threatened or not, this woman knows she is completely powerless to protect herself. Her sense of invulnerability is destroyed. The denial system that protects her from perpetual fear is no longer intact (i.e., ability to cross street without fear of being killed by a car). Depending on her value system and the severity of the physical trauma, there may be sexual consequences, including sexual aversion, dys-pareunia, vaginismus, and orgasmic dysfunction.

2. The quality of emergency management involves two categories: medical and psychological. Essential to the medical care is information regarding the possible medical consequences of rape: the various venereal diseases, pregnancy, and so on. Equally important is the prevention of these consequences where possible and close follow-up care. The quality of psychological management is critical at this point. The patient is herself a victim of the myth that there is invariably some degree of female complicity in the assault. She usually feels some degree of guilt and questions the appropriateness of her own behavior. She may be hysterical or withdrawn, hostile or apparently calm. The attitudes of the police and emergency staff treating her will have a marked effect on her later adjustment. Considerate, prompt attention to her medical and psychological needs is

paramount. Harsh indifference through ignorance and fear is terribly destructive.

3. Immediate and delayed reactions of family and friends play an important role in the length of recovery time. Initially, the family may be supportive, punitive, angry, or condemning, depending upon their mode of coping with severe stress. However, no matter how well motivated and supportive family and spouse are originally, few can sustain this posture for the months or years that may be involved in the patient's recovery. Sexual and emotional problems precipitated by the rape may cause or exaggerate relationship problems, leading to separation and divorce.

The physician, by being aware of the complex nature of the woman's posttraumatic rape syndrome, can ensure complete medical care with a focus on the medical and psychosexual sequelae; can direct her and her family for appropriate therapy; and can evaluate family and spouse regarding needs for direct care and counseling. A willingness to testify is psychologically reassuring to the patient, whether or not the case comes to trial.

The family can best help by seeking direct help themselves when they recognize stress and conflict within themselves and by encouraging the sexual assault victim to seek help.

Appropriate early therapeutic intervention can prevent the majority of psychological consequences that would otherwise occur.

BIBLIOGRAPHY

American College of Obstetrics and Gynecology (ACOG): Suspected rape, Technical Bulletin no. 14, July 1970 (revised, April 1972).

Amir, M.: Patterns of forcible rape, Chicago, 1971, University of Chicago Press.

Brooks, D.: Suspected rape medical guidelines, San Diego County Medical Society, May, 1975.

Brownmiller, S.: Against our will: men, women and rape, New York, 1975, Simon & Schuster.

Burgess, A. W., and Holmstrom, L. L.: Rape: victims of crisis, Bowie, Md., 1974, Robert J. Brady Co.

California penal code, felony section, Crimes against children, lewd and lascivious acts.

Chicago Hospital Council: Guidelines for the treatment of suspected rape victims, February 21, 1974, The Council.

Connell, N., and Wilson, C., editors: Rape: the first sourcebook for women, New York, 1974, The New American Library.

Crime in the United States, 1975, Uniform Crime Reports, FBI.

Dewing, S. A., et al.: Rape crisis intervention training manual, distributed by R.E.A.L. (Rape Emergency Assistance League), P.O. Box 468, El Cajon, California 92020.

Glover, D., Gerety, M., Bromberg, S., Fullam, S., DiVasto, P., and Kaufman, A.: Diethylstilbestrol in the treatment of rape victims, Western Journal of Medicine, October 1976, pp. 331-334.

Hillberman, E.: The rape victim, 1976, American Psychiatric Association, available by writing The American Psychiatric Association, 1700 18th St. N.W., Washington, D.C., 20009.

Horos, C. V.: Rape, New Canaan, Conn., 1974, Tobey Publishing Co.

Hospital Council of Southern California and Los Angeles County Department of Health Services Preventative Health Services: Guidelines for the emergency department for management of the forensic patient, February 1976.

Levitan, P.: Rape emergency care procedures manual (compiled and edited), Office of Emergency Medical Services, County of San Diego, San Diego, California, 1976.

MacDonald, J. M.: Rape: offenders and their victims, Springfield, Ill., 1971, Charles C Thomas, Publisher.

Medea, A., and Thompson, K.: Against rape, New York, 1974, Farrar, Strauss & Giroux.

Response to intrafamily violence and sexual assault, Advisory Board on the Status of Women, City of San Diego, vol. 1, issue 1, Oct. 1976.

Russell, D. E. H.: The politics of rape: the victim's perspective, New York, 1975, Stein & Day Publishers.

Schultz, L. G., editor: Rape victimology, Springfield, Ill., 1975, Charles C Thomas, Publisher.

"Taking care of yourself, a self help guide," prepared by the Sub-Committee on Sexual Assault and Intrafamily Violence, Advisory Board on Women, 1976, San Diego.

CHAPTER 32

Emergency care in infants and children

Alan E. Shumacher, M.D.

Recognition of a life-threatening situation in an infant or child demands continual alertness on the part of the emergency department or other first-line personnel. Once such a situation is recognized, the prompt institution of specific treatment may mean the difference between intact survival, survival with sequelae, or death.

In simplest terms, three organ systems are involved in the maintenance of life support. These are the following:

1. Cardiovascular system
2. Respiratory system
3. Central nervous system

The failure of any one of these systems may be lethal. Their functions are interlocked and the failure of a single system may be followed by failure of one or both of the other two. The approach to the child with a medical emergency must be a logical one if it is to have an optimal chance of success. Such a logical approach is presented below and gives first priority to functional assessment of these three systems.

THE CHILD WITH A MEDICAL EMERGENCY

History

In an urgent situation the history is taken concurrently with a physical examination directed toward the assessment of vital organ systems. Obvious abnormalities such as coma, cyanosis, traumatic injuries, or petechial rash should be the subject of questions to ascertain the following:

1. Time and nature of onset
2. Progression of symptoms
3. Duration of symptoms
4. Associated symptoms
   a. Fever
   b. Excess fluid or electrolyte loss
   c. Exposure to poison or toxin
5. History of prior illness or known chronic disease (e.g., diabetes, malignancy, cardiac disease)

Examination

General

1. Level of consciousness
2. Evidence of trauma—fractures, bleeding, ecchymosis, abrasions
3. Color—cyanosis, pallor, rash, other
4. Facial expression
5. Vital signs—pulse (rate and rhythm), respirations, blood pressure, temperature
6. Odor of breath or clothes

Head and neck

1. Evidence of trauma
2. Fontanelle in infants
3. Eyes, pupils—size, reaction, fundi

4. Cerebrospinal fluid otorrhea or rhinor-rhea, Battle's sign
5. Tracheal position
Chest
1. Respiratory distress, stridor, wheeze
2. Evidence of trauma
3. Cardiac examination—quality of sounds, rate, rhythm, neck veins, blood pressure (in legs as well as arms), murmur or rub
Abdomen
1. Distension
2. Masses
3. Tenderness
4. Organomegaly
5. Bowel sounds
6. Perineum
7. Back
8. Genitalia
Extremities
1. Position
2. Deformity
Neurologic examination
1. Cranial nerves
2. Reflexes

SPECIFIC EMERGENCIES
Shock in infants

Shock is a syndrome in which poor perfusion at the cellular level results in depressed function of one or more of the three vital systems. Hypotension is a characteristic feature. Shock in older children is similar to shock in adults, and the discussion here will be limited to the picture and treatment of shock in infants.

The infant in shock may appear lethargic and mottled with ashen or grayish color. This is associated with pallor and poor capillary filling. Tachycardia or tachypnea or both may be present. Blood pressure, which may be difficult to measure, is low.

The flush method for determining blood pressure is useful in infants. A hand or foot is squeezed firmly enough to cause blanching, and an appropriate size cuff is inflated proximally without releasing the pressure until inflation is above the anticipated systolic pressure. As pressure is slowly released, the hand or foot will flush with the influx of blood at a point corresponding to the systolic blood pressure.

Classifications. Causes of shock can be classified as follows:
1. Hypovolemic shock—hemorrhage, dehydration, or burns
2. Cardiogenic shock—decreased cardiac output or decreased venous return
3. Septic or endotoxic shock—peripheral vascular collapse causes diminished tissue perfusion
4. Neurogenic shock—loss of vascular tone causes relative hypovolemia
5. Anaphylactic shock—release of histamine and related compounds causes marked arteriolar dilatation

Management. General measures for immediate treatment of shock include the following:
1. Establishment of an airway and monitoring the heart
2. Administration of adequate amounts of oxygen
3. Establishment of an intravenous line; begin Ringer's lactate, 10 to 20 ml/kg
4. Placement of central venous and/or arterial catheters

The classification, pathophysiology, and treatment of specific types of shock are summarized in Table 32-1.

For the most part, replacement of lost volume is the single best method for the treatment of shock (other than cariogenic or anaphylactic). In the infant one must always remember that even moderate volume loss may cause profound hypoperfusion. Rapid infusion of hypertonic solutions such as 7.5% sodium bicarbonate may predispose to brain hemorrhage by drawing water into the vascular compartment from the brain. Maintenance of normal temperature is especially important to conserve calories and improve survival in shock. An infant warmer that provides radiant heat while allowing good access to the baby is a useful piece of equipment.

Assessment. Blood pressure and capillary filling are used to assess the adequacy of measures instituted to combat shock. Remember that the blood pressure determined in an extremity by flush or palpation may be 10 to 20 mm Hg lower than that determined directly from an arterial line or by a Doppler apparatus.

Capillary filling (peripheral perfusion) can be judged by the temperature of the hands and feet as a rough guide.

The mean systolic blood pressure in the newborn is approximately 60 mm Hg (by Doppler). By 3 months of age it is 70 to 80 mm Hg, and by 1 year of age it is 90 to 100 mm Hg.

Respiratory emergencies

Many pediatric emergency visits are necessitated by respiratory symptoms. The majority of these are associated with infection; but allergy, foreign body, and trauma are all possible causes of distress, cyanosis, and hypoxia.

Infection

Epiglottitis. Epiglottitis is a fulminating and potentially disastrous illness. Symptoms begin with the sudden onset of inspiratory stridor. Swallowing becomes difficult and painful very rapidly. The child often arrives in the emergency department with marked inspiratory stridor, drooling with the chin thrust forward, and an expression of extreme anxiety. If the child has begun to become hypoxic, restlessness and tachycardia are seen. Maintenance of the airway is of prime importance. No attempt to visualize the swollen, cherry-red epiglottis should be made unless personnel are prepared to intubate, perform a tracheostomy, or at least insert a large-bore needle through the cricothyroid membrane. This last technique is a temporary expedient and should only be used while an experienced physician is en route to perform a tracheostomy.

It is imperative that emergency department personnel perform these life-saving procedures before cyanosis and bradycardia indicate long-standing hypoxia. Adequate restraint of the intubated child who has recovered consciousness after relief of hypoxia is mandatory to prevent accidental extubation and potential tragedy.

Laryngotracheobronchitis (croup). Although somewhat less fulminating and dangerous than epiglottitis, croup is nevertheless capable of causing distress. Inspiratory stridor and a brassy cough can progress to obstruction of the airway. The use of 0.5 ml racemic epinephrine in 2.0 ml normal saline nebulized by IPPB via a tight mask may result in dramatic relief; but if not successful and early signs of hypoxia are

Table 32-1. Classification and treatment of shock in infancy

Classification	Pathophysiology	Treatment
Hypovolemic		
Hemorrhage	Decreased vascular volume, blood loss	Blood transfusion, correction of metabolic acidosis
Dehydration	Fluid and electrolyte loss	Ringer's lactate, 20-30 ml/kg/hr
Burns	Protein loss	Albumin, plasma, dextran 40, 10 ml/kg, Ringer's lactate, 10-20 ml/kg
Cardiogenic	Decreased cardiac output	Lidocaine, propranolol, isoproterenol, dopamine, digoxin, *no* vasodilators
Endotoxic (septic)	Splanchnic pooling	Increased vascular volume, isoproterenol, steroids, antibiotics, dopamine
Neurogenic	Decreased vascular tone, decreased cardiac output	Increased vascular volume, vasopressors, isoproterenol, dopamine
Anaphylactic	Arteriolar dilatation	Epinephrine, steroids, antihistamines

noted, the above remarks pertaining to airway obstruction in epiglottitis are equally true in this disease.

Bronchiolitis. Bronchiolitis commonly affects infants under 18 months of age and seldom is fulminant in onset. It most often begins with simple upper respiratory symptoms and progresses to dyspnea and wheezing because of edema of the lining of respiratory bronchioles. These infants can become severely ill, and the main role of the emergency department personnel is to recognize the potential severity of this illness so that the infant will be admitted for care.

Pneumonia. The complex of symptoms in childhood and infant pneumonia is a broad one. Emergency department physicians and nurses should be aware of the association between right upper lobe pneumonia and nuchal rigidity in small children. The presence of a stiff neck is, of course, an indication for lumbar puncture. In the absence of positive findings in the cerebrospinal fluid, a chest x-ray film may show right upper lobe pneumonia. There may be no detectable râles or other easily detectable physical findings in the chest. Even so, a consolidated lobe may be present and give rise to meningism as the presenting symptom.

Many small infants will have considerable difficulty in maintaining an airway clear of secretions. They may require admission for this reason alone.

Allergy

Bronchial asthma. The first drug used in treatment of the acute asthmatic attack is aqueous epinephrine 1:1000, 0.1 to 0.3 ml subcutaneously. This can be repeated at intervals of 15 to 20 minutes to a total of three doses. The child should be admitted if complete clearing does not occur.

Relief of the mild dehydration and acidosis accompanying an attack may enhance the response to epinephrine and to adjunctive drugs. Aminophylline, 4 mg/kg, can be given *slowly* intravenously over 20 to 30 minutes. Psychologic support and the use of IPPB may also be helpful.

Observance of the maxim "all that wheezes is not asthma" will remind emergency department personnel that foreign bodies can also cause wheezing.

Glossal, laryngeal, or angioneurotic edema. Epinephrine is the most useful drug in these conditions, but both antihistamines and steroids may be of help. Any of the allergic conditions may require that arterial punctures be done to assess respiratory function; intubation or tracheostomy may be necessary for airway maintenance.

Foreign bodies

The real emergencies in this category are usually caused by partially chewed meat, soft pieces of food, or vomitus. These are all capable of total airway obstruction in contradistinction to the metal or plastic toys, nuts, popcorn, pins, coins, and the like that cause problems but are not immediately life threatening. Many foreign bodies can be removed by the stimulation of coughing and turning the child upside down. The Heimlich maneuver appears to be worth a trial in toddlers and older children, but its value in infants is unclear. If these measures are unsuccessful, tracheostomy may be needed and should be done before critical hypoxia occurs.

Trauma

Airway obstruction can occur after burns, injury to the neck, or the ingestion or inhalation of caustics. Tracheostomy may be required.

Chest injuries causing pneumothorax are not uncommon. This can be relieved temporarily with a large gauge (No. 14) Medicut catheter.

Burns in children

Infants and children often present more difficult management problems when burned than do adults. The long-term therapy of burns will not be discussed here, only the immediate management of the burned child.

Shock. Shock is a common accompaniment to burns of even 5% to 10% of the body surface in children. Early treatment of a seemingly small burn may mean the difference between life and death. Proper early treatment may save a child from scarring or life-long disability.

Burns around the face should arouse the suspicion of airway burns, and in any case, evaluation of adequate airway is given first priority. The shock state usually noted in the burned patient is the result of both hypovolemia and neurogenic factors. An indwelling polyethylene or similar intravenous catheter (Medicut or Intracath) should be placed or a cutdown should be done. Blood can be drawn for complete blood cell count, electrolytes, BUN, total protein, and blood type and crossmatch.

Management. Neurogenic shock can be treated by giving meperidine (Demerol), 1 mg/kg *slowly* intravenously. Intramuscular or subcutaneous routes are unreliable in this situation.

The choice of initial fluids has been discussed widely for many years. Since the initial object of care is to restore plasma and extracellular fluid volume and to compensate for sodium and water losses into the cells, Ringer's lactate seems a good choice. The addition of 22 mEq (25 ml) of sodium bicarbonate to the first liter of fluid also helps to combat the concomitant metabolic acidosis. Low molecular weight dextran 40 may have the advantage of preventing intravascular sludging in injured vessels.

To determine the rate of fluid administration, the extent of second and third degree burns must be estimated. The "rule of nines" is satisfactory for all but the smallest infants.

The immediate local treatment of a burn is the rapid application of cold. This has usually been accomplished by the time the child arrives at the emergency department. All clothing should be removed and the burned areas protected from further contamination.

Any child with burns of the head, face, neck, hands, feet, or anogenital area should be hospitalized. The younger the child, the more imperative this becomes. Additionally, any 10% burn of other areas is best cared for on an inpatient basis.

Central venous pressure (CVP) monitoring can be a useful guide to the adequacy of volume replacement. The placement of a CVP line is not usually necessary in the emergency department, but personnel should be familiar with the techniques required.

Central nervous system emergencies

Coma

Midbrain hypoxia is the cause of coma. Any condition that interferes with acquisition, transport, or exchange of oxygen can cause unconsciousness. The treatment of coma depends on the cause. The following classification will be helpful.

Primary intracranial disorders

Trauma. Of all traumatic lesions of the brain causing unconsciousness, only two are surgical emergencies. These are the depressed skull fracture and the epidural hematoma, which is characterized by a fixed, dilated pupil with contralateral weakness. Acute cerebral edema constitutes a medical emergency. A combination of dexamethasone (Decadron), 4 to 8 mg, and mannitol, 1 to 2 g/kg, can be life saving.

Emergency department personnel should be well aware of the physical signs of nonaccidental injury (Chapter 33) and should remember that this is also a potential cause of coma.

Vascular disorders. Subdural hematoma is the most common vascular disorder. Spontaneous hemorrhage from an aneurysm or an angioma (previously unknown) has been described. Cerebral vascular thromboses are usually associated with febrile illness.

Infection. Meningitis, encephalitis, abscess, or sinus thrombosis can be the cause of coma.

Convulsions. The postictal state may be associated with idiopathic, posttraumatic, or febrile seizures.

Sytemic diseases affecting the central nervous system

Metabolic disease. Diabetes, hypoglycemia, anemia, and hyponatremia or hypernatremia can affect the central nervous system. Remember that glycosuria may occur with infection, cerebral injuries, or lead poisoning. A convulsion can cause a sharp rise in blood glucose levels.

Hemorrhagic diseases. Leukemia, aplastic anemia, or idiopathic thrombocytopenic purpura (ITP) are all capable of causing central nervous system bleeding because of thrombocytopenia. Hemophilia (either A or B) may present with intracranial bleeding.

Cardiovascular disease. Acute glomerulonephritis with hypertension may cause coma. Adams-Stokes attacks or carotid sinus syndrome are discussed in Chapter 27.

Intoxications and ingestions. Many agents are capable of producing unconsciousness.

Psychiatric causes. Hysteria may mimic many other causes of unconsciousness. Patients in hysterical coma often resist having their eyes opened by the examiner.

Treatment

The emergency treatment of coma consists of the following:

1. Cardiorespiratory support; maintenance of airway
2. Management of shock, if present
3. Determination of cause
4. Avoidance of drugs, if possible
5. Treatment of cerebral edema

Convulsions

Approximately 6% of infants and children suffer convulsions. Most common is the grand mal seizures, but psychomotor, focal, myoclonic, and petit mal seizures are all seen in children. Of specific pediatric interest, however, is the febrile convulsion. This occurs most commonly from 6 months to 3 years of age. After age 3 it is rare, and after age 5 it is almost unknown. The seizure is often associated with the rate of rise of fever rather than the height of the fever. Febrile seizures are of short duration, but the postictal state is commonly seen, and Todd's paralysis may also be seen.

The febrile seizure is often over by the time the patient arrives in the emergency department. Treatment consists of febrile control by tepid (not cold) water sponging if the temperature is over 39° C (103.4° F) (r) and the use of aspirin or acetaminophen suppositories, 60 mg per year of age. Phenobarbital, 6 mg/kg, may be used intramuscularly. A lumbar puncture should be done in *every* case of a first febrile seizure and in those children with a history of febrile seizures in whom no cause for fever is found on physical examination. Meningitis or encephalitis cannot be excluded without examination of the cerebral spinal fluid. To wonder whether to perform a lumbar puncture is often a valid indication to proceed with the tap.

The child with status epilepticus requires not only medication to terminate status, but certain general measures. These include the following:

1. Protection from injury
2. Removal or loosening of tight clothing
3. Avoidance of aspiration by keeping the patient on his or her side
4. Avoidance of anoxia

Termination of the seizure can be accomplished by administration of diazepam (Valium). This is given *slowly* intravenously until termination of the seizure, up to a maximum dose of 10 mg. The usual dosage is 3 to 10 mg. If the seizure should recur in 15 to 20 minutes, phenobarbital, 6 mg/kg, can be given intramuscularly, or the dosage of Valium may be repeated. Intramuscular paraldehyde, 1 ml per year of age is safe and effective. Emergency department personnel should be prepared to ventilate infants and children with status epilepticus if apnea occurs.

Cardiovascular emergencies

The scope of cardiovascular emergencies seen in children is vastly different from those seen in adults. The cause of the emergency is most often congenital, although infection, trauma, and acquired heart disease may also play a role.

Cardiac arrest. Cardiac arrest has been dealt with in Chapters 27 and 28 and will not be repeated here. Note only that effective external massage in the infant is best done with compression by both thumbs.

Arrhythmias. The following arrhythmias may occur in infants and children.

Paroxysmal atrial tachycardia (PAT). PAT is the most common arrhythmia of infancy and childhood other than those induced by digitalis toxicity. It is characterized by a rate of 250 to 300 beats per minute with an ECG showing a constant R-R interval and no distinct P waves. This may occur in the absence of any congenital or acquired heart disease, but hospitalization for further study is always indicated. Unilateral carotid sinus compression or supraorbital pressure should not be attempted in the infant but may infrequently terminate an attack in the older child. Failure of such vagal stimulatory methods calls for rapid digitalization. Further care is not within the province of emergency department personnel.

The effect of prolonged PAT is cardiac failure. Rates up to 200 beats per minute associated with crying or fever are not PAT.

Atrial flutter. Atrial flutter is uncommon. Rates run from 300 to 600 per minute, and abnormal "sawtooth" P waves are seen on the ECG. The treatment is digitalization. Hospitalization is always indicated.

Digitalis-induced arrhythmias. Any arrhythmia seen while the patient is receiving digitalis must be presumed to be the result of digitalis toxicity. These arrhythmias are diagnosed by ECG and call for hospitalization. First-degree atrioventricular block is a common therapeutic effect of digitalis and not necessarily a sign of toxicity.

Ventricular tachycardias. Ventricular tachycardias are rarely seen in childhood unless the patient is in a terminal state or has severe myocarditis. It often occurs before the onset of ventricular fibrillation.

Ventricular fibrillation. The clinical picture is that of circulatory arrest. If a regular rhythm—no matter how profound the tachycardia—is heard, ventricular fibrillation is not present. If fibrillation is present, defibrillation is used to convert as outlined elsewhere.

Congestive failure. Signs invariably present include tachycardia, tachypnea, and hepatomegaly with dull liver edge. A gallop rhythm may be heard. Edema may be seen only in the periorbital areas or on the dorsum of the hands and feet, but is seldom prominent. Cyanosis is notable only in the presence of a right to left shunt or severe hypoxemia due to pulmonary congestion. Cardiomegaly is seen on x-ray examination.

Historically, one may elicit a story of difficulty in feeding, poor growth, or lethargy. The treatment of congestive heart failure is not an emergency department function. Immediate care, however, may well include measures to document the underlying cause of failure. These include x-ray studies, ECG, arterial blood gas determinations, and, of course, complete physical examination with careful blood pressure determinations in arms and legs. Initial therapeutic measures include the administration of oxygen, placement in semi-Fowler's position, and the initiation of digitalis therapy with the possible use of morphine, 0.1 mg/kg SC.

To initiate digitalis therapy, an initial dose of 20 μg/kg (one half of the total digitalizing dose of 40 μg/kg) can be given intravenously. Digoxin for injection containing 100 μg/ml (rather than the older preparation containing 250 μg/ml) is an excellent choice.

A rare infant will appear in the emergency department in a moribund state. This will require ventilatory assistance as well as metabolic resuscitation with sodium bicarbonate or THAM. An isoproterenol drip (0.2 μg/kg/min) may also be of great value. This is made by adding 1 mg of isoproterenol to 100 ml of 5% dextrose, thus making a solution of 10 μg/ml. A drip of dopamine (5 to 100 μg/kg/min) can be made by adding 5 ml (200 mg) to 250 ml of 5% dextrose, obtaining a solution containing 800 μg/ml. This is useful in the treatment of shock in the presence of normal vascular volume.

Hypercyanotic spells. Hypercyanotic spells are episodes of acute hypoxemia in children with cyanotic congenital heart disease, especially tetralogy of Fallot. The child will exhibit increased cyanosis and dyspnea. The resultant increasing hypoxemia and acidosis can lead to alteration of consciousness and even death if not attended promptly. Placing the infant over the mother's shoulder or in the knee-chest position will be helpful. Morphine, 0.2 mg/kg SC, and the administration of oxygen (if it can be done without increasing the child's struggling) are effective. The treatment of acidosis with sodium bicarbonate intravenously is useful in the severe episodes. Other therapeutic measures may include the use of propranolol, a potent beta-adrenergic blocker, 0.1 to 0.5 mg/kg IV, or phenylephrine (Neo-Synephrine), an adrenergic stimulator.

These spells are a poor prognostic sign and point toward surgical intervention; therefore, admission and consultation are necessary.

Sickle cell crises

Pathophysiology and classification
Vaso-occlusive crises. Vaso-occlusive crises result from the occlusion of a vessel by masses of sickled red cells. Pain is the principal manifestation, and this represents the most common type of crisis. The symptom complex varies with the location of the occlusion. In infancy, painful swelling of the hands and feet (dactylitis) may be accompanied by fever. Older children may have joint and long bone symptoms. Abdominal pain may simulate intraabdominal

catastrophe and requires careful evaluation. Hepatic, pulmonary, or central nervous system involvement can, of course, also occur, each with its own symptomatology.

Aplastic crises. The child with sickle cell disease has a marrow already working at near capacity. Many common infections interfere with erythropoiesis and cause the aplastic crisis. Increasing anemia and decreasing reticulocytosis will be manifest by progressive weakness and pallor, especially after a viral infection.

Hemolytic crises. Acute infections may cause an increased rate of hemolysis due to shortened red blood cell survival. Weakness, pallor, increasing icterus, and increasing splenomegaly associated with a falling hematocrit and a rising reticulocyte count progress slowly over several weeks.

Acute splenic sequestration crises. The enlarged spleen of the young infant and child that has not yet become fibrotic from repeated infarction may sequester huge amounts of blood very suddenly. This fulminant splenomegaly can precipitate hypovolemia and shock and requires prompt transfusion.

Although the chronic splenic dysfunction that occurs in these children is not in itself an emergency, it is well to remember that an undue susceptibility to overwhelming sepsis with *Pneumococcus* exists; even infections that seem trivial at onset can rapidly become life threatening.

Management of crises. The administration of whole, fresh blood for sequestration crises or packed red blood cells for aplastic or hemolytic crises is of obvious value. In addition, infections must be searched for and appropriately treated when possible.

The vaso-occlusive crisis, however, requires treatment of pain with analgesics such as acetaminophen, propoxyphene (Darvon), or codeine and with sedation (chlorpromazine or promethazine). Measures that reduce sickling include the prevention and treatment of dehydration, the prevention of acidosis (a good reason to avoid aspirin), and the avoidance of hypoxia. Incremental transfusions of packed red blood cells will reduce the proportion of hemoglobin S.

The child with sickle cell disease deserves careful evaluation. In many instances a particular child who is not well known to emergency department personnel should be admitted for observation and specific therapy.

EMERGENCY DRUGS AND EQUIPMENT FOR PEDIATRIC USE
Drugs

Albumin 25%: 1 g/kg
Atropine sulfate: 0.01 mg/kg IV
Aminophylline: 3 to 4 mg/kg slow IV
Bicarbonate: 2 to 3 mEq/kg IV
Calcium gluconate: 100 to 200 mg/kg IV
Dextrose 25%: 2 to 4 ml/kg IV
Diazepam: 0.5 mg/kg slow IV (maximum 10 mg)
Dopamine: 5 to 100 μg/kg/min IV

Edrophonium: 0.1 to 0.2 mg/kg slow IV
Ethacrynic acid: 1 mg/kg
Furosemide: 1 to 2 mg/kg
Glucagon: 0.5 to 1 mg SC, IM, or IV
Hydrocortisone succinate: 50 mg/kg IV
Isoproterenol: 0.5 to 4.0 μg/kg/min IV
Levarterenol: 0.1 to 1.0 μg/kg/min IV
Lidocaine: 1 mg/kg slow IV
Mannitol: 1 g/kg IV
Methyldopa: 20 to 40 mg/kg (crisis dose)
Methylene blue: 0.1 to 0.2 mg/kg slow IV
Morphine: 0.1 to 0.2 mg/kg
Naloxone (Narcan): 5 to 10 μg/kg IM or IV
Propranolol: 0.025 to 0.1 mg/kg slow IV

Equipment

Endotracheal tubes (Portex): No. 2.5 and up with adapters and stylets
Suction catheters: No. 5 to 14 French with connectors

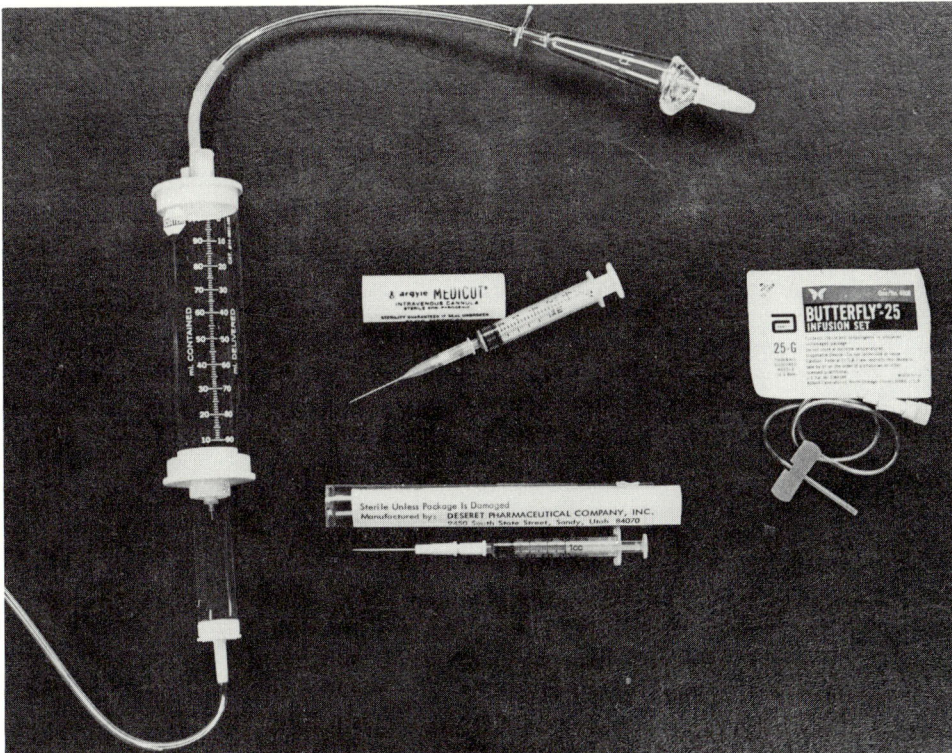

Fig. 32-1. *Left,* Volutrol (Cutter); *upper center,* Medicut (Argyle); *lower center,* intracath (Deseret); *right,* "scalp vein" needle.

Laryngoscope with Welch-Allen O, Miller 1, other larger

Medicut (or equivalent): No. 14 to 22 (Fig. 32-1)

Scalp vein needles No. 20 to 25 (Fig. 32-1)

Microdrips and Metrisets (Fig. 32-1)

Small arm boards

Small sandbags

Masks

Oral airways: 000 to 4

Pediatric electrodes for monitor

Pediatric defibrillator paddles

Intravenous fluids

   5% dextrose in water (D5W)

   Normal saline (N/S)

   Ringer's lactate

Masks: premature, newborn, infant, child

Breathing bags

Blood pressure cuffs

SUMMARY

The effective treatment of life-threatening emergencies demands that particular attention be paid to the cardiovascular, respiratory, and central nervous systems. History, physical examination, and laboratory and x-ray evaluation all help to assess the patient and the problem or problems.

ADDITIONAL READINGS

Green, M., and Haggerty, R. J.: Ambulatory pediatrics, Philadelphia, 1968, W. B. Saunders Co.

The Harriett Lane handbook, ed. 7, Chicago, 1975, Year Book Medical Publishers.

Smith, C. A.: The critically ill child, Philadelphia, 1968, W. B. Saunders Co.

Varga, C.: Handbook of pediatric medical emergencies, St. Louis, 1968, The C. V. Mosby Co.

CHAPTER **33**

Child abuse

Karen O. Butler, R.N., B.S.
David L. Chadwick, M.D.

Child abuse is the tragic product of family dysfunction in which an infant or child is injured, neglected, or emotionally damaged by the acts of caretakers. It is the responsibility of health professionals to recognize child abuse and to minimize the physical and mental damage it may do to families and children. It is common (perhaps one case per 500 population per year in the United States) and may be increasing. Many cases, especially severe ones, first surface in emergency departments, so the people there must learn to diagnose and manage the problem well. Child abuse is a condition in which early recognition can prevent major sequelae.

TYPES OF ABUSE

Child abuse may be divided into four basic categories: physical abuse, neglect, emotional maltreatment, and sexual abuse. Frequently several forms of abuse coexist in the same child, necessitating careful evaluation of all children suspected of being abused in any way.

Physical abuse

Physical abuse may be manifested in the child by obvious or occult injuries, ranging from fairly minor to life threatening. Injury that occurs from inadequate super-

vision in a potentially dangerous situation is also considered physical abuse or neglect.

Neglect

Defining what constitutes neglect is a difficult task, for to define neglect one must first describe acceptable child-rearing practices. What might be seen as a deviate form of behavior by one community's standards may be acceptable in another community. To allow for some variation, neglect is defined as "the withholding of emotional or physical support to a degree which threatens the child's ability to function normally."

Emotional maltreatment

The concept of emotional maltreatment is a relatively new one, and although over half of the states have reporting laws that include emotional maltreatment, the laws are not particularly helpful in describing this form of abuse.[1] The model Child Protective Services Act of 1976 attempts to clarify this type of abuse by referring to "mental injury," which is defined as "injury to the intellectual or psychological capacity of the child as evidenced by an observable and substantial impairment in his ability to function within a normal range of per-

487

formance and behavior, with due regard to his culture."

Sexual abuse

Sexual abuse includes not only sexual intercourse but any act designed to stimulate the child sexually, or to use the child for the sexual stimulation either of the perpetrator or of another person. As with other types of abuse, legal definitions vary from state to state, ranging from specific acts to broad interpretations. Estimates that reporting is especially low in this type of abuse include one study that estimates half of child-molesting incidents go unreported.[2]

IDENTIFICATION OF THE PHYSICALLY ABUSED AND NEGLECTED CHILD

The detection of abuse should be approached in the same logical fashion used for any other disease process. With the presence of a gross unexplained injury the diagnosis may be quite simple. The challenge is to detect the more subtle types of abuse early in the pathogenesis to protect the child from further injury and to assure effective early treatment.[3]

Bruises, abrasions, marks, and scars

Bruises by themselves are not often seen because children whose only sign of abuse is bruising are not usually brought for medical care. Bruises usually accompany a more serious problem such as a fracture or a head injury. They are also sometimes discovered on infants or children being examined for other complaints. While bruises are not usually serious or life threatening, they are often associated with more severe injuries.

Certain types of bruises can be considered nonaccidental at any age. These include the marks of a hand or fingers (usually on the face, arms, or buttocks), the patterns left by long limp objects like belts and doubled light cords, and the U-shaped marks of buckles and coat hangers. Extensive bruising of the buttocks is

almost always nonaccidental regardless of exact pattern or age. Bruising of the face (Fig. 33-1), including black eyes, in infants not yet walking is nonaccidental without a reliable history of an accidental blow. Bruising of the lips and lacerations under the tongue and in the mouth in young infants usually result from the rough or violent pushing of a nipple or a spoon into the mouth. The double crescent–shaped marks of human bites are easily recognized. Shorter but similar crescents, often on the scalp, can be produced by blows from the heels of women's shoes. Scratches on the thighs, abdomen, or buttocks made by diaper pins when carelessly or angrily handled are clues to the state of mind of the person caring for the infant.

Accidental bruises also demonstrate typically recognizable patterns such as those on the shins and knees of young children, and on the foreheads and faces of children learning to walk.

Some bruises will be difficult to classify and will not be objectively diagnosable. Whenever bruising is the chief sign of abuse it is necessary to exclude pathologic bruising by the performance of a blood count, prothrombin time, partial thromboplastin time, and an Ivy bleeding time.

Burns and burn scars

Hot water burns involving the buttocks, perineum, lower abdomen, and upper thighs are seen with some frequency and pose a major challenge. Such burns should always cause one to consider nonaccidental injury. They are usually seen in 2- to 4-year-old children who are already walking and often fairly agile; the history often given is that the child either got into the tub of hot water when the parent's back was turned or accidentally turned on the hot water while already in a tub partly filled with warm water. Since these burns are usually second-degree, the examiner should be aware that to cause them requires a three- to four-second immersion

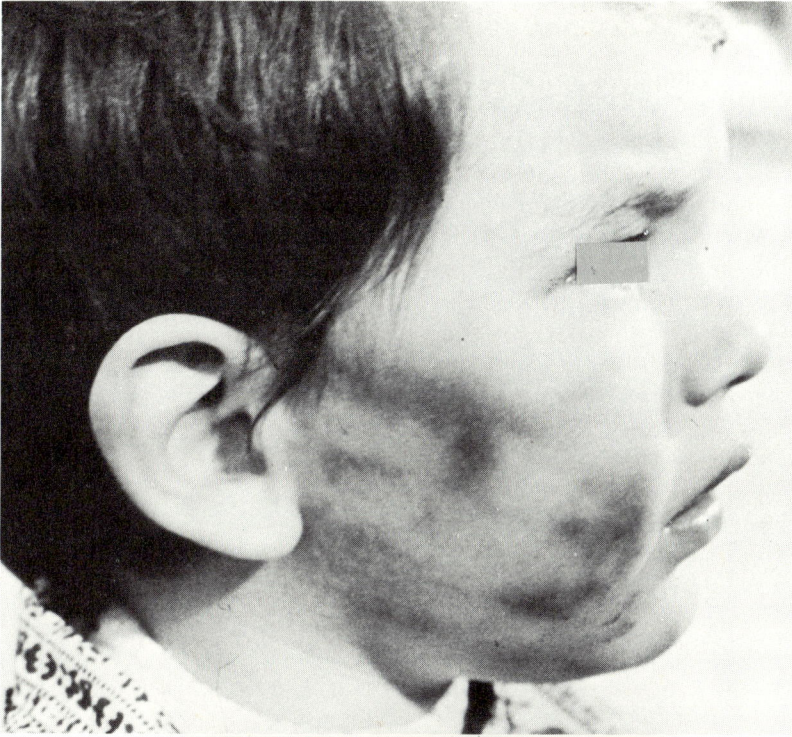

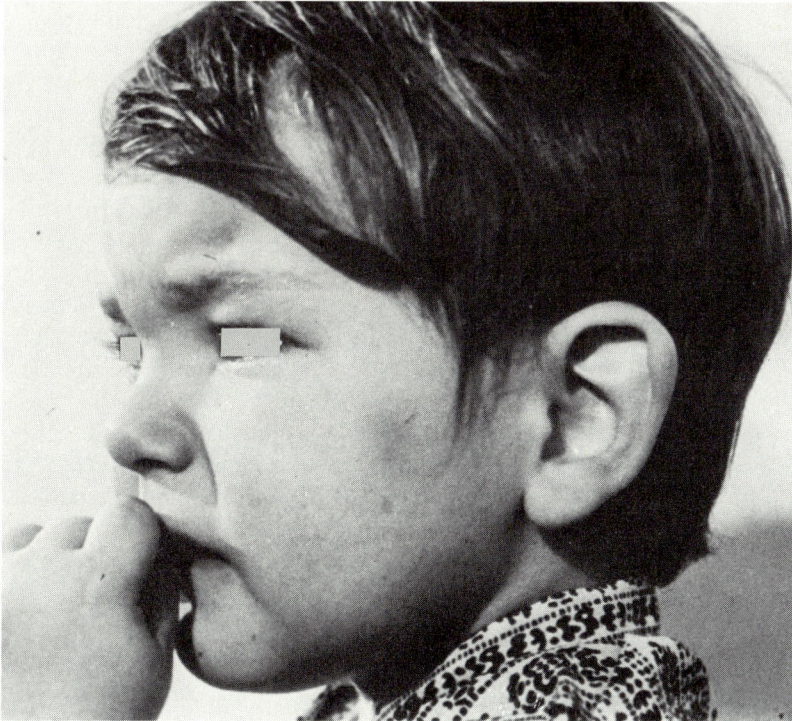

Fig. 33-1. Face of a 2½-year-old child with classic handprint bruise. **A,** Streaky bruises on right cheekbone conform to the fingers of an adult-sized left hand placed over his face. **B,** Small bruise on left cheekbone matches the thumb.

in 66° C (140° F) water, about the maximum temperature obtainable in a bathtub in most households. When the feet and lower legs are totally spared, the burn is almost certainly nonaccidental. The history of burning by the accidental addition of hot to warm water must be false in all case. When the feet and lower legs are involved along with the buttocks, accidental slipping into a tub in this position for the necessary length of time seems possible but rather improbable. Most likely, virtually all burns having this distribution are produced by parents who intend simultaneously to clean and punish their children after wetting or soiling and who use hot water in a tub for this purpose, holding the child in long enough to produce the burn.

Cigarette burns have a characteristic shape and size and, if multiple, can usually be recognized as nonaccidental. Burns from contact with radiators or floor furnaces must be evaluated in the light of the history given and the age and developmental status of the child.

Skeletal injuries

Injuries to bones can be documented radiologically and go through a fairly constant series of changes in the healing process that makes it possible to date them. In many cases bone injuries are the most reliable indicators of abuse, and x-ray films of the entire skeleton should be obtained when abuse is suspected in a child under 5 years of age. After 5 years of age, fractures are less commonly abusive.

Every fracture in infants less than 1 year of age should be considered nonaccidental, unless a documented history of accidental injury is available. Certain types of fractures are almost always nonaccidental. These include the so-called "corner" fractures on long bones, with or without accompanying periosteal new bone formation, rib fractures, and spiral fractures of the humerus, the tibia, or the femur. Any set

of two or more fractures of differing radiologic dates is likely to be nonaccidental. Skull fractures occurring alone offer the greatest diagnostic challenge since they can occur in accidental falls. The history given and the infant's age and developmental status must be carefully evaluated. Objective data are impossible to acquire, but physicians experienced in infants' and childrens' injuries are reluctant to accept a history of a 1½- to 2-foot fall from a couch or a bed to a carpet as likely to cause a skull fracture. Still, this may be the most common history given for an infant with a skull fracture.

Head injuries

Injuries to the head are the most serious manifestations of abuse and are the most common cause for the death and permanent physical disability that abuse produces. They usually occur in infants or very young children, and they present in a variety of ways with a variety of histories. Be alert for the infant brought in unconscious, apneic, or convulsing and always examine the retina when time permits. Retinal hemorrhages are signs of injury, and often their discovery will put an end to fruitless searches for medical causes of central nervous system disturbance. When central nervous system disturbance symptoms are accompanied by bruising or swelling about the head, the diagnosis is usually easy, but in many cases these signs are absent. Sometimes a skull x-ray film of an unconscious infant or child will show a fracture or signs of increased intracranial pressure that were not clinically obvious. However, severe brain damage may be present without damage to the skull or scalp. When intracranial pressure is elevated in infants, many clinicians perform subdural taps for both diagnostic and therapeutic reasons. If a bloody subdural or spinal fluid is obtained, its color and character should be recorded and the laboratory requested to record the color of the supernatant fluid after centrifugation. Any xanthochromia of the supernatant fluid after centrifugation indicates that blood has been mixed with CSF (cerebrospinal fluid) for at least a few hours, thereby precluding a traumatic tap as the source.

Nuclear and CAT scanning of the head may be useful in localizing intracranial bleeding. As yet these new methods shed little additional light on the original mechanisms of injury. The only condition other than trauma that causes intracranial bleeding in infancy is arteriovenous malformation. This is rarer than trauma by a factor of a few hundred and may be excluded by arteriography if the bleeding seems to have occurred spontaneously.

Visceral injuries

Visceral injuries such as lacerations of the liver or perforation of the bowel present with unmistakable signs of intraabdominal catastrophe. However, nonaccidental injury to the abdomen may produce visceral injury undetectable by physical examination. One of the most common injuries of this type is intramural duodenal hematoma. This is a challenge to the clinician since it can present subtly as a chronic low-grade upper-intestinal obstruction with vomiting of bile-stained material, but without physical findings such as abdominal distension or palpable masses. It usually seems to occur in 1- to 3-year-old children. They are rarely diagnosed in the emergency department but turn up on pediatric wards when a gastrointestinal series is done after a day or so of intravenous feedings and diagnostic evaluation.

Rib and chest wall injuries

Rib fractures, especially posterior rib fractures, generally indicate nonaccidental trauma. However, they are rarely seen acutely because the affected infants are infrequently brought in for the rib fracture alone. Rather, it is usually detected when the child is being examined for other medical reasons or as a result of a skeletal survey.

Neglect

Neglect takes myriad forms and merges into normal child care without a distinct boundary. It may accompany abuse or occur alone. Its long-term effects are often just as serious as those of abuse, and its recognition and proper management are just as important.

In infants and children less than 3 years of age, a common presenting syndrome is impaired weight gain and linear growth and delayed motor development. These problems occurring singly or together are often called failure to thrive, but no two writers use that term in the same way. Measurement of length and weight must be part of the assessment of an infant brought for care for any reason. Infants deprived of adequate feedings will usually first fail to gain while continuing to grow in length so they often look thin. Brain and head growth are maintained until undernutrition is severe. Infants who are denied love, affection, handling, and stimulation will sometimes fail to grow in all dimensions equally and will resemble infants dwarfed by medical problems.

Except in severe cases, it is quite difficult to determine the cause of developmental failure in a short time. Even though most neglected infants are not acutely ill, they require hospitalization on a well-run diagnostic pediatric service for approximately one week of observation and testing. Some fortunate communities contain crisis nurseries or other settings less expensive than the hospital in which infants can be placed while undergoing pediatric evaluation and which provide the type of nurturing care that will produce dramatic and diagnostic improvement in weight gain or growth. However, the large institutional infant shelters that many cities and counties provide are very poor places for these infants. Such institutions have high nosocomial infection rates, and infants placed in such shelters often wind up in a hospital within a few days because of respiratory or gastrointestinal infections.

Neglect may take the form of poor hygiene or of failure to seek medical care when most members of the culture would do so. A particularly common and recurrent medical neglect problem is that posed by refusal of care on religious grounds. Most juvenile courts are familiar with the problem and will take custody at any time of the day or night if necessary to save a child's life.

ASSESSMENT OF ABUSE AND NEGLECT

A diagnosis of suspected child abuse should be considered in any child who presents with an injury. For a diagnosis to be made, the health professional must be able to make the identification through a process of recognizing the effects of child abuse in children and the behavior patterns of their caretakers.

A careful, general examination is needed of all children who are admitted to the emergency department with any injury. Children with no apparent injuries but who exhibit some other indication of abuse, such as exceptional passivity, should also be thoroughly examined. Whenever possible a general assessment of an injured child should be conducted prior to a detailed examination of the local site of injury. Examination of the child as a whole will increase chances of detecting associated injuries, other injuries, or systemic manifestations of the observed injury.

A child who is admitted with serious injuries or with multiple injuries will obviously require an emergency medical assessment and appropriate intervention. Information regarding the treatment of life-threatening pediatric emergencies is contained in Chapter 32.

Careful assessment requires that all available information be recorded in as much detail as possible in order to document the conclusions. When the child is to be hospitalized, the record can be quite brief, with detailed descriptions left to those having more time to write them. When time or circumstances do not permit a meticulous examination, make it clear to the staff who take over care that your examination was incomplete.

Medical history

Information regarding the presenting problem may be obtained from the parents, other caretakers, and the child. The source or sources of the history should be recorded, including their relationship to the child. If the interviewer has the opportunity to talk with the same informant at different times, or with another informant, it is important to note any changes or contradictions in history from the same or different informants.

In addition to obtaining information about the child, interviewing the family members may help to determine whether there appears to be a potential for abuse. The behavior of the informants may provide important clues to the family's function. It is important to note anything that appears to interfere with that person's reliability, for example, apparent intoxication or other drug misuse, possible signs of mental illness, and overreaction or underreaction to the situation. Other behaviors of the caretaker that could be significant are the following: (1) being reluctant to provide information, (2) when questioned, appearing angry or anxious to leave, (3) displaying anger toward the child for being injured, or (4) not demonstrating concern for the child's injury, treatment, or prognosis.

Past and social histories

Past and social histories are exceedingly valuable in assisting families, but can rarely be obtained in the emergency department. Use of the social worker in emergency departments for this purpose has worked well in some hospitals and deserves further trial. The following information should be considered by someone within the hospital who is responsible for further assessment of family dysfunction.

Past history. Birth and developmental information may provide important clues to the family's potential for abuse. Was the pregnancy wanted? Did the pregnancy occur in a young mother? Have the parents relinquished other children? Was the child born prematurely? Was it a difficult labor or delivery?

How the parent perceives the child is also extremely important information. Often an abused child is seen as "different" by the family, either physically or behaviorally. Also, the parents may have unrealistic expectations of the child. This may be demonstrated by the parents' expecting a behavior before it is developmentally possible, such as being toilet trained during infancy. It may also be exhibited by the parents' expressing in some way that the child is not meeting their need for love or nurturing.

It is not uncommon for the child who is singled out for abuse to indeed be different in some way. The abused child may be hyperactive, physically handicapped, or mentally retarded or may in some other way place additional demand or stress on the family.

The child's past medical information should cover previous trauma, serious illness, emergency department visits, and hospitalizations. It is important to be alert for information that would indicate the child has been treated at various medical facilities. Often an abusing parent will avoid detection by changing physicians or hospitals.

Some communities have access to a central child-abuse file that is available to professionals for the purpose of checking for previous reports of abuse. Usually they are cross-filed by family so that information about incidents with siblings is also available.

Social history. When assessing family dysfunction, it is helpful to have informa-

tion about other persons living in the household and their relationship to the child. Information about other children should also include sex, age, and if possible any previous history of trauma, emergency department visits, and hospitalizations. Death of a sibling and the cause of death should be recorded.

How long the family has lived at their present address and their previous residence should be noted. Are there relatives living in the area? If the answer is "yes," do they see them regularly and get along with them? Abusing parents are often isolated and have no one to turn to in a crisis. Additional questions that may assist in identifying isolation are ones that would elicit information about their social contacts, whether they have help with child care or can afford child care, and whether they have access to a telephone and transportation.

Crisis within the family is closely associated with abuse. Information about financial burdens or special tensions, especially recent, should provide some insight into that possibility.

Other indicators of potential abuse are the parent or guardian's dwelling on his or her own needs and problems, showing detachment or lack of sensitivity to the child's needs, or showing evidence, or fear, of losing control in relation to the child.

Physical examination

As with all pediatric patients, the child who may have been abused needs age-appropriate preparation prior to examination and adequate support and reassurance throughout the process.

The following annotated format has been included to assist the professional in paying particular attention to signs that are commonly found in abused children.

General appearance: Describe in detail. Record the child's height, weight, body proportions, and percentiles. Look for surface signs of parental neglect, such as uncleanliness beyond acceptable standards for the parents' cultural and socioeconomic complex. Behavioral patterns are important to note.

The possibility of abuse should not be dismissed because the child's hygiene is good. The quality of child care should be questioned if there is neglected cradle cap, ammoniacal diaper dermatitis, or other signs of inadequate parenting.

An abused child's behavior is a function of a variety of factors including age, developmental level, pattern of parent-child interactions, the nature and extent of injury, and whether abuse is a chronic or an acute occurrence. Thus a wide range of behaviors may be noted in such a child. Abused children have been described in the following terms: indiscriminate and superficial in relationships, fearful, withdrawn, provocative, lacking trust, testing limits, clinging, and normal. Although description of significant behavior may provide helpful information in assessment, one must be careful about drawing conclusions from observed behavior for a brief period of time.

> Skin: Describe all lesions completely for size, color, texture, and distribution. Inspect all surface areas carefully, including the palms, soles, and scalp.

Familiarity with normal developmental capabilities of infants and toddlers and the diverse minor injuries common to active toddlers is indispensable in making appropriate assessments. For example, superficial injuries inflicted by abusing adults, just above elbows, knees and shins do not fit the clinical description of accidental injuries or of any dermatologic disease.[4]

> Head: Measure circumference under 2 years of age. Inspect and palpate for signs of injury.
> Eyes: Examine lids and sclerae for bruising or scratches. Funduscopic examination may disclose retinal hemorrhages, a detached retina, or traumatic cataracts.
> Ears: Examine for bruises on or behind the external ears and examine the drums for signs of rupture or middle ear bleeding. Ruptured

or hemorrhagic typanic membranes suggest slapping on the ears.
> Nose: Check for straightness and examine the inside of both nares for blood or clots.
> Mouth, throat, tongue: Examine for intactness of teeth and missing or fractured teeth. Check for traumatic lesions on and under the tongue or on mucous membranes. The frenulum of the upper lip is sometimes traumatized by rough feeding.
> Thorax: Examine as usual for heart and lungs, including palpation of the chest.
> Abdomen: Examine as usual being conscious of signs of duodenal obstruction or pancreatic injury.
> Genitalia: Inspect carefully (both sexes) for signs of injury. If oral, anal, or vaginal penetration is suspected, smears for gonorrhea, sperm, and appropriate evidence collection should be obtained. Appropriate management of the sexually abused child is included in the chapter on sexual assault; however, digital examination of the preadolescent vagina is usually contraindicated.
> Anus and rectum: Always inspect the anus. Digital examination may be omitted if it seems unlikely to add useful information or may be postponed in a child who may have a rectal injury but who is to be examined by a surgeon.
> Extremities: Palpate all bones and joints for swelling, tenderness, or deformity. Examine carefully for limitation of motion.
> Neurologic examination: Document in detail any signs of possible head injury and note any deficits in motor function.

Diagnosis and documentation

Throughout the process of obtaining the medical history and the physical examination, three important questions should be considered: (1) Are the injuries consistent with the child's age and developmental capability? (2) Does the set of injuries constitute a known syndrome of child abuse? (3) Are the findings consistent with the explanation offered?

Young children suspected of being neglected or abused should be admitted to the hospital for protection and further diagnostic evaluation. Older children should be admitted if medically indicated. Once the abuse has been reported, protective custody (without hospitalization) for the older child will usually be arranged through the community agency responsible for dependent children.

In the case of a child who demonstrates skin changes or other visible injuries, documentation can be reinforced with colored photographs. In instances requiring immediate attention, such as burns or other severe abuses, whenever possible the pictures should be taken before extensive medical treatment is performed.[5] If the skin shows recent changes, the color and intensity will not be so visible as in later stages. Therefore, follow-up photographs should be obtained on bruising within 48 hours.

DEALING WITH THE FAMILY

A well-recognized maxim of pediatric care is to view the child and family as a unit. Since interventions are normally directed toward maintaining and strengthening family ties, the appearance of an abused child in a medical care setting often presents a paradox for health professionals.[6]

The health professional who is most effective in intervening with abusing families is one who has the ability to proceed with shared concern for the child and parents. This approach conveys a therapeutic rather than a punitive tone and allows for a greater chance for communication with the family. Recognition that the majority of abusing parents have brought their child for care because of their concern may help the professional to avoid assigning guilt or acting out the anger he or she may feel toward the abusing parent.

Since the abused child often is seen initially in the emergency department, it is essential that someone be available to deal with the parents in a nonadversary way. Very often the health professional is the first of a variety of professionals who will be required to interact with the family. Depending upon the situation, that may include personnel from several social service agencies, law enforcement, the probation department, the juvenile justice system, and the office of the district attorney. If the initial interaction is perceived as negative or punitive by the abusing parent, he or she may be extremely reluctant to cooperate with others.

After the examiner is convinced that nonaccidental injury or neglect may be present and when the child's condition is stable enough to allow time for explanation, a brief meeting should be held with the parent(s) or other persons who accompanied the child. Whenever possible this should be done in an office in a comfortable confidential fashion. If a social worker is available, he or she should be present. The professional who has the responsibility to give information of this kind should be designated by the emergency department. Briefly and compassionately that person should state that the child has injuries the hospital is required by law to report and that the effect of the report will be to bring about an inquiry into how the injuries occurred. Decisions about the child's condition, the need for particular treatments or hospitalization, and statements about prognosis can be made at the same time. The professional must not convey anger or any feeling that a judgment has been made about who caused the injury. Immediately after this brief statement it is helpful if the services of a medical social worker can be offered. Usually this all takes place at about the time that the child is to be transferred to the hospital, thus ending (for the moment) the emergency department's responsibility.

LEGAL ASPECTS OF ABUSE AND NEGLECT
Reporting laws

Child-abuse and neglect reporting laws have been passed in every state requiring certain professionals, including health professionals, to report cases of suspected abuse and neglect to specified agencies.[1]

It is important to remember that the reporter is not required to prove the occurrence of abuse or neglect. Rather, the requirement is for reports to be made when the reporter has *reason to believe* or *reasonable cause* to suspect that abuse or neglect may be occurring.

The law specifies which local agencies are designated to receive reports, and these include law enforcement, welfare departments, probation departments, and health departments.

Immunity for reporter. Some potential reporters, particularly health professionals, may be reluctant to report suspected child abuse and neglect because they fear retaliatory lawsuits if the abuse or neglect is unconfirmed. However, every state's reporting law contains a provision for immunity to the reporter for all reports of suspected child abuse and neglect *made in good faith.* While reporting laws cannot prevent the filing of lawsuits against a reporter, they make the successful litigation of such suits impossible, provided the report was made in good faith.

Liability. State reporting laws usually contain provisions making it a crime knowingly to fail to report suspected child abuse and neglect.

Under the law of civil negligence, violation of a statutory duty, such as mandatory reporting of suspected child abuse and neglect, is negligence *per se.* That means that if it can be proved that a person willfully or negligently failed to report known or suspected child abuse or neglect, he or she can be sued for the injuries that occurred after the time when a report should have been made. This principle has recently been applied to cases in which reports of suspected abuse or neglect were not made. Two California cases in which a child suffered serious injuries from abuse subsequent to a hospital's failure to report its suspicions of possible child abuse have received considerable attention. A summary of one of those cases follows:

Eventually settled out of court for $600,000, this case involved a mother and a boyfriend who brought her young son to a hospital twice in a 12-hour period with severe injuries. Neither time did the hospital report abuse. A day later they brought the child to a second hospital with what turned out to be permanent brain damage. The boy's father sued the first hospital and others for negligence based on the hospital's failure to report the case.

Confidentiality and the doctor/patient privilege. In every state in which health professionals and social workers are required to report suspected child abuse or neglect, they must do so whether or not they have learned of the case as a result of confidential communications with their patient or client. Health professionals and social workers are also required by law to testify in child abuse and neglect cases when subpoenaed. Suspension of rules of confidentiality in child abuse and neglect cases exists even if no statutory privilege exists in a particular state.

Emergency detention of the child

In some situations a physician may feel that a child would be seriously endangered if released to the custody of the parent(s). In every state the law allows for emergency detention in such situations. In some states it may be necessary to obtain a court order prior to detention. In other states a police officer or a physician may be empowered to place the child in protective custody against the parents' wishes, provided that a written petition is filed with the juvenile court within 24 to 48 hours after the detention. According to California law a physician may call the probation department or local law enforcement agency to obtain legal hold on a child. The hold is valid for 48 hours, at which time a legal petition may be filed or the hold released. If medical treatment is required and the parents will not authorize it, the probation officer must request authorization for treatment from a judge.

Dealing with the police

When law enforcement agencies are the recipients of child abuse reports, the orientation and skill of the officers handling the cases vary widely. If the health professionals are experienced and confident they can often offer tactful guidance to the police and should not hesitate to do so as reports are made. Ideally, investigations of child abuse should be made by experienced police or probation officers accompanied by social workers with experience in managing family dysfunction, but few communities have achieved this system yet.

Serving as a medical witness

It was previously stated that in every state, child abuse and neglect reporting laws suspend confidentiality between health professionals and patients. Therefore, the physician is legally required to report, and if subpoenaed he or she is required to testify.

Medical records should always be subpoenaed in a child-abuse hearing, and the health professional should expect careful examination and cross-examination based on the information contained in the records. Prior to testifying, it is important to carefully review all records and notes relating to the case and be prepared to describe involvement with the case chronologically. Before the trial it is advisable to review the case with the attorney for the petitioner and discuss the need for certain witnesses or documents. If inexperienced as a medical witness, it may be helpful to discuss the types of questions to be asked and to role-play a few questions and answers with the attorney, for both direct examination and cross-examination.

Many health professionals are uncertain as to whether they are allowed to talk with the attorney for the parents or the attorney for the child prior to the hearing. Although not prohibited, the professional should be aware that he or she may be cross-examined by the attorney for the child or parents on any inconsistencies between what is said informally and what is testified to in court.

Arrangements can usually be made with the juvenile court for the physician to be placed on stand-by or on-call subpoena. This will allow the professional to remain in his or her setting until telephoned by the court, thus avoiding lengthy delays at the courthouse waiting to testify.

Direct examination. The medical witness presents evidence establishing the nature, extent, and seriousness of the injuries to the child and his or her opinion as to the cause of the injuries. The medical witness will *not* be expected to prove who caused the injuries to the child.

The use of medical records and other notes is allowed while giving testimony. The witness should be exact. For example, say "1:00 A.M.," instead of "around midnight," or "three fractures," instead of "several fractures." When medical terms are used in the testimony, it will be necessary to explain the terms in language that nonmedical persons will be able to understand.

Cross-examination. Cross-examination is usually the most difficult part of testifying for the health professional in child abuse and neglect cases. The key to effective performance during cross-examination is adequate preparation. The tactics of cross-examination often include attempts to discredit the witness by whatever techniques will work. These may include attempts at intimidation (if the witness acts timid) or attempts to anger (if the witness seems susceptible). There is simply no substitute for practice. The attorney for the petitioning agency should be able to assist the physician by pointing out likely questions that will be asked and by role-playing the cross-examination.

Health professionals are often questioned about the degree of certainty with which they are able to diagnose child abuse or neglect. Usually a physician is not in a position to be 100% certain of the diagnosis but can state reasons why in his or her best medical judgment, he or she believes the injuries resulted from abuse or neglect.

THE ROLE OF THE HOSPITAL

Prior planning and preparation for hospital care of the abused or neglected child will facilitate an appropriate response by staff members. This includes training of personnel involved with the problem and developing procedures for carrying out legal responsibilities.

Education of personnel

Preparation for the recognition of abuse and the responsibilities that are assumed when caring for an abused child is available from a variety of sources today. Awareness of the enormity of the problem has resulted in the inclusion of child abuse information in many initial and continuing education programs for health personnel. In areas that do not have readily available conferences, seminars, or other programs, hospital in-service programs are an excellent alternative. There is also a wealth of printed materials that covers the topic well. Additional readings are listed at the end of this chapter. Other references are available through libraries and the National Center on Child Abuse and Neglect.

Conducting an in-service program

Hospital programs should include all staff members who come in contact with children. Whenever possible they should be conducted or coordinated by someone who is well informed on the topic. Of particular value is participation by personnel from community agencies that are also involved with the abused child. Not only will this allow for mutual sharing of each agency's role, but hopefully will result in increased communication between the many disciplines that need to cooperate in order to meet the needs of troubled families.

Another advantage of hospital-based programs is the opportunity for the staff to explore their feelings and attitudes about working with abusing families. The effectiveness of interactions with abusing family members will depend largely on the ability of the contacting professional to deal with his or her responses and feelings in order to develop the necessary compassion. Certain personnel may display a great deal of anger in discussing child abuse. This is important to know when planning who will be responsible for providing information to abusing families.

Procedures in the emergency department

The development of a procedure manual or a placard summarizing pertinent information about physical indicators and suggested examinations is helpful for those who see abuse cases infrequently. Included in the information should be a summary of laws appropriate for the local areas. The following information should also be readily available: the names and phone numbers of agencies that receive phone reports and within what hours, and names of contact persons at the individual agencies. If reports are also required in writing, a supply of forms or a list of required data should also be available. The hospital also must determine which staff member will report child-abuse cases. Often it is the professional responsible for the child's medical treatment, but it may be a social worker or someone else designated to make the report.

In areas that permit photographs of abused children, careful attention should be given to local regulations regarding consent. If consent is required, provision for photographs could be included in the general treatment consent form. If law enforcement personnel are responsible for obtaining photographs, they may use their own form.

Community referral

Occasionally a family will come to the emergency department demonstrating behaviors or inadequate parenting skills that could eventually lead to child abuse or neglect. For the sake of prevention, intervention at this point is essential.

Knowledge of community resources, their services, and how referrals are made is the responsibility of all emergency departments. If uncertain about the appropriate referral for an "at risk" family, notifying the local public health nurse is a good first choice. Public health nurses are experienced in evaluating family problems and planning with the family to get appropriate help. Nurses also have the advantage of being considered healers and are often more successful at gaining access to troubled families than are other public agency personnel.

Hospital plan

The need for social service staff to be available for abusing families was mentioned earlier. If at all possible, someone should be on call throughout the day and evening hours. Social workers not only are important as providers of support and information but also can serve as a link between the family and other agencies or treatment resources.

For hospitals that see over 25 cases of abuse a year, a multidiscipline child abuse team should be formed.[7] The primary role of the team would be to review all cases and how they were managed and to prepare a treatment plan for the family. Makeup of the team should include one person each from the pediatric medical, nursing, social services, and psychiatry staffs. Often persons from community agencies who are working with the family participate in hospital case reviews. Some facilities also include the parents. Additional responsibilities of the team members would be to serve as consultants to hospital staff and to provide educational services.

Opportunities for prevention

Child abuse has complex roots in society, and complete prevention is beyond the capability of emergency departments and the scope of this chapter. Emergency medical personnel will have occasional opportunities to prevent abuse and should not overlook these chances.

For example, a mother may come to the hospital or call in saying that she thinks she is going to kill or injure her baby. Do not ignore such a remark. Use whatever resources are available, including the hospital if necessary, to allow the mother to separate temporarily from her infant and to get help.

A more subtle and more dangerous situation may present itself when a parent brings a child to the emergency department repeatedly with complaints of physical illness that are not confirmed by examination. If this happens twice in a few days it is a warning, and the third such visit within ten days is an absolute alarm signal. Something is very wrong in the relationship, and violence is likely.

These opportunities for primary prevention occur rarely compared to the opportunities for secondary prevention that occur when an infant or child with nonaccidental injuries appears and when recognition and management aim to prevent subsequent, more serious injury.

SUMMARY

Abused and neglected infants and children frequently appear in emergency departments. These children and their families require highly skilled management if ideal outcomes are to be achieved. The recognition of abuse in medical settings has been brought to a level where little, if any, abuse should go unrecognized. Family-oriented management aimed at the eventual safe return of the child to his family or permanent placement with another family should begin with the first medical contact.

REFERENCES

1. We Can Help . . . a curriculum on the identification, reporting referral and case management of child abuse and neglect, developed for the National Center on Child Abuse and Neglect (U.S. Children's Bureau, Office of Child Development, U.S. Department of Health, Education and Welfare) under contract No. HEW-105-75-1104 with Urban and Rural Systems Associates of San Francisco, California.
2. Gorham, C. W.: Not only the stranger—a study of the problem of child molestation in San Diego, California, J. Sch. Health 36:341-345, 1966.
3. Sanders, R. W.: Resistance to dealing with parents of battered children, Pediatrics **50:** 853, 1972.
4. Gregg, G. S.: Physician, child-abuse reporting laws, and injured child, Clin. Pediatr. **7**(12): 720-725, 1968.
5. Ford, R. J., Smistek, B. S., and Glass, J. T.: Photography of suspected child abuse and maltreatment, Biomedical Communications, 3(4): 12-16, 1975.
6. Neill, K., and Kauffman, C.: Care of the hospitalized abused child and his family: nursing implications, Am. J. Maternal Child Nurs. 1(2):117-123, 1976.
7. Helfer, R. E., and Kempe, C. H.: The battered child, ed. 2, Chicago, 1974, University of Chicago Press.

ADDITIONAL READINGS

Cameron, J. M., and Rae, L. J.: Atlas of the battered child, Edinburgh, 1975, Churchill Livingstone.

Helfer, R. E., and Kempe, C. H.: The battered child, ed. 2, Chicago, 1974, University of Chicago Press.

Kempe, C. H., and Helfer, R. E.: Child abuse: the family and the community, Cambridge, Mass., 1976, Ballinger Publishing Co.

Kempe, C. H., and Helfer, R. E.: Helping the battered child and his family, Philadelphia, 1972, J. B. Lippincott Co.

Index

Apathetic hyperthyroidism, 108-109
Aphasia, 322
Aplastic crises in children, 484
Apomorphine for emesis, 187, 260
Appendicitis, 434, 437-438
Apresoline; *see* Hydralazine
Apt test, 459
Aquatic emergencies, 287-314
    gastrointestinal, 308
Aquatic organisms; *see also* specific organism
    dangerous, 303-308
    poisonous, 308
    venomous, 303-308
Aramine; *see* Metaraminol
Arfonad, 120, 238
Arrest
    cardiac; *see* Heart, arrest of
    drug abuse and cardiopulmonary, 180-181
    sinus bradycardia with sinus, 408, 409
Arrhythmias, cardiac, 396-412
    in children, 483
    classification of, 396-397
    digitalis-induced, 404-405
        in children, 483
    drug-induced, 190
    in thyroid storm, 110
Arsenic
    antidote for, 261
    poisoning from, 259
Arterial aneurysm rupture, 440-441
Arterial blood pressure in shock, 81-82
Arterial hemorrhage, 73
Arterial lactate measurement in shock, 84-86
Arterial puncture technique, 133-135
    tray for, 135
Arteries, 215
    blunt trauma to, 233
    common femoral, 232
    embolus of, 235-236
    examination of, 230
    fracture-associated injury to, 233, 235
    injury to, 232-238
        comparison to venous injury, 241
        signs and symptoms of, 241
    insufficiency of, 233
    palpation of, 230
    penetrating injuries to, 232-233
    rupture of, 237
    thrombosis of, 233, 234, 235-236
Arteriography for solid viscus injury, 445
Arteriosclerotic aneurysm, 237
Arteriovenous fistula, 232-233
Arteriovenous malformation, 491
Artificial respiration for near-drowning victim, 290, 292
Arum family plants, poisoning with, 270-271
Asphyxia with near drowning, 288, 289
Aspiration
    of fluids
        near drowning with, 289-290
        near drowning without, 289
    of fresh water, 290, 291
    of salt water, 290, 291

Aspiration pneumonia, 177, 393-395, 427
Aspirin for extreme fevers, 192
Aspirin poisoning, 259, 262
Assault
    and battery, 15
    sexual; *see* Sexual assault
Assessment and triage, 45-57
    initial form for, 52, 53-55
    interview techniques for, 51-57
    questions in history taking during, 52-53
    trauma form for, 52, 53, 56-57
Assistance, financial, 33
Asthma in children, 480
Asthmatic reaction to street drugs, 177
Ataxia, cerebral, 111
Atrial fibrillation
    clinical presentation of, 402
    coarse, 403
    electrocardiographic recognition of, 401
    with sawtooth pattern, 402
    treatment of, 403-404
Atrial tachycardia, paroxysmal; *see* Paroxysmal atrial tachycardia
Atrioventricular dissociation and ventricular tachycardia, 406
Atropine, 409
    absorption by charcoal, 261
    as antidote, 262
    for children, 485
    for cholinesterase inhibitor poisoning, 268
    combined hallucinogen overdose with, 163
    dilation of pupils by, 185, 420
    for mushroom poisoning, 270
    poisoning from, 259, 264
    for slow heart rhythm, 424
Auscultation
    for bowel sounds, 436
    for bruits, 230-231
Australia antigen, 125
Autonomic nervous system drug poisoning, 264
Autopsy, legal considerations of, 14
Auxiliary facilities for emergency medical care, 8
Avulsion laceration, 65

B
Bacitracin for burns, 254
Bacitracin sensitization, 362
Back strain, 382
Bacterial endocarditis with drug use, 178
Bacterial pneumonia, 393
Bag-valve-masks, 426, 427
B.A.L. as antidote, 262
Barbiturates, 158, 400
    abdominal pain from, 437
    alkalinization of urine for overdose of, 188
    antidote for, 261
    intoxication from, 176
    poisoning from, 259, 263-265
Barotrauma, pulmonary, 300-303
Bartholin's gland abscess, 455-456
Basilar skull fractures, 321, 327
Battering, spouse, 31
Battery, 15

Harvest of blood, 122
Hash oil intoxication, 202
Hashish intoxication, 202
Head
  examination of, 320-321
  injuries to, 162, 315-330, 331
    child abuse and, 490-491
    definition of, 315-319
    diagnosis of, 321-326
    management of, 326-330
Headaches, 146-150
  assessment of, 146-148
  characteristics of serious, 147
  diagnosis of, 148-149
  intervention in, 149-150
  symptoms of, 147
Healing of wounds, 59-61
Health professional and child abuse cases, 495
Hearing, loss of, from "squeeze," 300
Heart
  arrest of
    after chemotherapy, 158
    in children, 483
    life support for, 416-420
    mechanisms of, 414-416
    prevention of, 416
    unconsciousness from, 141
  arrhythmias of, 396-412
    classification of, 396-397
    drug-induced, 190
  compression of, external, 420
    complications of, 421
  contusion of, 370
  failure of, congestive, in children, 483-484
  monitoring of, 423
  output of, in shock, 82
  tamponade of, 87-89
Heart block
  clinical presentation of, 409
  complete, 410-411
  incomplete, 409-410
Heat burns, 249-250; *see also* Burns
Heimlich maneuver, 418-419
  for children, 480
Helicopters and emergency medical care, 7
Heloderma horridum, 280; *see also* Gila monsters
Heloderma suspectum, 280; *see also* Gila monsters
Hemangioma, 355
Hematoma, 323
  epidural, 318
  intracerebral, 318
  intracranial
    diagnosis of, 324-326
    treatment of, 326, 328-330
    unconsciousness from, 142-143, 144
  intramural duodenal, from child abuse, 491
  scalp, 315, 321, 326
  subdural, 147, 148, 149-150, 318
  subungual, 72-73
  treatment of, 328-330
Hematochezia, 434
Hemiparesis, 322, 324
Hemofil, 129

Hemolysis, profound signs of, 123
Hemolytic crises in children, 484
Hemolytic reactions to transfusion, 123-124
Hemophilia, transfusion for, 128-129
Hemophilia B, transfusion for, 129
Hemorrhage, 73-74, 318
  in abdomen, 441-442
  bowel, lower, 442
  brain, in children, 481
  from chest injuries, 365, 366
  from ear, 352-353
  in facial injuries, control of, 332
  gastrointestinal, upper, 441-442
  in hemophilia, 128-129
  from hypopharynx, 354-355
  intracranial, 140, 146, 147, 148, 149
  intraluminal, 441-442
  from larynx, 355
  from mouth, 354-355
  multiunit transfusion after, 125
  from nose, 353
  with oral anticoagulants, 129-130
  postnasal, 353-354
  postpartum, 457, 460-461
  retroorbital, 332
  subconjunctival, 344
  from surface trauma, 58-74
  from throat, 354-355
  tilt test for, 74
  from tonsils, 355
  vaginal, 448-454
Hemorrhagic diseases in children, 482
Hemothorax, 366
Hemotympanum, 321
Heparin
  for amniotic fluid embolism, 460
  for amputations, 218
  for arterial puncture, 133
  in missed abortion, 451
  for pelvic thrombophlebitis, 451
  for pulmonary embolism, 395
  for thrombophlebitis, 250
Hepatic disorders causing hypoglycemia, 103
Hepatitis, 125, 130, 435, 436
  from transfusion, 125
Hernias, 434
Herniation, transtentorial, 318-319
Heroin, abuse of, 170
Heroin and respiratory depression, 189
Herpes simplex
  eye infection caused by, 346-347
  virus infection, 456
Herpes zoster causing abdominal pain, 437
High output low resistance shock, 89
High output shock syndrome, 82
Hinged half-ring splint, 222
Hinged splints, 220-221
Hip
  dislocations of, splinting of, 226
  fractures of
    in children, 226
    occult, 225
    splinting of, 225

Phlegmasia cerulea dolens, 239-240
Phobias, school, 164
Phosphate insecticide, antidote for, 262
Phosphates for hypercalcemia, 116-117
Phosphorus poisoning, 259, 261
Phospho-Soda cathartic, 261
Photophobia from iritis, 347
Physical abuse of children, 487
Physician, personal, requests for, 23
Physician triage, 49
Physostigmine
    as antidote, 183, 190, 262, 264, 265
    for fever, 192
    poisoning from, 264
Picrotoxin, contraindication of, with central nervous system depression, 261
Pill taking by children, 207
Pilocarpine
    for eyes, 340
    for glaucoma, 340
    poisoning from, 264
Pinprick sensitivity, 231
Pit vipers
    anatomy of, 272-273
    bite of; *see* Snakes, bites of
    fangs of, 273
    striking mechanism of, 273
    venom of, 273-274
Pitocin for incomplete abortion, 450; *see also* Oxytocin
Pitressin; *see* Vasopressin
Placenta, separation of, 461
Placenta accreta, 457
Placenta praevia, 456-457
Placidyl and substance abuse, 184
Plants, poisoning from, 259, 270
Plasma
    expansion of, 190
    potassium-laden, transfusion of, 125
    thyroid hormone in, 111
    whole, transfusion of, 128
Plaster splints, 232
Platelets
    transfusions of, 127
    typing of, 127
Pneumococcal pneumonia, 393
Pneumonia
    aspiration, 177, 393-395, 427
        treatment of, 394-395
    bacterial, 393
    in children, 480
    lipid, 269
    nonbacterial, 393
    symptoms of, 393
    treatment of, 393
Pneumonitis
    as cause of diabetic coma, 97
    chemical, 393
Pneumothorax, 365-366
    preferred drainage sites for, 371-372
    from pulmonary barotrauma, 301, 302
    and respirator, 374
    spontaneous, 366

Poisoning; *see also* Poisons
    acetanilid, 259
    acetophenetidin, 262
    acid, 259, 269-270
    alcohol, 259
    aldrin, 267
    alkali, 259, 270
    Amanita, 270
    aminophylline, 265
    amitriptyline, 265
    amphetamine, 259, 264
    analgesic, 262
    anesthetic, 262-263
    with aniline dyes, 259
    with antidepressants, 265
    with antihistamines, 259
    with antiseptics, 265
    arsenic, 259
    with Arum family plants, 270-271
    aspirin, 259, 262
    atropine, 259, 264
    with autonomic nervous system drugs, 264
    barbiturate, 259, 263-265
    belladonna, 259, 264, 271
    benzene, 259, 269
    bethanechol, 264
    with bleaching agents, 267
    bromide, 259
    by calla lily, 270-271
    camphor, 259
    carbon dioxide, 259
    carbon monoxide, 259, 265
        in underwater swimming, 295, 298
    with cardiovascular drugs, 265-266
    with castor beans, 270
    with caustics, 265
    chlordane, 267, 268
    chloroform, 259
    chlorpromazine, 264
    with cholinesterase inhibitors, 268
    ciguatera, 308
    cocaine, 259, 262-263
    codeine, 263
    with corrosives, 259, 269-270
    creosote, 265
    DDT, 267-268
    definition of, 168
    with depressants, 263-265
    dextropropoxyphene, 259
    by dieffenbachia, 270-271
    Dieldrin, 267-268
    digitalis, 259, 265
    diphenhydramine, 264
    diphenoxylate, 259, 263
    disulfiram, 265
    edrophonium, 264
    Endrin, 267-268
    ephedrine, 259, 264
    epinephrine, 264
    EPN, 268
    ethanol, 259
    ether, 259
    fluoride, 259

Radios, hospital, 5-6
Radius, fractures of, splinting of, 224
Rape, 31, 32, 464, 465
  assessment of, 467
  dealing with victim of, 474
  homosexual, 465
  laboratory specimen chart for, 475
  objectives of care after, 467-468
  physical injury and trauma from, 465-466
  protocol, 467-474
    evidence collection in, 471-472, 475
    follow-up in, 474
    medical examination in, 470-471
    medical procedures in, 472-474, 475
    procedures prior to medical examination in, 468-470
Rapid transfusions, 126
Rattlesnakes; *see* Pit vipers
Reactions, drug, 175-178
Reactions to emergencies, 29-31
Reactive hypoglycemia, 103, 104
Receptor sites of drugs, 169
Recompression, 300
  for decompression sickness, 302-303
  for pulmonary barotrauma, 302
Records, patient, legal responsibility for, 15
Rectum, examination of, 435
Rectus muscles, spasm of, 435-436
Red cells, packed, 126-127
Red eyes, causes of, 346-347
Red tides, 309
Reed's classification of coma, 183-184
Referral services, 32-33
Referrals in child abuse cases, 499
Referred pain in abdomen, 432
Refractory shock, 92
Regional anesthesia, 61-62
Regional enteritis, 438
Regitine; *see* Phentolamine
Rejection by lover or spouse, 164
Relapse, cyclic, following drug overdose, 192
Release, affectual, 155
Religious beliefs and child neglect, 492
Religious practices, respect for, 21
Renal embolus, 236
Renal failure, 261
Reporting laws for child abuse and neglect, 495-496
Reptiles, poisonous, 272-286
Res ipsa loquitur, 15
Resistance, peripheral, reduction of, 416
Respirations
  artificial, for near-drowning victim, 290, 292
  checking, in head-injured patient, 320
  in children, 428
  Kussmaul, in diabetic coma, 98
Respirators
  IPPB, 427
  pneumothorax and, 374
  pressure cycled, 392, 427
  volume cycled, 392
Respiratory centers, depression of, 414

Respiratory emergencies, 385-395
  in children, 479-480
Respiratory excretion for drug overdose, 188
Respiratory failure, 326, 416
Respiratory infections in children, 479-480
Respiratory insufficiency causing unconsciousness, 141, 416
Respiratory trauma in children, 480
Respondeat superior, 14-15
Resuscitation
  cardiopulmonary; *see* Life support
  expired air, 419
  mouth-to-mouth, 417-418
  mouth-to-nose, 418
  after near drowning, 290, 292
  post, 429
Reticular activating system, 317, 318-319
Retinal detachment, 347
Retrodisplacement of maxilla, 332
Retrodisplacement of tongue, 331
Retroorbital hemorrhage, 332
Reversible shock, 76-77, 93
Rh antigen system, 122-123
Rhinorrhea with skull fracture, 321
RhoGam, 452, 453, 461
Rib injuries from child abuse, 491
Ribs, fractured, 371, 421
Ricin, 270
Rigid splints, 220-222
  application of, 222
Rigidity, nuchal, 140, 142
Ring, removal of, without cutting, 72
Ring splint, Thomas, for fractures of lower extremities, 226
Ritalin and amphetamine psychosis, 200; *see also* Methylphenidylacetate
Robaxin for spinal injury, 382
Robinul; *see* Glycopyrrolate
Rotating tourniquets, 73
Rovsing's sign, 435
Rupture
  of abdominal aneurysm, 440
  of aorta, 233
  arterial, 237
  of arterial aneurysm, pain in, 440-441
  of blebs, 366
  of bronchus, 369
    treatment of, 375
  of diaphragm, 370-371
  of lung, 374
  of ovarian follicle, 436
  of spleen, 444
  of tendons, 218
  uterine, 460
Rust ring in eye, 341

S

Sadness as reaction to emergency, 31
Salicylates
  absorption of, 258, 260
  alkalinization of urine for overdose of, 188
  elimination of, 261
  poisoning by, 185, 258, 259, 260, 262